Nanotechnology in Drug Delivery and Pharmaceuticals

Nanotechnology in Drug Delivery and Pharmaceuticals

Editor: Toby Cabral

AMERICAN
MEDICAL PUBLISHERS
www.americanmedicalpublishers.com

AMERICAN
MEDICAL PUBLISHERS
www.americanmedicalpublishers.com

Cataloging-in-Publication Data

Nanotechnology in drug delivery and pharmaceuticals / edited by Toby Cabral.
p. cm.
Includes bibliographical references and index.
ISBN 979-8-88740-291-8
1. Drug delivery systems. 2. Nanotechnology. 3. Nanotechnology--Therapeutic use.
4. Nanoparticles. 5. Pharmaceutical technology. 6. Pharmaceutical biotechnology.
I. Cabral, Toby.
RS199.5 .N36 2023
615.6--dc23

American Medical Publishers,
41 Flatbush Avenue,
1st Floor, New York,
NY 11217, USA

ISBN 979-8-88740-291-8 (Hardback)

Contents

Preface VII

Chapter 1 **Polydopamine-Functionalized CA-(PCL-*ran*-PLA) Nanoparticles for Target Delivery of Docetaxel and Chemo-Photothermal Therapy of Breast Cancer** 1
Na Kong, Mei Deng, Xiu-Na Sun, Yi-Ding Chen and Xin-Bing Sui

Chapter 2 **H_2O_2-Responsive Nanoparticle Based on the Supramolecular Self-Assemble of Cyclodextrin** 15
Zhenqiang Dong, Yang Kang, Qijuan Yuan, Manli Luo and Zhipeng Gu

Chapter 3 **Topical Use of Quercetin-Loaded Chitosan Nanoparticles Against Ultraviolet B Radiation** 25
Wenhao Nan, Li Ding, Houjie Chen, Fahim U. Khan, Lu Yu, Xinbing Sui and Xiaojun Shi

Chapter 4 **Optimization of the Linker Length of Mannose-Cholesterol Conjugates for Enhanced mRNA Delivery to Dendritic Cells by Liposomes** 36
Fazhan Wang, Wen Xiao, Mostafa A. Elbahnasawy, Xingting Bao, Qian Zheng, Linhui Gong, Yang Zhou, Shuping Yang, Aiping Fang, Mohamed M. S. Farag, Jinhui Wu and Xiangrong Song

Chapter 5 **Facile Fabrication of Reduction-Responsive Supramolecular Nanoassemblies for Co-delivery of Doxorubicin and Sorafenib toward Hepatoma Cells** 50
Qingqing Xiong, Mangmang Cui, Ge Yu, Jian Wang and Tianqiang Song

Chapter 6 **Controlled Drug Delivery by Polylactide Stereocomplex Micelle for Cervical Cancer Chemotherapy** 61
Kai Niu, Yunming Yao, Ming Xiu, Chunjie Guo, Yuanyuan Ge and Jianmeng Wang

Chapter 7 **Effects of Chitosan Oligosaccharides on Human Blood Components** 73
Xi Guo, Tong Sun, Rui Zhong, Lu Ma, Chao You, Meng Tian, Hao Li and Chengwei Wang

Chapter 8 **Enhanced Anti-Tumor of Pep-1 Modified Superparamagnetic Iron Oxide/PTX Loaded Polymer Nanoparticles** 83
Baoyan Wang, Weijun Wu, Hongjin Lu, Zhi Wang and Hongliang Xin

Chapter 9 **Nanoliposome-Encapsulated Brinzolamide-Hydropropyl-β-Cyclodextrin Inclusion Complex: A Potential Therapeutic Ocular Drug-Delivery System** 92
Fazhan Wang, Xingting Bao, Aiping Fang, Huili Li, Yang Zhou, Yongmei Liu, Chunling Jiang, Jinhui Wu and Xiangrong Song

Chapter 10 **A Robust Nanoparticle Platform for RNA Interference in Macrophages to Suppress Tumor Cell Migration** 101
Shi Liang, Junmeng Zheng, Wei Wu, Quan Li, Phei Er Saw, Jianing Chen, Xiaoding Xu, Herui Yao and Yandan Yao

Chapter 11 **Poly(Ethylene Glycol)-Polylactide Micelles for Cancer Therapy** 111
Jixue Wang, Shengxian Li, Yuping Han, Jingjing Guan, Shirley Chung, Chunxi Wang and Di Li

Chapter 12 **DACHPt-Loaded Nanoparticles Self-assembled from Biodegradable Dendritic Copolymer Polyglutamic Acid-*b*-D-α-Tocopheryl Polyethylene Glycol 1000 Succinate for Multidrug Resistant Lung Cancer Therapy** 126
Hsiang-I Tsai, Lijuan Jiang, Xiaowei Zeng, Hongbo Chen, Zihuang Li, Wei Cheng, Jinxie Zhang, Jie Pan, Dong Wan, Li Gao, Zhenhua Xie, Laiqiang Huang, Lin Mei and Gan Liu

Chapter 13 **Ceramide-Graphene Oxide Nanoparticles Enhance Cytotoxicity and Decrease HCC Xenograft Development: A Novel Approach for Targeted Cancer Therapy** 136
Shi-Bing Wang, Ying-Yu Ma, Xiao-Yi Chen, Yuan-Yuan Zhao and Xiao-Zhou Mou

Chapter 14 **Dual-Responsive Core Cross-Linking Glycopolymer-Drug Conjugates Nanoparticles for Precise Hepatocarcinoma Therapy** 147
Jing Wu, Jiayi Yuan, Baotong Ye, Yaling Wu, Zheng Xu, Jinghua Chen and Jingxiao Chen

Chapter 15 **Significant Suppression of Non-Small-Cell Lung Cancer by Hydrophobic Poly(ester amide) Nanoparticles with High Docetaxel Loading** 159
Xing Chen, Lili Zhao, Yang Kang, Zhiyu He, Fei Xiong, Xiang Ling and Jun Wu

Chapter 16 **Icariin Activates Autophagy via Down-Regulation of the NF-κB Signaling-Mediated Apoptosis in Chondrocytes** 170
Bobin Mi, Junqing Wang, Yi Liu, Jing Liu, Liangcong Hu, Adriana C. Panayi, Guohui Liu and Wu Zhou

Chapter 17 **Lipid Nanoparticles-Encapsulated YF4: A Potential Therapeutic Oral Peptide Delivery System for Hypertension Treatment** 182
Shengnan Zhao, Jinhua Li, Yang Zhou, Lingjing Huang, Yanfei Li, Juanjuan Xu, Chunmei Fu, Xia Guo and Jian Yang

Chapter 18 **Polypeptide Nanogels with Different Functional Cores Promote Chemotherapy of Lung Carcinoma** 192
Kai Niu, Nan Li, Yunming Yao, Chunjie Guo, Yuanyuan Ge and Jianmeng Wang

Chapter 19 **Human Albumin Fragments Nanoparticles as PTX Carrier for Improved Anti-Cancer Efficacy** 207
Liang Ge, Xinru You, Jun Huang, Yuejian Chen, Li Chen, Ying Zhu, Yuan Zhang, Xiqiang Liu, Jun Wu and Qian Hai

Chapter 20 **Tumor-Associated Fibronectin Targeted Liposomal Nanoplatform for Cyclophilin A siRNA Delivery and Targeted Malignant Glioblastoma Therapy** 216
Phei Er Saw, Ao Zhang, Yan Nie, Lei Zhang, Yingjie Xu and Xiaoding Xu

Permissions

List of Contributors

Index

Preface

Nanotechnology refers to the branch of engineering and science, focused on the design, production, and usage of systems, devices and structures through the manipulation of molecules and atoms at the nano scale. It facilitates the production of better products and it has applications in medicine for combating various diseases. The capability to manipulate systems at the atomic level enables the production of nanomaterials. They can be used as probes, sensors, or vehicles for the transportation of biomolecules in biological systems. Implementation of nanotechnology in medicine involves designing mechanisms and technologies so that nanoparticles and nanodevices can interact with the body at sub-cellular or molecular level with extreme precision. Nanotechnology can be used within the field of pharmaceuticals for site specific and target oriented delivery of medicines. It can help in reducing the drug consumption and side effects by specifically targeting the morbid region. This book explores all the important aspects of nanotechnology and its significance in drug delivery and pharmaceuticals in the present day scenario. It elucidates new techniques and their applications in a multidisciplinary manner. This book will help the readers in keeping pace with the rapid changes in this field.

The information contained in this book is the result of intensive hard work done by researchers in this field. All due efforts have been made to make this book serve as a complete guiding source for students and researchers. The topics in this book have been comprehensively explained to help readers understand the growing trends in the field.

I would like to thank the entire group of writers who made sincere efforts in this book and my family who supported me in my efforts of working on this book. I take this opportunity to thank all those who have been a guiding force throughout my life.

Editor

1

Polydopamine-Functionalized CA-(PCL-*ran*-PLA) Nanoparticles for Target Delivery of Docetaxel and Chemo-Photothermal Therapy of Breast Cancer

Na Kong[1,2†], Mei Deng[3†], Xiu-Na Sun[1,2], Yi-Ding Chen[3*] and Xin-Bing Sui[4,5,6*]

[1] *Sir Run Run Shaw Hospital, Zhejiang University School of Medicine, Hangzhou, China,* [2] *Institute of Translational Medicine, Zhejiang University, Hangzhou, China,* [3] *Department of Surgical Oncology, The Second Affiliated Hospital, Zhejiang University School of Medicine, Hangzhou, China,* [4] *Department of Medical Oncology, Holistic Integrative Oncology Institutes and Holistic Integrative Cancer Center of Traditional Chinese and Western Medicine, The Affiliated Hospital of Hangzhou Normal University, College of Medicine, Hangzhou Normal University, Hangzhou, China,* [5] *Department of Cancer Pharmacology, Holistic Integrative Pharmacy Institutes, College of Medicine, Hangzhou Normal University, Hangzhou, China,* [6] *Key Laboratory of Elemene Class Anti-cancer Chinese Medicine of Zhejiang Province and Engineering Laboratory of Development and Application of Traditional Chinese Medicine from Zhejiang Province, Hangzhou Normal University, Hangzhou, China*

Correspondence:
Xin-Bing Sui
hzzju@zju.edu.cn
Yi-Ding Chen
ydchen@zju.edu.cn

† These authors have contributed equally to this work.

Current limitations of cancer therapy include the lack of effective strategy for target delivery of chemotherapeutic drugs, and the difficulty of achieving significant efficacy by single treatment. Herein, we reported a synergistic chemo-photothermal strategy based on aptamer (Apt)-polydopamine (pD) functionalized CA-(PCL-*ran*-PLA) nanoparticles (NPs) for effective delivery of docetaxel (DTX) and enhanced therapeutic effect. The developed DTX-loaded Apt-pD-CA-(PCL-*ran*-PLA) NPs achieved promising advantages, such as (i) improved drug loading content (LC) and encapsulation efficiency (EE) initiated by star-shaped copolymer CA-(PCL-*ran*-PLA); (ii) effective target delivery of drugs to tumor sites by incorporating AS1411 aptamers; (iii) significant therapeutic efficacy caused by synergistic chemo-photothermal treatment. In addition, the pD coating strategy with simple procedures could address the contradiction between targeting modification and maintaining formerly excellent bio-properties. Therefore, with excellent bio-properties and simple preparation procedures, the DTX-loaded Apt-pD-CA-(PCL-*ran*-PLA) NPs effectively increased the local drug concentration in tumor sites, minimized side effects, and significantly eliminated tumors, indicating the promising application of these NPs for cancer therapy.

Keywords: polydopamine coating, star-shaped copolymer, aptamer, target delivery, chemo-photothermal therapy

INTRODUCTION

Breast cancer, the leading type of cancer for deaths among women worldwide, has caused over an estimated 2,421,698 deaths for the year 2015 (Global Burden of Disease Cancer Collaboration, 2017). Current approaches for breast cancer therapy are still limited by the level of our medical technology. For example, chemotherapy, which is one of the most common clinical methods for breast cancer therapy, is non-specific and always accompanied with serious side effects because of lacking effective carriers (Tao et al., 2013, 2015a; Shi J. et al., 2017; Zeng et al., 2017). Nano-biotechnology has shown promising prospects for changing the landscape of pharmaceutical and biomedical industries fundamentally (Shi et al., 2010; Tao et al., 2015b, 2017b,d; He et al., 2016; Wang et al., 2016, 2017; Hofmann et al., 2017; Niu et al., 2017; Qi et al., 2017; Shi B. et al., 2017; Shi J. et al., 2017; Xu et al., 2017a,b). The key to solve the side effects caused by cytotoxic anticancer drugs is to increase the local effective drug concentrations in the tumor sites, which could be addressed by employing polymeric nanoparticles (NPs) as highly promising target drug delivery systems (Kamaly et al., 2016; Kakkar et al., 2017; Nie et al., 2017; Tao et al., 2017c; Xu et al., 2017). In addition, due to the molecular complexity of cancers, treatment based on monotherapies is suboptimal and can not effective eliminated tumors (Greco and Vicent, 2009; Sun et al., 2011). By combining two or more therapies with different therapeutic mechanisms in one nano-system (e.g., chemotherapy and photothermal therapy), a promising strategy could be achieved to significantly enhance the therapeutic efficacy and have a better long-term prognosis (Cheng et al., 2017; Tao et al., 2017d). Thus, developing multifunctional target delivery platforms that intelligently integrated with different therapeutic approaches is urgently needed for effective cancer therapy.

Aptamers, which are essentially single-stranded DNA or RNA oligonucleotides and have specific 3D structures, are able to bind various biological targets on cancer cells with unique specificity and high affinity (Farokhzad et al., 2004; Dhar et al., 2008; Xu et al., 2016). Aptamers possess distinct advantages over antibodies. Examples include easier production without the use of animal, smaller size, readily availability, lower molecular weights, non-immunogenicity, higher targeting efficacy and *in vivo* stability (Jiang et al., 1996; Sun et al., 2014). Therefore, aptamers have been widely used as effective targeting agents for cancer therapy and diagnosis (Zhu D. et al., 2016). As one of the most commonly used DNA aptamers, AS1411 is able to effectively target a wide variety of cancer cells including breast cancer cells (MCF-7) (Keefe et al., 2010). Because of the excellent performance on the targeting efficacy, AS1411 can be incorporated in the surface modification of NPs as an effective targeting ligand for breast cancer therapy. Nevertheless, major concerns still exist for NPs prepared by pre-functionalized polymers. For example, the synthesis of AS1411 aptamer-polymer conjugates could be inefficient, possibly altering the chemical properties, lengthy with high cost, and at a risk of compromising the ability for drug encapsulation of polymers (Ho and Leclerc, 2004). Another method to conjugate AS1411 on the surface of NPs is surface modification of prepared NPs, but this will be cumbersome for NPs lacking reactive functional groups, which still require reacting with reactive linkers or coupling agents followed by exhaustive purification processes in order to remove excess reactants and catalysts (Takahashi et al., 2010).

In order to address these issues, a simple and versatile surface modification strategy based on polydopamine (pD) was adopted in this study. As reported by Park et al., surface modification with pD is applicable to various NP-based drug carriers no matter what the types of ligands (e.g., small molecules, peptides, or polymers) and how is the chemical reactivity of NPs (Park et al., 2014). Briefly, dopamine catechol could be oxidized to quinone followed by reactions with other quinones or catechols to form pD in weak alkaline conditions, gradually forming a water-insoluble polymeric film on NP surface during the process (Jiang et al., 2011; Chang et al., 2016). Afterward, ligands possessing amine or thiol groups could be simply conjugated on the surface of pD-coated NPs via Michael addition or Schiff base reactions (Lee et al., 2007, 2009; Tao et al., 2016). Besides the function of surface modification, pD and its derivatives have been widely reported as effective photothermal agents, which could contribute to phtotothermal therapy of breast cancer in the meantime. As phtotothermal therapy is a potent technique for cancer therapy because of its high selectivity and minimal invasiveness (Huang et al., 2013; Miao et al., 2016; Song et al., 2016; Tao et al., 2017a), it will be rather promising to initiate a synergistic target chemo-photothermal strategy (Tao et al., 2017d).

It has been reported that star-shaped copolymers possess many unique advantages for developing NP-based drug delivery platforms (Mei et al., 2013). To build the core of the NPs, a star-shaped co-polymer cholic acid functionalized poly(ε-caprolactone-*ran*-lactide) [CA-(PCL-*ran*-PLA)] was successfully synthesized according to a previous report (Tao et al., 2014), which has been demonstrated with many advantages such as improved bioavailability (i.e., solubility, stability, and permeability) of anticancer drugs, increased drug loading content (LC) and encapsulation efficiency (EE), controlled drug release profiles, and excellent antitumor efficacy. Herein, we used a nano-precipitation method to prepare CA-(PCL-*ran*-PLA NPs, coated the developed NPs with pD layer [pD-CA-(PCL-*ran*-PLA) NPs], and target functionalizing the pD-coated NPs with AS1411 aptamers [Apt-pD-CA-(PCL-*ran*-PLA) NPs]. The newly developed NPs were characterized by surface morphology, LC and EE, stability, photothermal properties and drug release profiles. The *in vitro* and *in vivo* targeting effect of these NPs were also accessed. With excellent biocompatibility, the docetaxel (DTX)-loaded Apt-pD-CA-(PCL-*ran*-PLA) NPs were demonstrated with a significant antitumor efficacy through a target chemo-photothermal strategy.

MATERIALS AND METHODS

Materials

Colic acid, D,L-Lactide (3,6-dimethyl-1,4-dioxane-2,5-dione, $C_6H_8O_4$), 4-(dimethylamino)pyridine (DMAP), 1,3-diisopropylcarbodiimide (DCC), 2-(3,4-dihydroxyphenyl) ethylamine (dopamine) hydrochloride, 3-(4,5-dimethylthiazol-2-yl)-2,5-diphenyltetrazolium bromide (MTT), and Stannous octoate $[Sn(Oct)_2]$ were purchased from Sigma (St. Louis, MO, United States). ε-caprolactone (CL) was purchased from Acros Organics (Geel, Belgium). Commercial Taxotere® and docetaxel (DTX) were provided by Shanghai Jinhe Bio-tech Co., Ltd (Shanghai, China). Methanol and acetonitrile were provided by EM Science (ChromAR, HPLC grade, Mallinckrodt Baker, United States). All other agents used were of analytical reagent grade. Boon Environmental Tech. Industry Co., Ltd (Tianjin, China) provided the ultrahigh pure water utilized throughout all the studies. Human breast cancer cell line MCF-7 was purchased from American Type Culture Collection (ATCC, Rockville, MD, United States).

Synthesis of DTX/Apt-pD-CA-(PCL-*ran*-PLA) NPs

Preparation of DTX/CA-(PCL-*ran*-PLA) NPs

The star-shaped random copolymer CA-(PCL-*ran*-PLA) was synthesized through the ring opening copolymerization, and provided by Prof. Lin Mei's group at Tsinghua University (Tao et al., 2014). We adopted a modified nanoprecipitation method with water/acetone system to develop DTX-loaded CA-(PCL-*ran*-PLA) NPs (DTX/CA-(PCL-*ran*-PLA) NPs) (Zeng et al., 2013a, 2015a; Zhang et al., 2014a,b, 2015; Wang et al., 2015; Wu et al., 2015). In brief, 200 mg of CA-(PCL-*ran*-PLA) copolymers and 20 mg of DTX were dissolved in 16 mL of acetone. The solution was then titrated into 200 mL of 0.03% (w/v) TPGS aqueous solution with continuous stirring. After stirring overnight at a speed of 800 rpm to remove acetone, the pure DTX/CA-(PCL-*ran*-PLA) NPs were obtained by centrifugation at a speed of 20,000 rpm (4°C) for 20 min, followed by three times washing in 20 mL of deionized water to remove TPGS emulsifier and unencapsulated DTX. Finally, pre-calculated amount of the obtained DTX/CA-(PCL-*ran*-PLA) NPs were weighted for pD coating, while the left NPs were dispersed in deionized (DI) water and lyophilized 2 days for further use.

Surface Modification with pD Layers

The DTX/pD-CA-(PCL-*ran*-PLA) NPs were prepared by incubating DTX/CA-(PCL-*ran*-PLA) NPs in 0.1 mg/mL dopamine hydrochloride/10 mM Tris buffer solution (pH 8.5) under magnetic stirring at room temperature. After 6 h of reaction, the suspensions gradually turned darker, indicating that dopamine was successfully polymerized. The obtained DTX/pD-CA-(PCL-*ran*-PLA) NPs were centrifuged (12,000 rpm, 30 min) and lyophilized for conjugation of targeting AS1411 aptamers.

Conjugation of Targeting AS1411 Aptamers

The sequence of AS1411 aptamers used in this study contains 10 extra T bases at the 3-terminus (5′-GGT GGT GGT GGT TGT GGT GGT GGT GGT TTT TTT TTT-thiol-3′). The SH-terminated aptamers were conjugated on the surface of pD-coated NPs through a Michael addition reaction (Park et al., 2014). Briefly, the DTX/pD-CA-(PCL-*ran*-PLA) NPs were dissolved in the Tris buffer (pH 8.0) containing aptamers with final concentrations of NPs and AS1411 aptamers at 1 and 0.5 mg/mL, respectively. After 2 h of magnetic stirring at room temperature, the resulting DTX/Apt-pD-CA-(PCL-*ran*-PLA) NPs were centrifuged (12,000 rpm, 30 min), washed three times with deionized water and lyophilized 2 days for further use.

All the fluorescent coumarin-6 (C6)-loaded NPs (i.e., C6/CA-(PCL-*ran*-PLA) NPs, C6/pD-CA-(PCL-*ran*-PLA) NPs, and C6/Apt-pD-CA-(PCL-*ran*-PLA) NPs) were prepared with the same method at each of the 3 steps described above.

Characterization of DTX/Apt-pD-CA-(PCL-*ran*-PLA) NPs

The size of DTX/CA-(PCL-*ran*-PLA) NPs, DTX/pD-CA-(PCL-*ran*-PLA) NPs, and DTX/Apt-pD-CA-(PCL-*ran*-PLA) NPs were performed by Malvern Mastersizer 2000 (Zetasizer Nano ZS90, Malvern Instruments Ltd., United Kingdom). The transmission electron microscopy (TEM, Tecnai G2 F30, FEI Company, Hillsboro, OR, United States) was used to access the surface morphology of these NPs. The photothermal properties of these NPs were determined by recording the temperature changes of various solutions with different concentrations of NPs (62.5, 125, 250, and 500 μg/mL) under the irradiation of an 808 nm NIR laser (Shanxi Kaisite Electronic Technology Co., Ltd., Xi'an, China) at a power density of 1.0 W/cm^2. To study the effect of power density on the photothermal effect of DTX/Apt-pD-CA-(PCL-*ran*-PLA) NPs, NP solution at the concentration of 500 μg/mL was irradiated by different power densities (0.5–2.0 W/cm^2) and the changes of temperature were recorded. The temperatures were monitored by an infrared thermal imaging camera (TI100 Infrared Camera FLK-TI100 9HZ, FLUKE).

Drug Loading Content (LC) and Encapsulation Efficiency (EE)

The LC and EE of the DTX/CA-(PCL-*ran*-PLA) NPs, DTX/pD-CA-(PCL-*ran*-PLA) NPs, and DTX/Apt-pD-CA-(PCL-*ran*-PLA) NPs were determined by HPLC (LC 1200, Agilent Technologies, Santa Clara, CA, United States). In brief, 5 mg of NPs were dissolved in 1 mL of DCM under vigorous vortexing, and the prepared solution was transferred to 5 mL of mobile phase containing acetonitrile and DI water (50:50, v/v). In order to get a clear solution for HPLC, a nitrogen stream was used to evaporate DCM for 15 min. A reverse-phase C-18 column (150 × 4.6 mm, 5 μm, C18, Agilent Technologies, Santa Clara, CA, United States) was utilized at 35°C, and the flow rate of mobile phase was set at 1.0 mL/min. A UV/VIS detector was used to detect the column effluent at 227 nm. The drug LC and EE of these NPs were calculated by the following equations respectively ($n = 3$).

$$\text{LC}(\%) = \frac{\text{Weight of DTX in NPs}}{\text{Weight of NPs}} \times 100\%$$

$$\text{EE}(\%) = \frac{\text{Weight of DTX in NPs}}{\text{Weight of the feeding DTX}} \times 100\%.$$

In Vitro Drug Release Profiles

In order to study the *in vitro* DTX release profiles, 5 mg of the lyophilized NPs were dispersed in 5 mL of PBS (pH 7.4, containing 0.1% w/v Tween 80). Tween 80 was used to increase the solubility of DTX while avoid the binding of DTX on the tube wall. Afterward, the NP suspension was transferred into a dialysis membrane bag (MWCO = 3,500, Shanghai Sangon, China) which immersed in 15 mL of fresh PBS in a centrifuge tube. The whole tube was then transferred into an orbital water bath and shaken at a speed of 120 rpm (37°C). At designated time points, 10 mL of release medium was picked out for HPLC analysis. After changing 15 mL of fresh PBS solution, the tuber was transferred back to the shaker for continuous tests. The cumulative release of DTX from the DTX/CA-(PCL-*ran*-PLA) NPs, DTX/pD-CA-(PCL-*ran*-PLA) NPs, and DTX/Apt-pD-CA-(PCL-*ran*-PLA) NPs was plotted against time.

Cellular Uptake of Fluorescent NPs

MCF-7 cells were cultured in Dulbecco's Modified Eagle's Medium (DMEM) supplemented with 10% fetal bovine serum (FBS), 100 mg/mL streptomycin, and 100 U/mL penicillin in 5% CO_2 at 37°C. The cell culture was stayed in 95% air humidified atmosphere. The cells were incubated with 250 μg/mL C6/CA-(PCL-*ran*-PLA) NPs, C6/pD-CA-(PCL-*ran*-PLA) NPs, or C6/Apt-pD-CA-(PCL-*ran*-PLA) NPs for 2 h, washed with cold PBS three times, and fixed by cold methanol for 20 min. After that, the nuclei were counterstained with DAPI for 10 min and washed twice with PBS. In order to visualize the cells, the chambers were mounted onto the confocal laser scanning microscope (CLSM, Olympus Fluoview FV-1000, Tokyo, Japan) with a blue channel excited at 340 nm and a green channel excited at 485 nm.

For quantitative analysis, MCF-7 cells were plated in 96-well black plates and incubated overnight at its initial density of 1×10^4 cells/well. Then the cells were equilibrated with Hank's buffered salt solution (HBSS) for 1 h at 37°C, and C6/CA-(PCL-*ran*-PLA) NPs, C6/pD-CA-(PCL-*ran*-PLA) NPs, or C6/Apt-pD-CA-(PCL-*ran*-PLA) NPs were added at concentrations of 100, 250, and 500 μg/mL, respectively. After 2 h of incubation, the medium was removed and the wells were washed three times with 50 μL of cold PBS. Finally, 50 μL of 0.5% Triton X-100 in 0.2 N sodium hydroxide was added to each sample to lyse the MCF-7 cells.

For flow cytometric (FCM) experiments, MCF-7 cells were seeded in 6-well plates (at a density of 1×10^5 cells/well), and treated with 500 μg/mL of C6/CA-(PCL-*ran*-PLA) NPs, C6/pD-CA-(PCL-*ran*-PLA) NPs, or C6/Apt-pD-CA-(PCL-*ran*-PLA) NPs for 1 h at 37°C, respectively. After removing the cell culture medium, the cells were washed with PBS twice, digested by trypsin, and harvested by centrifugation. Finally, the fluorescence intensity of C6 was detected by a flow cytometer (BD Biosciences, San Jose, CA, United States) at an excitation wavelength of 488 nm and an emission wavelength of 530 nm.

In Vitro Cell Viability Studies

In order to evaluate the biocompatibility of drug-free NPs and the *in vitro* antitumor efficacy of the DTX-loaded NPs, MCF-7 cells were seeded in 96-well plates (at a density of 5,000 cells/well) and incubated overnight.

For the biocompatibility studies, the MCF-7 cells were incubated with drug-free CA-(PCL-*ran*-PLA) NPs, pD-CA-(PCL-*ran*-PLA) NPs, or Apt-pD-CA-(PCL-*ran*-PLA) NPs at different NP concentrations (25, 125, 250, and 500 μg/mL) and incubation time (24 and 48 h). Afterward, the previous mediums were changed with MTT-contained DMEM (5 mg/mL) and the cells were incubated for an additional 4 h. Then MTT was removed and DMSO was added to dissolve the formazan crystals (2 h, dark, 37°C). The absorbance at 570 nm was measured using a microplate reader (Bio-Rad Model 680, United Kingdom). Control group with untreated cells was used as 100% of viability, and cells incubated with MTT-free medium were utilized as blank to calibrate the spectrophotometer to zero absorbance.

For the *in vitro* antitumor efficacy studies, (i) Chemotherapy groups: the MCF-7 cells were incubated with commercial Taxotere®, DTX/CA-(PCL-*ran*-PLA) NPs, DTX/pD-CA-(PCL-*ran*-PLA) NPs, or DTX/Apt-pD-CA-(PCL-*ran*-PLA) NPs at 0.25, 2.5, 12.5, and 25 μg/mL equivalent DTX concentrations for 24 h and 48 h, respectively. (ii) Irradiation groups: DTX/CA-(PCL-*ran*-PLA) NPs, DTX/pD-CA-(PCL-*ran*-PLA) NPs, or DTX/Apt-pD-CA-(PCL-*ran*-PLA) NPs at 0.25, 2.5, 12.5, and 25 μg/mL equivalent DTX concentrations were added into the medium of MCF-7 cells and immediately irradiated with an 808 nm NIR laser for 10 min at a power density of 1.5 W/cm^2. Afterward, MCF-7 cells from all the groups were further cultured for 24 and 48 h, respectively. Untreated cells only received NIR laser irradiation were used as controls. The same MTT method was used to test the cell viability of cells from all these groups in order to access the *in vitro* antitumor efficacy.

Xenograft Breast Tumor Model

The 4–5 weeks old of female severe combined immunodeficient (SCID) nude mice were purchased from the Institute of Laboratory Animal Sciences, Chinese Academy of Medical Science. The Administrative Committee on Animal Research in Zhejiang University approved the protocols for animal studies. A total volume of 200 μL MCF-7 cells in PBS were implanted subcutaneously on the backs of mice at a dosage of 2×10^6 cells per mouse. The tumor growth in each mouse was observed at frequent intervals. The tumor size was measured by a vernier caliper, and tumor volume (V) was calculated by this formulation: $4\pi/3 \times (\text{length}/2) \times (\text{width}/2)^2$. About 95% of the mice developed a tumor with an average volume of about 100 mm^3 after 2 weeks.

In Vivo Photothermal Imaging and *in Vivo* Antitumor Efficacy

The photothermal imaging studies were performed when tumor size reached about 400 mm^3. The mice were intravenously (i.v.) injected with Saline, DTX/pD-CA-(PCL-*ran*-PLA) NPs, and DTX/Apt-pD-CA-(PCL-*ran*-PLA) NPs at the same volume and dose. After 12 h of injection, NIR laser irradiation was performed (808 nm, 1.5 W/cm^2, 10 min) at tumor sites. The temperature changes of tumor sites, as well as infrared thermographic maps, were recorded by an infrared thermal imaging camera (TI100 Infrared Camera FLK-TI100 9HZ, FLUKE).

For *in vivo* antitumor efficacy studies, Apt-pD-CA-(PCL-*ran*-PLA) NPs were chosen based on their excellent performance on *in vitro* cellular targeting, *in vitro* antitumor efficacy, and *in vivo* tumor targeting. Different treatments were performed when the tumor volume reached approximately 100 mm^3. The tumor-bearing mice were randomly divided into five groups

($n = 5$), and different treatments were performed on Day 0, 4, 8, and 12: (1) Saline, (2) Taxotere®, (3) DTX/Apt-pD-CA-(PCL-*ran*-PLA) NPs, (4) Apt-pD-CA-(PCL-*ran*-PLA) NPs + NIR, and (5) DTX/Apt-pD-CA-(PCL-*ran*-PLA) NPs + NIR. All the formulations were i.v. injected. Taxotere® and DTX/Apt-pD-CA-(PCL-*ran*-PLA) NPs were injected at a same DTX dose of 10 mg/kg in 100 μL PBS. Apt-pD-CA-(PCL-*ran*-PLA) NPs were injected at a same NP dose with DTX/Apt-pD-CA-(PCL-*ran*-PLA) NPs. NIR laser irradiation was performed (808 nm, 10 min, 1.5 W/cm^2) after 12 h injection of NPs. The tumor size and body weights were recorded every 2 days. After 14 days of treatment, the mice were humanely executed. Tumor growth profiles were recorded to evaluate the antitumor efficacy in this study.

Another batch of SCID mice bearing MCF-7 tumor xenograft were further used to access the antitumor efficacy of the mice through recording their survival time after receiving the same treatments mentioned above. The mice with similar physical status (i.e., age, body weight, and 100 mm^3 of tumor volume) were randomly divided into five groups ($n = 5$). The survival results were presented as Kaplane–Meier plots and evaluated using a log-rank test.

Statistical Methodology

All tests were performed at least three times in all studies unless otherwise stated. The results are expressed as mean ± SD, and the statistical significance of the results was determined by the Student's t-test. The results were considered to be statistically significant if $P < 0.05$.

RESULTS AND DISCUSSION

Preparation of DTX/Apt-pD-CA-(PCL-*ran*-PLA) NPs

The star-shaped random copolymer CA-(PCL-*ran*-PLA) was synthesized through a the ring opening copolymerization of ε-caprolactone (CL) and D,L-lactide (LA) with colic acid (CA) as an initiator (**Figure 1A**) (Tao et al., 2014). The fabrication of DTX-loaded Apt-pD-CA-(PCL-*ran*-PLA) NPs (DTX/Apt-pD-CA-(PCL-*ran*-PLA) NPs) was illustrated in **Figure 1B**: (i) First, a modified nano-precipitation method, which is a mild and effective way to prepare drug-loaded NPs (Zeng et al., 2013a, 2015b), was applied to prepare DTX/CA-(PCL-*ran*-PLA) NPs. (ii) Second, the prime-coating of pD layer was achieved through an oxidative polymerization reaction (pH 8.5) to prepare DTX/pD-CA-(PCL-*ran*-PLA) NPs. (iii) Finally, conjugation of aptamers on the surface of DTX/pD-CA-(PCL-*ran*-PLA) NPs could be fulfill via a Michael addition reaction in a weak alkaline solution (pH 8.0). The suspensions gradually turned darker in the second step after dopamine hydrochloride was added, indicating the formation of pD layer. A 26-mer SH-terminated DNA aptamer-AS1411, which possesses a thiol group at the 3′- end for effective conjugation to the pD layer, was applied to provide high affinity to interact with breast cancer cells (Cao et al., 2009).

Characterization of DTX/Apt-pD-CA-(PCL-*ran*-PLA) NPs

The size and surface properties of polymeric NPs, which play a vital role on their drug release, endocytosis and *in vivo* pharmacokinetics (Tao et al., 2016; Behzadi et al., 2017; Ding et al., 2017), have been well-characterized in this study. As shown in **Figures 2a–c**, the surface morphology of DTX/CA-(PCL-*ran*-PLA) NPs, DTX/pD-CA-(PCL-*ran*-PLA) NPs, and DTX/Apt-pD-CA-(PCL-*ran*-PLA) NPs was characterized through TEM images. It could be obviously observed that spherical films have been deposited on the surface of DTX/pD-CA-(PCL-*ran*-PLA) NPs and DTX/Apt-pD-CA-(PCL-*ran*-PLA) NPs, which is quite different from bare DTX/CA-(PCL-*ran*-PLA) NPs and gives direct evidences on the formation of pD layers. The average size distribution in TEM images is about 80 nm for DTX/CA-(PCL-*ran*-PLA) NPs, and about 95 nm for DTX/pD-CA-(PCL-*ran*-PLA) NPs and DTX/Apt-pD-CA-(PCL-*ran*-PLA) NPs (**Figures 2d–f**). As presented in **Table 1**, the average DLS size of DTX/CA-(PCL-*ran*-PLA) NPs was 103.4 ± 3.3 nm (PDI 0.126), while that of DTX/pD-CA-(PCL-*ran*-PLA) NPs was 120.3 ± 4.6 nm (PDI 0.115) and that of DTX/Apt-pD-CA-(PCL-*ran*-PLA) NPs was 124.6 ± 5.1 nm (PDI 0.123). The increased DLS size of DTX/pD-CA-(PCL-*ran*-PLA) NPs and DTX/Apt-pD-CA-(PCL-*ran*-PLA) NPs could be attributed to the thickness of pD layers formed on the surface of DTX/CA-(PCL-*ran*-PLA) NPs, which also indicates the successful modification of pD layers through the oxidative polymerization reaction. With the mean hydrodynamic size of NPs ranging from about 100–120 nm in diameter, they are perfectly fit for high accumulation in tumor vasculature driven by the influence of the enhanced permeability and retention (EPR) effect (Zhu et al., 2015; Zhu X. et al., 2016, 2017; Liu et al., 2017). The smaller size obtained from TEM images (compared with DLS testing) may be contributed to the shrink and collapse of NPs when in the dry state (Tao et al., 2013). The stability of NPs was accessed by monitoring particle size in PBS over a span of 2 weeks (**Figure 3A**). The average size of all the NPs hardly changed during the testing period, indicating a great stability of the NPs.

As shown in **Table 1**, the absolute value of zeta potential of DTX/Apt-pD-CA-(PCL-*ran*-PLA) NPs (−19.2 ± 5.2 mV) increased slightly or kept similarly compared to DTX/pD-CA-(PCL-*ran*-PLA) NPs (−18.6 ± 3.6 mV) and DTX/CA-(PCL-*ran*-PLA) NPs (−17.8 ± 3.9 mV). The negative charge of NPs could benefit the blood compatibility and passive accumulation of the NPs in tumor sites through reducing clearance by the reticuloendothelial system (RES) including liver. Moreover, **Table 1** also showed that the LC and EE of DTX/Apt-pD-CA-(PCL-*ran*-PLA) NPs (9.73 ± 0.46%, 94.18 ± 2.76%) were almost the same as those of DTX/pD-CA-(PCL-*ran*-PLA) NPs (9.98 ± 0.39%, 94.31 ± 1.98%) and DTX/CA-(PCL-*ran*-PLA) NPs (10.02 ± 0.28%, 95.01 ± 2.16%), indicating this strategy is facile and does not affect the effectiveness of drug LC and EE.

In Vitro Drug Release Kinetics

Figure 3B showed the *in vitro* DTX release from DTX/CA-(PCL-*ran*-PLA) NPs, DTX/pD-CA-(PCL-*ran*-PLA) NPs, and

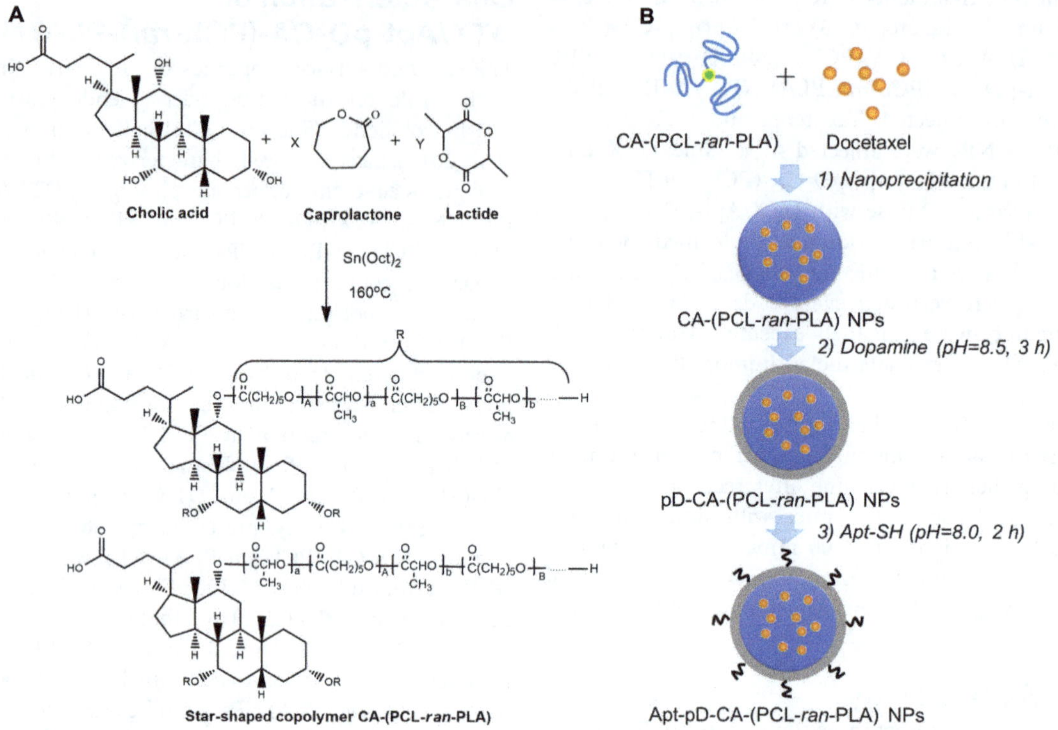

FIGURE 1 | Illustration for the synthesis of **(A)** star-shaped CA-(PCL-*ran*-PLA) copolymer, and **(B)** DTX/Apt-pD-CA-(PCL-*ran*-PLA) NPs.

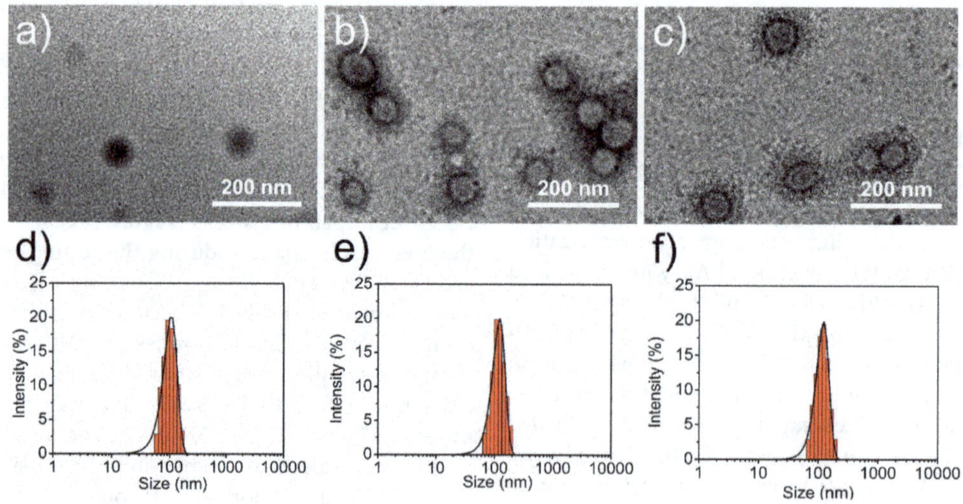

FIGURE 2 | Surface morphology (TEM images) of **(a)** DTX/CA-(PCL-*ran*-PLA) NPs, **(b)** DTX/pD-CA-(PCL-*ran*-PLA) NPs, and **(c)** DTX/Apt-pD-CA-(PCL-*ran*-PLA) NPs. Size distribution of **(d)** DTX/CA-(PCL-*ran*-PLA) NPs, **(e)** DTX/pD-CA-(PCL-*ran*-PLA) NPs, and **(f)** DTX/Apt-pD-CA-(PCL-*ran*-PLA) NPs.

TABLE 1 | Characterization of DTX/CA-(PCL-*ran*-PLA) NPs, DTX/pD-CA-(PCL-*ran*-PLA) NPs and DTX/Apt-pD-CA-(PCL-*ran*-PLA) NPs.

Samples (n = 3)	Size (nm)	PDI	ZP (mV)	LC (%)	EE (%)
DTX/CA-(PCL-*ran*-PLA) NPs	103.4 ± 3.3	0.126	−17.8 ± 3.9	10.02 ± 0.28	95.01 ± 2.16
DTX/pD-CA-(PCL-*ran*-PLA) NPs	120.3 ± 4.6	0.115	−18.6 ± 3.6	9.98 ± 0.39	94.31 ± 1.98
DTX/Apt-pD-CA-(PCL-*ran*-PLA) NPs	124.6 ± 5.1	0.123	−19.2 ± 5.2	9.73 ± 0.46	94.18 ± 2.76

PDI, polydispersity index; ZP, zeta potential; LC, loading content; EE, encapsulation efficiency, n = 3.

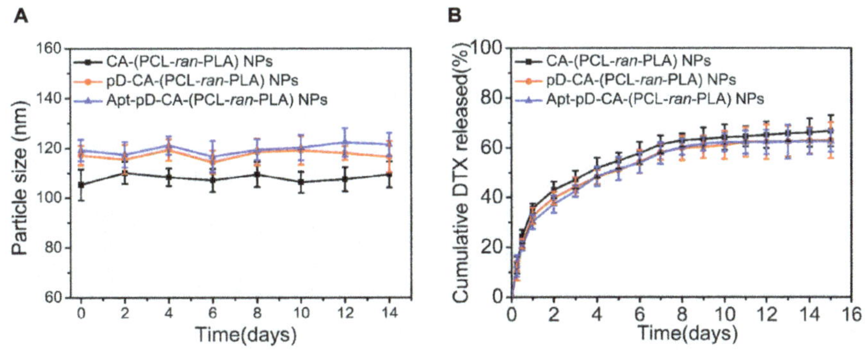

FIGURE 3 | (A) Particle stability of DTX/CA-(PCL-*ran*-PLA) NPs, DTX/pD-CA-(PCL-*ran*-PLA) NPs, and DTX/Apt-pD-CA-(PCL-*ran*-PLA) NPs in PBS, respectively. **(B)** *In vitro* drug release profiles of DTX/CA-(PCL-*ran*-PLA) NPs, DTX/pD-CA-(PCL-*ran*-PLA) NPs, and DTX/Apt-pD-CA-(PCL-*ran*-PLA) NPs.

DTX/Apt-pD-CA-(PCL-*ran*-PLA) NPs in the release medium (pH 7.4, PBS containing 0.1% w/v Tween 80) at 37°C. An initial burst release of DTX could be observed within the first 48 h, as about 40% of the loaded drugs were released in all kinds of NPs. At the end of our release studies (Day 15), about 66.8, 63.2, and 62.8% of DTX were released from DTX/CA-(PCL-*ran*-PLA) NPs, DTX/pD-CA-(PCL-*ran*-PLA) NPs, and DTX/Apt-pD-CA-(PCL-*ran*-PLA) NPs, respectively. Notably, the release rates from DTX/CA-(PCL-*ran*-PLA) NPs, DTX/pD-CA-(PCL-*ran*-PLA) NPs, and DTX/Apt-pD-CA-(PCL-*ran*-PLA) NPs were quite similar, which means the pD modification and AS1411 functionalization did not actually change the drug release properties of the prepared NPs. Therefore, Apt-pD-CA-(PCL-*ran*-PLA) NPs may be a promising drug delivery platform in nano-biotechnology and nanomedicines.

In Vitro Photothermal Properties of DTX/Apt-pD-CA-(PCL-*ran*-PLA) NPs

The photothermal properties of DTX/Apt-pD-CA-(PCL-*ran*-PLA) NPs was accessed by testing the temperature changes under the irradiation of an 808-nm NIR laser. **Figures 4A,E** showed a rapid temperature increase of ~20°C was achieved by DTX/pD-CA-(PCL-*ran*-PLA) NPs and DTX/Apt-pD-CA-(PCL-*ran*-PLA) NPs (500 μg/mL) after 10 min of irradiation with the NIR laser (1.0 W/cm^2). However, DI water and the DTX/CA-(PCL-*ran*-PLA) NPs showed little temperature change at totally the same conditions, demonstrating the superior photothermal effect of these NPs was majorly attributed to the pD layers. As shown in **Figure 4B**, the photothermal effect of DTX/Apt-pD-CA-(PCL-*ran*-PLA) NPs had a concentration-dependent relationship. The solutions of DTX/Apt-pD-CA-(PCL-*ran*-PLA) NPs also exhibited a laser power intensity-dependent manner as the temperatures increased with the rise of laser power intensity (**Figure 4C**). Moreover, the temperature changes did not exhibit noticeable difference during five cycles of "laser on"-"laser off" (**Figure 4D**), indicating an excellent photo-stability of DTX/Apt-pD-CA-(PCL-*ran*-PLA) NPs. Therefore, DTX/Apt-pD-CA-(PCL-*ran*-PLA) NPs have a good photothermal effect and a superior photostability, which could be applied in cancer photothermal therapy.

Endocytosis of Fluorescent NPs and *in Vitro* Cellular Targeting

Since the endocytosis and sustained retention of NPs acts as a critical and final step on the therapeutic efficacy of NPs (Xu et al., 2012; Behzadi et al., 2017), the endocytosis of Apt-pD-CA-(PCL-*ran*-PLA) NPs was carefully investigated. We replaced the loaded DTX with a fluorescent molecule, coumarin-6 (C6), in order to study the endocytosis of all the developed NPs in MCF-7 cells. The CLSM images of MCF-7 cells after 2 h of incubation with 250 μg/mL of C6/CA-(PCL-*ran*-PLA) NPs, C6/pD-CA-(PCL-*ran*-PLA) NPs, and C6/Apt-pD-CA-(PCL-*ran*-PLA) NPs in DMEM are provided in **Figure 5A**. As could be observed from this figure, the fluorescence intensity (i.e., representing cellular uptake efficiency) within the MCF-7 cells did not show much difference between C6/CA-(PCL-*ran*-PLA) NPs and C6/pD-CA-(PCL-*ran*-PLA) NPs. Notably, the fluorescence intensity increased significantly within the MCF-7 cells incubated with C6/Apt-pD-CA-(PCL-*ran*-PLA) NPs, demonstrating the presence of AS1411 aptamers on NP surface may lead to high levels of *in vitro* cellular targeting efficacy.

In order to quantitatively verify the significant role of AS1411 aptamers during the endocytosis of NPs, MCF-7 cells were incubated with C6/CA-(PCL-*ran*-PLA) NPs, C6/pD-CA-(PCL-*ran*-PLA) NPs, and C6/Apt-pD-CA-(PCL-*ran*-PLA) NPs at the concentration of 100, 250, and 500 μg/mL, respectively. As shown in **Figure 5B**, the cellular uptake efficiency of C6/CA-(PCL-*ran*-PLA) NPs did not show much difference compared to that of C6/pD-CA-(PCL-*ran*-PLA) NPs at all concentrations. However, the cellular uptake efficiency of C6/Apt-pD-CA-(PCL-*ran*-PLA) NPs was 1.37-, 1.53-, and 1.91-fold of that of C6/CA-(PCL-*ran*-PLA) NPs at the concentration of 100, 250, and 500 μg/ml, respectively. In addition, similar results could also be confirmed by FCM assays (**Figure 5C**). Taken all together, the specific interactions between AS1411 aptamers and MCF-7 cells reinforcing the endocytosis of targeted C6/Apt-pD-CA-(PCL-*ran*-PLA) NPs compared to

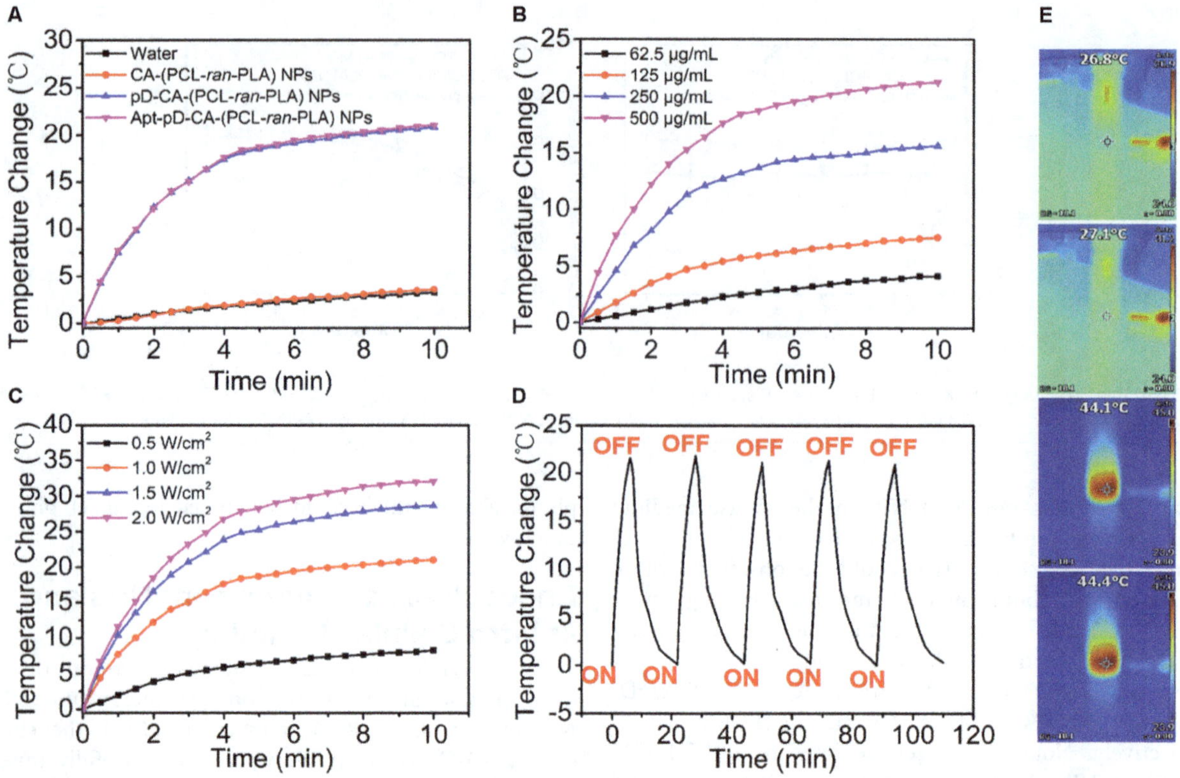

FIGURE 4 | (A) Photothermal heating curves of DI water, DTX/CA-(PCL-*ran*-PLA) NPs, DTX/pD-CA-(PCL-*ran*-PLA) NPs, and DTX/Apt-pD-CA-(PCL-*ran*-PLA) NPs solution under an 808 nm laser irradiation (1.0 W/cm^2) for 10 min. **(B)** Photothermal heating curves of the DTX/Apt-pD-CA-(PCL-*ran*-PLA) NPs solution with different concentrations (62.5, 125, 250, and 500 μg/mL). **(C)** Photothermal heating curves of the DTX/Apt-pD-CA-(PCL-*ran*-PLA) NPs solution with different power intensities of irradiation (0.5, 1.0, 1.5, and 2.0 W/cm^2). **(D)** Heating of a suspension of the DTX/Apt-pD-CA-(PCL-*ran*-PLA) NPs in water for five laser on/off cycles with an 808 nm NIR laser (1.0 W/cm^2). **(E)** IR thermal image of DI water, DTX/CA-(PCL-*ran*-PLA) NPs, DTX/pD-CA-(PCL-*ran*-PLA) NPs, and DTX/Apt-pD-CA-(PCL-*ran*-PLA) NPs (from top to bottom) solution under continuous NIR laser irradiation (1.0 W/cm^2) for 10 min.

non-targeted C6/CA-(PCL-*ran*-PLA) NPs and C6/pD-CA-(PCL-*ran*-PLA).

Effects of the Developed NPs on Cell Viability

MTT assays were carried out to evaluate the cytotoxicity of all the developed NPs. We first checked the *in vitro* toxicity of drug-free CA-(PCL-*ran*-PLA) NPs, pD-CA-(PCL-*ran*-PLA) NPs, and Apt-pD-CA-(PCL-*ran*-PLA) NPs at different concentrations (25, 125, 250, and 500 μg/mL) and after different incubation time (24 and 48 h). As shown in **Figures 6A,B**, none of these drug free NPs showed any functionalization of NPs (pD modification and aptamer conjugation) were biocompatible and non-toxic. Furthermore, the *in vitro* therapeutic efficacy of DTX/CA-(PCL-*ran*-PLA) NPs, DTX/pD-CA-(PCL-*ran*-PLA) NPs, and DTX/Apt-pD-CA-(PCL-*ran*-PLA) NPs without (i.e., chemotherapy groups) and with (i.e., chemo-photothermal therapy groups) the irradiation of NIR laser (808 nm, 10 min, 1.5 W/cm^2) was performed in MCF-7 cells. Taxotere®, which is a clinical DTX formulation, was chosen as a reference. Group treated with only NIR laser were also chosen as a reference. MCF-7 cells were treated at 0.25, 2.5, 12.5, and 25 μg/mL of equivalent DTX concentrations for 24 and 48 h. For the chemo-photothermal therapy groups, NIR laser irradiation was performed immediately after adding different NPs before 24 or 48 h of incubation. It could be concluded from **Figure 6C**: (i) the cell viability decreased as the incubation time increased for both Taxotere® and NP groups, indicating a time-dependent and dose-dependent effect; (ii) the DTX/Apt-pD-CA-(PCL-*ran*-PLA) NPs showed better *in vitro* therapeutic efficacy than Taxotere®, DTX/CA-(PCL-*ran*-PLA) NPs, DTX/pD-CA-(PCL-*ran*-PLA) NPs, and DTX/Apt-pD-CA-(PCL-*ran*-PLA) NPs. For instance, the cell viability of MCF-7 cells (48 h, at the DTX concentration of 12.5 μg/mL) was 48.2% for Taxotere®, 42.3% for DTX/CA-(PCL-*ran*-PLA) NPs, 39.4% for DTX/pD-CA-(PCL-*ran*-PLA) NPs, and 25.9% for DTX/Apt-pD-CA-(PCL-*ran*-PLA) NPs; (iii) the NIR laser irradiation did not change the viability of MCF-7 cells treated with DTX/CA-(PCL-*ran*-PLA) NPs. However, the cell viability significantly decreased for groups treated with DTX/pD-CA-(PCL-*ran*-PLA) NPs and DTX/Apt-pD-CA-(PCL-*ran*-PLA) NPs after the irradiation of NIR laser. For example, the cell viability of MCF-7 cells (48 h, at the DTX concentration of 12.5 μg/mL) was 42.8% for DTX/CA-(PCL-*ran*-PLA) NPs + NIR, 27.9% for DTX/pD-CA-(PCL-*ran*-PLA) NPs + NIR, and 16.2% for DTX/Apt-pD-CA-(PCL-*ran*-PLA)

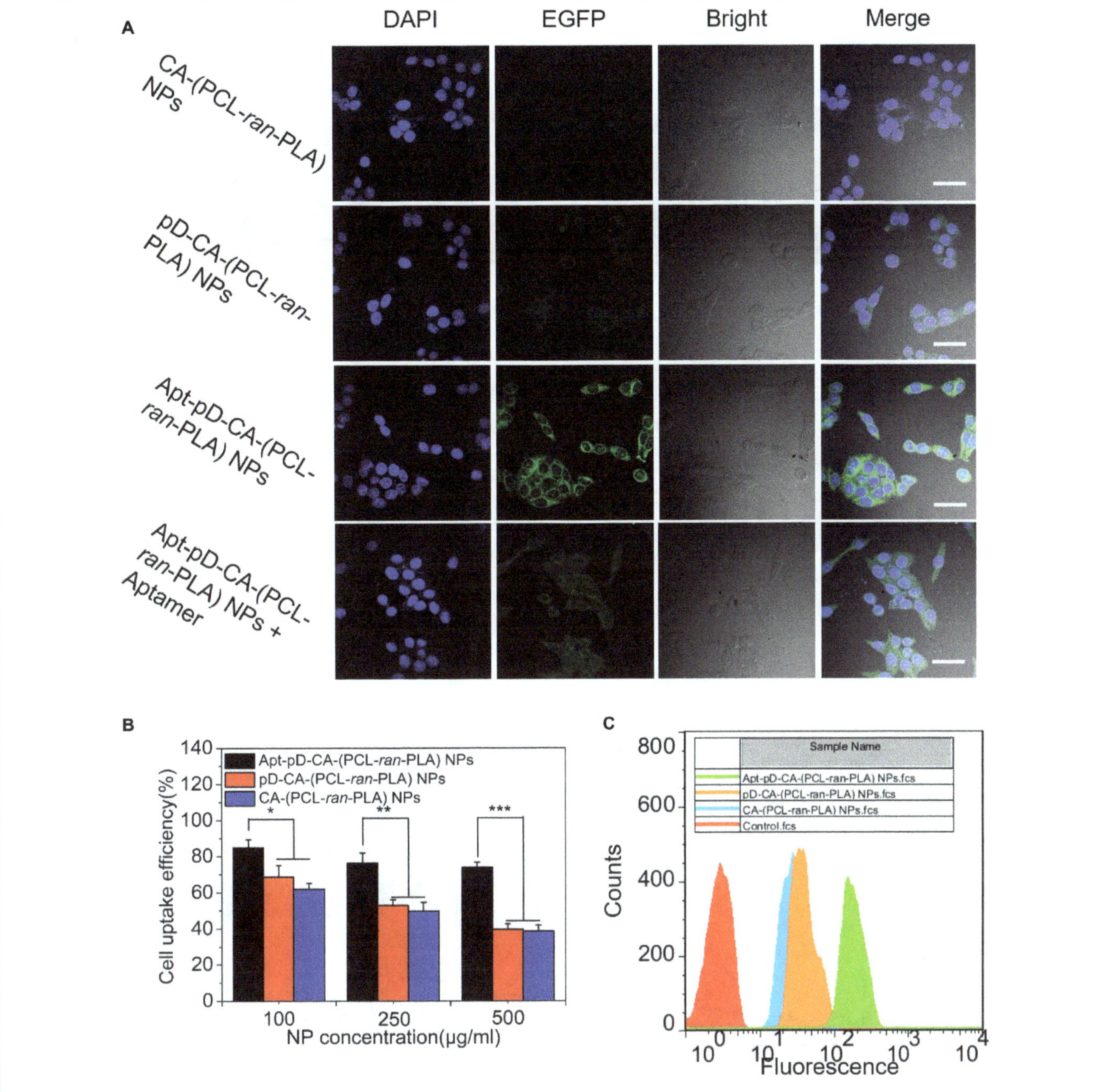

FIGURE 5 | Cell uptake of coumarin 6-loaded CA-(PCL-*ran*-PLA) NPs, pD-CA-(PCL-*ran*-PLA) NPs and Apt-pD-CA-(PCL-*ran*-PLA) NPs. **(A)** CLSM images of MCF-7 cells after 2 h-incubation (scale bar: 40 μm). **(B)** Cellular uptake efficiency of different NPs in MCF-7 cells after 2 h-incubation. **(C)** FCM histograms for different NPs in MCF-7 cells after 1 h-incubation. (*t*-test, $^{*}P < 0.05$, $^{**}P < 0.01$, $^{***}P < 0.001$).

NPs + NIR. (iv) the DTX/CA-(PCL-*ran*-PLA) NPs and DTX/pD-CA-(PCL-*ran*-PLA) NPs showed similar viability at various concentrations, further demonstrating the surface coating of pD layers is biocompatible and non-toxic. In a word, AS1411 aptamers may have an effective targeting efficacy for NPs and the synergistic chemo-photothermal strategy showed the most significant therapeutic efficacy. Therefore, DTX/Apt-pD-CA-(PCL-*ran*-PLA) NPs could be employed as promising targeted drug delivery systems for effective chemo-photothermal cancer therapy.

In Vivo Photothermal Imaging of DTX/Apt-pD-CA-(PCL-*ran*-PLA) NPs

Based on the promising *in vitro* targeting and therapeutic efficacy, we performed *in vivo* photothermal imaging of mice after intravenous (i.v.) injection of saline,

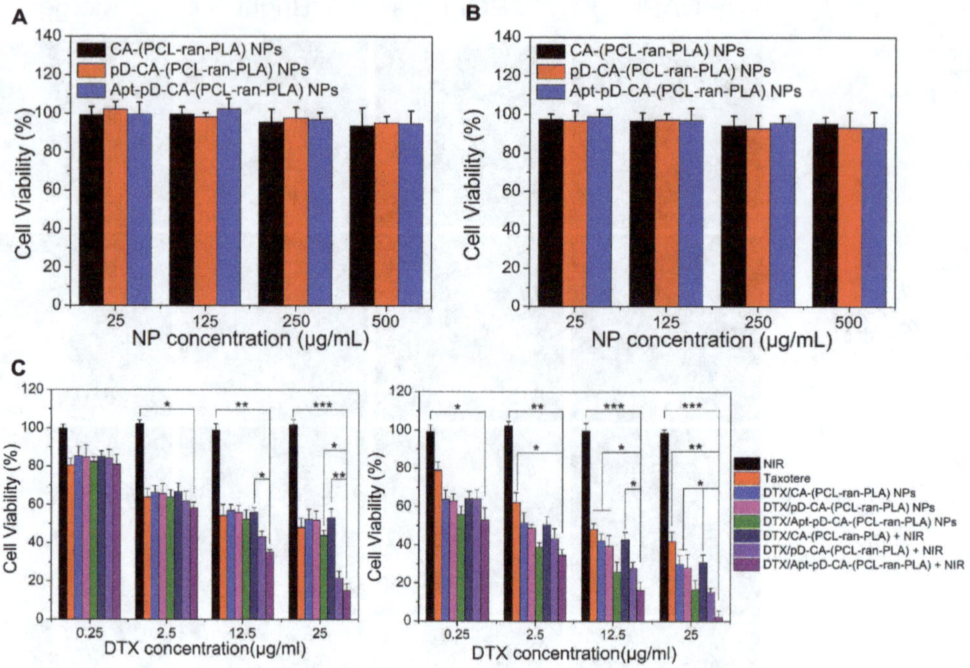

FIGURE 6 | *In vitro* cytotoxicity of drug-free CA-(PCL-*ran*-PLA), drug-free pD-CA-(PCL-*ran*-PLA), and drug-free Apt-pD-CA-(PCL-*ran*-PLA) NPs after different incubation time: **(A)** 24 h, and **(B)** 48 h. **(C)** Viability of MCF-7 cells after various treatments at different DTX concentrations. The cells were cultured with DTX-loaded NPs in comparison with that of Taxotere® at the same DTX dose for 24 h (left) and 48 h (right). NIR laser irradiation (808 nm, 10 min, 1.5 W/cm^2) was performed immediately after adding different NPs before different incubation time (*t*-test, $^*P < 0.05$, $^{**}P < 0.01$, $^{***}P < 0.001$).

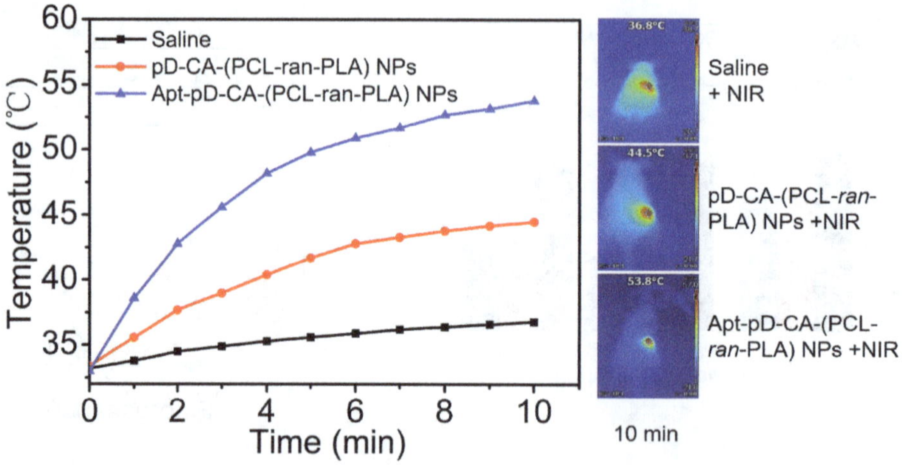

FIGURE 7 | Time-dependent temperature changes of the tumor sites recorded by an IR camera under an 808 nm NIR laser (1.5 W/cm^2). Saline, DTX/pD-CA-(PCL-*ran*-PLA) NPs and DTX/Apt-pD-CA-(PCL-*ran*-PLA) NPs were intravenous injected at the same volume and dose. After 12 h of injection, NIR laser irradiation was performed. Inset: Photothermal imaging after 10 min of irradiation.

DTX/pD-CA-(PCL-*ran*-PLA) NPs, and DTX/Apt-pD-CA-(PCL-*ran*-PLA) NPs respectively to further access the *in vivo* targeting efficacy. After 12 h of i.v. injection, NIR laser irradiation (808 nm, 10 min, 1.5 W/cm^2) was performed at tumor sites. As shown in **Figure 7**, the temperature increments in the tumor sites of the mice treated with DTX/Apt-pD-CA-(PCL-*ran*-PLA) NPs and DTX/pD-CA-(PCL-*ran*-PLA) NPs were 20.8°C and 11.1°C respectively, reaching a temperature of 53.8°C and 44.5°C after irradiation. DTX/Apt-pD-CA-(PCL-*ran*-PLA) NPs group exhibited a higher temperature increment than DTX/pD-CA-(PCL-*ran*-PLA) NPs group, which could be explained by the active tumor targeting effect of AS1411 aptamers and higher accumulation of DTX/Apt-pD-CA-(PCL-*ran*-PLA) NPs in tumor sites. However, the tumor site temperature of mice

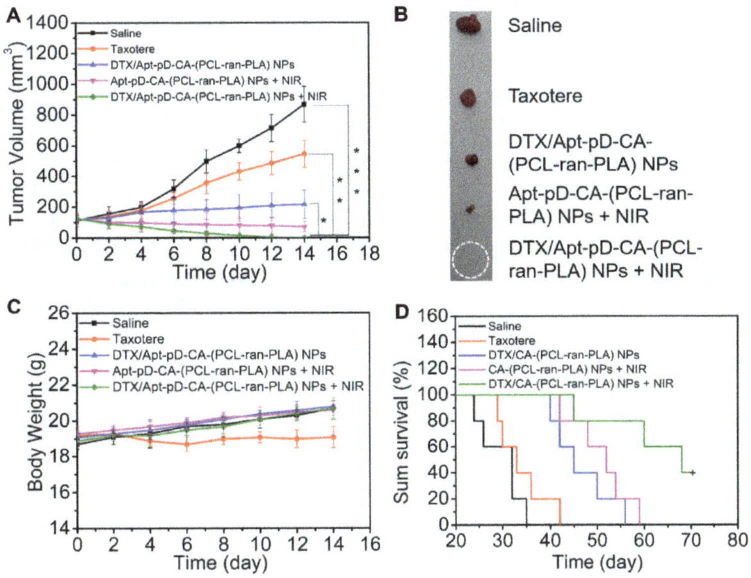

FIGURE 8 | Anti-tumor efficacy of different treatments on the nude mice bearing MCF-7 xenograft. Taxotere® and DTX/Apt-pD-CA-(PCL-*ran*-PLA) NPs were injected at the same DTX dose. After 12 h of injection, NIR laser irradiation was performed (808 nm, 10 min, 1.5 W/cm^2). **(A)** Tumor growth curve after different treatments (*t*-test, $^*P < 0.05$, $^{**}P < 0.01$, $^{***}P < 0.001$). **(B)** Images of tumors from each group at the end point of study. **(C)** Body weight curves of the nude mice during the treatment period. **(D)** Kaplan–Meier survival log-rank analysis of the nude mice bearing MCF-7 xenograft after different treatments.

received i.v. injection of saline did not show much increment with a highest temperature of 36.8°C, which was not enough for tumor ablation.

In Vivo Antitumor Effects of NPs

The blood circulation time was firstly accessed by *in vivo* pharmacokinetic studies before *in vivo* antitumor studies. As shown in Supplementary Figure S1, all the prepared NPs have extended the blood circulation time of the DTX compared to Taxotere®, which may contribute to effective delivery of DTX *in vivo*. On the basis of the above *in vitro* cell experiments and *in vivo* targeting imaging studies, DTX/Apt-pD-CA-(PCL-*ran*-PLA) NPs were chosen to further verify the *in vivo* antitumor efficacy of this targeting chemo-photothermal strategy. As shown in **Figures 8A,B**, both commercial Taxotere® and NP treatment groups could inhibit the tumor growth. In detail, all the NP treatment groups, i.e., DTX/Apt-pD-CA-(PCL-*ran*-PLA) NPs (target chemotherapy group), Apt-pD-CA-(PCL-*ran*-PLA) NPs + NIR (target photothermal group), and DTX/Apt-pD-CA-(PCL-*ran*-PLA) NPs + NIR (target chemo-photothermal therapy group), showed better *in vivo* antitumor efficacy than Taxotere®. The synergistic chemo-photothermal therapy group showed the highest therapeutic efficacy which significantly eliminated the tumors. These results were consistent with the above cellular experiments and *in vivo* targeting studies. Moreover, the body weight of the mice in all the NP treatment groups did not show any difference compared to the control group receiving saline, which that of Taxotere® showed slightly weight loss, indicating the potential *in vivo* biocompatibility of DTX/Apt-pD-CA-(PCL-*ran*-PLA) NPs (**Figure 8C**). Another batch of nude mice were used to access the survival data of nude mice receiving different treatments (**Figure 8D**). As could be concluded from this figure, the survival time of "DTX/Apt-pD-CA-(PCL-*ran*-PLA) NPs + NIR" group was at least extended by 35, 28, 14, and 11 days compared to "Saline" group, "Taxotere®" group, "DTX/Apt-pD-CA-(PCL-*ran*-PLA) NPs" group, and "Apt-pD-CA-(PCL-*ran*-PLA) NPs + NIR" group. These results further demonstrated the significant therapeutic efficacy of this target chemo-photothermal therapy strategy based on DTX/Apt-pD-CA-(PCL-*ran*-PLA) NPs, indicating these NPs are able to be applied as promising targeting drug delivery systems for synergistic chemo-photothermal therapy of breast cancer.

CONCLUSION

In this study, we for the first time reported the successful synthesis of robust DTX/Apt-pD-CA-(PCL-*ran*-PLA) NPs with star shaped CA-(PCL-*ran*-PLA) copolymers, which could be applied as promising targeting drug delivery systems for synergistic chemo-photothermal therapy of breast cancer. By surface modification with facile dopamine polymerization method, AS1411 aptamers were able to be simply conjugated on the surface of NPs for target delivery of drugs. The DTX/Apt-pD-CA-(PCL-*ran*-PLA) NPs were well characterized by surface morphology, LC and EE, stability, photothermal properties and drug release profiles. The *in vitro* and *in vivo* targeting effect of these NPs were also accessed. The *in vitro* cytotoxicity assays by MTT showed that DTX/Apt-pD-CA-(PCL-*ran*-PLA) NPs together with NIR laser irradiation (target chemo-photothermal therapy) could significantly inhibit cell proliferation compared with all other groups. The *in vivo* antitumor assays, as well as the improved survival time and reduced side effects, further confirmed the significant therapeutic effects of this target chemo-photothermal therapy strategy. All the results observed from the *in vivo* studies were consist with the *in vitro* assays, suggesting the robust DTX/Apt-pD-CA-(PCL-*ran*-PLA) NPs are promising in target delivery of drugs and synergistic chemo-photothermal therapy of breast cancer.

AUTHOR CONTRIBUTIONS

NK, MD, Y-DC, and X-BS conceived the idea and designed the study. NK and MD performed all the experiments and analyzed the data. X-NS helped in nanoparticle preparation and *in vitro* experimental assays. Y-DC and X-BS provided the technical support and corrections of the manuscript. NK wrote the manuscript and revised it according to the comments of Y-DC and X-BS.

FUNDING

This research was supported by grants from National Natural Science Foundation of China (Grant No. 81672932), Zhejiang Provincial Natural Science Foundation of China for Distinguished Young Scholars (Grant No. LR18H160001), Zhejiang Province Medical Science and Technology Project (Grant No. 2017RC007), Talent Project of Zhejiang Association for Science and Technology (Grant No. 2017YCGC002), and Zhejiang Province Science and Technology Project of TCM (Grant No. 2015ZB033).

REFERENCES

Behzadi, S., Serpooshan, V., Tao, W., Hamaly, M. A., Alkawareek, M. Y., Dreaden, E. C., et al. (2017). Cellular uptake of nanoparticles: journey inside the cell. *Chem. Soc. Rev.* 46, 4218–4244. doi: 10.1039/c6cs00636a

Cao, Z., Tong, R., Mishra, A., Xu, W., Wong, G. C. L., Cheng, J., et al. (2009). Reversible cell-specific drug delivery with aptamer-functionalized liposomes. *Angew. Chem. Int. Ed.* 48, 6494–6498. doi: 10.1002/anie.200901452

Chang, D., Gao, Y., Wang, L., Liu, G., Chen, Y., Wang, T., et al. (2016). Polydopamine-based surface modification of mesoporous silica nanoparticles as pH-sensitive drug delivery vehicles for cancer therapy. *J. Colloid Interface Sci.* 463, 279–287. doi: 10.1016/j.jcis.2015.11.001

Cheng, W., Nie, J., Gao, N., Liu, G., Tao, W., Xiao, X., et al. (2017). A multifunctional nanoplatform against multidrug resistant cancer: merging the best of targeted chemo/gene/photothermal therapy. *Adv. Funct. Mater.* 27:1704135. doi: 10.1002/adfm.201704135

Dhar, S., Gu, F. X., Langer, R., Farokhzad, O. C., and Lippard, S. J. (2008). Targeted delivery of cisplatin to prostate cancer cells by aptamer functionalized Pt(IV) prodrug-PLGA-PEG nanoparticles. *Proc. Natl. Acad. Sci. U.S.A.* 105, 17356–17361. doi: 10.1073/pnas.0809154105

Ding, L., Zhu, X., Wang, Y., Shi, B., Ling, X., Chen, H., et al. (2017). Intracellular fate of nanoparticles with polydopamine surface engineering and a novel strategy for exocytosis-inhibiting, lysosome impairment-based cancer therapy. *Nano Lett.* 17, 6790–6801. doi: 10.1021/acs.nanolett.7b03021

Farokhzad, O. C., Jon, S., Khademhosseini, A., Tran, T. N., Lavan, D. A., and Langer, R. (2004). Nanoparticle-aptamer bioconjugates: a new approach for targeting prostate cancer cells. *Cancer Res.* 64, 7668–7672. doi: 10.1158/0008-5472.CAN-04-2550

Global Burden of Disease Cancer Collaboration (2017). Global, regional, and national cancer incidence, mortality, years of life lost, years lived with disability, and disability-adjusted life-years for 32 cancer groups, 1990 to 2015: a systematic analysis for the global burden of disease study. *JAMA Oncol.* 3, 524–548. doi: 10.1001/jamaoncol.2016.5688

Greco, F., and Vicent, M. J. (2009). Combination therapy: opportunities and challenges for polymer–drug conjugates as anticancer nanomedicines. *Adv. Drug Deliv. Rev.* 61, 1203–1213. doi: 10.1016/j.addr.2009.05.006

He, C.-F., Wang, S.-H., Yu, Y.-J., Shen, H.-Y., Zhao, Y., Gao, H.-L., et al. (2016). Advances in biodegradable nanomaterials for photothermal therapy of cancer. *Cancer Biol. Med.* 13, 299–312. doi: 10.20892/j.issn.2095-3941.2016.0052

Ho, H. A., and Leclerc, M. (2004). Optical sensors based on hybrid aptamer/conjugated polymer complexes. *J. Am. Chem. Soc.* 126, 1384–1387. doi: 10.1021/ja037289f

Hofmann, C. L., O'Sullivan, M. C., Detappe, A., Yu, Y., Yang, X., Qi, W., et al. (2017). NIR-emissive PEG-b-TCL micelles for breast tumor imaging and minimally invasive pharmacokinetic analysis. *Nanoscale* 9, 13465–13476. doi: 10.1039/c7nr02363d

Huang, P., Lin, J., Li, W., Rong, P., Wang, Z., Wang, S., et al. (2013). Biodegradable gold nanovesicles with an ultrastrong plasmonic coupling effect for photoacoustic imaging and photothermal therapy. *Angew. Chem. Int. Ed.* 52, 13958–13964. doi: 10.1002/anie.201308986

Jiang, F., Kumar, R. A., Jones, R. A., and Patel, D. J. (1996). Structural basis of RNA folding and recognition in an AMP–RNA aptamer complex. *Nature* 382, 183–186. doi: 10.1038/382183a0

Jiang, J., Zhu, L., Zhu, L., Zhu, B., and Xu, Y. (2011). Surface characteristics of a self-polymerized dopamine coating deposited on hydrophobic polymer films. *Langmuir* 27, 14180–14187. doi: 10.1021/la202877k

Kakkar, A., Traverso, G., Farokhzad, O. C., Weissleder, R., and Langer, R. (2017). Evolution of macromolecular complexity in drug delivery systems. *Nat. Rev. Chem.* 1:0063. doi: 10.1038/s41570-017-0063

Kamaly, N., Yameen, B., Wu, J., and Farokhzad, O. C. (2016). Degradable controlled-release polymers and polymeric nanoparticles: mechanisms of controlling drug release. *Chem. Rev.* 116, 2602–2663. doi: 10.1021/acs.chemrev.5b00346

Keefe, A. D., Pai, S., and Ellington, A. (2010). Aptamers as therapeutics. *Nat. Rev. Drug Discov.* 9, 537–550. doi: 10.1038/nrd3141

Lee, H., Dellatore, S. M., Miller, W. M., and Messersmith, P. B. (2007). Mussel-inspired surface chemistry for multifunctional coatings. *Science* 318, 426–430. doi: 10.1126/science.1147241

Lee, H., Rho, J., and Messersmith, P. B. (2009). Facile conjugation of biomolecules onto surfaces via mussel adhesive protein inspired coatings. *Adv. Mater.* 21, 431–434. doi: 10.1002/adma.200801222

Liu, G., Tsai, H. I., Zeng, X., Zuo, Y., Tao, W., Han, J., et al. (2017). Phosphorylcholine-based stealthy nanocapsules enabling tumor microenvironment-responsive doxorubicin release for tumor suppression. *Theranostics* 7, 1192–1203. doi: 10.7150/thno.17881

Mei, L., Jiang, Y., and Feng, S.-S. (2013). Star-shaped block polymers as a molecular biomaterial for nanomedicine development. *Nanomedicine* 9, 9–12. doi: 10.2217/nnm.13.180

Miao, W., Kim, H., Gujrati, V., Kim, J. Y., Jon, H., Lee, Y., et al. (2016). Photo-decomposable organic nanoparticles for combined tumor optical imaging and multiple phototherapies. *Theranostics* 6, 2367–2379. doi: 10.7150/thno.15829

Nie, J., Cheng, W., Peng, Y., Liu, G., Chen, Y., Wang, X., et al. (2017). Co-delivery of docetaxel and bortezomib based on a targeting nanoplatform for enhancing cancer chemotherapy effects. *Drug Deliv.* 24, 1124–1138. doi: 10.1080/10717544.2017.1362677

Niu, Y.-Q., He, T., Song, J., Chen, S.-P., Liu, X.-Y., Chen, Z.-G., et al. (2017). A new AIE multi-block polyurethane copolymer material for subcellular microfilament imaging in living cells. *Chem. Commun.* 53, 7541–7544. doi: 10.1039/C7CC02555F

Park, J., Brust, T. F., Lee, H. J., Lee, S. C., Watts, V. J., and Yeo, Y. (2014). Polydopamine-based simple and versatile surface modification of polymeric nano drug carriers. *ACS Nano* 8, 3347–3356. doi: 10.1021/nn405809c

Qi, R., Wang, Y., Bruno, P. M., Xiao, H., Yingjie, Y., Li, T., et al. (2017). Nanoparticle conjugates of a highly potent toxin enhance safety and circumvent platinum resistance in ovarian cancer. *Nat. Commun.* 8:2166. doi: 10.1038/s41467-017-02390-7

Shi, B., Zheng, M., Tao, W., Chung, R., Jin, D., Ghaffari, D., et al. (2017). Challenges in DNA delivery and recent advances in multifunctional polymeric DNA delivery systems. *Biomacromolecules* 18, 2231–2246. doi: 10.1021/acs.biomac.7b00803

Shi, J., Kantoff, P. W., Wooster, R., and Farokhzad, O. C. (2017). Cancer nanomedicine: progress, challenges and opportunities. *Nat. Rev. Cancer* 17, 20–37. doi: 10.1038/nrc.2016.108

Shi, J., Votruba, A. R., Farokhzad, O. C., and Langer, R. (2010). Nanotechnology in drug delivery and tissue engineering: from discovery to applications. *Nano Lett.* 10, 3223–3230. doi: 10.1021/nl102184c

Song, J., Wang, F., Yang, X., Ning, B., Harp, M. G., Culp, S. H., et al. (2016). Gold nanoparticle coated carbon nanotube ring with enhanced raman scattering and photothermal conversion property for theranostic applications. *J. Am. Chem. Soc.* 138, 7005–7015. doi: 10.1021/jacs.5b13475

Sun, H., Zhu, X., Lu, P. Y., Rosato, R. R., Tan, W., and Zu, Y. (2014). Oligonucleotide aptamers: new tools for targeted cancer therapy. *Mol. Ther. Nucleic Acids* 3:e182. doi: 10.1038/mtna.2014.32

Sun, T. M., Du, J. Z., Yao, Y. D., Mao, C. Q., Dou, S., Huang, S. Y., et al. (2011). Simultaneous delivery of siRNA and paclitaxel via a "two-in-one" micelleplex promotes synergistic tumor suppression. *ACS Nano* 5, 1483–1494. doi: 10.1021/nn103349h

Takahashi, M., Yoshino, T., and Matsunaga, T. (2010). Surface modification of magnetic nanoparticles using asparagines-serine polypeptide designed to control interactions with cell surfaces. *Biomaterials* 31, 4952–4957. doi: 10.1016/j.biomaterials.2010.02.048

Tao, W., Ji, X., Xu, X., Islam, M. A., Li, Z., Chen, S., et al. (2017a). Antimonene quantum dots: synthesis and application as near-infrared photothermal agents for effective cancer therapy. *Angew. Chem. Int. Ed.* 56, 11896–11900. doi: 10.1002/anie.201703657

Tao, W., Ji, X., Xu, X., Islam, M. A., Li, Z., Chen, S., et al. (2017b). Inside cover: antimonene quantum dots: synthesis and application as near-infrared photothermal agents for effective cancer therapy. *Angew. Chem. Int. Ed.* 56, 11656–11656. doi: 10.1002/anie.201707385

Tao, W., Liu, G., Zeng, X., and Mei, L. (2017c). Multi-functionalized polymeric nanoparticles realized enhanced drug loading efficiency, extended circulation time, and significant in vivo tumor targeting effect. *J. Control. Release* 259, e133–e134. doi: 10.1016/j.jconrel.2017.03.272

Tao, W., Zeng, X., Liu, T., Wang, Z., Xiong, Q., Ouyang, C., et al. (2013). Docetaxel-loaded nanoparticles based on star-shaped mannitol-core PLGA-TPGS diblock copolymer for breast cancer therapy. *Acta Biomater.* 9, 8910–8920. doi: 10.1016/j.actbio.2013.06.034

Tao, W., Zeng, X., Wu, J., Zhu, X., Yu, X., Zhang, X., et al. (2016). Polydopamine-based surface modification of novel nanoparticle-aptamer bioconjugates for in vivo breast cancer targeting and enhanced therapeutic effects. *Theranostics* 6, 470–484. doi: 10.7150/thno.14184

Tao, W., Zeng, X., Zhang, J., Zhu, H., Chang, D., Zhang, X., et al. (2014). Synthesis of cholic acid-core poly(ε-caprolactone-ran-lactide)-b-poly(ethylene glycol) 1000 random copolymer as a chemotherapeutic nanocarrier for liver cancer treatment. *Biomater. Sci.* 2, 1262–1274. doi: 10.1039/C4BM00134F

Tao, W., Zhang, J., Zeng, X., Liu, D., Liu, G., Zhu, X., et al. (2015a). Blended nanoparticle system based on miscible structurally similar polymers: a safe, simple, targeted, and surprisingly high efficiency vehicle for cancer therapy. *Adv. Healthc. Mater.* 4, 1203–1214. doi: 10.1002/adhm.201400751

Tao, W., Zhang, J., Zeng, X., Liu, D., Liu, G., Zhu, X., et al. (2015b). Pharmaceutical Nanotechnology: Blended nanoparticle system based on miscible structurally similar polymers: a safe, simple, targeted, and surprisingly high efficiency vehicle for cancer therapy. *Adv. Healthc. Mater.* 4, 1260–1260. doi: 10.1002/adhm.201570050

Tao, W., Zhu, X., Yu, X., Zeng, X., Xiao, Q., Zhang, X., et al. (2017d). Black phosphorus nanosheets as a robust delivery platform for cancer theranostics. *Adv. Mater.* 29:1603276. doi: 10.1002/adma.201603276

Wang, J., Tao, W., Chen, X., Farokhzad, O. C., and Liu, G. (2017). Emerging advances in nanotheranostics with intelligent bioresponsive systems. *Theranostics* 7, 3915–3919. doi: 10.7150/thno.21317

Wang, S., Shang, L., Li, L., Yu, Y., Chi, C., Wang, K., et al. (2016). Metal–organic-framework-derived mesoporous carbon nanospheres containing porphyrin-like metal centers for conformal phototherapy. *Adv. Mater.* 28, 8379–8387. doi: 10.1002/adma.201602197

Wang, T., Zhu, D., Liu, G., Tao, W., Cao, W., Zhang, L., et al. (2015). DTX-loaded star-shaped TAPP-PLA-b-TPGS nanoparticles for cancer chemical and photodynamic combination therapy. *RSC Adv.* 5, 50617–50627. doi: 10.1016/j.actbio.2015.08.016

Wu, Y., Wang, Z., Liu, G., Zeng, X., Wang, X., Gao, Y., et al. (2015). Novel simvastatin-loaded nanoparticles based on cholic acid-core star-shaped PLGA for breast cancer treatment. *J. Biomed. Nanotechnol.* 11, 1247–1260. doi: 10.1166/jbn.2015.2068

Xu, A., Yao, M., Xu, G., Ying, J., Ma, W., Li, B., et al. (2012). A physical model for the size-dependent cellular uptake of nanoparticles modified with cationic surfactants. *Int. J. Nanomed.* 7, 3547–3554. doi: 10.2147/IJN.S32188

Xu, G., Yu, X., Zhang, J., Sheng, Y., Liu, G., Tao, W., et al. (2016). Robust aptamer-polydopamine-functionalized M-PLGA-TPGS nanoparticles for targeted delivery of docetaxel and enhanced cervical cancer therapy. *Int. J. Nanomed.* 11, 2953–2965. doi: 10.2147/IJN.S103513

Xu, X., Saw, P. E., Tao, W., Li, Y., Ji, X., Bhasin, S., et al. (2017). ROS-responsive polyprodrug nanoparticles for triggered drug delivery and effective cancer therapy. *Adv. Mater.* 29. doi: 10.1002/adma.201700141 [Epub ahead of print].

Xu, X., Saw, P. E., Tao, W., Li, Y., Ji, X., Yu, M., et al. (2017a). Tumor microenvironment-responsive multistaged nanoplatform for systemic RNAi and cancer therapy. *Nano Lett.* 17, 4427–4435. doi: 10.1021/acs.nanolett.7b01571

Xu, X., Wu, J., Liu, Y., Saw, P. E., Tao, W., Yu, M., et al. (2017b). Multifunctional envelope-type siRNA delivery nanoparticle platform for prostate cancer therapy. *ACS Nano* 11, 2618–2627. doi: 10.1021/acsnano.6b07195

Zeng, X., Liu, G., Tao, W., Ma, Y., Zhang, X., He, F., et al. (2017). A drug-self-gated mesoporous antitumor nanoplatform based on pH-sensitive dynamic covalent bond. *Adv. Funct. Mater.* 27:1605985. doi: 10.1002/adfm.201605985

Zeng, X., Tao, W., Mei, L., and Feng, S.-S. (2015a). Docetaxel-loaded nanoparticles of dendrimer-like amphiphilic copolymer for cancer therapy. *J. Control. Release* 213:e119. doi: 10.1016/j.jconrel.2015.05.200

Zeng, X., Tao, W., Wang, Z., Zhang, X., Zhu, H., Wu, Y., et al. (2015b). Docetaxel-loaded nanoparticles of dendritic amphiphilic block copolymer H40-PLA-b-TPGS for cancer treatment. *Part. Part. Syst. Char.* 32, 112–122. doi: 10.1002/ppsc.201400048

Zeng, X., Tao, W., Mei, L., Huang, L., Tan, C., and Feng, S. S. (2013a). Cholic acid-functionalized nanoparticles of star-shaped PLGA-vitamin E TPGS copolymer for docetaxel delivery to cervical cancer. *Biomaterials* 34, 6058–6067. doi: 10.1016/j.biomaterials.2013.04.052

Zhang, J., Tao, W., Chen, Y., Chang, D., Wang, T., Zhang, X., et al. (2015). Doxorubicin-loaded star-shaped copolymer PLGA-vitamin E TPGS nanoparticles for lung cancer therapy. *J. Mater. Sci. Mater. Med.* 26:165. doi: 10.1007/s10856-015-5498-z

Zhang, X., Dong, Y., Zeng, X., Liang, X., Li, X., Tao, W., et al. (2014a). The effect of autophagy inhibitors on drug delivery using biodegradable polymer nanoparticles in cancer treatment. *Biomaterials* 35, 1932–1943. doi: 10.1016/j.biomaterials.2013.10.034

Zhang, X., Yang, Y., Liang, X., Zeng, X., Liu, Z., Tao, W., et al. (2014b). Enhancing therapeutic effects of docetaxel-loaded dendritic copolymer nanoparticles by co-treatment with autophagy inhibitor on breast cancer. *Theranostics* 4, 1085–1095. doi: 10.7150/thno.9933

Zhu, D., Tao, W., Zhang, H., Liu, G., Wang, T., Zhang, L., et al. (2016). Docetaxel (DTX)-loaded polydopamine-modified TPGS-PLA nanoparticles as a targeted drug delivery system for the treatment of liver cancer. *Acta Biomater.* 30, 144–154. doi: 10.1016/j.actbio.2015.11.031

Zhu, X., Tao, W., Liu, D., Wu, J., Guo, Z., Ji, X., et al. (2017). Surface De-PEGylation controls nanoparticle-mediated siRNA delivery in vitro and in vivo. *Theranostics* 7, 1990–2002. doi: 10.7150/thno.18136

Zhu, X., Wu, J., Shan, W., Tao, W., Zhao, L., Lim, J. M., et al. (2016). Polymeric nanoparticles amenable to simultaneous installation of exterior targeting and interior therapeutic proteins. *Angew. Chem. Int. Ed.* 55, 3309–3312. doi: 10.1002/anie.201509183

Zhu, X., Xu, Y., Solis, L. M., Tao, W., Wang, L., Behrens, C., et al. (2015). Long-circulating siRNA nanoparticles for validating Prohibitin1-targeted non-small cell lung cancer treatment. *Proc. Natl. Acad. Sci. U.S.A.* 112, 7779–7784. doi: 10.1073/pnas.1505629112

2

H_2O_2-Responsive Nanoparticle Based on the Supramolecular Self-Assemble of Cyclodextrin

Zhenqiang Dong[1,2†], Yang Kang[3†], Qijuan Yuan[1], Manli Luo[4] and Zhipeng Gu[1]*

[1] Key Laboratory of Sensing Technology and Biomedical Instrument of Guangdong Province, School of Engineering, Sun Yat-sen University, Guangzhou, China, [2] College of Chemical and Material Engineering, Quzhou University, Quzhou, China, [3] Key Laboratory of Mountain Ecological Restoration and Bioresource Utilization, Chengdu Institute of Biology, Chinese Academy of Sciences, Chengdu, China, [4] Guangdong Provincial Key Laboratory of Malignant Tumor Epigenetics and Gene Regulation, Sun Yat-sen Memorial Hospital, Sun Yat-sen University, Guangzhou, China

***Correspondence:**
Zhipeng Gu
guzhp@mail.sysu.edu.cn

† These authors have contributed equally to this work.

Designing stimuli responsive, controllable and biocompatible multifunctional nanoparticles is an important progress in the current quest for drug delivery systems. Herein, we devoted to developing a β-cyclodextrin (β-CD) based drug delivery nanoparticles (NPs) that release Bovine serum albumin (BSA) via glucose-responsive gate. The design involves synthesis of sodium alginate with β-CD modified (Alg-β-CD) and methoxypolyethylene glycol (mPEG-Fc) containing ferrocene (Fc) uncharged end-capping. When α-cyclodextrin (α-CD) was added with these two segments, the stable non-covalent supramolecular structure of Alg-β-CD/mPEG-Fc/α-CD can be self-assembled into NPs in aqueous solution. BSA loaded Alg-β-CD/mPEG-Fc/α-CD also has been prepared. Interestingly, these supramolecular Alg-β-CD/mPEG-Fc/α-CD/BSA NPs showed uniform sphere structure and constant BSA loading content. Also, this new kind of NPs can disassemble in the present of hydrogen peroxide (H_2O_2). Since glucose oxidase (GOD) can oxidize glucose and produce H_2O_2, so this kind of polymeric NPs can also have glucose responsive behavior in the GOD containing environment. Developed functional Alg-β-CD/mPEG-Fc/α-CD might be a promising drug delivery strategy for diabetes or immunotherapy with more efficiency.

Keywords: responsive, cyclodextrin, self-assemble, nanoparticle, BSA

INTRODUCTION

For the past decades, stimuli responsive nanoparticles (NPs) based delivery technique have emerged as a promising strategy for controllable drug delivery, especially for protein delivery due to ingenious design (Tao et al., 2013; Wu et al., 2014; Kuang et al., 2016; Ding et al., 2017; Kang et al., 2017b). As smart vehicles, these ideal NPs can undergo reversible physical or chemical changes to control drug release in response to external stimuli such as pH, light, temperature, redox and molecules (Kang et al., 2015; Tao et al., 2016, 2017a,b; Rosenblum et al., 2018; Zhu et al., 2018). For cancer therapy, diverse intracellular and extracellular endogenous stimuli within

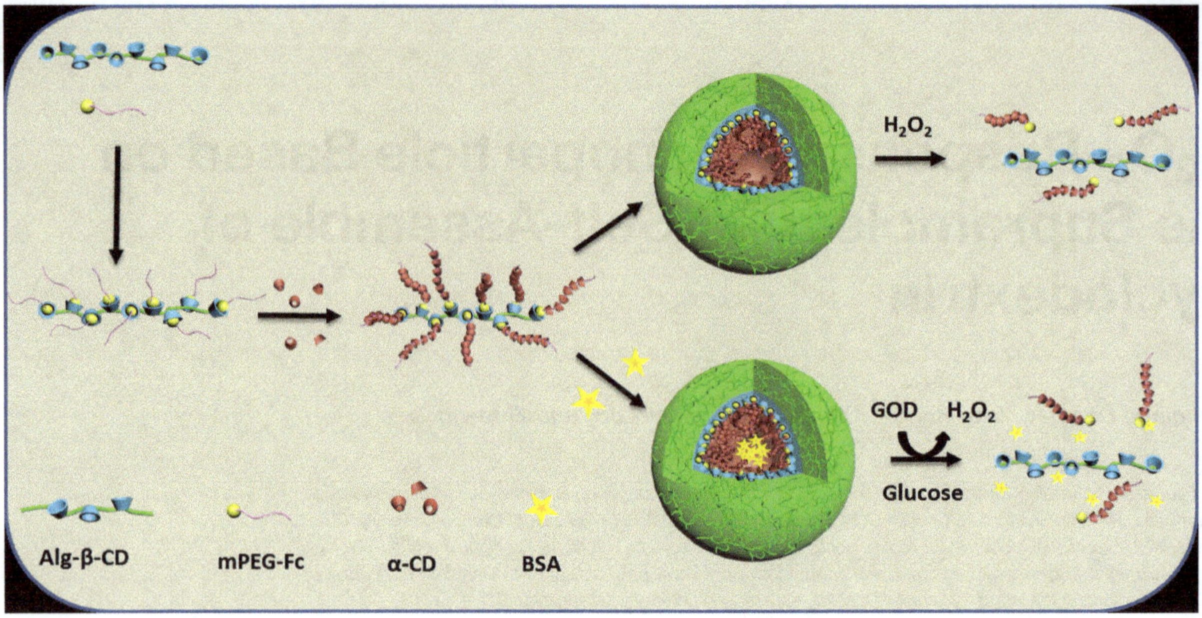

FIGURE 1 | Schematic illustration of the formation of Alg-β-CD/mPEG-Fc/α-CD nanoparticles and their enzyme encapsulation and controlled release behavior.

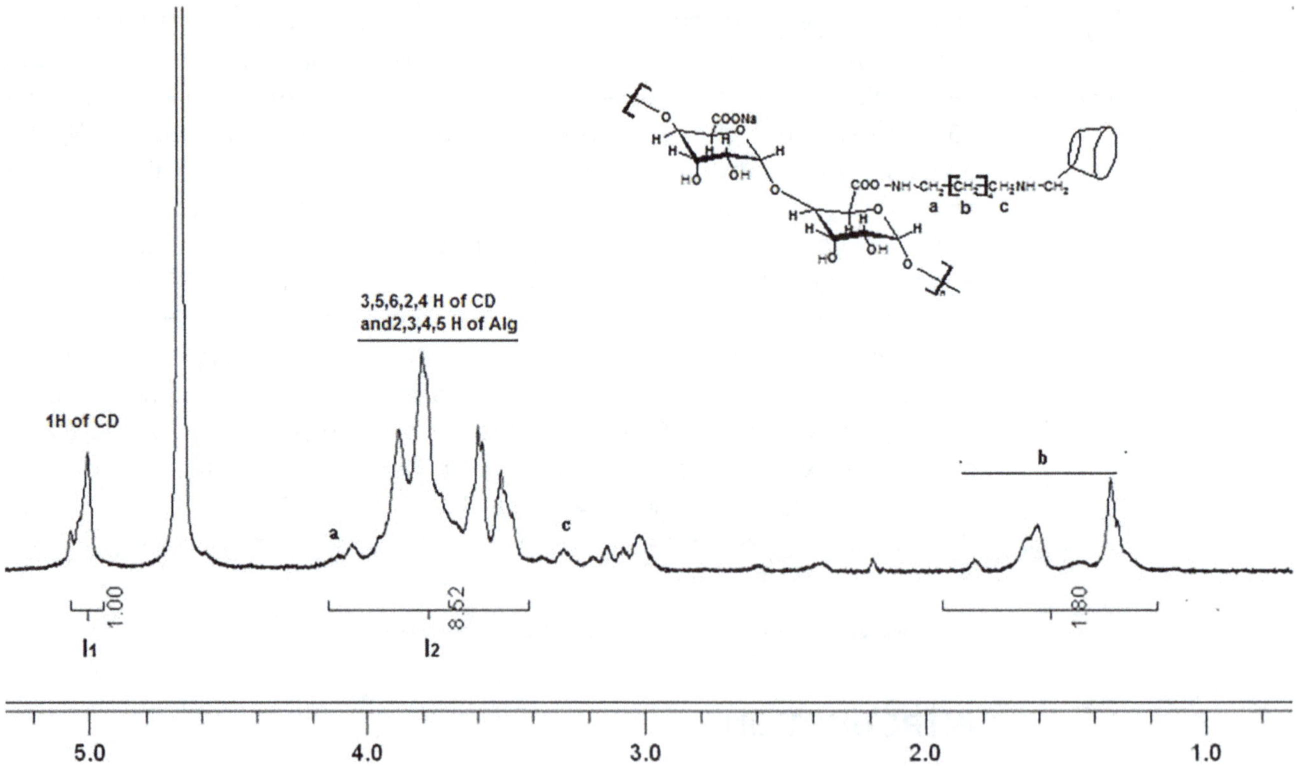

FIGURE 2 | ^{1}HNMR spectrum of sodium alginate with β-CD (Alg-β-CD) in D_2O. a–f mean the different H of the molecule structure.

tumor microenvironment, such as low pH value, hypoxia, enzymes and reactive oxygen species (ROS) have been widely investigated in stimuli responsive NPs and explored as the stimuli to selectively trigger drug control release or transfer prodrug systems into active form (Chen et al., 2015; Ruan et al., 2015, 2016; Liao et al., 2016; Wang et al., 2017b).

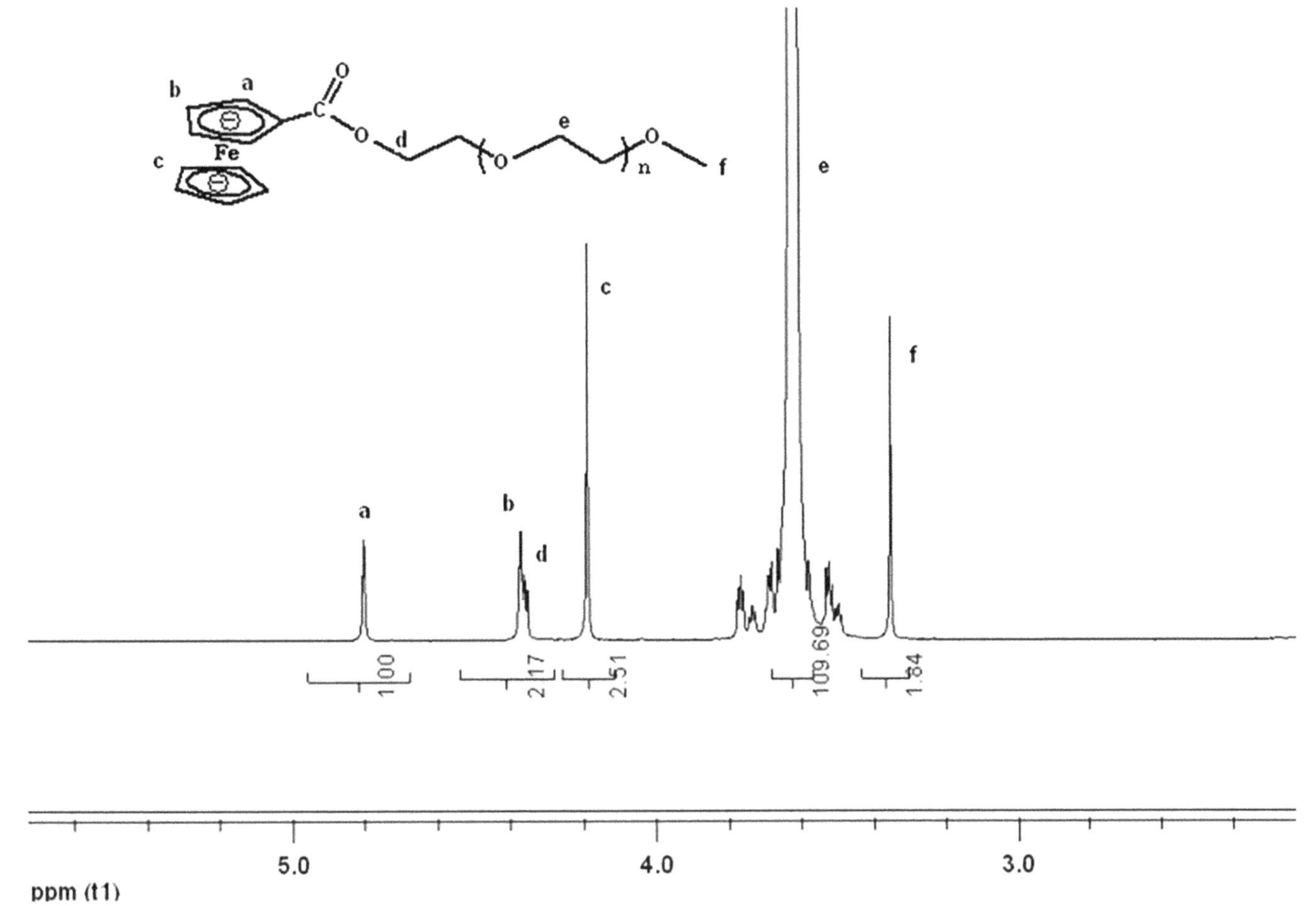

FIGURE 3 | ^{1}H NMR spectrum of mPEG-Fc in $CDCl_3$. a-f mean the different H of the molecule structure.

As an important hallmark, it should be noticed that various studies have demonstrated that hydrogen peroxide (H_2O_2) could be used as a second messenger in intracellular signaling cascades and would be generated in multiple skin lesions, initiating aging cells and the tumoral tissue (Miao et al., 2015). In this regard, H_2O_2-responsive NPs would be a promising therapeutic strategy for the treatment of specific disease.

At present, block copolymer approaches for H_2O_2-responsive NPs has been widely used and rapidly developed. For instance, a tyrosol incorporated copolyoxalate (TPOX) NPs have been developed by Kim et al. (2017), which demonstrated that TPOX NPs released entrapped nile red through the degradation under H_2O_2 stimulation and could be used as H_2O_2-responsive therapeutic NPs for the treatment and inflammatory. Recently, Gu group have designed a glucose-responsive mechanism directly utilizing H_2O_2-sensitive polymeric vesicles by using polyethylene glycol (PEG) and phenylboronic ester (PBE)-conjugated polyserine for smart insulin delivery (Hu et al., 2017). Apart from stimuli-responsive polymeric NPs via cleavable covalent bonds to control their properties, supramolecular based NPs via non-covalent bonds have also been widely studied due to that functional ligands and environmental responsive bonds can be conveniently incorporated through host-guest interaction, $\pi-\pi$ interaction, hydrogen bonding interaction and so on (Wang et al., 2015, 2017a). Cyclodextrin (CD), as a most common case of supermolecules, which has been demonstrated that can bind some specific hydrophobic guest molecules into its cavities to construct stable host-guest complex (Yuan et al., 2013). CDs are also considered as a good choice for drug delivery strategy due to their adjustable water solubility, good biocompatibility, and non-toxicity toward biological systems (Kang et al., 2014). In the previous studies, various stimuli-responsive CDs NPs based on host-guest interactions between CDs and different guest molecules [such as azobenzene, ferrocene (Fc), and adamantine] have been widely developed. For instance, Guo and Lei (2015) have developed a kind of redox-responsive cationic supramolecular polymers based on the host-guest interaction between β-CD and Fc, which indicated the potential application for gene nanocarrier. To conduct the redox-stimuli in an effect way, Kang et al. (2017a) have designed a kind of dual redox-responsive micelles which fabricated by methoxypolyethylene glycol conjugated β-CD (mPEG-β-CD) and Fc conjugated camptothecin (Fc-SS-CPT)

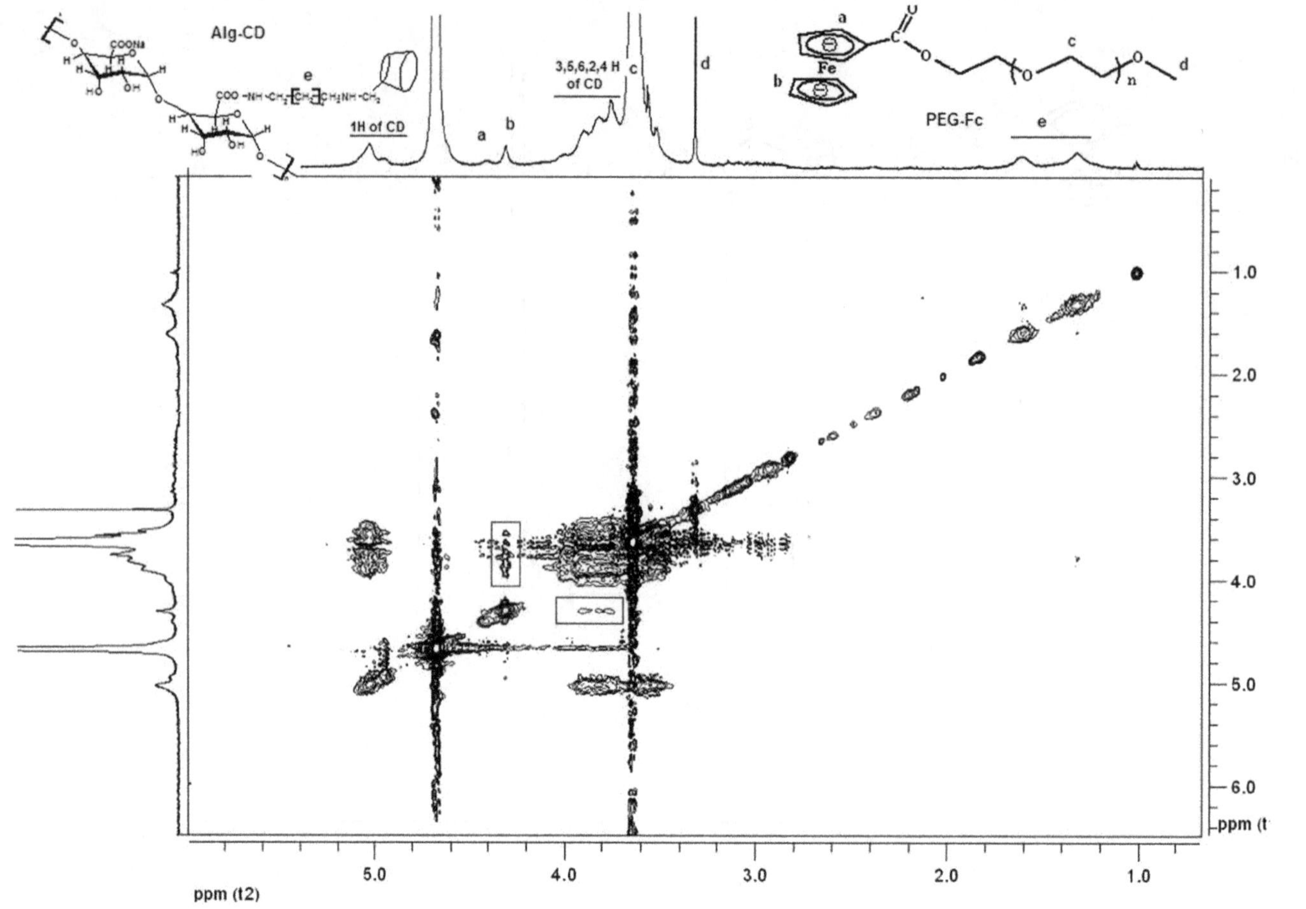

FIGURE 4 | 2D-NOESY-NMR spectrum of mixture of Alg-β-CD and PEG-Fc inclusion complex in D_2O. a-f mean the different H of the molecule structure.

segments for achieving dual ROS and glutathione responsive. It is reasonable to design H_2O_2-sensitive NPs based on CD, which can load and controllable releasing drugs for treatment of specific disease.

In this paper, a novel oxidation responsive rod-coil polymeric NPs have been prepared using water as the self-assemble solvent (**Figure 1**) Firstly, sodium alginate with β-CD end-decoration (Alg-β-CD) and mPEG conjugated with Fc (mPEG-Fc) were designed and synthesized, and then the self-assembly behavior of them in water was studied in detail. This supramolecular copolymer grows up to form comb shaped polymer in aqueous solution by the terminal host-guest inclusion. When adding certain amount of α-CD to this solution, the PEG will form inclusion complex with α-CD to form the rod section while sodium alginate form the coil section. This kind of structure will self-assemble into rod-coil NPs in water and load Bovine serum albumin (BSA). This new kind of NPs can disassemble in the present of H_2O_2. Since glucose oxidase (GOD) can oxidize glucose and produce H_2O_2, so this kind of polymeric nanosphere can also have glucose responsive behavior in the GOD containing environment. This will make it very promising to use in biomedical application field in body environment.

MATERIALS AND METHODS

Materials and Reagents

β-cyclodextrin (β-CD), α-Cyclodextrin (α-CD) was purchased from Sigma and dried in a vacuum before use. Sodium alginate (Alg) was purchased from Tianjin Yuanhang Chemicals Co., Ltd., China. Methoxypolyethylene glycol (mPEG, Mw = 2000) was purchased from Shanghai Jingchunshiye Co., Ltd., China. Glucose oxidase was purchased from Aspergillus Niger (GOD, lyophilized powder protein, Mw = 186 000, catalase <4%). BSA was purchased from Aoke Biological Co., Ltd., China. Carboxyferrocene (Fc-COOH), morpholinoethanesulfonic acid (MES), dicyclohexylcarbodiimide (DCC), 4-(dimethylamino) pyridine (DMAP), *N*-hydroxysuccinimide (NHS), 1-ethyl-3-[3-(dimethylamino)propyl]carbodiimide hydrochloride (EDCI), and other reagents were purchased from Chengdu Kelong Co., Ltd., China.

Synthesis of Alg-β-CD and mPEG-Fc

Sodium alginate with β-CD was synthesized in two steps with slight modification. Firstly, the mono-6-(*p*-tolylsulfonyl)-β-cyclodextrin (6-β-CD-OTs) and

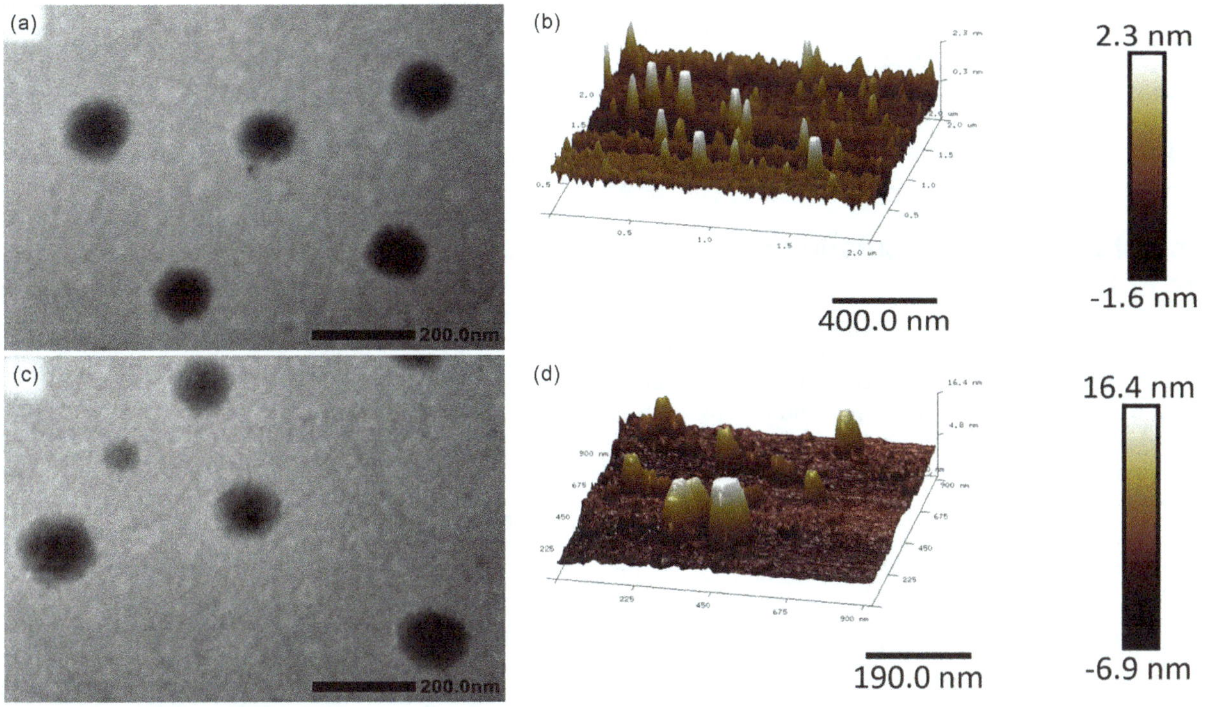

FIGURE 5 | (a) Transmission electron microscopy (TEM) micrograph of Alg-β-CD/PEG-Fc/α-CD NPs; **(b)** Atomic force microscopy (AFM) macrograph of Alg-β-CD/PEG-Fc/α-CD NPs; **(c)** TEM micrograph of Alg-β-CD/PEG-Fc/α-CD NPs entrapped Bovine serum albumin (BSA); **(d)** AFM macrograph of Alg-β-CD/PEG-Fc/α-CD NPs entrapped BSA.

mono-6-deoxy-6-hexamethylenediamine-β-CD (6-β-CD-HDA) were synthesized according to the method reported in the previous study (Quan et al., 2010). Briefly, β-CD was grafted onto the sodium alginate backbone via amido link condensation reaction. 1% sodium alginate solution (w/v) was prepared in MES buffer solution (0.1 M) and NaCl (0.5 M), and the pH was adjusted to 6.0. After 29 mg NHS and 95 mg EDC (molar ration of EDC: NHS: COO- = 1: 0.5: 1) were added to 40 mL above alginate solution, the solution was then agitated for 30 min to obtain a homogeneous solution followed by the addition of 10 mL 3.08 % 6-β-CD-HDA MES solution (w/v). The reaction was then continuing at 4°C for 24 h. Alg-β-CD was obtained after the resulting mixture dialyzed against pure water and then freeze dried. The degree of β-CD substitution (DS) to alginate was calculated according to the followed equation:

$$\frac{I_1}{I_2 - 6I_1 - \frac{2}{7}I_2} = \frac{7}{4}\mathrm{DS}$$

where I_1 is the digital integration of anomeric protons of β-CD, I_2 is the total digital integration of 3.4–4.2 ppm. The final degree of substitution (DS) of Alg-β-CD was 25.6 % by this calculated method. ^{1}HNMR (400 MHz, D_2O) were shown in **Figure 2**.

mPEG-Fc was synthesized with one pot method. DMAP (0.183 g) and DCC (1.12 g) were added successively to a solution of mPEG (3.0 g) and carboxyferrocene (0.69 g) in dry chloroform ($CHCl_3$, 100 mL) for 24 h at room temperature. After removing dicyclohexylurea (DCU) by filtration, the filtrate was concentrated in a vaccum and purified by dissolving in deionized water and extracting with diethyl ether four times. Subsequently, the product was further purified by using gel column with methanol and water as the solvent to remove the unreacted carboxyferrocene and catalyst residue. Finally, the dark red product was concentrated in a vaccum and dried in the vacuum oven for 2 days. The final DS of PEG-Fc used was 95.4% which was calculated though the integral ratio between H_d and H_f. ^{1}HNMR (400 MHz, $CDCl_3$) were shown in **Figure 3**.

Preparation of Alg-β-CD/mPEG-Fc/α-CD and Alg-β-CD/PEG-Fc/α-CD/BSA NPs

PEG-Fc (6.6 mg) and Alg-β-CD (8.4 mg) were added to 3 mL deionized water and kept stirring for 5 h to get a transparent solution. Then α-CD (0.2 g) was added to the above solution and continued to stir over night. For BSA loading, 1.5 mg BSA was added with stirring for 10 min before the addition of α-CD. The solution changes from transparent to turbid gradually indicating the formation of the Alg-β-CD/PEG-Fc/α-CD and Alg-β-CD/PEG-Fc/α-CD/BSA NPs.

Characterization of the Alg-β-CD/mPEG-Fc/α-CD and Alg-β-CD/mPEG-Fc/α-CD/BSA NPs

The product was characterized by ^1H–^1H (2D) NOESY NMR spectroscopy which recorded on an Advance Bruker 600 NMR spectrometer. The transmission electron microscopy (TEM) images were taken by using a JEOL JEM-100CX instrument operating at an accelerating voltage of 80 kV. Each sample were prepared and imaged by Atomic force microscopy (AFM) in tapping mode with a Nanoscope IIIa Digital Instrument. X-ray powder diffraction (XRD) patterns of the samples were recorded by using Cu-Kα irradiation source with X' Pert MPD (20 kV; 35 mA; 2°theta/min) to determine the crystalline structures.

Self-Assembly NPs Encapsulation and Leakage of BSA

Self-assembly NPs encapsulated BSA were prepared and then their encapsulation efficiency was determined as follows. The BSA loaded NPs (0.5 mg BSA, 0.5%) was centrifuged for 20 min at 12,000 rpm to completely separate the free and encapsulated BSA and the supernatant was analyzed by determined by UV spectrophotometry. The BSA encapsulation efficiency was calculated as follows (1):

$$\text{Bovine serum albumin encapsulation efficiency (\%)} = \frac{\text{mass of BSA used in formulation} - \text{mass of free BSA}}{\text{mass of BSA used in formulation}} \times 100$$

Then the NPs were continuing stored in aqueous solution for 48 h to evaluate leakage of BSA. The mixture was again separated by centrifugation and the supernatant was analyzed for determination of BSA leakage efficiency as above method (2):

$$\text{Bovine serum albumin leakage efficiency (\%)} = \frac{\text{mass of BSA in the supernatant}}{\text{mass of BSA encapsulated}} \times 100$$

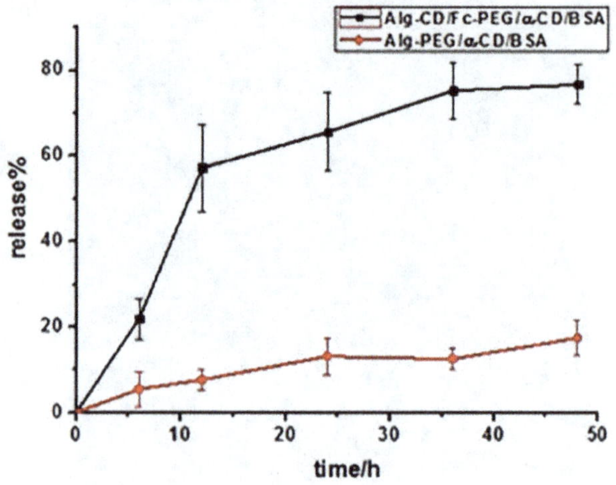

FIGURE 8 | Bovine serum albumin release from Alg-β-CD/PEG-Fc/α-CD/BSA and Alg-PEG/α-CD/BSA nanoparticles at 37°C in 12 mL 0.1 M glucose and 10 mg GOD containing solution.

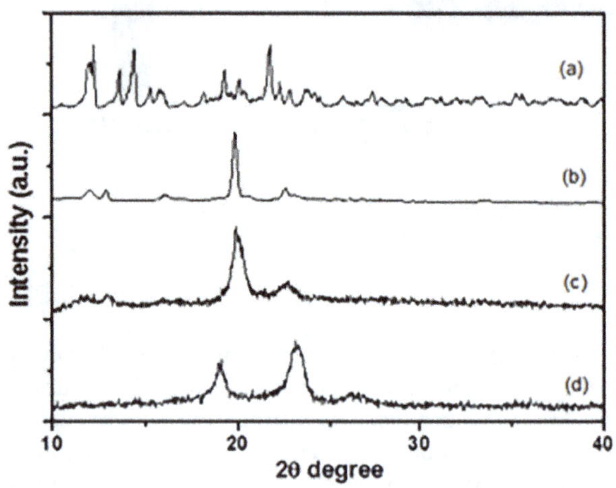

FIGURE 6 | X-ray diffraction patterns of **(a)** α-CD, **(b)** PEG/α-CD inclusion complex, **(c)** Alg-β-CD/PEG-Fc/α-CD particles, **(d)** Alg-β-CD/PEG-Fc.

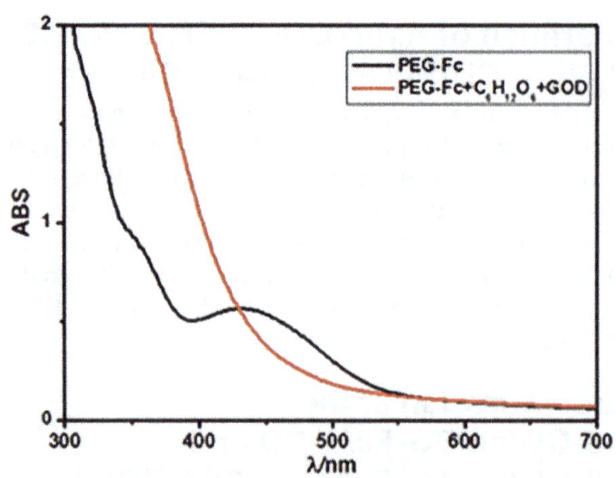

FIGURE 7 | UV-vis spectra of the PEG-Fc in 12 mL 0.1 M glucose before and after 10 mg glucose oxidase (GOD) was added after 12 h.

In Vitro Release Studies

The Alg-β-CD/PEG-Fc/α-CD self-assembly NPs encapsulated BSA was prepared and centrifuged for *in vitro* BSA release study (12,000 rpm, 20 min). The lower sediment was added 12 mL 0.1 M glucose solution and 10 mg GOD and kept stirring for 10 min. The solution was placed in a constant temperature incubator and kept the temperature at 37°C during the whole release process. 2 mL solution had been taken out and centrifugation at 12,000 rpm for 20 min every 6 h. The amount of BSA released in the supernate was collected and determined by UV spectrometry at specified time. The BSA release was quantified when the standard curve was plotted using a standard BSA solution.

In Vitro Cell Studies

Methyl tetrazolium (MTT) assay was carried out on murine colon carcinoma cells (CT26) as the cell line for biocompatibility evaluation of the self-assembly NPs. 5 × 10^3 cells were culture for

24 h to attach in 96-well plates. Then the cells were treated with fresh medium containing 1 mg/mL Alg-β-CD/mPEG-Fc/α-CD NPs and Alg-β-CD/mPEG-Fc/α-CD/BSA NPs. The cell viability was measured after incubation for desired time duration (48 h). The cells without treatment were used as the control. Each group was repeated in triplicate.

Further, confocal laser scanning microscopy (CLSM) was used for monitoring the *in vitro* endocytosis. Briefly, self-assembly NPs encapsulated Dil were prepared and incubated with CT26 cells at 37°C for 4 h. After incubation, all samples were stained with LysoTracker Green (Life Technologies, Carlsbad, CA, United States) and 10 μg/mL of Hoechst 33342 (Life Technologies, Carlsbad, CA, United States).

Statistical Analysis

All the results obtained in this study were expressed as mean ± standard deviation unless otherwise noted. Comparisons between two groups were made using two-tailed student's *t*-test and between multiple groups were made using one-way analysis of variance (ANOVA). Statistical analyses were performed using SPSS 21.0 and considered statistically significance when $^*p < 0.05$.

RESULTS AND DISCUSSION

According to the previous, it has demonstrated that inclusion complexes would form when β-CD interact with Fc group (Tomatsu et al., 2010). Further, the formation of complexation between the Fc groups on mPEG-Fc and β-CD groups on Alg-β-CD could be observed by using 2D NMR NOESY spectra. As shown in **Figure 4**, the peaks of β-CD group were in accordance with the resonance of the Fc groups could be found in the 2D NOESY spectrum of Alg-β-CD/PEG-Fc, which indicating that the Fc groups threaded through the cavity of β-CD to form an inclusion complex.

The resulting Alg-β-CD/PEG-Fc was hydrophilic copolymers, which could form transparency solution in water. By adding α-CD to the aqueous solution of Alg-β-CD/PEG-Fc at room temperature, the solution gradually became turbid gradually when the aggregates were formed. The morphology of these aggregates has been observed by TEM and atomic force microscope (AFM). TEM micrographs of **Figure 5a** revealed that the Alg-β-CD/PEG-Fc/α-CD aggregates appeared round line shapes and their diameters were about 100 nm. In the AFM micrographs of **Figure 5c**, Alg-β-CD/PEG-Fc/α-CD self-assembly NPs also showed rounded line shapes with a horizontal length about 100 nm. Particularly, it is noted that most height of the aggregates (<5 nm) was about 20 times smaller than horizontal length. The main reason for such size differences between horizontal and vertical direction might be the collapsing of this NPs. Further, the height of NPs increased about threefold when BSA was encapsulated, which demonstrated that the BSA has been successfully encapsulated into the Alg-β-CD/PEG-Fc/α-CD NPs (**Figures 5b,d**).

The XRD patterns of the α-CD (**Figure 6a**), PEG/α-CD inclusion complex (**Figure 6b**), Alg-β-CD/PEG-Fc/α-CD (**Figure 6c**), and Alg-β-CD/PEG-Fc (**Figure 6d**) has been shown in **Figure 6**. As an important index to evaluate the inclusion structures formation of CD based complex. The pattern of Alg-β-CD/PEG-Fc/α-CD showed in the figure was differs from that of free Alg-β-CD/PEG-Fc or α-CD. It was also found that the homo-PEG crystalline peaks (2 theta = 19.2° and 23.3°) and α-CD crystalline peak (2 theta = 21.5°) were absent. According to the previous study, the peak at 2 theta = 19.9° is a typical peak of PEG-α-CD channel-type crystallites that demonstrated the inclusion structures of Alg-β-CD/PEG-Fc/α-CD contained PEG-α-CD (Lautens et al., 1990). Meanwhile, the NPs would

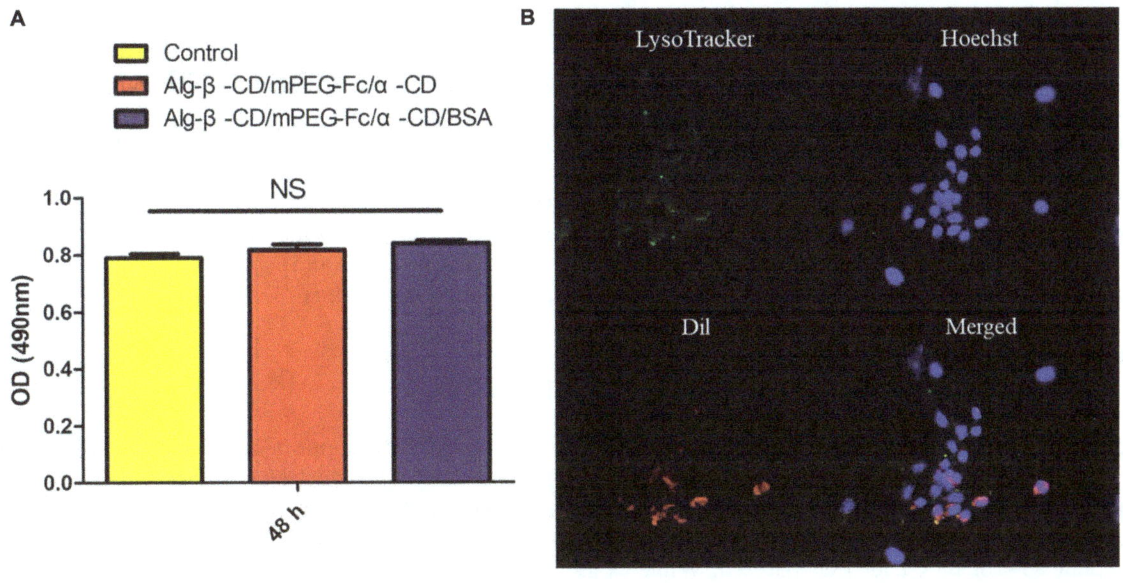

FIGURE 9 | (A) The *in vitro* cytotoxicity of Alg-β-CD/PEG-Fc/α-CD NPs with and without BSA; **(B)** The cellular uptake of Alg-β-CD/PEG-Fc/α-CD NPs.

form an inner rod-like PEG-α-CD inclusion block surrounded by a protonated coil-like Alg shell when insoluble PEG-α-CD inclusion blocks formed and water became a selective solvent for the Alg-β-CD/PEG-Fc/α-CD. This rod-like block in rod-coil system preferred parallel packing which may result in the formation of hollow NPs promoted by efficient space-filling has been investigated (Jenekhe and Chen, 1999).

As mentioned in the literature and our previous study, the Alg-β-CD/PEG-Fc/α-CD self-assemble NPs were connected by the Fc-β-CD inclusions. These NPs could release BSA through their collapse after the dissociation of Fc-β-CD. To achieve this goal, the oxidization Fc to Fc^+ is an efficacy way while β-CD could not form complex with Fc derivatives in their oxidized state (Matsue et al., 1985). To get a clear vision, hydrogen peroxide (H_2O_2) was chosen as the oxidant in this study. After the addition of H_2O_2 (1 mL, 30%, H_2O_2 solution) to Alg-β-CD/PEG-Fc/α-CD hollow NPs (10 mL, 1%), the system became unstable and produced polyrotaxane precipitate in 5 min. The possible mechanism of this phenomenon can be seen in **Figure 7**. The addition of H_2O_2 dissociated Fc-β-CD inclusion complex and leaving the rod-like hydrophobic PEG-Fc/α-CD part precipitated out of water.

Nowadays, one of the most widely used applications of the stimuli-responsive NPs is in the on demand drug-release field (Tao et al., 2015). It requires the micelle system release the aim drugs gradually to achieve the long-term drug action. Since H_2O_2 could be produce in a rather sustained way through oxidization of glucose by glucose oxidase (GOD) so that can oxidize Fc to its oxidation state gradually. **Figure 7** shows the UV-vis spectra of the PEG-Fc in 0.1 M glucose before and after 10 mg GOD was added. After adding GOD for 12 h, the absorption peak around 450 nm due to Fc groups d–d transition peak (in reduced form) almost disappeared indicating that the Fc groups in the PEG-Fc could be oxidized to ferrocenium as anticipated (Yamamoto et al., 2000). Tan et al. (2012) have been developed the glucose sensitive hydrogel using the GOD and glucose interaction to produce hydrogen peroxide to disintegrate the ICs of Fc and β-CD. Therefore, it is possible to get glucose sensitive Alg-β-CD/PEG-Fc/α-CD micelles by adding GOD to the Alg-β-CD/PEG-Fc/α-CD system.

Otherwise, serum albumins, as a major soluble protein, have got much attention and been widely used due to their physiological functions. It has been applied in the nanomedicine field because of they serve as a depot protein and as a transport protein for a variety of compounds. BSA has been one of the most extensively member used as a protein drug model, particularly because of its structural homology with human serum albumin (Papadopoulou et al., 2005). The incorporation of BSA into Alg-β-CD/PEG-Fc/α-CD particles had been studied. The encapsulation efficiency and leakage efficiency was 71.4 and 6.6%, respectively. The *in vitro* release profile of BSA from Alg-β-CD/PEG-Fc/α-CD/BSA and Alg-PEG/α-CD/BSA particles was presented in **Figure 8**. In Alg-β-CD/PEG-Fc/α-CD/BSA particles group, the BSA appeared to be released in a continuous way. After 48 h, about 80% of BSA had been released. While as a counterpart, the Alg-PEG/α-CD/BSA group (BSA encapsulation efficiency was 66.7%), under the same condition, there was less than 20% of BSA had been released which is much less than the Alg-β-CD/PEG-Fc/α-CD/BSA group. This result further confirmed that in glucose and GOD containing environment the Alg-β-CD/PEG-Fc/α-CD/BSA particle achieved BSA delayed release behavior through the β-CD-Fc inclusion complex as redox trigger.

The biocompatibility of NPs is of critical importance to their eventual success (Tao et al., 2014). As shown in **Figure 9A**, the results demonstrate the non-toxic of Alg-β-CD/PEG-Fc/α-CD and Alg-β-CD/PEG-Fc/α-CD/BSA NPs, which could be used as the biocompatible drug delivery system. The performance of NPs cellular internalization through the observation of NPs encapsulated Dil interaction with labeling CT26 cells (**Figure 9B**). The results indicated that large numbers of Alg-β-CD/PEG-Fc/α-CD NPs entered the cells after 4 h and some of them began to enter into cell nucleus.

CONCLUSION

In summary, Alg-β-CD/PEG-Fc/α-CD rod-coil hollow NPs have been prepared through the supramolecular self-assemble. The rod-part PEG-α-CD and the coil-part Alg were connected through β-CD-Fc inclusion complex. The BSA enzyme was successfully encapsulated in Alg-β-CD/PEG-Fc/α-CD hollow sphere in aqueous solution. These Alg-β-CD/PEG-Fc/α-CD hollow NPs showed good H_2O_2 sensitivity. Further study showed that this nanoparticle encapsuled BSA can achieve BSA delayed drug-release behavior in the glucose containing environment at the existence of GOD. Therefore, this study exhibits that using the host-guest interactions would be a general, useful and effective way for fabricating stimuli-responsive drug delivery NPs. Furthermore, the glucose mediated H_2O_2 sensitive behavior of the Alg-β-CD/PEG-Fc/α-CD NPs may benefit its application in more and more fields such as enzyme immobilization, drug delivery and micro-reactors.

AUTHOR CONTRIBUTIONS

ZG designed experiments, supervised the experiments, and revised and finalized the manuscript. ZD and YK performed the experiments, analyzed the data, and prepared the figures and the manuscript. QY performed the cell culture. ML contributed to the results discussion and paper writing. All authors reviewed and approved the final paper.

FUNDING

This study was supported by the funding and generous support of the National Natural Science Foundation of China (21704104), West Light Foundation of the Chinese Academy of Sciences (2016XBZG_XBQNXZ_B_003). Meanwhile, we also want to sincerely acknowledge the funding from the Guangdong Province Key Laboratory of Malignant Tumor Epigenetics and Gene Regulation (2017B030314026).

REFERENCES

Chen, J., Cun, X., Ruan, S., Wang, Y., Zhang, Y., He, Q., et al. (2015). Glioma cell-targeting doxorubicin delivery and redox-responsive release using angiopep-2 decorated carbonaceous nanodots. *RSC Adv.* 5, 57045–57049. doi: 10.1039/C5RA08245E

Ding, L., Zhu, X., Wang, Y., Shi, B., Ling, X., Chen, H., et al. (2017). Intracellular fate of nanoparticles with polydopamine surface engineering and a novel strategy for exocytosis-inhibiting, lysosome impairment-based cancer therapy. *Nano Lett.* 17, 6790–6801. doi: 10.1021/acs.nanolett.7b03021

Guo, W., and Lei, Z. (2015). Redox-responsive supramolecular polymer based on β-cyclodextrin and ferrocene-decorated main chain of PAA. *J. Mater. Res.* 30, 3201–3210. doi: 10.1557/jmr.2015.284

Hu, X., Yu, J., Qian, C., Lu, Y., Kahkoska, A. R., Xie, Z., et al. (2017). H2O2-responsive vesicles integrated with transcutaneous patches for glucose-mediated insulin delivery. *ACS Nano* 11, 613–620. doi: 10.1021/acsnano.6b06892

Jenekhe, S. A., and Chen, X. L. (1999). Self-assembly of ordered microporous materials from rod-coil block copolymers. *Science* 283, 372–375. doi: 10.1126/science.283.5400.372

Kang, Y., Guo, K., Li, B. J., and Zhang, S. (2014). Nanoassemblies driven by cyclodextrin-based inclusion complexation. *Chem. Commun.* 50, 11083–11092. doi: 10.1039/c4cc03131h

Kang, Y., Ju, X., Ding, L. S., Zhang, S., and Li, B. J. (2017a). Reactive oxygen species and glutathione dual redox-responsive supramolecular assemblies with controllable release capability. *ACS Appl. Mater. Interfaces* 9, 4475–4484. doi: 10.1021/acsami.6b14640

Kang, Y., Ju, X., Wang, L., Ding, L. S., Liu, G. T., Zhang, S., et al. (2017b). pH and glutathione dual-triggered supramolecular assemblies as synergistic and controlled drug release carriers. *Polym. Chem.* 8, 7260–7270. doi: 10.1039/C7PY01644A

Kang, Y., Ma, Y., Zhang, S., Ding, L. S., and Li, B. J. (2015). Dual-stimuli-responsive nanoassemblies as tunable releasing carriers. *ACS Macro Lett.* 4, 543–547. doi: 10.1021/acsmacrolett.5b00171

Kim, A., Ha, J. H., and Park, S. N. (2017). Selective release system for antioxidative and anti-inflammatory activities using H2O2-responsive therapeutic nanoparticles. *Biomacromolecules* 18, 3197–3206. doi: 10.1021/acs.biomac.7b00844

Kuang, T. R., Liu, Y. R., Gong, T. T., Peng, X. F., Hu, X. L., and Yu, Z. Q. (2016). Enzyme-responsive nanoparticles for anticancer drug delivery. *Curr. Nanosci.* 12, 38–46. doi: 10.2174/15734137116661506241 70518

Lautens, M., Abdelaziz, A. S., and Schmidt, G. (1990). Synthesis and epoxidation of cis-enriched polydeltacyclene. *Macromolecules* 23, 89–132. doi: 10.1021/ma00212a038

Liao, W., Lai, T., Chen, L., Fu, J., Sreenivasan, S. T., Yu, Z., et al. (2016). Synthesis and characterization of a walnut peptides–zinc complex and its antiproliferative activity against human breast carcinoma cells through the induction of apoptosis. *J. Agric. Food Chem.* 104, 849–859. doi: 10.1021/acs.jafc.5b04924

Matsue, T., Evans, D. H., Osa, T., and Kobayashi, N. (1985). Cheminform abstract: electron-transfer reactions associated with host-guest complexation. Oxidation of ferrocenecarboxylic acid in the presence of β-cyclodextrin. *Chem. Inform.* 16.

Miao, P., Wang, B. D., Yin, J., Chen, X. F., and Tang, Y. G. (2015). Electrochemical tracking hydrogen peroxide secretion in live cells based on autocatalytic oxidation reaction of silver nanoparticles. *Electrochem. Commun.* 53, 37–40. doi: 10.1016/j.elecom.2015.02.007

Papadopoulou, A., Green, R. J., and Frazier, R. A. (2005). Interaction of flavonoids with bovine serum albumin: a fluorescence quenching study. *J. Agric. Food Chem.* 53, 158–163. doi: 10.1021/jf048693g

Quan, C. Y., Chen, J. X., Wang, H. Y., Li, C., Chang, C., Zhang, X. Z., et al. (2010). Core-shell nanosized assemblies mediated by the alpha-beta cyclodextrin dimer with a tumor-triggered targeting property. *ACS Nano* 4, 4211–4219. doi: 10.1021/nn100534q

Rosenblum, D., Joshi, N., Tao, W., Karp, J. M., and Peer, D. (2018). Progress and challenges towards targeted delivery of cancer therapeutics. *Nat. Commun.* 9:1410. doi: 10.1038/s41467-018-03705-y

Ruan, S., Hu, C., Xian, T., Cun, X., Wei, X., Shi, K., et al. (2016). Increased gold nanoparticle retention in brain tumors by in situ enzyme-induced aggregation. *ACS Nano* 10, 10086–10098. doi: 10.1021/acsnano.6b05070

Ruan, S., Yuan, M., Zhang, L., Hu, G., Chen, J., Cun, X., et al. (2015). Tumor microenvironment sensitive doxorubicin delivery and release to glioma using angiopep-2 decorated gold nanoparticles. *Biomaterials* 37, 425–435. doi: 10.1016/j.biomaterials.2014.10.007

Tan, L., Liu, Y., Ha, W., Ding, L. S., Peng, S. L., Zhang, S., et al. (2012). Stimuli-induced gel-sol transition of multi-sensitive supramolecular β-cyclodextrin grafted alginate/ferrocene modified pluronic hydrogel. *Soft Matter* 8, 5746–5749. doi: 10.1039/c2sm25084e

Tao, W., Ji, X., Xu, X., Ariful Islam, M., Li, Z., Chen, S., et al. (2017a). Antimonene quantum dots: synthesis and application as near-infrared photothermal agents for effective cancer therapy. *Angew. Chem. Int. Ed.* 56, 11896–11900. doi: 10.1002/anie.201703657

Tao, W., Zhu, X., Yu, X., Zeng, X., Xiao, Q., Zhang, X., et al. (2017b). Black phosphorus nanosheets as a robust delivery platform for cancer theranostics. *Adv. Mater.* 29:1603276. doi: 10.1002/adma.201603276

Tao, W., Zeng, X., Liu, T., Wang, Z., Xiong, Q., Ouyang, C., et al. (2013). Docetaxel-loaded nanoparticles based on star-shaped mannitol-core PLGA-TPGS diblock copolymer for breast cancer therapy. *Acta Biomater.* 9, 8910–8920. doi: 10.1016/j.actbio.2013.06.034

Tao, W., Zeng, X., Wu, J., Zhu, X., Yu, X., Zhang, X., et al. (2016). Polydopamine-based surface modification of novel nanoparticle-aptamer bioconjugates for in vivo breast cancer targeting and enhanced therapeutic effects. *Theranostics* 6, 470–484. doi: 10.7150/thno.14184

Tao, W., Zeng, X., Zhang, J., Zhu, H., Chang, D., Zhang, X., et al. (2014). Synthesis of cholic acid-core poly (ε-caprolactone-ran-lactide)-b-poly (ethylene glycol) 1000 random copolymer as a chemotherapeutic nanocarrier for liver cancer treatment. *Biomater. Sci.* 2, 1262–1274. doi: 10.1039/C4BM00134F

Tao, W., Zhang, J., Zeng, X., Liu, D., Liu, G., Zhu, X., et al. (2015). Blended nanoparticle system based on miscible structurally similar polymers: a safe, simple, targeted, and surprisingly high efficiency vehicle for cancer therapy. *Adv. Healthc. Mater.* 4, 1203–1214. doi: 10.1002/adhm.201400751

Tomatsu, I., Hashidzume, A., and Harada, A. (2010). Redox-responsive hydrogel system using the molecular recognition of < I > -cyclodextrin. *Macromol. Rapid Commun.* 27, 238–241. doi: 10.1002/marc.200500793

Wang, H., Chen, J., Xu, C., Shi, L., Tayier, M., Zhou, J., et al. (2017a). Cancer nanomedicines stabilized by π-π stacking between heterodimeric prodrugs enable exceptionally high drug loading capacity and safer delivery of drug combinations. *Theranostics* 7, 3638–3652. doi: 10.7150/thno.20028

Wang, H., Lu, Z., Wang, L., Guo, T., Wu, J., Wan, J., et al. (2017b). New generation nanomedicines constructed from self-assembling small molecule prodrugs alleviate cancer drug toxicity. *Cancer Res.* 77, 6963–6974. doi: 10.1158/0008-5472.CAN-17-0984

Wang, H., Xie, H., Wang, J., Wu, J., Ma, X., Li, L., et al. (2015). Self-assembling prodrugs by precise programming of molecular structures that contribute distinct stability, pharmacokinetics, and antitumor efficacy. *Adv. Funct. Mater.* 25, 4956–4965. doi: 10.1002/adfm.201501953

Wu, J., Kamaly, N., Shi, J., Zhao, L., Xiao, Z., Hollett, G., et al. (2014). Development of multinuclear polymeric nanoparticles as robust protein nanocarriers. *Angew. Chem.* 53, 8975–8979. doi: 10.1002/anie.201404766

Yamamoto, T., Takashi Morikita, A., Maruyama, T., Kubota, K., and Katada, M. (2000). Poly(aryleneethynylene) type polymers containing a ferrocene unit in the π-conjugated main chain. preparation, optical properties, redox behavior, and mössbauer spectroscopic analysis. *Macromolecules* 30, 5390–5396. doi: 10.1021/ma9704368

Yuan, Q. J., Wang, Y. F., Li, J. H., Li, B. J., and Zhang, S. (2013). pH-Switchable macroscopic assembly through host-guest inclusion. *Macromol. Rapid Commun.* 34, 1174–1180. doi: 10.1002/marc.201300289

Zhu, X., Ji, X., Kong, N., Chen, Y., Mahmoudi, M., Xu, X., et al. (2018). Intracellular mechanistic understanding of 2D MoS2 nanosheets for anti-exocytosis-enhanced synergistic cancer therapy. *ACS Nano* 12, 2922–2938. doi: 10.1021/acsnano.8b00516

3

Topical Use of Quercetin-Loaded Chitosan Nanoparticles Against Ultraviolet B Radiation

Wenhao Nan[1,2†], Li Ding[1,2†], Houjie Chen[1,2], Fahim U. Khan[1,2], Lu Yu[3], Xinbing Sui[4,5] and Xiaojun Shi[1,2*]*

[1] School of Life Sciences, Tsinghua University, Beijing, China, [2] Graduate School at Shenzhen, Tsinghua University, Shenzhen, China, [3] Shenzhen Modo Biotech Co., Ltd., Shenzhen, China, [4] Department of Medical Oncology, Holistic Integrative Oncology Institutes and Holistic Integrative Cancer Center of Traditional Chinese and Western Medicine, The Affiliated Hospital of Hangzhou Normal University, College of Medicine, Hangzhou Normal University, Hangzhou, China, [5] Department of Cancer Pharmacology, Holistic Integrative Pharmacy Institutes, College of Medicine, Hangzhou Normal University, Hangzhou, China

***Correspondence:**
Xinbing Sui
hzzju@zju.edu.cn
Xiaojun Shi
shixj@sz.tsinghua.edu.cn

† These authors have contributed equally to this work.

Ultraviolet radiation is a major risk factor for human skin damage, especially solar ultraviolet-B (UVB) which can induce inflammation, photoaging, and skin cancer. Quercetin (Qu), one of flavonoid family members, has showed protective effects against UVB radiation. However, its application for topical use is limited by low hydrophilicity and poor percutaneous absorption. Herein, we found that Qu, if entrapped into TPP-Chitosan nanoparticles (TCs), can be efficiently uptake by HaCaT cells and easily permeate through the epidermis layer, meanwhile display better stability and low cytotoxicity. We also found that Qu-loaded TCs (QTCs) could notably enhance the effect of Qu on inhibiting the NF-kB/COX-2 signaling pathway as well as ameliorating the skin edema caused by UVB radiation. Therefore, this study provided a method to get rid of Qu's low hydrophilicity, enhance its percutaneous absorption and retention in the skin, and further improve its anti-UVB effect, and demonstrated that Qu-loaded chitosan nanoparticles can be used as the therapeutic agent for topical use against UVB radiation.

Keywords: Quercetin, chitosan, nanoparticles, topical use, anti-UVB radiation, skin damaging

INTRODUCTION

Previous studies have reported that the ultraviolet radiation (UVR) harms the human skin, particularly in fair skin populations (Madronich and Gruijl, 1993; Gallagher and Lee, 2006; Morganroth et al., 2013). Currently, due to gradual depletion of the ozone layer caused by chemical compounds containing gaseous chlorine or bromine from industries or human in atmosphere, the solar ultraviolet-B (UVB; 280–315 nm) radiation significantly penetrates to Earth's surface resulting in skin diseases including erythema, sunburn, inflammation, photoaging, oxidative stress, DNA damage, immunosuppression, and even skin cancer (Kerr and Mcelroy, 1993; Pal et al., 2015).

One of the most important mechanisms involved in UVB radiation caused skin damage is the activation of NF-κB/cyclooxygenase-2 (COX-2) signaling pathway. COX-2 one of the enzyme plays a key role in converting arachidonic acid (AA) into prostaglandins (PGE2) which increases the vascular permeability and promotes edema (Kim et al., 2005; Liu et al., 2009; Hur et al., 2010;

Pal et al., 2015; Tang et al., 2017). In addition, high COX-2 level are frequently correlated with skin inflammation and cancer development (Pentland et al., 1999; Tang et al., 2008; Mccarty, 2012; Jiao et al., 2014). Once our skin suffers from UVB radiation, IkB-α is phosphorylated through a family of serine/threonine kinases known as IKK, and subsequently falls off from NF-κB protein complex, which drives NF-κB translocating from the cytoplasm to the nucleus. Furthermore, this kind of NF-κB translocation enhances the expression of COX-2 (Kim et al., 2005; Liu et al., 2009; Hur et al., 2010; Pal et al., 2015; Tang et al., 2017).

Many flavonoids including Quercetin (Qu) play a vital role in regulating NF-κB/COX-2 signaling pathway (Serafini et al., 2010; de Alencar Filho et al., 2016). Qu is one representative flavonoid with anti-oxidant, anti-inflammation, and anti-tumor properties (Formica and Regelson, 1995). Previous research has revealed that Qu is very effective against UVB radiation through downregulating COX-2 level *in vitro* (Steerenberg et al., 1997). However, *in vivo* application of Qu is limited by its low hydrophilicity and poor percutaneous absorption (Hung et al., 2012). Therefore, many researchers managed to seek for new dosage forms of Qu to solve this problem, including Qu-loaded liposome or nanoparticles (NPs) (Hatahet et al., 2016). Our previous study has also reported using PLGA-TPGS NPs to load Qu (Zhu et al., 2016). However, although the application of PLGA-TPGS NPs significantly enhanced the protective effect of Qu, we think it is still not ideal preparation of Qu considering the natural disadvantages of PLGA-TPGS NPs. That is, PLGA-TPGS NPs, owing negative surface charge, will no doubt impede the nano-bio interaction with skin cell cytomembrane which also negatively charged (Yang et al., 2009).

Chitosan (CS), an abundant linear cationic biopolymer, has several favorable biological characteristics such as biodegradability, non-toxicity, biocompatibility, and anti-pathogen (Enríquez et al., 2006). Most importantly, CS NPs (CSs) can increase the cellular uptake due to their positive surface charge which can enhance the interaction with negatively surface charged cytomembrane (Schipper et al., 1997; Huang et al., 2002). Another advantage of CSs is its enhancement of the skin permeation of hydrophobic drugs and promotion of the retention of drugs in the epidermis, due to its interaction with the skin surface which will change the morphology of the stratum corneum and break the close conjugation of the corneocyte layers (Tan et al., 2011). Thus, theoretically Qu, if loaded into CSs, may efficiently overcome the shortcomings of Qu for topical use to protect skin from UVB radiation damage.

In this work, we compared the protective effects of Qu and Qu-loaded TPP-Chitosan NPs (QTCs) against UVB radiation *in vitro* and *in vivo*, using HaCaT cells and C57BL/6 mice models. We found that QTCs which displayed better stability and low cytotoxicity could be uptake by HaCaT cells efficiently and easily permeate through stratum corneum and epidermis. Besides, the application of CSs carrier enhanced the effect of Qu on inhibiting the NF-κB/COX-2 signaling pathway, further ameliorating the skin edema induced by UVB radiation. In this study, we firstly showed the advantages of Qu-loaded CS NPs for topical use against UVB radiation-induced skin damage.

MATERIALS AND METHODS

Chemicals

Quercetin and coumarin-6 were purchased from Sigma-Aldrich (St. Louis, MO, United States). Chitosan (deacetylation degree ≥ 95%, viscosity 100–200 mpa.s, biotechnology level) and sodium tripolyphosphate (TPP) were purchased from Macklin (Shanghai, China). 4',6-Diamidino-2-phenylindole dihydrochloride (DAPI) and dimethyl sulfoxide (DMSO) were purchased from Sangon Biotech (Shanghai, China). Wheat Germ Agglutinin Alexa Fluor 594 conjugate (WGA-594) were purchased from Thermo Fisher Scientific (Eugene, OR, United States). All other chemicals and reagents of the highest quality were commercially available and used as received. Antibodies against p-IkB-α, NF-κB, COX-2, GAPDH, β-actin and lamin A/C were purchased from Cell Signaling Technology.

Formulation and Characterization of NPs

The preparation of TPP-Chitosan NPs (TCs) was based on ionic gelation of chitosan with TPP anions reported before (Zhang et al., 2008), but with some modifications. Under magnetic stirring at room temperature, 20 mg CS was dissolved into 10 ml 1% (V/V) acetum and adjusted the pH to 5.5, then 3.5 ml TPP with the concentration of 2 mg/ml was dropwise added into CS solution. Opalescent and transparent solution was formed after transient sonication. Qu loaded TPP-Chitosan NPs (QTCs) were formed by dropwise adding 1 ml Qu ethanol solution with the concentration of 3 mg/ml into CS solution before adding TPP. The NPs were centrifuged at 8,000 rpm, 4°C for 30 min, the supernatant was collected for HPLC and the precipitation was suspended after washed three times by ddH_2O, and finally lyophilized.

The hydrodynamic diameter and zeta potential of NPs were measured by Dynamic Light Scattering Zetasizer (Zetasizer Nano ZS90, Malvern Instruments Ltd., Malvern, United Kingdom). The morphology of NPs was showed by transmission electron microscopy (TEM, Tecnai G20, FEI Company, Hillsboro, OR, United States).

Measurement of Drug Encapsulation Efficiency and Drug Loading Content

The drug encapsulation efficiency (EE) and drug loading content (LC) of the QTCs were measured by HPLC (LC 1200, Agilent Technologies, Santa Clara, CA, United States). The mobile phase of HPLC was 0.2% phosphoric acid solution and MeOH with the volume ratio of 55:45. The flow rate of mobile phase was 1 ml/min. The UV detection wavelength was 360 nm. A C-18 column (150 mm × 4.6 mm, GL Science Inc., Tokyo, Japan) was used. The supernatant of QTCs after centrifugation was used for HPLC to detect the concentration of Qu in the supernatant; therefore, we can detect the amount of Qu in supernatant (W_1). We named the weight of lyophilized precipitation as

W_2 and the amount of Qu added in the preparation of QTC as W_3.

$$EE = (W_3 - W_1)/W_3 \times 100\%$$

$$LC = (W_3 - W_1)/W_2 \times 100\%$$

Cell Culture

HaCaT cells were cultured in Dulbecco's modified Eagle's medium (DMEM; Gibco BRL, United States) supplemented with 10% fetal bovine serum (FBS, Gibco) at 37°C with 5% CO_2.

Cellular Uptake of Coumarin-6-Loaded TCs and Its Efficiency

Coumarin-6 was used as the fluorescent probe which was entrapped into TCs to show the cellular uptake of QTCs. HaCaT cells were seeded in 12-well plate containing cover glasses in the bottom. After the cells adhered to the glasses, 100 μg/ml coumarin-6-loaded TCs was added to the culture medium and incubated at 37°C for 3 h. Then removed the culture medium and washed with PBS three times. Next added WGA-594 diluted by PBS to the wells and incubated at 37°C for 20 min to stain the cytomembrane, then washed with PBS three times and fixed with 4% paraformaldehyde for 20 min, finally, cells were stained with DAPI for 15 min and washed with PBS three times. Thereafter, cells were investigated by confocal laser scanning microscope (CLSM, Olympus Fluoview FV-1000, Tokyo, Japan).

To quantitatively measure the cellular uptake efficiency of coumarin-6-loaded TCs, 100 μg/ml coumarin-6-loaded TCs were incubated with HaCaT cells in 12-well plate at 3, 6, 12, 24 (each group, n = 3), and the quantitative ratio of coumarin-6 fluorescence in cytoplasm were measured by detecting the absorbance value at 320 nm.

Cytotoxicity and UVB Protective Experiment *in Vitro*

Cytotoxicity was evaluated by MTT assay. Cells were seeded in 96-well plate, after the cell attachment rate reached 60∼70%, replaced the culture medium to new culture medium mixed with or without different concentrations of Qu (mixed with DMSO, at the concentration of no influence on cells), QTCs, TCs and incubated for another 24 h. Then removed the culture medium, added new culture medium mixed with MTT (0.5 mg/ml) and incubated 4 h. Finally, the absorbance value of 490 nm was detected.

The method to investigate the UVB protective effects of Qu, QTCs, and TCs *in vitro* were almost the same as cytotoxicity experiment. The difference was the time of incubation with different concentrations of Qu, QTCs, and TCs been cut to 8 h, then removed the culture medium and irradiated using a microprocessor-controlled UV Crosslinker (XL-1000, SPECTROLINKER™, United States) of 12 mJ/cm^2. After the radiation, cells were added new drug free culture medium and returned to the incubator immediately.

Immunoblotting

Cell and tissue lysates were separated by 12% SDS-PAGE and analyzed by immunoblotting using P-IkB-α, NF-κB, COX-2 antibodies, followed by enhanced chemiluminescence (ECL) detection. Isolation of nuclear protein was conducted using the manufacturer's protocol (Abcam, Cambridge, MA, United States).

Immunocytochemical Staining of NF-κB

Cell culture and UVB radiation were the same as the UVB radiation treatment mentioned before. 10 h after UVB radiation, the cells were fixed and immunofluorescence stained with NF-κB antibody. After stained with DAPI, the cells were detected by CLSM.

Percutaneous Absorption and Retention Study of QTCs and Qu Aqueous Solution

All animal experiment protocols were approved by the Administrative Committee on Animal Research in the Graduate School at Shenzhen, Tsinghua University. Female C57BL/6 mice (aged 6 weeks, weighing about 20 g) were purchased from Guangdong Medical Laboratory Animal Center. After execution, the dorsal skin was carefully shaved with electric clippers and then carefully cut down the dorsal skin. Scrape the subcutaneous tissue completely and carefully by using a knife, and then fixed the skin on the V-C diffusion cell to investigate the percutaneous absorption of QTCs aqueous solution and Qu aqueous solution (each group, n = 3). Take samples regularly on 2, 4, 6, 8, 12, and 24 h for HPLC. The preparation of QTCs aqueous solution was mentioned before, and the preparation of Qu aqueous solution was by dropwise adding 1 ml Qu ethanol solution (5 mg/ml) to 9 ml ddH_2O under magnetic stirring.

Skin Permeation of QTCs and Its Mechanism

Coumarin-6-loaded TCs was applied to represent skin permeation of QTCs visually. After the mice dorsal skin was carefully shaved with electric clippers, Coumarin-6-loaded TCs aqueous solution (80 mg/20 ml) was applied every 3 h, and after 12 h the treated skin was excised for frozen section to observe the skin permeation of Coumarin-6-loaded TCs. Divided the dorsal skin shaved mice into three groups (one group was for control with no treatment) and used the same method to treat shaved dorsal skin by H_2O and QTCs aqueous solution, then the treated skin was excised and the paraffin section was processed for hematoxylin and eosin (HE) staining to observe the difference of stratum corneum between different treated skins.

UVB Radiation on Animal, Staining, and Histopathological Analysis

After anesthesia with chloral hydrate, the dorsal skin of C57BL/6 mice was carefully shaved with electric clippers, depilated with depilatory paste (Veet®) and divided into five groups (one group was for control), then ddH_2O, 10 mg/20 ml Qu aqueous solution and 80 mg/20 ml QTCs and TCs aqueous solution were applied to the dorsal skin every 8 h. Three days later, UVB radiation was applied at the intensity of 400 mJ/cm^2. After radiation, the four kinds of aqueous solutions were applied every 8 h. After 48 h, the mice were executed. The aqueous solution treated areas were excised, cut into small pieces, part of which were prepared paraffin sections and protein extraction. The protein extraction was used for immunoblotting, and the paraffin sections were used for HE and Masson staining which were further used for histopathological analysis. The other part of treated skin pieces was used for detecting the content of PGE2. Respectively weigh 100 mg different treated skin pieces, added into 1 ml PBS (pH 7.2) after cut into small pieces with intermittent ultrasonic for 1 h and then detected the absorbance value at 278 nm, Using the absorbance value per gram of skin (A/g) to represent the content of PGE2.

Statistical Analysis

All data are presented as the mean ± SEM of no less than three independent experiments. Comparisons were performed using a two-tailed paired Student's test ($^*P < 0.05$, $^{**}P < 0.01$, $^{***}P < 0.001$, $^{****}P < 0.0001$).

RESULTS

Preparation and Characterization of NPs

We prepared the QTCs using the published protocol, but with minor modification (Zhang et al., 2008). As we presented in **Figures 1A–C**, Qu can firstly adhere to CS based on similarity-intermiscibility theory, and then formed nanospheres through TPP-CS crosslinking under continuously stirring condition.

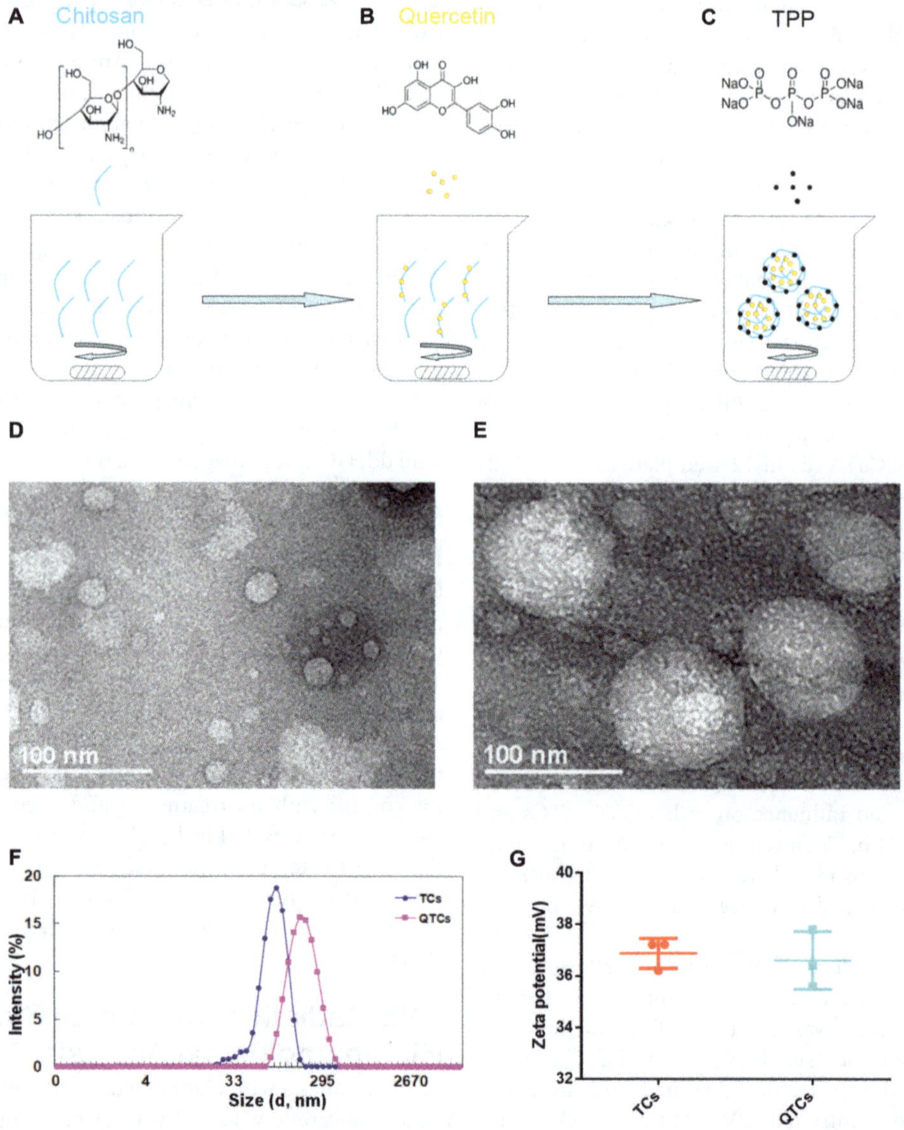

FIGURE 1 | Preparation and characterization of QTCs. **(A–C)** Scheme of preparation of QTCs. **(D)** TEM image of TCs and **(E)** QTCs. **(F)** DLS size distribution of TCs and QTCs. **(G)** Zeta potential of TCs and QTCs.

Next, the morphologies of QTCs and TCs were observed. From the TEM image, QTCs and TCs were all nearly spherical in shape, but the size between each was quite different (**Figures 1D,E**). The dynamic light scattering (DLS) assay showed that the average size of TCs was about 89.48 ± 2.03 nm while QTCs was about 183.63 ± 1.52 nm in **Figure 1F**, consistent with the results of TEM. Moreover, zeta potential, an essential index in the stability of NPs in suspension through electrostatic repulsion between the NPs, had been tested. As the result presented in **Figure 1G**, both QTCs and TCs showed almost the same zeta potential, about 37 mV in average. This data implied that both QTCs and TCs were highly stable in suspension. Then the drug EE and LC of QTCs were measured by HPLC. EE and LC of QTCs were 90.98 ± 1.66% and 13.15 ± 0.77%, respectively, indicating the excellent drug carrier ability of QTCs.

Cellular Uptake, Cytotoxicity, and UVB Protective Effect of QTCs *in Vitro*

Many studies have been reported that CSs could enhance cellular uptake because their positive surface charge can promote the bio-nano interaction with the cytoplasmic-membrane which has negative surface charge (Schipper et al., 1997; Huang et al., 2002), which is also the reason why CSs have been often used as gene delivery carrier (Özbaş-Turan and Akbuğa, 2011). In our study, the enhancement UVB protective effect of QTCs depends on the successful internalization and sustained retention by skin cells. Therefore, we used coumarin-6 which is a kind of fluorescent dye, instead of Qu in order to visually investigate the cellular uptake of QTCs and its efficiency. HaCaT cells, the most commonly used human skin cells, were chosen as representative cells. **Figure 2A** showed the confocal images of HaCaT cells after incubation with coumarin-6-loaded TCs for 3 h. The data suggested coumarin-6-loaded TCs can be ingested by HaCaT cells and internalized into the cytoplasm. Moreover, to investigate the cellular uptake efficiency of QTCs, we measured the quantitative ratio of coumarin-6 fluorescence in cytoplasm at indicated times after incubation of coumarin-6-loaded TCs with HaCaT cells. The result showed that HaCaT cells could almost consistently uptake coumarin-6-loaded TCs in 24 h. The cellular uptake efficiency was gradually increased and reached at about 50% at 24 h (**Figure 2B**).

Next, we evaluated the cytotoxicity of Qu and QTCs in HaCaT cells. **Figure 2C** showed the *in vitro* cell viability of the drug formulated in QTCs and Qu at equivalent concentrations of 5, 10, 20, 40 μg/ml, respectively. High dose free Qu showed obvious cytotoxicity compared with QTCs at the same equivalent concentration at 24 h, which indicated that QTCs can significantly reduce cytotoxicity of high dose Qu. Additionally, the TCs did not show any obvious toxicity against HaCaT cells. After verifying the safety of QTCs, we furthermore tried to investigate the protective effect of QTCs compared to Qu on HaCaT cells under UVB radiation.

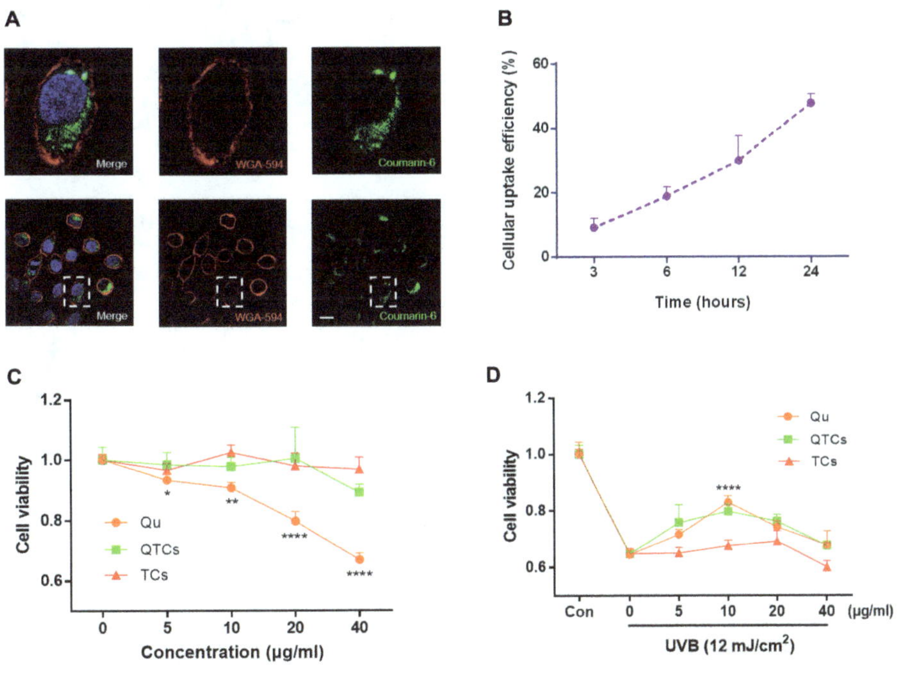

FIGURE 2 | Cellular uptake, cytotoxicity, and UVB protective effect of QTCs *in vitro*. **(A)** Cellular uptake of coumarin-6-loaded TCs (100 μg/ml) was tested by CLSM after 3 h incubation with HaCaT cells. The images above are the enlarged ones in the white box on the below images. Cytomembrane was labeled with WGA-594 (red). Scale bar: 10 μm. **(B)** The cellular uptake efficiency of coumarin-6-loaded TCs (100 μg/ml) was measured at indicated times. **(C)** Cytotoxicity evaluation of Qu, QTCs, and TCs after 24 h incubation with HaCaT cells. **(D)** UVB protective effect evaluation of Qu, QTCs, and TCs. HaCaT cells were firstly incubated with Qu, QTCs or TCs, respectively, for 8 h and then treated with 12 mJ/cm² UVB radiation. Concentration of QTCs was at the same drug dose compared to Qu, and that the TCs was at the same nanoparticles concentration with QTCs (*$P < 0.05$, **$P < 0.01$, ****$P < 0.0001$).

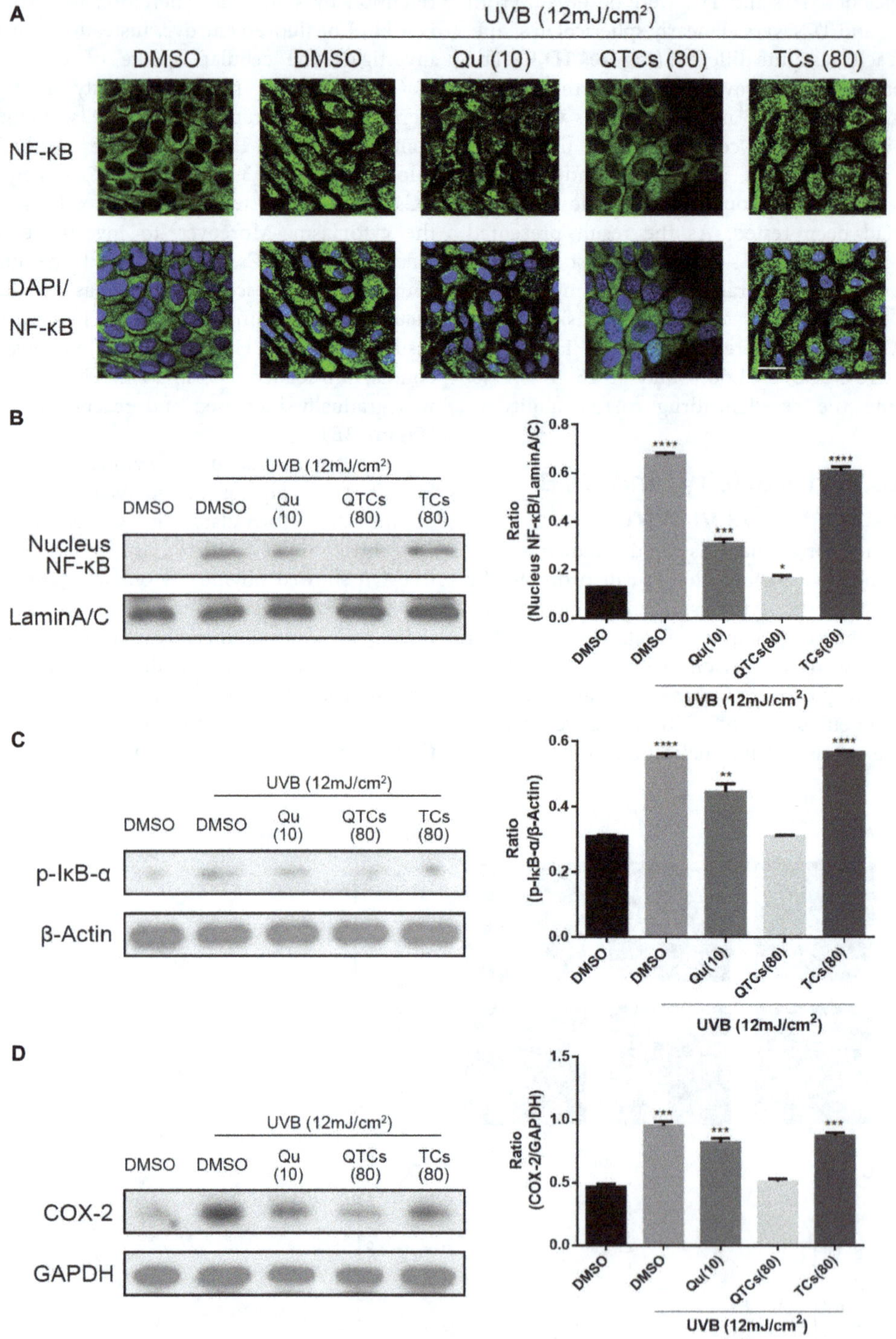

FIGURE 3 | QTCs enhance the inhibition effect of Qu on the NF-κB/COX-2 signaling pathway *in vitro*. **(A)** Effect of Qu, QTCs, and TCs on the translocation of NF-κB from cytoplasm to the nuclei was visually illustrated by CLSM. Scale bar: 20 μm. **(B)** Immunoblotting analysis of the effect of Qu, QTCs, and TCs on the expression of NF-κB in nucleus. **(C)** Immunoblotting analysis of the effect of Qu, QTCs, and TCs on the phosphorylation of IkB-α. **(D)** Immunoblotting analysis of the effect of Qu, QTCs, and TCs on the expression of COX-2. Histograms represent quantitative analysis of the immunoblotting results (**P* < 0.05, ***P* < 0.01, ****P* < 0.001, *****P* < 0.0001).

We found that QTCs had same protective effects on HaCaT cells as Qu after 12 mJ/cm^2 UVB radiation (**Figure 2D**). At the equivalent concentration of 10 μg/ml of Qu, both QTCs and Qu showed the highest protective efficiency on UVB radiation. Meanwhile, TCs showed no significant protective effect on UVB radiation.

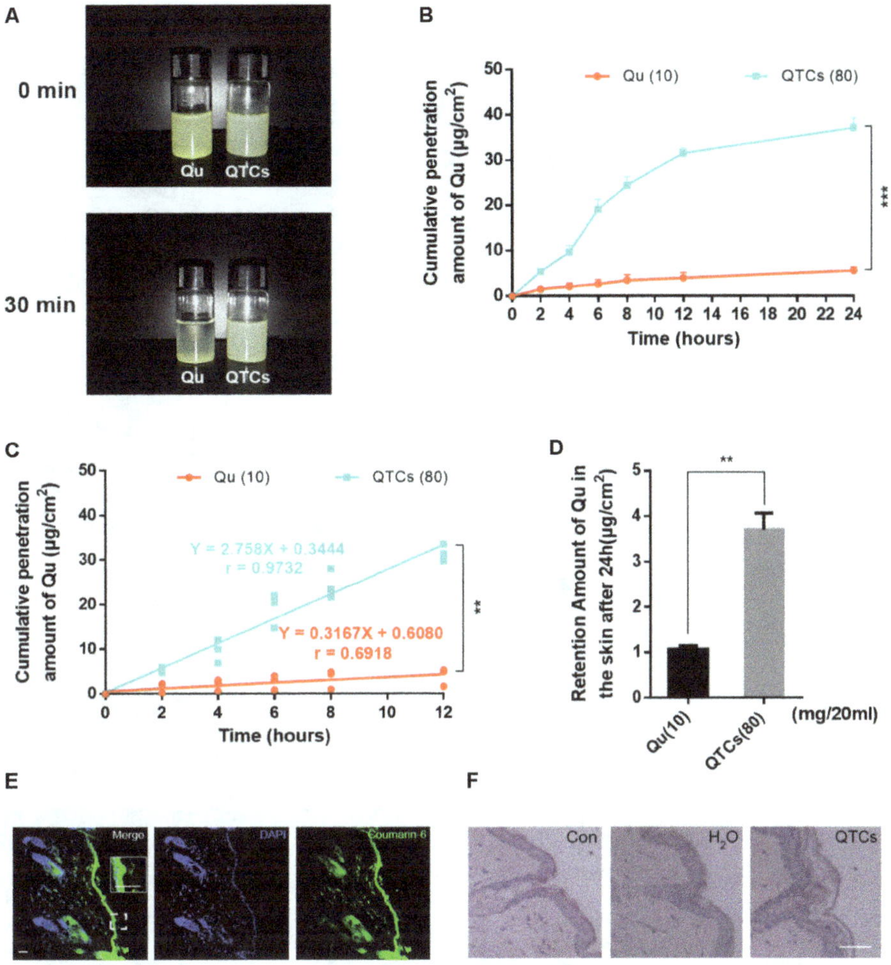

FIGURE 4 | QTCs enhance the percutaneous absorption of Qu and its mechanism. **(A)** Comparison of stability between Qu aqueous solution and QTCs aqueous solution. **(B)** Cumulative penetration amount curves of Qu and QTCs in 24 h. **(C)** Cumulative penetration amount curves of Qu and QTCs in 12 h. **(D)** Retention amount of Qu in the skin after 24 h. (**$P < 0.01$, ***$P < 0.001$). **(E)** Coumarin-6-loaded TCs permeated and deposited in mice skin. The image in the white box is enlarged vision of the small white box below. **(F)** HE staining of normal, H_2O and QTCs aqueous solution treated mice skin. Scale bars: 50 μm.

QTCs Enhance the Inhibition Efficacy of Qu on the NF-κB/COX-2 Signaling Pathway *in Vitro*

Many pharmacological researches have revealed that Qu is very effective against UVB radiation *via* downregulating COX-2 level *in vitro* through NF-κB/COX-2 signaling pathway (13, 14). In non-stimulated cells, the NF-κB dimer binds to one of the three inhibitors (IkBα, IkBβ, and IkBε) and exists in an inactive state. Various signals activate NF-κB by degrading one or more of these three inhibitors (DiDonato et al., 1997). Therefore, the hallmark of NF-κB activation is that the activated NF-κB protein will enter the nucleus, and then binds to DNA in the nucleus to upregulate COX-2 level. In order to further evaluate the protective effect of QTCs, we observed immunofluorescent staining of NF-κB protein in HaCaT cells with UVB radiation in different treatment groups. As can be seen in **Figure 3A**, after 12 mJ/cm^2 UVB radiation, NF-κB protein was translocated from the cytoplasm to the nucleus. But when pre-treatment with 10 μg/ml Qu, the NF-κB protein in the nucleus reduced. And the pre-treatment 80 μg/ml QTCs (consistent drug dose with 10 μg/ml Qu) showed more reduction compared with free Qu. TCs showed no obvious influence on this process. What must be mentioned was that the nucleus size of UVB irradiated HaCaT cells was smaller compared to normal HaCaT cells, and the morphology of UVB irradiated cells also changed to be abnormal, whereas the HaCaT cells pretreated with QTCs looked nearly normal condition after UVB irradiation. Representative western blotting image of nucleus NF-κB protein level also showed the same conclusion (**Figure 3B**). Furthermore, pre-treatment with 10 μg/ml Qu or 80 μg/ml QTCs (consistent drug dose with 10 μg/ml Qu) can also inhibit the over-phosphorylation of IkB-α caused by UVB radiation (**Figure 3C**). As a result, COX-2 protein expression level stayed relatively low in Qu or QTCs pre-treatment group (**Figure 3D**). Similarly, the effect of QTCs on these proteins was much stronger than free Qu. All of these data has proved that QTCs not only just remains the Qu-like inhibition effect on the

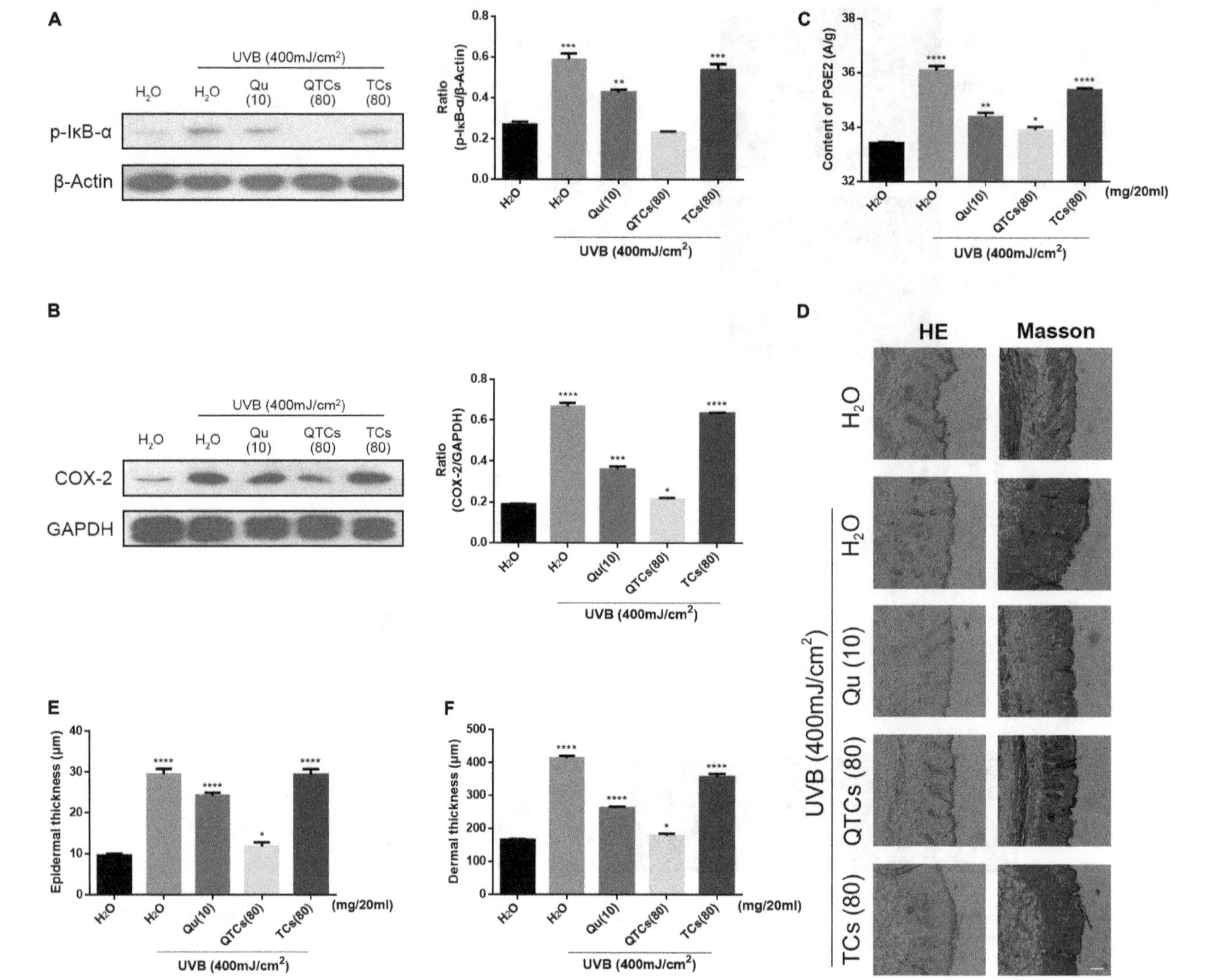

FIGURE 5 | QTCs enhance the protective effect of Qu on UVB induced skin damages *in vivo*. **(A)** Immunoblotting analysis of the effect of Qu, QTCs, and TCs on the phosphorylation of IkB-α and **(B)** COX-2. Histograms represent quantitative analysis of the immunoblotting results. **(C)** The content of PGE2 in the mice skin under different treatments. **(D)** HE and Masson staining represents the alteration of epidermis and dermis, especially the thickness. Scale bar: 50 μm. **(E)** The epidermal thickness of differently treated mice. **(F)** The dermal thickness of differently treated mice. (**P* < 0.05, ***P* < 0.01, ****P* < 0.001, *****P* < 0.0001).

NF-κB/COX-2 signaling pathway *in vitro*, but also enhances its therapeutic efficacy.

QTCs Enhance the Percutaneous Absorption and Retention of Qu

The efficiency of an external dosage form mostly depends on the percutaneous absorption. As we mentioned before, CSs is reported as nanomaterials with the advantages of enhancement of the skin permeation of hydrophobic drugs and promotion of the retention of drugs in the epidermis, due to its interaction with the skin surface will change the morphology of the stratum corneum and break the close conjugation of the corneocyte layers (Tan et al., 2011). Therefore, we next checked the contribution of CSs on percutaneous absorption and retention of Qu *in vitro*. Firstly, we conducted the percutaneous absorption experiment of QTCs and Qu and compared the efficiency of percutaneous absorption in different groups. The results shown in **Figure 4A** indicated that Qu aqueous solution was very unstable and would precipitate within 30 min because of the low hydrophilicity of Qu. And the cumulative penetration amount of Qu in aqueous solution was very small even after 24 h (**Figure 4B**). On the contrary, QTCs showed better stability in aqueous solution (**Figure 4A**) and the cumulative penetration amount of Qu in QTCs shown higher level after 24 h (**Figure 4B**). Moreover, the cumulative penetration amount of Qu in QTCs presented an upward tendency in a linear line within 12 h, as showed in **Figure 4C** the *r*-value was 0.9732 which approaches to 1, demonstrating that QTCs can significantly improve the percutaneous absorption efficiency of Qu *in vitro*. Further result

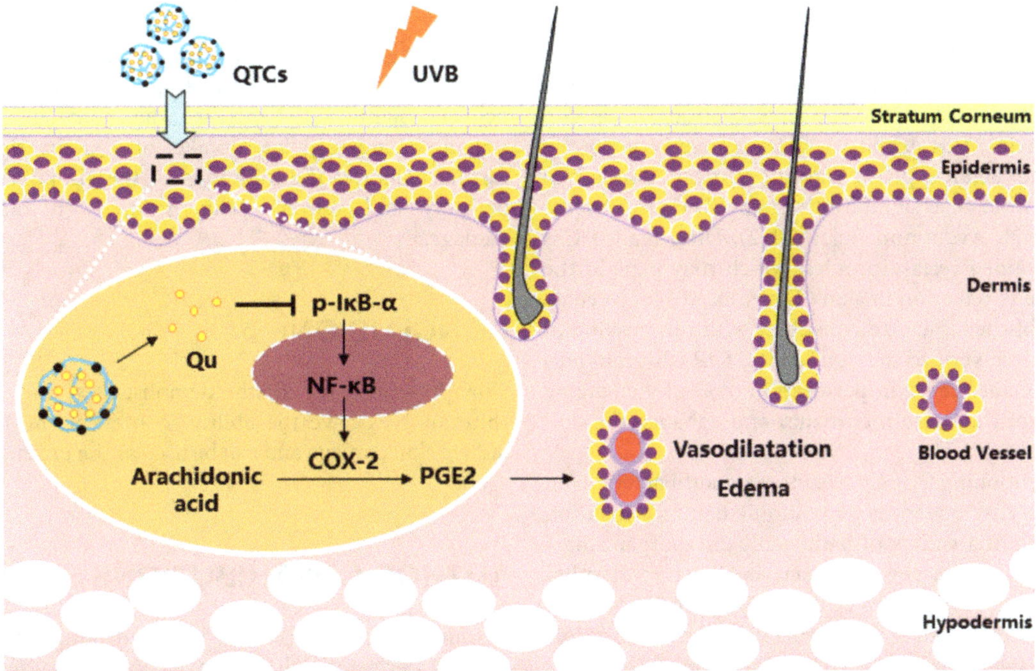

FIGURE 6 | Mechanism of QTCs on enhancing the protective effect of Qu on UVB induced skin vasodilatation and edema.

shown QTCs helped the retention of Qu in skin after 24 h (**Figure 4D**).

Then, to visually show the skin permeation of QTCs *in vivo*, we also used coumarin-6-loaded TCs to represent QTCs. As showed in **Figure 4E**, after application of coumarin-6-loaded TCs aqueous solution on the shaved mice skin after 12 h, we found the coumarin-6-loaded TCs permeated and stored in the skin. Furthermore, we compared the HE staining of normal, ddH_2O treated and QTCs aqueous solution treated mice skin, and the results showed in **Figure 4F**. The stratum corneum of QTCs aqueous solution treated mice skin was more swelling and had larger pore space than normal and ddH_2O treated skin. This result was consistent with the enlarged vision in the white box in **Figure 4E**, which also showed that the stratum corneum of coumarin-6-loaded TCs aqueous solution treated skin was swelling. These results proved that QTCs can also significantly improve the percutaneous absorption efficiency of Qu *in vivo*.

In Vivo Study of the Protective Effects of QTCs on UVB-Induced Skin Damage

We further investigated the protective effects of QTCs *in vivo* after UVB radiation. We compared the effects of four different aqueous solution containing ddH_2O, 10 mg/20 ml Qu, 80 mg/20 ml QTCs, and 80 mg/20 ml TCs in mice after UVB radiation. The immunoblotting results were shown in **Figures 5A,B**. From the results, it was obvious that QTCs had a significant enhancement effect on inhibiting NF-κB/COX-2 signaling pathway by downregulating the phosphorylation of IkB-α and the expression of COX-2 when compared with Qu. However, TCs had no notably influence on NF-κB/COX-2 signaling pathway after UVB radiation.

Moreover, PGE2 can be significantly increased after UVB radiation due to the activation of NF-kB/COX-2 signaling pathway, which can induce the increase of the vascular permeability and promotes skin edema (Kim et al., 2005; Liu et al., 2009; Hur et al., 2010; Pal et al., 2015; Tang et al., 2017). Herein, we quantificationally compared the content of PGE2 in different treated skins. Mice skin treated with QTCs showed less amount of PGE2 (**Figure 5C**). And the HE and Masson staining results in **Figure 5D**, which could help to intuitively see the alteration of mice skin after UVB radiation, also suggested the slighter disorder of collagen fiber and edema of the epidermis and dermis in mice skin treated with QTCs. The thickness of epidermis and dermis of mice also varied from different treatment. Consistent with the previous results, the status of QTCs-treated mice was most close to the normal mice skin (**Figures 5E,F**). However, TCs also had no significant difference compared with non-external preparation treatment group. With all these results, we can conclude that QTCs significantly enhanced the effect of Qu on the inhibition of the increase of PGE2 and inhibition of the edema of skin, which was closer to the normal skin, compared to Qu and TCs.

DISCUSSION

The pH of skin surface ranges from 5.4 to 5.9 (Eberleinkönig et al., 2000; Ali and Yosipovitch, 2013). Interestingly, the surface charge of CSs is positive in this pH, which could increase the interaction between CSs and negatively charged stratum corneum.

The interaction between CSs and stratum corneum changes the morphology of the stratum corneum and breaks the close conjugation of the corneocyte layers, which means CSs could notably enhance the skin permeation of hydrophobic drugs (Tan et al., 2011). What's more, due to the large quantities of amino groups on its chains, CSs exhibits a pH-sensitive behavior, so CSs can undergo volume phase transitions from swollen to collapsed states, which can significantly change the drug release capacity (Seda Tığlı Aydın and Pulat, 2012). Drug-loaded CSs demonstrate sustained release profiles, which may explain the promotion of drug's retention in skin (Tan et al., 2011; Hu et al., 2014). These published data are consistent with our results. In this study, we indeed verified that Qu-loaded TPP-Chitosan NPs (QTCs) could enhance the skin permeation of Qu by changing the morphology of the stratum corneum and enhance the skin retention of Qu.

It is worth mentioning that CS has inherent antibacterial and antimycotic properties due to its polycationic nature, which can inhibit the growth of a variety of pathogenic microorganisms – Gram-positive and Gram-negative bacteria, yeasts and other fungi (Rabea et al., 2003; Ignatova et al., 2013). Furthermore, CSs could also inhibit the growth of various bacteria, including *E. coli*, *S. choleraesuis*, *S. typhimurium*, and *S. aureus* (Qi et al., 2004).

Owing to these advantages, CSs can be an ideal carrier for topical drug and gene delivery (Özbaş-Turan and Akbuğa, 2011; Yang et al., 2013). Our study firstly elucidates the advantage of using Qu-loaded CSs for topical use to prevent UVB radiation-induced skin damage. As displayed in **Figure 6**, our finding showed that the UVB radiation stimulates the phosphorylation of IkB-α and subsequent degradation of IkB-α-NF-κB complex, which makes the activated NF-κB translocate to the nucleus from the cytoplasm. Nucleus NF-κB then activates the expression of COX-2, the key enzyme converting AA into prostaglandins (PGE2). Excess PGE2 increases the vascular permeability and promotes edema and further damage. Qu is well-known for inhibiting NF-κB/COX-2 pathway, but its topical use is largely restricted by its natural disadvantages of low hydrophilicity and poor percutaneous absorption. However, in QTCs drug delivery system, TCs contributes to overcome the natural disadvantages of Qu, resulting in better hydrophilicity and low cytotoxicity of QTCs drug delivery system, and also help to significantly increase the percutaneous absorption, retention and cellular uptake of Qu in the skin, which further enhances the inhibition of the NF-κB/COX-2 signaling pathway and prevents skin from UVB radiation-induced damage.

CONCLUSION

Our present study firstly demonstrates that the Qu-loaded chitosan NPs have the ability to prevent the UVB radiation-induce skin damage and can be used as the promising therapeutic agent.

AUTHOR CONTRIBUTIONS

XjS and WN conceived the idea and designed the study. WN and LD performed all the experiments, analyzed the data, and co-wrote the paper. HC and LY provided technical support. FK helped correcting the manuscript. XjS and XbS provided reagents and conceptual advice.

FUNDING

This work was supported by grants from National Natural Science Foundation of China (Grant No. 81730108), Key Project of Zhejiang province Ministry of Science and Technology (Grant No. 2015C03055), Key Project of Hangzhou Ministry of Science and Technology (Grant Nos. 20162013A07 and 20142013A63), and Shenzhen Science and Technology Program (Grant Nos. JCYJ20170412153453623 and JCYJ20130402145002433).

REFERENCES

Ali, S. M., and Yosipovitch, G. (2013). Skin pH: from basic science to basic skin care. *Acta Derm. Venereol.* 93, 261–267. doi: 10.2340/00015555-1531

de Alencar Filho, J. M. T., Sampaio, P. A., Valenccedil, E. C., Pereira, A., Gonccedil, R., Juacute, A. D. O., et al. (2016). Flavonoids as photoprotective agents: a systematic review. *J. Med. Plants Res.* 10, 848–864. doi: 10.5897/JMPR2016.6273

DiDonato, J. A., Hayakawa, M., Rothwarf, D. M., Zandi, E., and Karin, M. (1997). A cytokine-responsive IκB kinase that activates the transcription factor NF-κB. *Nature* 388, 548–554. doi: 10.1038/41493

Eberleinkönig, B., Schäfer, T., Hussmarp, J., Darsow, U., Möhrenschlager, M., Abeck, D., et al. (2000). Skin surface pH, stratum corneum hydration, trans-epidermal water loss and skin roughness related to atopic eczema and skin dryness in a population of primary school children. *Acta Derm. Venereol.* 80, 188–191. doi: 10.1080/000155500750042943

Enríquez, D. S. A., Diebold, Y., Calonge, M., García-Vazquez, C., Callejo, S., Vila, A., et al. (2006). Chitosan nanoparticles as a potential drug delivery system for the ocular surface: toxicity, uptake mechanism and in vivo tolerance. *Invest. Ophthalmol. Vis. Sci.* 47, 1416–1425. doi: 10.1167/iovs.05-0495

Formica, J. V., and Regelson, W. (1995). Review of the biology of Quercetin and related bioflavonoids. *Food Chem. Toxicol.* 33, 1061–1080. doi: 10.1016/0278-6915(95)00077-1

Gallagher, R. P., and Lee, T. K. (2006). Adverse effects of ultraviolet radiation: a brief review. *Prog. Biophys. Mol. Biol.* 92, 119–131. doi: 10.1016/j.pbiomolbio.2006.02.011

Hatahet, T., Morille, M., Hommoss, A., Devoisselle, J. M., Müller, R. H., and Bégu, S. (2016). Quercetin topical application, from conventional dosage forms to nanodosage forms. *Eur. J. Pharm. Biopharm.* 108, 41–53. doi: 10.1016/j.ejpb.2016.08.011

Hu, X., Wang, Y., and Peng, B. (2014). Chitosan-capped mesoporous silica nanoparticles as pH-responsive nanocarriers for controlled drug release. *Chem. Asian J.* 9, 319–327. doi: 10.1002/asia.201301105

Huang, M., Ma, Z., Khor, E., and Lim, L. Y. (2002). Uptake of FITC-chitosan nanoparticles by A549 cells. *Pharm. Res.* 19, 1488–1494. doi: 10.1023/A:1020404615898

Hung, C. F., Fang, C. L., Alsuwayeh, S. A., Yang, S. Y., and Fang, J. Y. (2012). Evaluation of drug and sunscreen permeation via skin irradiated with UVA and UVB: comparisons of normal skin and chronologically aged skin. *J. Dermatol. Sci.* 68, 135–148. doi: 10.1016/j.jdermsci.2012.09.005

Hur, S., Lee, Y. H., Yang, J. H., and Kim, T. Y. (2010). Homoisoflavanone inhibits UVB-induced skin inflammation through reduced cyclooxygenase-2 expression and NF-kappaB nuclear localization. *J. Dermatol. Sci.* 59, 163–169. doi: 10.1016/j.jdermsci.2010.07.001

Ignatova, M., Manolova, N., and Rashkov, I. (2013). Electrospun antibacterial chitosan-based fibers. *Macromol. Biosci.* 13, 860–872. doi: 10.1002/mabi.201300058

Jiao, J., Mikulec, C., Ishikawa, T. O., Magyar, C., Dumlao, D. S., Dennis, E. A., et al. (2014). Cell-type-specific roles for COX-2 in UVB-induced skin cancer. *Carcinogenesis* 35, 1310–1319. doi: 10.1093/carcin/bgu020

Kerr, J. B., and Mcelroy, C. T. (1993). Evidence for large upward trends of ultraviolet-b radiation linked to ozone depletion. *Science* 262, 1032–1034. doi: 10.1126/science.262.5136.1032

Kim, S. O., Kundu, J. K., Shin, Y. K., Park, J. H., Cho, M. H., Kim, T. Y., et al. (2005). [6]-Gingerol inhibits COX-2 expression by blocking the activation of p38 MAP kinase and NF-kappaB in phorbol ester-stimulated mouse skin. *Oncogene* 24, 2558–2567. doi: 10.1038/sj.onc.1208446

Liu, X. J., Shi, S. T., Ye, J. L., Liu, L. Q., Sun, M., and Wang, C. B. (2009). Effect of polypeptide from *Chlamys farreri* on UVB-induced ROS/NF-kappaB/COX-2 activation and apoptosis in HaCaT cells. *J. Photochem. Photobiol. B Biol.* 96, 109–116. doi: 10.1016/j.jphotobiol.2009.04.010

Madronich, S., and Gruijl, F. R. D. (1993). Skin cancer and UV radiation. *Nature* 366:23. doi: 10.1038/366023a0

Mccarty, M. F. (2012). Minimizing the cancer-promotional activity of cox-2 as a central strategy in cancer prevention. *Med. Hypotheses* 78, 45–57. doi: 10.1016/j.mehy.2011.09.039

Morganroth, P. A., Lim, H. W., and Burnett, C. T. (2013). Ultraviolet radiation and the skin: an in-depth review. *Am. J. Lifestyle Med.* 7, 168–181. doi: 10.1177/1559827612460499

Özbaş-Turan, S., and Akbuğa, J. (2011). Plasmid DNA-loaded chitosan/TPP nanoparticles for topical gene delivery. *Drug Deliv.* 18, 215–222. doi: 10.3109/10717544.2010.544688

Pal, H. C., Athar, M., Elmets, C. A., and Afaq, F. (2015). Fisetin inhibits UVB-induced cutaneous inflammation and activation of PI3K/AKT/NFκB signaling pathways in SKH-1 hairless mice. *Photochem. Photobiol.* 91, 225–234. doi: 10.1111/php.12337

Pentland, A. P., Schoggins, J. W., Scott, G. A., Khan, K. N., and Han, R. (1999). Reduction of UV-induced skin tumors in hairless mice by selective COX-2 inhibition. *Carcinogenesis* 20, 1939–1944. doi: 10.1093/carcin/20.10.1939

Qi, L., Xu, Z., Jiang, X., Hu, C., and Zou, X. (2004). Preparation and antibacterial activity of chitosan nanoparticles. *Carbohydr. Res.* 339, 2693–2700. doi: 10.1016/j.carres.2004.09.007

Rabea, E. I., Badawy, E. T., Stevens, C. V., Smagghe, G., and Steurbaut, W. (2003). Chitosan as antimicrobial agent: applications and mode of action. *Biomacromolecules* 4, 1457–1465. doi: 10.1021/bm034130m

Schipper, N. G., Olsson, S., Hoogstraate, J. A., Deboer, A. G., Vårum, K. M., and Artursson, P. (1997). Chitosans as absorption enhancers for poorly absorbable drugs 2: mechanism of absorption enhancement. *Pharm. Res.* 14, 923–929. doi: 10.1023/A:1012160102740

Seda Tığlı Aydın, R., and Pulat, M. (2012). 5-Fluorouracil encapsulated chitosan nanoparticles for pH-stimulated drug delivery: evaluation of controlled release kinetics. *J. Nanomater.* 2012:313961. doi: 10.1155/2012/313961

Serafini, M., Peluso, I., and Raguzzini, A. (2010). Flavonoids as anti-inflammatory agents. *Proc. Nutr. Soc.* 69, 273–278. doi: 10.1017/S002966511000162X

Steerenberg, P. A., Garssen, J., Dortant, P. M., Vliet, H. V. D., Geerse, E., Verlaan, A. P. J., et al. (1997). The effect of oral quercetin on UVB-induced tumor growth and local immunosuppression in SKH-1. *Cancer Lett.* 114, 187–189. doi: 10.1016/S0304-3835(97)04659-4

Tan, Q., Liu, W., Guo, C., and Zhai, G. (2011). Preparation and evaluation of quercetin-loaded lecithin-chitosan nanoparticles for topical delivery. *Int. J. Nanomed.* 6, 1621–1630. doi: 10.2147/IJN.S22411

Tang, S. C., Liao, P. Y., Hung, S. J., Ge, J. S., Chen, S. M., Lai, J. C., et al. (2017). Topical application of glycolic acid suppresses the UVB induced IL-6, IL-8, MCP-1 and COX-2 inflammation by modulating NF-κB signaling pathway in keratinocytes and mice skin. *J. Dermatol. Sci.* 86, 238–248. doi: 10.1016/j.jdermsci.2017.03.004

Tang, X., Kim, A. L., Kopelovich, L., Bickers, D. R., and Athar, M. (2008). Cyclooxygenase-2 inhibitor nimesulide blocks ultraviolet B-induced photocarcinogenesis in SKH-1 hairless mice. *Photochem. Photobiol.* 84, 522–527. doi: 10.1111/j.1751-1097.2008.00303.x

Yang, R., Shim, W. S., Cui, F. D., Cheng, G., Han, X., Jin, Q. R., et al. (2009). Enhanced electrostatic interaction between chitosan-modified PLGA nanoparticle and tumor. *Int. J. Pharm.* 371, 142–147. doi: 10.1016/j.ijpharm.2008.12.007

Yang, Y., Bugno, J., and Hong, S. (2013). Nanoscale polymeric penetration enhancers in topical drug delivery. *Polym. Chem.* 4, 2651–2657. doi: 10.1016/j.xphs.2016.08.022

Zhang, Y., Yang, Y., Tang, K., Hu, X., and Zou, G. (2008). Physicochemical characterization and antioxidant activity of quercetin-loaded chitosan nanoparticles. *J. Appl. Polym. Sci.* 107, 891–897. doi: 10.1002/app.26402

Zhu, X., Zeng, X., Zhang, X., Cao, W., Wang, Y., Chen, H., et al. (2016). The effects of quercetin-loaded PLGA-TPGS nanoparticles on ultraviolet B-induced skin damages in vivo. *Nanomedicine* 12, 623–632. doi: 10.1016/j.nano.2015.10.016

4

Optimization of the Linker Length of Mannose-Cholesterol Conjugates for Enhanced mRNA Delivery to Dendritic Cells by Liposomes

Fazhan Wang[1†], Wen Xiao[1†], Mostafa A. Elbahnasawy[2†], Xingting Bao[1], Qian Zheng[1], Linhui Gong[1], Yang Zhou[1], Shuping Yang[1], Aiping Fang[1], Mohamed M. S. Farag[2], Jinhui Wu[1*] and Xiangrong Song[1*]*

[1] State Key Laboratory of Biotherapy, Geriatrics and Cancer Center, West China Hospital, and Collaborative Innovation Center for Biotherapy, Sichuan University, Chengdu, China, [2] Department of Botany and Microbiology, Faculty of Science, Al-Azhar University, Cairo, Egypt

***Correspondence:**
Xiangrong Song
songxr@scu.edu.cn
Jinhui Wu
wujinhui@scu.edu.cn
Mohamed M. S. Farag
mohamed.farag@azhar.edu.eg

† These authors have contributed equally to this work

Liposomes (LPs) as commonly used mRNA delivery systems remain to be rationally designed and optimized to ameliorate the antigen expression of mRNA vaccine in dendritic cells (DCs). In this study, we synthesized mannose-cholesterol conjugates (MP_n-CHs) by click reaction using different PEG units (PEG_{100}, PEG_{1000}, and PEG_{2000}) as linker molecules. MP_n-CHs were fully characterized and subsequently used to prepare DC-targeting liposomes (MP_n-LPs) by a thin-film dispersion method. MP_n-LPs loaded with mRNA (MP_n-LPX) were finally prepared by a simple self-assembly method. MP_n-LPX displayed bigger diameter (about 135 nm) and lower zeta potential (about 40 mV) compared to MP_n-LPs. The *in vitro* transfection experiment on DC2.4 cells demonstrated that the PEG length of mannose derivatives had significant effect on the expression of GFP-encoding mRNA. MP_{1000}-LPX containing MP_{1000}-CH can achieve the highest transfection efficiency (52.09 ± 4.85%), which was significantly superior to the commercial transfection reagent Lipo 3K (11.47 ± 2.31%). The optimal DC-targeting MP_{1000}-LPX showed an average size of 132.93 ± 4.93 nm and zeta potential of 37.93 ± 2.95 mV with nearly spherical shape. Moreover, MP_{1000}-LPX can protect mRNA against degradation in serum with high efficacy. The uptake study indicated that MP_{1000}-LPX enhanced mRNA expression mainly through the over-expressing mannose receptor (CD206) on the surface of DCs. In conclusion, mannose modified LPs might be a potential DC-targeting delivery system for mRNA vaccine after rational design and deserve further study on the *in vivo* delivery profile and anti-tumor efficacy.

Keywords: mRNA vaccine, dendritic cell targeting liposomes, mannose conjugates, linker length, click reaction

INTRODUCTION

Messenger RNA (mRNA) has recently generated great attention as one of promising therapeutics with the potential for cancer immunotherapy and vaccines because the *in vitro*-transcribed (IVT) mRNA does not need to enter the nucleus and induces only transient protein expression without the risk of genomic integration compared with the widely investigated DNA (Sahin et al., 2014; Pardi et al., 2018). Some mRNA vaccines have been demonstrated to be effective in the preclinical mouse models of cancer (Kreiter et al., 2015;

Oberli et al., 2017; Sayour et al., 2017). Nevertheless, the anionic character of mRNA does not facilitate its penetration into cells, resulting in low antigen expression and curative effect. It has been shown that the cellular uptake rate of naked mRNA is less than 1 in 10,000 molecules (Sahin et al., 2014). Moreover, mRNA is prone to degradation by RNases present everywhere (Tsui et al., 2002). Thus, sufficiently efficacious delivery system is urgently required to target antigen presentation cells (APCs) and protect mRNA from nuclease degradation, which will be beneficial for the clinical application of more mRNA vaccines (Pardi et al., 2018).

Non-viral vectors such as lipids, lipid-like materials, polymer or hybrid systems are widely studied for delivery of mRNA vaccines, which have low unwanted immune responses in contrast to the viral systems including adeno- associated viruses, lentiviruses and the Sendai virus (Giacca and Zacchigna, 2012; Midoux and Pichon, 2015; Hajj and Whitehead, 2017). Liposomes (LPs) are the most appealing and commonly used non-viral carriers of mRNA vaccines (Markov et al., 2015; Kranz et al., 2016; Persano et al., 2017; Verbeke et al., 2017). The mRNA loaded LPs namely RNA-LPX for cancer immunotherapy have been in phase I dose-escalation trial (Kranz et al., 2016). RNA-LPX protected mRNA from RNases and the encoded antigen can be efficiently expressed in the specialized APCs, like DCs (Kranz et al., 2016). Furthermore, the antigen-specific T-cell responses were also induced in melanoma patients. However, only 1 in 3 patients showed regression of a suspected metastatic thoracic lymph node lesion. The limited antitumor efficacy of RNA-LPX indicated that the LPs were worthy of being further reformed by functionalization of particles with ligands targeting DCs.

Dendritic cells express several mannose residue-recognizing membrane lectins like CD206 (mannose receptor, MR), CD209 (DC-SIGN) and CD207 (langerin) (Caminschi et al., 2012; Le Moignic et al., 2018). Macrophages as also expressed CD206 receptor (Chen et al., 2016; Kim et al., 2017) with the ability to present antigens (Malissen et al., 2014). They can mediate endocytosis of cargos encapsulated in mannose-modified nano-preparations (Li et al., 2013; Chen et al., 2014; Wang C. et al., 2014). Of note, enhanced *in vivo* anticancer efficacy via mannose modification on the nano-preparations has been widely reported in the literatures (Lai et al., 2018; Le Moignic et al., 2018; Yang et al., 2018). LPs can be easily modified because phospholipids and cholesterol are typically included (Hua and Wu, 2013). These lipophilic molecules can conjugate with various moieties binding to surface receptors of the target cells with high selectivity. Our previous studies demonstrated that folic acid-conjugating LPs can specifically deliver DNA into folate receptor-overexpressing tumor (He Z.Y. et al., 2013; Yang et al., 2016). The targeting molecule folic acid was linked to cholesterol, which efficiently kept its binding specificity to folate receptor (He Z. et al., 2013). Taking into account of these, mannosylated cholesterol derivatives were designed and synthesized to prepare mannosylated LPs to help delivery to DCs in this study.

According to literatures, the length and flexibility of the space between ligand molecules and the surface of particles might be important parameters for efficient recognition of receptors (Engel et al., 2003; Stefanick et al., 2013; Jeong et al., 2014). A short linker may restrict the translational freedom of ligand, while the longer one might bury a large fraction of the conjugated ligand (Stefanick et al., 2013). The optimal linker provides a more effective ligand-receptor interaction (Stefanick et al., 2013; Jeong et al., 2014). Thus, a rational design of the targeting LPs is crucial to enhanced mRNA delivery to DCs.

In our study, MP_n-CHs containing different PEG units were firstly synthesized and then used to prepare the MP_n-LPs by a typical thin-film dispersion method. The mRNA encapsulating liposomes (MP_n-LPX) were constructed by complexing the obtained MP_n-LPs and mRNA. The preferable MP_n-LPX were picked out according to the *in vitro* transfection efficiency of GFP-encoding mRNA on DCs. The pharmaceutical properties and preliminary cytotoxicity of the optimal delivery system were also assessed to favor its potential application for mRNA delivery.

MATERIALS AND METHODS

Materials

1,2,3,4,6-Penta-*O*-acetyl-alpha-D-mannopyranoside was obtained from Jinan Samuel Pharmaceutical Co., Ltd. (Shandong, China). Cholesterol was supplied from Shanghai Yuanju Biology Technology Company (Shanghai, China). Cholesterol-PEG_{2000}-N_3 was purchased by Shanghai Ponsure Biotech, Inc (Shanghai, China). 1,2-dioleoyl-3-trimethylammonium-propane (DOTAP) and 1,2-dioleoyl-sn-glycero-3-phosphoethanolamine (DOPE) was provided by Shanghai A.V.T. Pharmaceutical Co., Ltd. (Shanghai, China). GFP-mRNA was obtained from TriLink (San Diego, CA, United States). DMEM and fetal bovine serum (FBS) were purchased from Gibco. All the other chemical reagents were of analytical grade or better without further purification unless otherwise stated.

Cell Culture

DC2.4 cells were cultured in DMEM medium supplemented with 10% FBS and 1% penicillin/streptomycin with 5% CO_2 at 37°C in a humidified atmosphere.

Synthesis and Characterization of MP_n-CH

Synthesis of MP_{100}-CH

As shown in **Figure 1A**, MP_{100}-CH was obtained with similar procedures as described previously (Kim et al., 2012; Nguyen et al., 2016). In brief, Diethylene glycol (5.0 eq), paratoluensulfonyl chloride (TosCl, 1.0 eq) and triethylamine (TEA, 1.1 eq) were dissolved in anhydrous dichloromethane (DCM) and stirred for 24 hours (h) at room temperature (rt). The crude product was purified by silica gel with a mixed solvent system of DCM and methanol to harvest compound **1**. 1,2,3,4,6-Penta-*O*-acetyl-alpha-D-mannopyranoside (1.5 eq), compound 1 (1.0 eq) and $BF_3{\cdot}Et_2O$ (1.5 eq) were dissolved in anhydrous DCM. Compound **2** was acquired and purified by column chromatography. Compound 2 (1.0 eq) and sodium

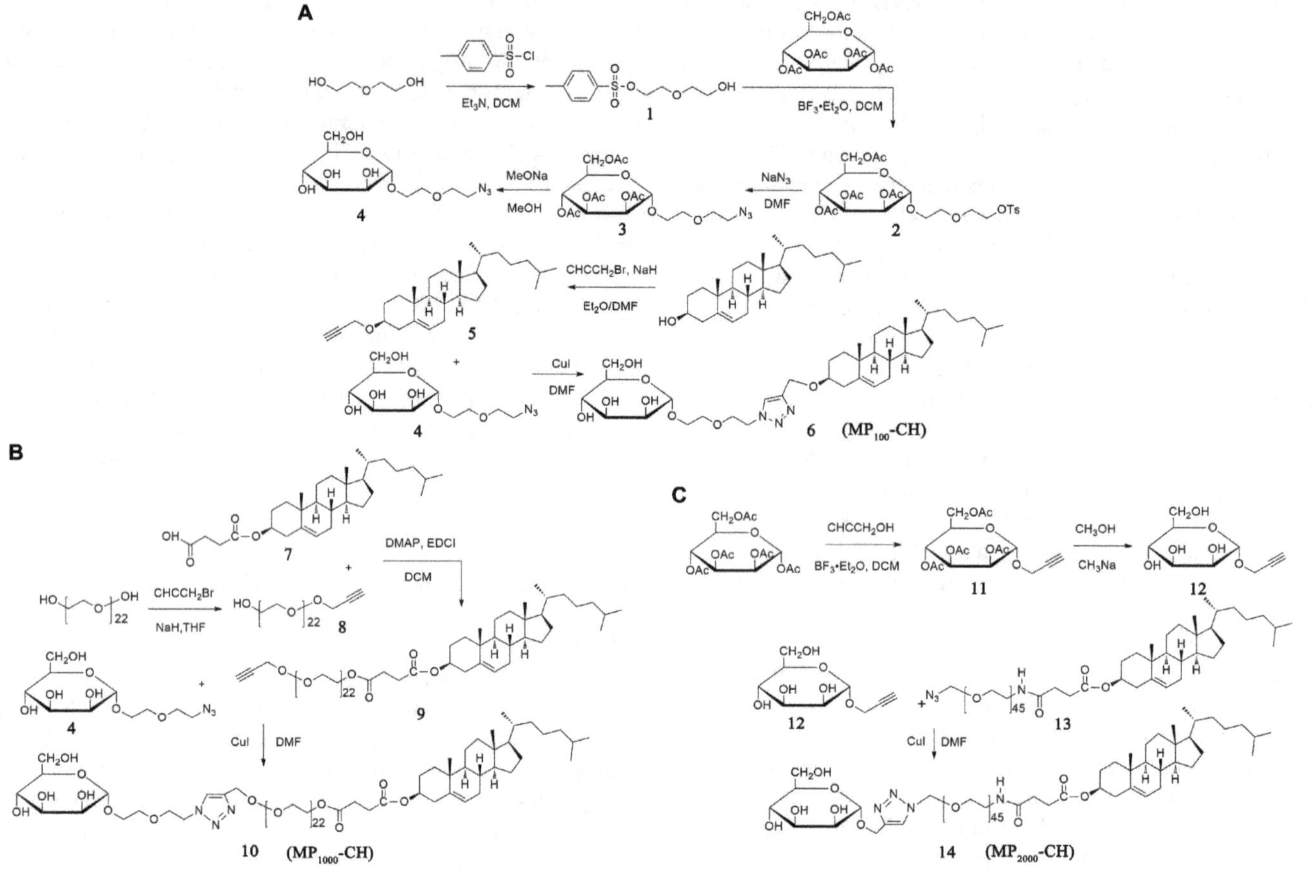

FIGURE 1 | Synthesis of MP_n-CHs. Schematic of the synthetic steps for MP_{100}-CH **(A)**, MP_{1000}-CH **(B)**, and MP_{2000}-CH **(C)**, respectively.

azide (5.0 eq) were added into anhydrous N, *N*-dimethyl-Formamide (DMF) and stirred suitably for 24 h at 60°C to prepare compound **3**. Subsequently, deacetylation of compound 3 was performed in methanol solution (HPLC grade) of sodium methoxide (NaOMe) (10:1, v/v). Then the reaction system was treated with (H+) resin to get product named compound **4**. Compound **5** was prepared as described previously (Rull-Barrull et al., 2016). In brief, Cholesterol (1.0 eq) and 3-bromopropyne (2.0 eq) were dissolved in component solvent containing anhydrous ether and anhydrous DMF (1:1, v/v). Sodium hydride (NaH, 5.0 eq) was added mildly and the solution was stirred at rt for 24 h. Finally, compound 4, compound 5 and copper iodide were mixed in equal molar ratio and dissolved in anhydrous DMF. The mixture was reacted for 24 h at rt and concentrated to obtained compound **6** (MP_{100}-CH) via column chromatography.

Synthesis of MP_{1000}-CH

The synthetic scheme was shown in **Figure 1B** and specific experimental steps were as follows. Compound **7** was prepared and purified according to our previously reported method (He Z.Y. et al., 2010). PEG_{1000} (5.0 eq), propargyl bromide (2.0 eq) and hydrogenated sodium (NaH, 3.0 eq) were dissolved in anhydrous tetrahydrofuran (THF). The mixture was stirred at rt overnight. Compound **8** was purified by column chromatography. Compound 7 (1.2 eq), 8 (1.0 eq), DMAP (0.5 eq), and EDCI (2.0 eq) were dissolved in DCM and stirred at rt for 24 h. Compound **9** was obtained after the crude product was purified by column chromatography. Similar to the synthetic method of compound 6, compound 4 was connected to compound 9, and compound **10** (MP_{1000}-CH) was obtained.

Synthesis of MP_{2000}-CH

Compound 14 were prepared according to the scheme showed in **Figure 1C**. Briefly, compound **11** was prepared according to the synthesis method of compound 2 but replace the compound 1 with propargyl alcohol. Subsequently, compound **12** was acquired using the similar synthesis method of compound 4. Compound **14** (MP_{2000}-CH) was obtained with the similar synthesis method of compound 10 after column chromatography.

General Characterization of Prepared Compounds

^{1}H-NMR spectra of MP_n-CH and other prepared compounds dissolved in $CDCl_3$, D_2O or Dimethyl Sulfoxide-D_6 containing TMS were recorded on a Unity Inova-400 (400 MHz) (Varian Inc., Palo Alto, CA, United States). Chemical shifts were analyzed in ppm relative to the residual solvent peaks of TMS. The mass spectra of various compounds were obtained using a Waters Q-TOF Premier (Milford, MA, United States) equipped with the ion spray source and using N_2 as nebulization gas. In addition, the identity of the conjugate was also verified by Fourier Transform infrared spectroscopy (FTIR) using a Vector 22 spectrometer (Bruker, Ettlingen, Switzerland). The purity and retention time of MP_n-CHs and other cholesterol derivatives were evaluated by high performance liquid chromatography (HPLC, Waters, Milford, MA, United States) at 201 nm. The mobile phase, at 1 mL/min flow rate, was composed of 100% chromatographic methanol. The retention time and purity of cholesterol derivatives were summarized in **Table 1**.

Preparation and Characterization of MP_n-LPX

Preparation of MP_n-LPs

The cationic LPs were prepared using a thin-film dispersion method with some modifications (Wang F. et al., 2018). Briefly, cationic lipid DOTAP, the helper lipid DOPE, CH and MP_n-CHs at a molar ratio of 50:10:35:5 or 50:10:40:0 (**Table 2**) were dissolved in a mixture solvent of chloroform/ethanol (1:1, v/v) to prepare MP_n-LPs and LPs, respectively. The organic solvents were evaporated using a rotary evaporator at 37°C for 2 h. The lipid film was rehydrated with 2 mL RNase-free water at 60°C for 40 min to obtain a suspension with the final lipid concentration of 6 mM. Subsequently, the above suspension was sonicated at 80 W for 3 min and filtered with a 0.22 μm sterilized filter for the following experiment. The coumarin-6 (Cou-6) loaded LPs were acquired using the similar procedure with the addition of Cou-6 into the chloroform/ethanol (1:1 v/v) solvent mixture. The fluorescent intensity of Cou-6 loaded particles was measured using CyrationTM3 (BioTek Instruments, Inc, United States).

Preparation of MP_n-LPX

In our study, MP_n-LPX was composed of DOTAP contained LPs and mRNA at N/P ratio of 3, 5 or 7, named MP_n-LPX NP 3, MP_n-LPX NP 5 or MP_n-LPX NP 7, respectively. MP_n-LPX were prepared according to previous reported methods with some modifications (Kranz et al., 2016). Briefly, mRNA was diluted by water and 1.5 M NaCl followed by adding corresponding MP_n-LPs diluted with water to reach the desired ratio of N/P with the final concentration of NaCl of 150 mM. After incubated at rt for 15 min, MP_n-LPX were finally obtained.

Size and Zeta Potential Measurements

The average particle size, size distribution (polydispersity index, PDI) and zeta potential of different formulations were recorded by Zetasizer Nano ZS90 (Malvern Instruments, Malvern, United Kingdom). All measurements were carried out using diluted samples at 25°C and were conducted in triplicate.

Cellular Transfection of MP_n-LPX

To optimize the appropriate ratio of N/P, DC2.4 cells in the logarithmic growth period were seeded in 24 well plates at 4×10^5 cells/well and incubated for 24 h at 37°C, followed by incubation with different N/P of LPX (0.5 μg GFP-mRNA per well) in triplicate from 3 to 7. Before transfection, the culture medium was replaced with 500 μL FBS-free DMEM. Subsequently, LPX were added. After 4 h of incubation, 500 μL complete medium was added, and the cells were incubated for another 20 h. Expression of GFP by DC2.4 cells was visualized using a fluorescence microscope (Olympus Corp., Tokyo, Japan) and transfection efficiency was obtained based on the percentage of GFP positive cells from the live cell population by flow cytometry. Additionally, mean GFP fluorescence intensity of individual cells from GFP positive cells population after transfection was measured using FlowJo software (Li et al., 2017b).

To further investigate the transfection efficiency of MP_n-LPX, DC2.4 cells in 24 well plates were incubated with MP_n-LPX with the N/P of 5 following the same procedure described above. Transfection efficiency and mean fluorescence intensity (MFI) of GFP positive DC2.4 cells were evaluated by flow cytometry. In brief, DC2.4 cells were captured via forward scatter (FSC) and side scatter (SSC). Live DC2.4 cells were gated as shown in Region 1 (R1), of which GFP positive cells were selected (R2). Transfection efficiency (% GFP^+ cells) was auto displayed with R2. MFI of GFP expression in GFP positive cells was acquired using FlowJo software. MFI was calculated after subtraction of background values of untreated DC2.4 cells. To further elaborate the kinetics of mRNA transfection *in vitro*, transfection efficiency of MP_{1000}-LPX NP 5 on DC2.4 cells from 12 to 72 h has also been studied.

TABLE 1 | The retention time and purity of cholesterol derivatives was evaluated by HPLC.

	Peak 1		Peak 2		Peak 3	
	Time (min)	Purity (%)	Time (min)	Purity (%)	Time (min)	Purity (%)
Compound **6**	**9.743**	**97.948**	10.493	1.996	–	–
Compound **9**	7.14	2.9	11.557	2.204	**16.692**	**94.881**
Compound **10**	7.548	1.627	11.556	1.878	**13.122**	**96.495**
Compound **13**	–	–	10.278	8.749	13.662	91.251
Compound **14**	**6.907**	**91.532**	10.896	2.321	13.796	6.147

Bold values represents the retention time and purity of each compound.

TABLE 2 | Formulation component and relative molar content used in the manuscript.

	LPs	MP_{100}-LPs	MP_{1000}-LPs	MP_{2000}-LPs
DOTAP	50	50	50	50
DOPE	10	10	10	10
CH	40	35	35	35
MP_{100}-CH	0	5	0	0
MP_{1000}-CH	0	0	5	0
MP_{2000}-CH	0	0	0	5

Characterization of Optimal MP_{1000}-LPX

Microscopy Investigation

The appearance and Tyndall effect of MP_{1000}-LX were recorded by a digital camera. The morphology of MP_{1000}-LPX NP 5 was examined by transmission electron microscopy (TEM, H-600, Hitachi, Japan). Briefly, 100 μL of MP_{1000}-LPX suspension was added onto copper electron microscopy grids. Subsequently, they were negatively stained with 2% phosphotungstic acid for observation.

Gel Electrophoresis Retardation Assay

To evaluate the complexation of mRNA and MP_{1000}-LPs, 1 μg free mRNA and MP_{1000}-LPX (containing 1 μg mRNA) were diluted with RNase-free water. Then NorthernMax® formaldehyde load dye containing ethidium bromide (50 μg/mL) was added and mixed. After incubating the samples for 10 min in 65°C, the samples were loaded into a 1% denaturing formaldehyde agarose gel in precooled MOPS buffer. The gel was run for 20 min at 180 V and analyzed using a molecular imager, ChemiDocTM 219 XRS system (Bio-Rad, United States). RNA Millennium™ markers (Ambion) with bands at a range of 0.5–9 kb was included to provide size determination of the mRNA.

Stability Assay

For storage stability experiments, prepared MP_n-LPX NP 5 were stored at 4°C for 1 and 3 days and another 1 h at rt before particle size and transfection efficiency measurement following the similar procedure described previously (Kranz et al., 2016).

To evaluate the serum stability, 1 μg free mRNA and MP_n-LPX NP 5 (containing 1 μg mRNA) were incubated in parallel with 150 mM NaCl supplemented with or without FBS at 50% final concentration at 37°C for 2 h, respectively. To release mRNA from LPX, 1 μL of 10% Triton X-100 was added to 10 μL of MP_{1000}-LPX samples and incubated at rt for 10 min. After mixed with NorthernMax® formaldehyde load dye, samples were treated and visualized using the similar process as described in Section "Gel Electrophoresis Retardation Assay."

Cytotoxicity Assay

To test potential cytotoxicity, DC2.4 cells were treated with MP_{1000}-LPX according to the transfection procedure. Cell viability was investigated using an Apoptosis Detection Kit according to the manufacturer's protocol by flow cytometry. Three independent cytotoxicity assays were performed in duplicate.

Cellular Uptake of MP-LPX

Cellular uptake study was performed using Cou-6 as previously reported (Xu et al., 2016). DC2.4 cells in the logarithmic growth period were collected and seeded at a density of 8×10^5 cells/well in a 24-well plate and incubated for 24 h at 37°C. To screen the appropriate incubation time, DC2.4 cells were treated with LPX (Cou-6, 5 ng/mL) in triplicate by different time from 0.5 h to 6 h. At the end of the study, the cells were collected and washed three times with cold phosphate buffer saline. The MFI of cells was quantified by BD FACS. To further screen the uptake concentration of Cou-6, DC2.4 cells were treated in triplicate by different concentrations of Cou-6 from 2.5 μg/mL to 20 μg/mL for 2 h.

To investigate the MR mediate uptake of MP_{1000}-LPX (Cou-6, 10 ng/mL), DC2.4 cells were pre-treated with or without 0.16 mol/L of mannose solution for 30 min followed by incubation with LPX and MP_{1000}-LPX at 37°C, respectively. For binding assays, DC2.4 cells were incubated at 4°C for 30 min. Subsequently, LPX and MP_{1000}-LPX were added and incubated for 2 h at 4°C.

Statistical Analysis

The data were presented as mean ± SEM unless otherwise noted. Statistical analysis was performed using Graphpad Prism 5.0. Data of two or multiple groups were analyzed using Student's *t*-test or non-parametric one-way ANOVA, respectively. The *p*-values < 0.05 were considered statistically significant.

RESULTS

Characterization of MP_n-CH

Characterization of MP_{100}-CH

We construct MP_{100}-CH (compound **6**) according to reasonable design as shown in **Figure 1A**. The structure of compounds **1**, **2**, **3**, **4**, and **5** were validated in **Supplementary Figures S1–S5**, respectively. As shown in **Figure 2A**, the ^1H NMR spectra of compounds **4, 5** and **6** were recorded. The single peaks at δ5.33 (s) were attributed to the protons of olefinic bond (-CH_2-CH = C-) in cholesterol. The single peak at δ8.01 (s) came from the protons of olefinic bond (N-CH = C-N) in coupled places. The peaks at δ3.15-3.88 (m) were attributed to the protons from the glycol unit (-O-CH_2-CH_2-O-CH_2–) in PEG chain. These results indicated that MP_{100}-CH has been successfully synthesized. As seen in **Figure 2B**, the mass spectrum of MP_{100}-CH showed a peak at 740.49 (product + Na^+), which was consistent with the expected molecular weight of MP_{100}-CH. In addition, compound **6** was further confirmed by FTIR spectroscopy with of the following principal peaks: ν-OH (3700–3400 cm^{-1}), ν-CH_3 and ν-CH_2 (2960–2850 cm^{-1}), ν-CH_2-O-CH_2- (1210–1050 cm^{-1}) presence but ν-N = N-N- (2100–2270 cm^{-1}) attributed to compound 4, ν-CH (about 3300 cm^{-1}) attributed to compound 5 absence in compounds **6** (**Figure 2C**). Finally, as shown in **Figure 2D**, the spectrum of HPLC exhibited a characteristics absorption peak of MP_{100}-CH at 9.743 min (201 nm). According to the method of area normalization, the purity of MP_{100}-CH is 97.948%.

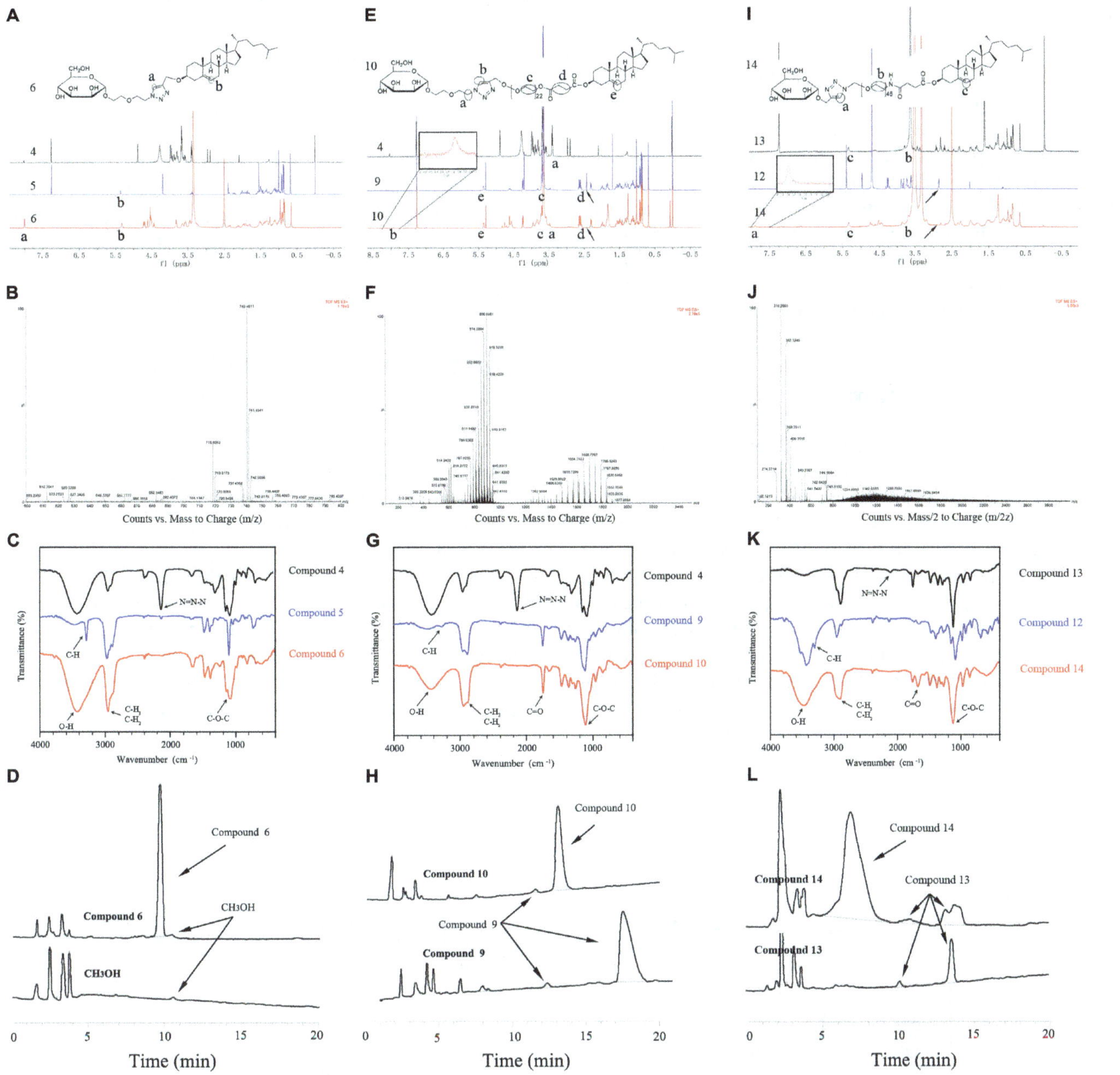

FIGURE 2 | Characterization of MP_n-CHs. **(A)** Comparison of the ^{1}H NMR spectra of compounds **4**, **5**, and **6**. The protons of olefinic bond (N-CH = C-N) in coupled places were shown in compounds 6. **(B)** Mass spectrum of MP_{100}-CH was shown as $(M + Na)^+$, m/z: 740.4911. **(C)** FTIR spectrum of compounds **4**, **5**, and **6**. **(D)** High purity (97.984%) of MP_{100}-CH was confirmed using HPLC. **(E)** Comparison of the ^{1}H NMR spectra of compounds **4**, **9**, and **10** in $CDCl_3$. **(F)** Mass spectrum of compounds 10 was shown as $(M+Na)^+$, m/z: 1484.8359 to 1830.8468. **(G)** FTIR spectrum of compounds **4**, **9**, and **10**. **(H)** HPLC spectra was used to evaluate the purity of MP_{1000}-CH (95.621%). ^{1}H NMR spectra **(I)** and FTIR spectrum **(K)** of compounds **12**, **13**, and **14**. **(J)** Mass spectrum of MP_{2000}-CH was shown as $(M/2+Na)^+$, m/z. **(L)** The purity of MP_{2000}-CH was evaluated (91.532%).

Characterization of MP_{1000}-CH

To construct MP_{1000}-CH (compound **10**), compound 4 was jointed to compound 9 via click reaction as shown in **Figure 1B**. The structure of compounds **8** and **9** were firstly confirmed in **Supplementary Figures S6, S7**, respectively. The ^{1}H NMR spectra of compounds **4, 9** and **10** were recorded in $CDCl_3$. The principal proton peaks at δ2.42-2.45 (t) attributed to the protons of alkynyl group (-CH) in compounds **9** were disappeared in compounds **10** as in shown **Figure 2E**. Similar to MP_{100}-Chol (presence of single peak at δ8.01), the successful synthesis of MP_{1000}-Chol has also been validated. The mass spectrum of MP_{1000}-Chol showed broad peaks from 1484.8359 to 1830.8468 (**Figure 2F**) while that of compound 9 were from 1185.8085 to 1480.0358 (**Supplementary Figure S8**). The increased molecular weight coincided with the molecular weight of compounds **4**, which also confirmed the structure of compound 10 referring to previously report (Li et al., 2014). The FIIR spectroscopy of compounds 10 (**Figure 2G**) was similar to compounds 4 but the presence of unique ν-CH_2-CO-O- of compounds 10 at around 1740 cm^{-1}. Additionally, the characteristics absorption peak (201 nm) of compounds **10** and compounds **9** were at 13.122 min with the purity of 96.595% (**Figure 2H**) and 16.692 min with the purity of 94.881%, respectively. Consistent with expectation, the hydrophilicity of compound 10 was increased and the retention time was decreased when compared with compound 9. All of the results of ^{1}H NMR spectra, mass spectrum, FTIR spectroscopy and HPLC confirmed the successful synthesis of compounds **10**.

Characterization of MP_{2000}-CH

Similar to compound **10**, compound **14** was acquired according to our designed strategies (**Figure 1C**) and authenticated via ^{1}H-NMR (**Figure 2I**), electrospray ionization mass spectrometry (ESI-MS) (**Figure 2J**), FTIR (**Figure 2K**), and HPLC (**Figure 2L**). The structure of compounds **11** and **12** were firstly confirmed in **Supplementary Figures S9**, **S10**, respectively. Of note, the measured molecular weight of compound **12** was 241.07 (product + Na^+) (**Supplementary Figure S11**), which was consistent with the expected molecular weight. When compared mass spectrum of compound 14 (**Figure 2J**) with compound 13 (**Supplementary Figure S12**), nearly 200 molecular weight were increased. The retention time at 201 nm of compound 14 and compound 13 were at 6.907 min with the purity of 91.532% and 13.662 min with the purity of 91.251% (**Figure 2L**), respectively.

Particle Size and Zeta Potential Measurement

The size and zeta potential of all formulations in this study were evaluated. There was no statistical difference between the particle size and zeta potential among different MP_n-LPs or MP_n LPX formulations. The particle size and zeta potential of all different MP_n-LPs was about 60 nm (**Figure 3A**) and 50 mV (**Figure 3B**), respectively. In addition, the particle size and zeta potential of all different LPX was about 135 nm (**Figure 3C**) and 40 mV (**Figure 3D**), respectively. The PDI were all less than 0.3. As was shown, the size of MP_n-LPX was larger and the zeta potential was lower than the corresponding MP_n-LPs formulations.

In vitro Transfection of MP_n-LPX

To investigate the *in vitro* transfection efficacy of MP_n-LPX in DC2.4 cells, the appropriate ratio of N/P of LPX was optimized firstly. GFP expression on DC2.4 cells with different treatment were observed and recorded by fluorescence microscope (**Supplementary Figures S13A–H**). As shown in **Supplementary Figure S13I**, both LPX NP 7 and LPX NP 5 achieved significant increment in transfection efficiency compared with LPX NP 3. What's more, LPX NP 5 with similar transfection efficiency to LPX NP 7 exhibited dramatically enhanced GFP fluorescence intensity (mean GFP expression level per cell) (**Supplementary Figure S13J**). By the way, calculation of MFI and GFP positive cells was shown in **Supplementary Figure S14**. Thus, MP_n-LPX were prepared by setting the N/P ratio at 5:1. The GFP expression was subsequently observed by fluorescence microscope (**Figure 4A**). As shown in **Figure 4B**, MP_{1000}-LPX induced the most GFP positive cells and the

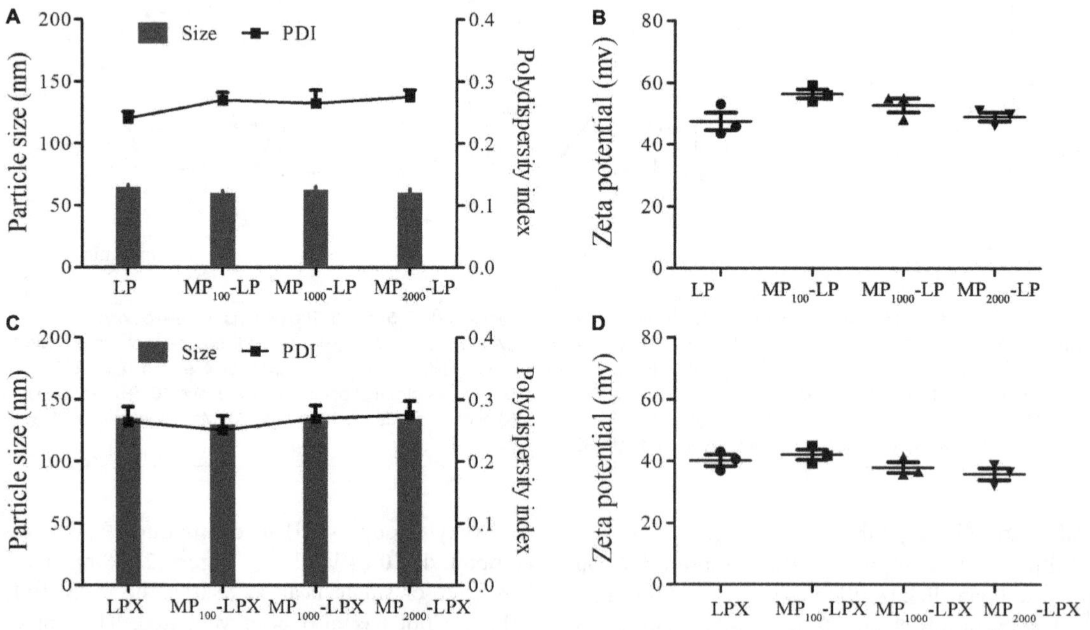

FIGURE 3 | Physicochemical properties of MP_n-LPs and MP_n-LPX. Size **(A)** and zeta potential **(B)** of MP_n-LPs with different PEG linkers. Size **(C)** and zeta potential **(D)** of different formulations loaded with mRNA.

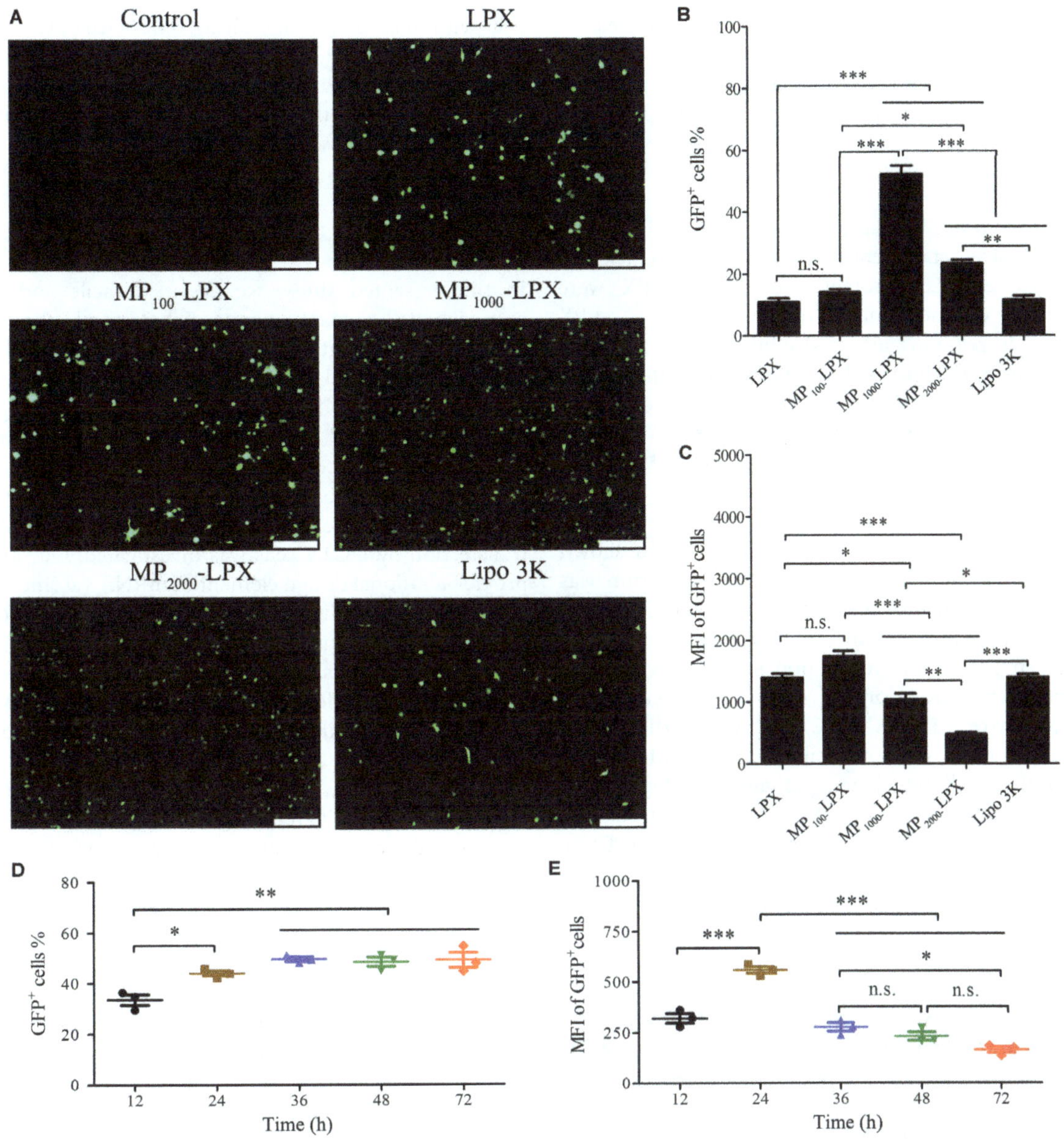

FIGURE 4 | Transfection of MP_n-LPX with different PEGs length on DC2.4 cells at N/P 5. **(A)** GFP expression by DC2.4 cells observed by a fluorescence microscope. Transfection efficiency (%GFP^+ cells) **(B)** and MFI of GFP^+ cells **(C)** were quantified. Kinetics of MP_{1000}-LPX NP 5 transfection efficiency **(D)** and MFI of GFP positive cells **(E)** on DC2.4 cells from 12 h to 72 h. Scale bars, 200 μm. $^*p < 0.05$; $^{**}p < 0.01$; $^{***}p < 0.001$.

percentage was up to 52%, which was significantly higher than any other groups ($p < 0.001$). However, the MFI of the GFP positive cells of MP_{1000}-LPX NP 5 was not the best among these groups (**Figure 4C**). Taking into account of transfection efficiency and MFI, MP_{1000}-LPX with the highest transfection efficiency and moderate MFI were selected for further study in this manuscript.

The kinetics of MP_{1000}-LPX NP 5 transfection on DC2.4 cells was studied. As shown in **Figures 4D,E**, transfection efficiency first increased and then reached a plateau with the increase of the incubation time (from 12 to 72 h) while the MFI of GFP positive cells first increased and then decreased. In summary, the transfection efficiency achieved the maximum at 24 h and MFI was also the strongest at 24 h.

Further Study on the Optimal MP_{1000}-LPX

Morphology Examination

The appearance and morphological studies of MP_{1000}-LPX were conducted. The colloidal solution was colorless and transparent (**Figure 5A**). Overt Tyndall effect of MP_{1000}-LPs and MP_{1000}-LPX colloidal solution were observed compared with water as was shown in **Figure 5B**. Representative images of size and zeta potential of MP_{1000}-LP(X) were shown in **Figures 5C–F**, respectively. As shown in **Figure 5G**, the morphological of MP_{1000}-LPX was observed distinct lipid membrane structure with nearly spherical in shape. Moreover, complete complexation of the mRNA with MP_{1000}-LPs was confirmed when the N/P ratio of 3 and 5 (**Figure 5H**).

Stability Assessment

The preliminary storage stability of the MP_{1000}-LPX was determined by the size, zeta potential and transfection efficiency. The particle size and zeta potential of MP_{1000}-LPX were determined at predetermined time of storage at 4°C. MP_{1000}-LPX displayed a little decrease in particle size but not zeta potential (**Figure 6A**) As shown in **Figure 6B**, the transfection efficiency of MP_{1000}-LPX remained about 50% when stored at 4°C for 3 days. Additionally, MP_{100}-LPX (**Supplementary Figure S15A**) and MP_{2000}-LPX (**Supplementary Figure S15B**) performed excellent storage stability in the preliminary test.

For serum stability, 5 μL of fresh MP_{1000}-LPX were diluted in FBS (1:1, v/v) and incubated for 2 h at 37°C. As shown in **Figure 6C**, the signal of naked mRNA band in serum was completely disappeared (lane 3) compared to naked mRNA alone (lane 1). MP_{1000}-LPX did not dissociate after incubation in 50% serum (lane 5) similar to that incubation in NaCl of 150 mM (lane 4). When the free mRNA or MP_{1000}-LPX were treated with Triton X-100, the free mRNA (lane 2) and mRNA dissociated from MP_{1000}-LPX (lane 4) were visible in line with mRNA treated without Triton X-100 (lane 1) as shown in **Figure 6D**. Similarly, MP_{100}-LPX and MP_{2000}-LPX exerted good stability in the presence of serum (**Supplementary Figure S15C**). These results confirmed the adequate protection of the mRNA against degradation.

Cytotoxicity Assay

After incubation with indicated formulations for 24 h, cytotoxicity analysis was performed by flow cytometry. Representative figure of each condition was showed in **Figure 7A**. The percentage of living DC2.4 cells were found to be 86.7 ± 3.6 %, 86.4 ± 1.7%, and 90.1 ± 1.2% (**Figure 7B**) for control (treated with equal volume of medium), MP_{1000}-LPX and Lipo 3K group, respectively. None significant percentage difference of living cells, early apoptosis, late apoptosis or necrosis was found among these three groups indicating that MP_{1000}-LPX might do no harm to DC2.4 cells. Overall, MP_{1000}-LPX NP 5 performed good safety *in vitro*. Considering the excellent transfection efficacy, MP_{1000}-LPX might be one of good candidates for DC-targeting mRNA nanovaccine for *in vivo* application.

In vitro Uptake

In the preliminary uptake experiment, incubation time and concentration of Cou-6 were optimized. According to the results in **Supplementary Figures S16A,B**, 2 h and 10 ng/mL were selected for future cellular uptake experiment, respectively. To evaluate the potency of MP_{1000}-LPX NP 5 on targeted delivery into DC2.4 cells, the fluorescent of Cou-6 internalized by cells was assayed by BD FACS. The results in **Figure 7C** indicated that intracellular uptake of MP_{1000}-LPX was significantly higher than that of LPX at 37 and 4°C, respectively. When pretreated the cells with mannose, no significant difference of Cou-6 in cellular uptake between MP_{1000}-LPX and LPX was observed. Moreover, intracellular uptake of LPX and MP_{1000}-LPX was significantly lower at 4°C than that at 37°C, indicating that uptake of LPs loaded with mRNA was energy dependent.

DISCUSSION

In the presented study, we designed facile and inexpensive approach to prepare mannose-cholesterol conjugates with various linker length as synthetic ligands applied to mRNA nanovaccine. MP_n-LPs were prepared by a modified thin-film dispersion method. Subsequently, the DCs targeting MP_n-LPX were prepared by complexing MP_n-LPs with mRNA. No significant difference in size and zeta potential was observed among MP_n-LPX comprised MP_n-CH with different PEG units. The effect of linker length of mannose derivatives in MP_n-LPX on transfection by DC2.4 cells was investigated. Our results might provide a rational design element of mRNA vaccine.

Linker length of ligand exerted significantly effect on targeting cellular uptake (Engel et al., 2003; Stefanick et al., 2013; Jeong et al., 2014). Thus, a proper linker length of the ligands was essential for effective receptor recognize and binding. For recognition and binding to MR, linker length of mannose should consist of at least two PEG units according to previously report (Jeong et al., 2014). In our study, mannose-cholesterol conjugates with different linker length were designed and constructed by facile strategies utilizing the click reaction. In detail, mannose derivatives have been conjugated to cholesterol derivatives modified with PEG of different lengths (PEG_{100}, PEG_{1000}, or PEG_{2000}). Each target product was fully characterized by ^{1}H-NMR, ESI-MS, FTIR to confirm the successful of synthesis. HPLC was used to evaluate the purity and the successful synthesis of the products as previously reported (Shariat et al., 2014). The synthetic strategies designed here offered some overt advantages over the previously reported methods for Man-C_4-chol (Kawakami et al., 2000) and Man-C_6-chol (Li et al., 2013), because our target products were easily to synthesis, purify and characterize. What's more, the length of PEG-linkers could be varied with desired length, resulting in many other analogous compounds with MR targeting function.

We constructed MP_n-LPs with various linker lengths between cholesterol and mannose using different length of PEG linker. All MP_n-LPs were constructed with the same molar ratio of mannose modified cholesterol. The MP_n-LPs had similar average size and surface charge despite of the introduction of MP_n-CHs with different linker lengths of PEG. We then prepared MP_n-LPX and performed cellular transfection studies in DC2.4 cells with the evaluated parameters of transfection efficiency and MFI of GFP positive cells, respectively. Transfection efficiency and MFI of LPX was preliminary optimized to find optimal ratio of N/P. Our results showed no significant difference in transfection efficiency of LPX NP 5 and LPX NP 7, while both exhibited significantly higher transfection efficiency than LPX NP 3. However, MFI of the GFP positive cells of LPX NP 5

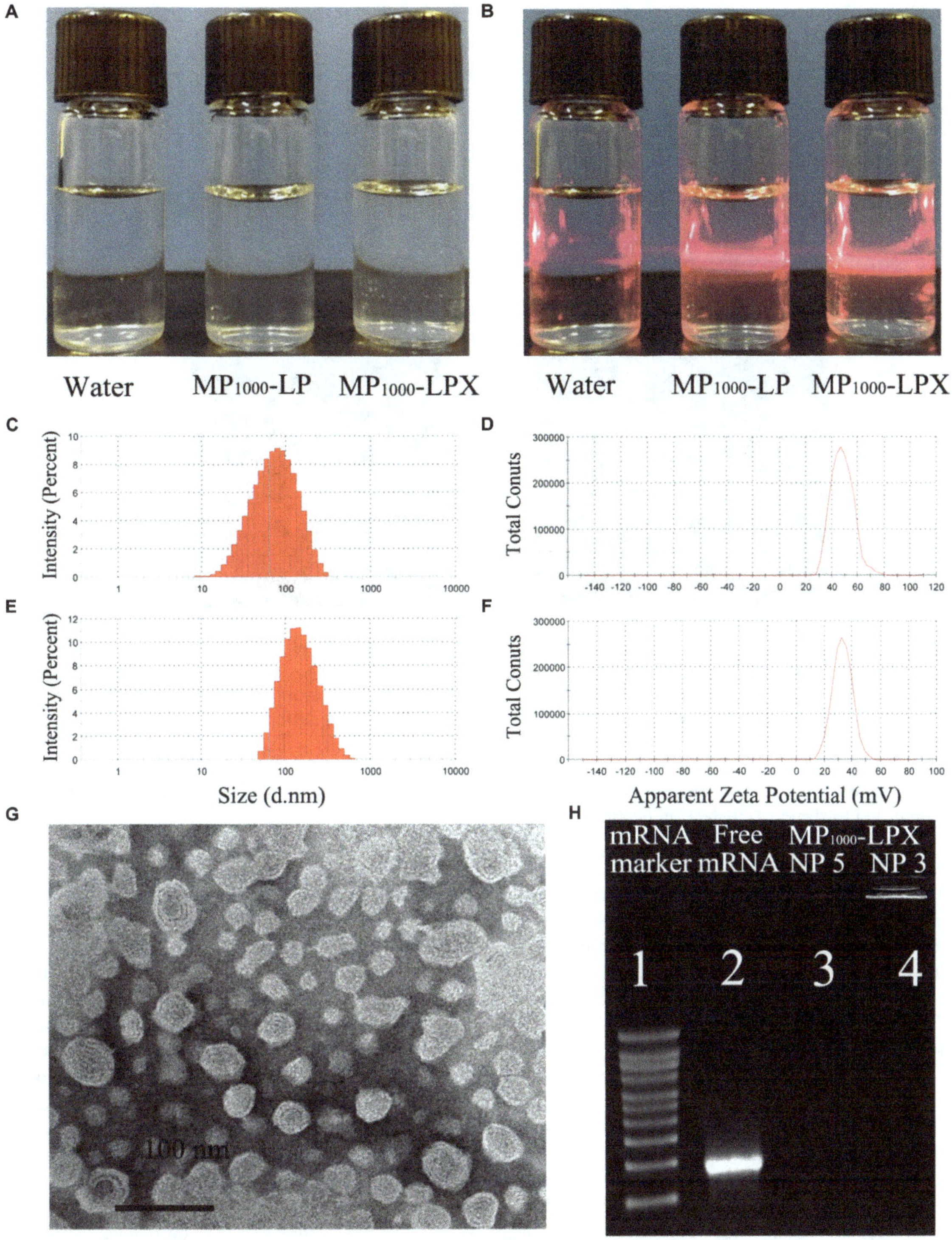

FIGURE 5 | Characterization of MP_{1000}-LPX. Appearance **(A)** and Tyndall effect **(B)** of MP_{1000}-LPX. Size **(C)** and zeta potential **(D)** of MP_{1000}-LP were recorded by Zetasizer Nano ZS90, and representative images were showed. Representative images of size **(E)** and zeta potential **(F)** of MP_{1000}-LPX. **(G)** TEM images of the MP_{1000}-LPX NP 5. **(H)** Agarose gel electrophoresis image of mRNA maker, Free mRNA, MP_{1000}-LPX (N/P 5) and MP_{1000}-LPX (N/P 3).

was significantly higher compared to that of LPX NP 7. Taken the transfection efficiency and MFI of the GFP positive cells into consideration, the ratio of N/P of 5 was selected for future studies. The difference between the percentage of transfected cells and the MFI of transfected cells was consistent with previously reported results (McLenachan et al., 2013; Avci-Adali et al., 2014;

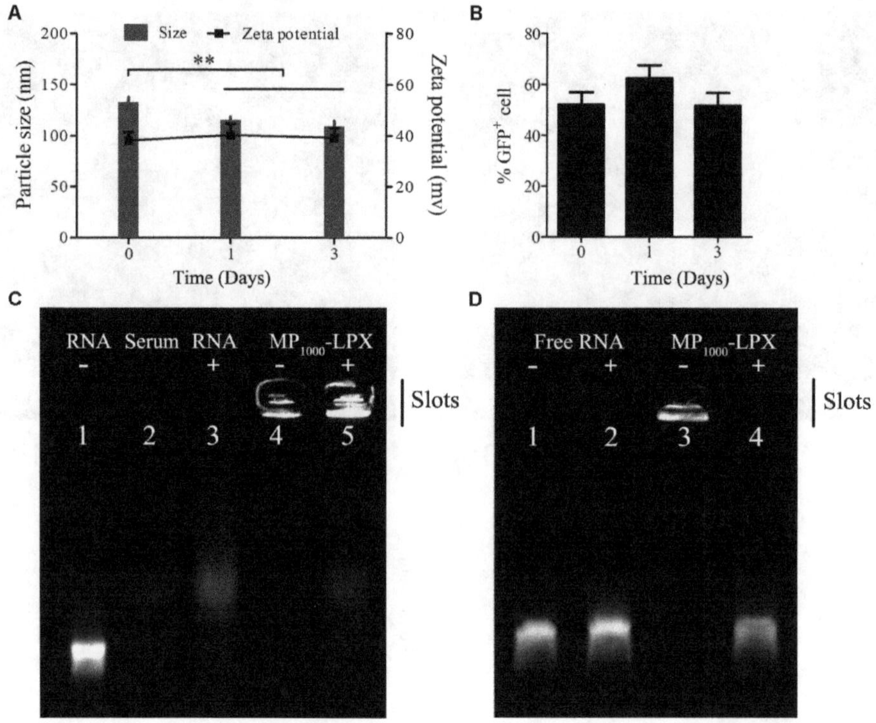

FIGURE 6 | Stability of MP_{1000}-LPX. **(A)** Size and zeta potential measurements of MP_{1000}-LPX at 0, 1, and 3 days stored at 4°C. **(B)** Transfection efficiency of MP_{1000}-LPX at 0, 1, and 3 days stored at 4°C. **(C,D)** Gel electrophoresis retardation assay of MP_{1000}-LPX (N/P:5:1) to test serum stability. **(C)** Free RNA (lane 1), Serum (lane 2), Serum + RNA (lane 3), MP_{1000}-LPX (lane 4) and Serum + MP_{1000}-LPX (lane 5). **(D)** Free RNA in 150 mM NaCl treated without (lane 1) or with Triton X-100 (lane 2). MP_{1000}-LPX in 150 mM NaCl treated without (lane 3) and or with Triton X-100 (lane 4). $^{**}p < 0.01$.

Lee et al., 2015; Li et al., 2017a). Transfection using the same transfection reagent led to similar transfection efficiency but not the MFI (**Figures 4D,E**) with the increase of the incubation time, which was consistent with previously report (Avci-Adali et al., 2014). In addition, increasing the amount of mRNA can significantly increase the average fluorescence intensity without affecting the transfection efficiency within a certain range (Avci-Adali et al., 2014). Moreover, MFI values showed the strength of the fluorescence intensity. Higher MFI values reflected a higher production of GFP by individual cell but not higher percentage of GFP positive cells.

According to literatures, upon interaction with serum, nanocarriers rapidly absorbed protein and formed a corona (Bertrand et al., 2017; Pan et al., 2017). It was the nanocarrier–corona complex, rather than the nanocarrier, that interacted with biological systems, here with a cell membrane receptor (CD206), which might partially obscure the role of target ligands (Monopoli et al., 2012). To reduce this effect, culture medium without serum was used at initial and complete culture medium with serum were added 4 h after the adding of LPX. As was known, the fate of nano-preparations in serum (mimic the *in vivo* environment) was very important to predict its potential therapeutic efficacy. Our preliminary test showed that the presence serum significantly affected the transfection of MP_{1000}-LPX. We were still working on this. Hopefully, we would show the data of mRNA delivery in the presence of serum *in vitro* and expression of the nano-preparations *in vivo* in our future work.

MP_{1000}-LPX exhibited a higher level of transfection efficiency than LPX, MP_{100}-LPX, MP_{2000}-LPX and positive control Lipo 3K. No size and charge variation were found in the vectors then no inference can be made on the transfection efficiency correlation with size and charge. The excellent transfection efficiency of MP_{1000}LPX was most likely attributed to the appropriate linker length used to conjugate mannose and cholesterol. However, MP_{1000}LPX exerted the highest transfection efficiency but moderate MFI. The inconsistency of cellular transfection efficiency and MFI observed in the field of targeted mannose modified LPX partially resulted from differences in the types of cell, incubation time, the amount of mRNA, ability of lysosome escape and types of lipid mannose modified (Kim et al., 2012; Li et al., 2013; Avci-Adali et al., 2014; Chen et al., 2015; Wang C. et al., 2015). The best effect of MP_{1000}-LPs conjugates may be related to the above factors. However, most likely it was attributed to the linkers used to conjugate mannose and the other different component of targeting formulations (Kim et al., 2012; Wang N. et al., 2014; Wang C. et al., 2015). There are many other known and unknown factors for ligand receptor affinity beside linker length of ligand. Moreover, the intracellular metabolism of mRNA nanovaccine might also affect the expression of protein encoded by mRNA. Accurately, we cannot declare that the linker length

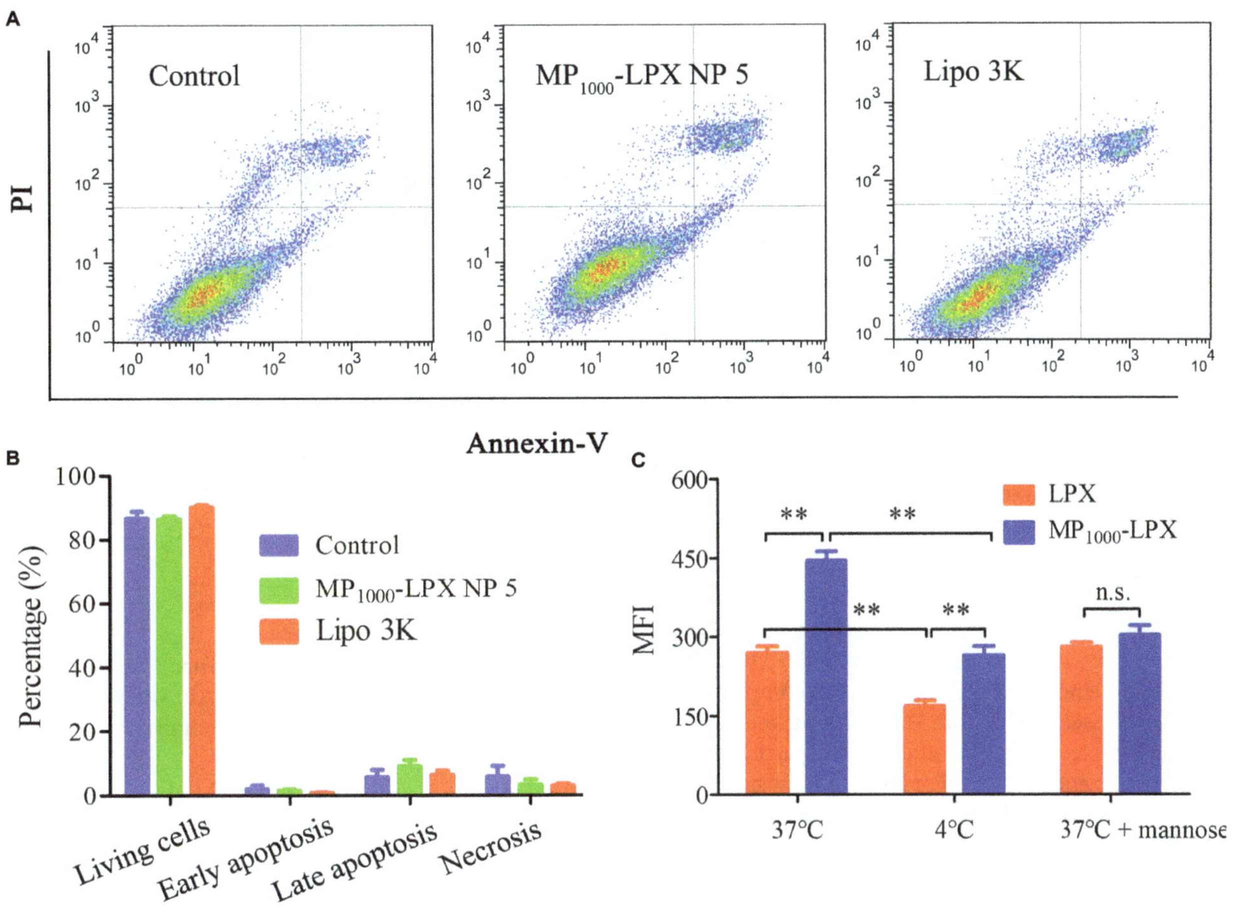

FIGURE 7 | Cytotoxicity and uptake assay of MP_{1000}-LPX on DC2.4 cells. **(A,B)** Flow cytometry measurement of cell apoptosis induced by MP_{1000}-LPX NP 5 and Lipo3K on DC2.4 cells. The data showed mean ± SEM from a representative experiment from three independent experiments. **(C)** Cellular uptake mediated by mannose receptor at different conditions, including incubated at 4, 37, or 37°C with free mannose. *$p < 0.05$; **$p < 0.01$.

of MP_{1000}-LPX is optimal for transfection by DC2.4 cells but selected MP_{1000}-LPX as a representative formulation from our result for further investigation.

The pharmaceutical properties including particle size, zeta potential, storage stability and the ability to protect mRNA against serum degradation of optimal MP_{1000}-LPX were then characterized systemically. MP_{1000}-LPX displayed bigger diameter and lower zeta potential compared to MP_{1000}-LPs, indicating the complexation of MP_{1000}-LPs with mRNA. We were surprised to find that particle size measurement results of MP_{1000}-LPX by Zetasizer Nano ZS90 was much larger than that by TEM although some other researchers also observed the similar phenomenon (Wang K. et al., 2018; Yang et al., 2018). The larger size distribution by Zetasizer than TEM observed in the field of size measurement partially resulted from the interference of the dispersant into the hydrodynamic diameter. Complete complexation of the mRNA with MP_{1000}-LPs was also validated according to the results of gel electrophoresis retardation assay. The preliminary storage stability experiment revealed that MP_{1000}-LPX could maintain its excellent transfection efficiency at least for 3 days at 4°C, which might benefit from the protection of the mRNA against degradation. It has been reported that triMN-LPR with high zeta potential (about 35 mV) could better target human and murine dendritic cells, result in higher recruitments of DCs to draining lymph nodes, and induced significant antitumor responses (Le Moignic et al., 2018). Additionally, Folate modified cationic LPs loaded with DNMT1 gene with positive charge (>30 mV) exerted excellent *in vitro* targeted genome editing and *in vivo* antitumor effects (He et al., 2018). However, there seemed to be much cationic charge in the MP_{1000}-LPX. Further formulation optimization will be done to balance the transfection efficiency and the high positive zeta potential in our future work.

The cellular cytotoxicity and uptake mechanism of MP_{1000}-LPX were also evaluated. MP_{1000}-LPX presented good safety *in vitro* according to the data of cell apoptosis and might be a safe formulation for *in vivo* application. It has been reported that the presence of free mannose could decrease the uptake of mannose modified preparations (Li et al., 2013; Wang C. et al., 2014). The amount of free mannose in this study was used according to a previously reported literature (Wang C. et al., 2014). Moreover, the experiment design was similar to previous reports (Li et al., 2013; Wang C. et al., 2014). When DC2.4 cells were pretreated with free mannose as an inhibitor, no significant effect on uptake by LPX was observed, while uptake by MP_{1000}-LPX was significantly decreased. This difference in uptake indicated that the enhanced uptake and transfection were mainly through the MR on DC2.4 cells in line with previous reports (Li et al., 2013; Wang C. et al., 2014). Taken together, our results of uptake *in vitro* confirmed that the enhanced transfection of MP_{1000}-LPX occurs mainly via a MR-mediated mechanism and the linker length of mannose exerts a crucial role. Although MP_{1000}-LPX exhibited higher level of transfection efficiency through the MR than MP_{100}-LPX and MP_{2000}-LPX, we could not exclude that other linker length of mannose modified cholesterol would exhibit more effective transfection in DC2.4 cells through MR. Nevertheless, a rational design element was proposed and more detailed future studies will be indispensable to facilitate the progression of mRNA nanovaccine.

CONCLUSION

In summary, MP_n-CHs with different linker molecules (PEG_{100}, PEG_{1000}, and PEG_{2000}) were successfully synthesized by a simple and cost-efficient method. The DC-targeting LPs complexed with mRNA were self-assembled using MP_n-CHs as the targeting lipids. The linker molecules had no effect on the particle size and zeta potential of LPs and mRNA-complexed LPs but significantly affected the transfection efficiency of GFP-encoding mRNA. Unexpectedly, PEG_{1000} rather than PEG_{100} or the commonly used PEG_{2000} as the linker achieved the maximal level of GFP expression. MP_{1000}-LPX containing MP_{1000}-CH displayed good profiles including small size with nearly spherical shape, good stability in serum and little cytotoxicity, indicating a hopeful DCs-targeting delivery system for mRNA vaccine.

AUTHOR CONTRIBUTIONS

XS conceived the project. MF and JW designed the experiments. FW, WX, and XB conducted most of the experiments. WX and QZ further performed and analyzed the transfection and characterization of formulations. FW, ME, and WX drafted the manuscript. LG and SY performed the ^{1}H-NMR and HPLC analysis. QZ and YZ performed the some preliminary experiments. WX, QZ, and AF participated in literature searching. XS and MF finished the manuscript editing. All authors reviewed and approved the manuscript.

FUNDING

This work was financially supported by National Key S&T Special Projects (2018ZX09201018-024) and Sichuan Province Science and Technology Support Program (2015SZ 0234).

REFERENCES

Avci-Adali, M., Behring, A., Keller, T., Krajewski, S., Schlensak, C., and Wendel, H. P. (2014). Optimized conditions for successful transfection of human endothelial cells with in vitro synthesized and modified mRNA for induction of protein expression. *J. Biol. Eng.* 8:8. doi: 10.1186/1754-1611-8-8

Bertrand, N., Grenier, P., Mahmoudi, M., Lima, E. M., Appel, E. A., Dormont, F., et al. (2017). Mechanistic understanding of in vivo protein corona formation on polymeric nanoparticles and impact on pharmacokinetics. *Nat. Commun.* 8:777. doi: 10.1038/s41467-017-00600-w

Caminschi, I., Maraskovsky, E., and Heath, W. R. (2012). Targeting dendritic cells in vivo for cancer therapy. *Front. Immunol.* 3:13. doi: 10.3389/fimmu.2012.00013

Chen, D., Koropatnick, J., Jiang, N., Zheng, X., Zhang, X., Wang, H., et al. (2014). Targeted siRNA silencing of indoleamine 2, 3-dioxygenase in antigen-presenting cells using mannose-conjugated liposomes: a novel strategy for treatment of melanoma. *J. Immunother.* 37, 123–134. doi: 10.1097/CJI.0000000000000022

Chen, J., Son, H. N., Hill, J. J., Srinivasan, S., Su, F. Y., Stayton, P. S., et al. (2016). Nanostructured glycopolymer augmented liposomes to elucidate carbohydrate-mediated targeting. *Nanomedicine* 12, 2031–2041. doi: 10.1016/j.nano.2016.05.001

Chen, J. L., Luo, J., Zhao, Y., Pu, L. Y., Lu, X. J., Gao, R., et al. (2015). Increase in transgene expression by pluronic L64-mediated endosomal/lysosomal escape through its membrane-disturbing action. *ACS Appl. Mater. Interfaces* 7, 7282–7293. doi: 10.1021/acsami.5b00486

Engel, A., Chatterjee, S. K., Al-arifi, A., Riemann, D., Langner, J., and Nuhn, P. (2003). Influence of spacer length on interaction of mannosylated liposomes with human phagocytic cells. *Pharm. Res.* 20, 51–57. doi: 10.1023/A:1022294624256

Giacca, M., and Zacchigna, S. (2012). Virus-mediated gene delivery for human gene therapy. *J. Control. Release* 161, 377–388. doi: 10.1016/j.jconrel.2012.04.008

Hajj, K. A., and Whitehead, K. A. (2017). Tools for translation: non-viral materials for therapeutic mRNA delivery. *Nat. Rev. Mater.* 2:17056. doi: 10.1038/natrevmats.2017.56

He, Z., Yu, Y., Zhang, Y., Yan, Y., Zheng, Y., He, J., et al. (2013). Gene delivery with active targeting to ovarian cancer cells mediated by folate receptor alpha. *J. Biomed. Nanotechnol.* 9, 833–844. doi: 10.1166/jbn.2013.1587

He, Z. Y., Wei, X. W., Luo, M., Luo, S. T., Yang, Y., Yu, Y. Y., et al. (2013). Folate-linked lipoplexes for short hairpin RNA targeting claudin-3 delivery in ovarian cancer xenografts. *J. Control. Release* 172, 679–689. doi: 10.1016/j.jconrel.2013.10.015

He, Z. Y., Zhang, Y. G., Yang, Y. H., Ma, C. C., Wang, P., Du, W., et al. (2018). In Vivo Ovarian Cancer Gene Therapy Using CRISPR-Cas9. *Hum. Gene Ther.* 29, 223–233. doi: 10.1089/hum.2017.209

He, Z. Y., Zheng, X., Wu, X. H., Song, X. R., He, G., Wu, W. F., et al. (2010). Development of glycyrrhetinic acid-modified stealth cationic liposomes for gene delivery. *Int. J. Pharm.* 397, 147–154. doi: 10.1016/j.ijpharm.2010.06.029

Hua, S., and Wu, S. Y. (2013). The use of lipid-based nanocarriers for targeted pain therapies. *Front. Pharmacol.* 4:143. doi: 10.3389/fphar.2013.00143

Jeong, H. S., Na, K. S., Hwang, H., Oh, P. S., Kim, D. H., Lim, S. T., et al. (2014). Effect of space length of mannose ligand on uptake of mannosylated liposome in RAW 264.7 cells: in vitro and in vivo studies. *J. Biomed. Mater. Res. A* 102, 4545–4553. doi: 10.1002/jbm.a.35112

Kawakami, S., Sato, A., Nishikawa, M., Yamashita, F., and Hashida, M. (2000). Mannose receptor-mediated gene transfer into macrophages using novel mannosylated cationic liposomes. *Gene Ther.* 7, 292–299. doi: 10.1038/sj.gt.3301089

Kim, H., Kim, B. H., Huh, B. K., Yoo, Y. C., Heo, C. Y., Choy, Y. B., et al. (2017). Surgical suture releasing macrophage-targeted drug-loaded nanoparticles for an enhanced anti-inflammatory effect. *Biomater. Sci.* 5, 1670–1677. doi: 10.1039/c7bm00345e

Kim, H. K., Wei, H., Kulkarni, A., Pogranichniy, R. M., and Thompson, D. H. (2012). Effective targeted gene delivery to dendritic cells via synergetic interaction of mannosylated lipid with DOPE and BCAT. *Biomacromolecules* 13, 636–644. doi: 10.1021/bm2014119

Kranz, L. M., Diken, M., Haas, H., Kreiter, S., Loquai, C., Reuter, K. C., et al. (2016). Systemic RNA delivery to dendritic cells exploits antiviral defence for cancer immunotherapy. *Nature* 534, 396–401. doi: 10.1038/nature18300

Kreiter, S., Vormehr, M., van de Roemer, N., Diken, M., Lower, M., Diekmann, J., et al. (2015). Mutant MHC class II epitopes drive therapeutic immune responses to cancer. *Nature* 520, 692–696. doi: 10.1038/nature14426

Lai, C., Duan, S., Ye, F., Hou, X., Li, X., Zhao, J., et al. (2018). The enhanced antitumor-specific immune response with mannose- and CpG-ODN-coated liposomes delivering TRP2 peptide. *Theranostics* 8, 1723–1739. doi: 10.7150/thno.22056

Le Moignic, A., Malard, V., Benvegnu, T., Lemiegre, L., Berchel, M., Jaffres, P. A., et al. (2018). Preclinical evaluation of mRNA trimannosylated lipopolyplexes as therapeutic cancer vaccines targeting dendritic cells. *J. Control. Release* 278, 110–121. doi: 10.1016/j.jconrel.2018.03.035

Lee, K., Yu, P., Lingampalli, N., Kim, H. J., Tang, R., and Murthy, N. (2015). Peptide-enhanced mRNA transfection in cultured mouse cardiac fibroblasts and direct reprogramming towards cardiomyocyte-like cells. *Int. J. Nanomed.* 10, 1841–1854. doi: 10.2147/IJN.S75124

Li, L., Li, X., Wu, Y., Song, L., Yang, X., He, T., et al. (2017a). Multifunctional nucleus-targeting nanoparticles with ultra-high gene transfection efficiency for in vivo gene therapy. *Theranostics* 7, 1633–1649. doi: 10.7150/thno.17588

Li, L., Song, L., Liu, X., Yang, X., Li, X., He, T., et al. (2017b). Artificial virus delivers CRISPR-Cas9 system for genome editing of cells in mice. *ACS Nano* 11, 95–111. doi: 10.1021/acsnano.6b04261

Li, P., Chen, S., Jiang, Y., Jiang, J., Zhang, Z., and Sun, X. (2013). Dendritic cell targeted liposomes-protamine-DNA complexes mediated by synthetic mannosylated cholesterol as a potential carrier for DNA vaccine. *Nanotechnology* 24:295101. doi: 10.1088/0957-4484/24/29/295101

Li, X. Y., Zhao, Y., Sun, M. G., Shi, J. F., Ju, R. J., Zhang, C. X., et al. (2014). Multifunctional liposomes loaded with paclitaxel and artemether for treatment of invasive brain glioma. *Biomaterials* 35, 5591–5604. doi: 10.1016/j.biomaterials.2014.03.049

Malissen, B., Tamoutounour, S., and Henri, S. (2014). The origins and functions of dendritic cells and macrophages in the skin. *Nat. Rev. Immunol.* 14, 417–428. doi: 10.1038/nri3683

Markov, O. V., Mironova, N. L., Shmendel, E. V., Serikov, R. N., Morozova, N. G., Maslov, M. A., et al. (2015). Multicomponent mannose-containing liposomes efficiently deliver RNA in murine immature dendritic cells and provide productive anti-tumour response in murine melanoma model. *J. Control. Release* 213, 45–56. doi: 10.1016/j.jconrel.2015.06.028

McLenachan, S., Zhang, D., Palomo, A. B., Edel, M. J., and Chen, F. K. (2013). mRNA transfection of mouse and human neural stem cell cultures. *PLoS One* 8:e83596. doi: 10.1371/journal.pone.0083596

Midoux, P., and Pichon, C. (2015). Lipid-based mRNA vaccine delivery systems. *Expert Rev. Vaccines* 14, 221–234. doi: 10.1586/14760584.2015.986104

Monopoli, M. P., Aberg, C., Salvati, A., and Dawson, K. A. (2012). Biomolecular coronas provide the biological identity of nanosized materials. *Nat. Nanotechnol.* 7, 779–786. doi: 10.1038/nnano.2012.207

Nguyen, H., Katavic, P., Bashah, N. A. H., and Ferro, V. (2016). Synthesis of mannose-cholesterol conjugates for targeted liposomal drug delivery. *ChemistrySelect* 1, 31–35. doi: 10.1002/slct.201600007

Oberli, M. A., Reichmuth, A. M., Dorkin, J. R., Mitchell, M. J., Fenton, O. S., Jaklenec, A., et al. (2017). Lipid nanoparticle assisted mRNA delivery for potent cancer immunotherapy. *Nano Lett.* 17, 1326–1335. doi: 10.1021/acs.nanolett.6b03329

Pan, Z., Fang, D., Song, N., Song, Y., Ding, M., Li, J., et al. (2017). Surface distribution and biophysicochemical properties of polymeric micelles bearing gemini cationic and hydrophilic groups. *ACS Appl. Mater. Interfaces* 9, 2138–2149. doi: 10.1021/acsami.6b14339

Pardi, N., Hogan, M. J., Porter, F. W., and Weissman, D. (2018). mRNA vaccines - a new era in vaccinology. *Nat. Rev. Drug Discov.* 17, 261–279. doi: 10.1038/nrd.2017.243

Persano, S., Guevara, M. L., Li, Z., Mai, J., Ferrari, M., Pompa, P. P., et al. (2017). Lipopolyplex potentiates anti-tumor immunity of mRNA-based vaccination. *Biomaterials* 125, 81–89. doi: 10.1016/j.biomaterials.2017.02.019

Rull-Barrull, J., d'Halluin, M., Le Grognec, E., and Felpin, F. X. (2016). Harnessing the dual properties of thiol-grafted cellulose paper for click reactions: a powerful reducing agent and adsorbent for Cu. *Angew. Chem. Int. Ed Engl.* 55, 13549–13552. doi: 10.1002/anie.201606760

Sahin, U., Kariko, K., and Tureci, O. (2014). mRNA-based therapeutics–developing a new class of drugs. *Nat. Rev. Drug Discov.* 13, 759–780. doi: 10.1038/nrd4278

Sayour, E. J., De Leon, G., Pham, C., Grippin, A., Kemeny, H., Chua, J., et al. (2017). Systemic activation of antigen-presenting cells via RNA-loaded nanoparticles. *Oncoimmunology* 6:e1256527. doi: 10.1080/2162402X.2016.1256527

Shariat, S., Badiee, A., Jalali, S. A., Mansourian, M., Yazdani, M., Mortazavi, S. A., et al. (2014). P5 HER2/neu-derived peptide conjugated to liposomes containing MPL adjuvant as an effective prophylactic vaccine formulation for breast cancer. *Cancer Lett.* 355, 54–60. doi: 10.1016/j.canlet.2014.09.016

Stefanick, J. F., Ashley, J. D., Kiziltepe, T., and Bilgicer, B. (2013). A systematic analysis of peptide linker length and liposomal polyethylene glycol coating on cellular uptake of peptide-targeted liposomes. *ACS Nano* 7, 2935–2947. doi: 10.1021/nn305663e

Tsui, N. B., Ng, E. K., and Lo, Y. M. (2002). Stability of endogenous and added RNA in blood specimens, serum, and plasma. *Clin. Chem.* 48, 1647–1653.

Verbeke, R., Lentacker, I., Wayteck, L., Breckpot, K., Van Bockstal, M., Descamps, B., et al. (2017). Co-delivery of nucleoside-modified mRNA and TLR agonists for cancer immunotherapy: restoring the immunogenicity of immunosilent mRNA. *J. Control. Release* 266, 287–300. doi: 10.1016/j.jconrel.2017.09.041

Wang, C., Liu, P., Zhuang, Y., Li, P., Jiang, B., Pan, H., et al. (2014). Lymphatic-targeted cationic liposomes: a robust vaccine adjuvant for promoting long-term immunological memory. *Vaccine* 32, 5475–5483. doi: 10.1016/j.vaccine.2014.07.081

Wang, C., Liu, P., Zhuang, Y., Li, P., Jiang, B., Pan, H., et al. (2015). Lymphatic-targeted cationic liposomes: a robust vaccine adjuvant for promoting long-term immunological memory. *J. Control. Release* 213:e16. doi: 10.1016/j.jconrel.2015.05.022

Wang, F., Bao, X., Fang, A., Li, H., Zhou, Y., Liu, Y., et al. (2018). Nanoliposome-encapsulated Brinzolamide-hydropropyl-beta-cyclodextrin inclusion complex: a potential therapeutic ocular drug-delivery system. *Front. Pharmacol.* 9:91. doi: 10.3389/fphar.2018.00091

Wang, K., Wen, S., He, L., Li, A., Li, Y., Dong, H., et al. (2018). Minimalist" nanovaccine constituted from near whole antigen for cancer immunotherapy. *ACS Nano* 12, 6398–6409. doi: 10.1021/acsnano.8b00558

Wang, N., Wang, T., Zhang, M., Chen, R., Niu, R., and Deng, Y. (2014). Mannose derivative and lipid A dually decorated cationic liposomes as an effective cold chain free oral mucosal vaccine adjuvant-delivery system. *Eur. J. Pharm. Biopharm.* 88, 194–206. doi: 10.1016/j.ejpb.2014.04.007

Xu, B., Jin, Q., Zeng, J., Yu, T., Chen, Y., Li, S., et al. (2016). Combined tumor- and neovascular-"dual targeting" gene/chemo-therapy suppresses tumor growth and angiogenesis. *ACS Appl. Mater. Interfaces* 8, 25753–25769. doi: 10.1021/acsami.6b08603

Yang, R., Xu, J., Xu, L., Sun, X., Chen, Q., Zhao, Y., et al. (2018). Cancer cell membrane-coated adjuvant nanoparticles with mannose modification for effective anticancer vaccination. *ACS Nano* doi: 10.1021/acsnano.7b09041 [Epub ahead of print].

Yang, Y., He, L., Liu, Y., Xia, S., Fang, A., Xie, Y., et al. (2016). Promising nanocarriers for PEDF gene targeting delivery to cervical cancer cells mediated by the over-expressing FRalpha. *Sci. Rep.* 6:32427. doi: 10.1038/srep32427

Facile Fabrication of Reduction-Responsive Supramolecular Nanoassemblies for Co-delivery of Doxorubicin and Sorafenib toward Hepatoma Cells

Qingqing Xiong [1], Mangmang Cui [1,2], Ge Yu [1], Jian Wang [3] and Tianqiang Song [1]**

[1] Department of Hepatobiliary Cancer, National Clinical Research Center for Cancer, Key Laboratory of Cancer Prevention and Therapy, Tianjin's Clinical Research Center for Cancer, Tianjin Medical University Cancer Institute and Hospital, Tianjin, China, [2] Hebei province Cangzhou Hospital of Integrated Traditional and Western Medicine, Cangzhou, China, [3] Department of Immunology, National Clinical Research Center for Cancer, Key Laboratory of Cancer Prevention and Therapy, Tianjin's Clinical Research Center for Cancer, Tianjin Medical University Cancer Institute and Hospital, Tianjin, China

***Correspondence:**
Jian Wang
wangjian112358@163.com
Tianqiang Song
tjchi@hotmail.com

Combination of doxorubicin with sorafenib (SF) was reported to be a promising strategy for treating hepatocellular carcinoma (HCC). In this study, we designed a reduction-responsive supramolecular nanosystem based on poly (ethylene glycol)-β-cyclodextrin (PEG-CD) and a disulfide-containing adamantine-terminated doxorubicin prodrug (AD) for efficient co-delivery of doxorubicin and sorafenib. PEG-CD/AD supramolecular amphiphiles were formed through host-guest interaction between cyclodextrin and adamantine moieties, and then self-assembled into regular spherical nanoparticles with a uniform size of 166.4 nm. Flow cytometry analysis and confocal laser scanning microscopy images showed that PEG-CD/AD nanoparticles could be successfully taken up by HepG2 cells and then released doxorubicin into the cell nuclei. Moreover, sorafenib could be facilely encapsulated into the hydrophobic cores to form PEG-CD/AD/SF nanoparticles with a slightly larger size of 186.2 nm. PEG-CD/AD/SF nanoparticles sequentially released sorafenib and doxorubicin in a reduction-response manner. *In vitro* cytotoxicity assay showed that PEG-CD/AD/SF nanoparticles had an approximately 4.7-fold decrease in the IC_{50} value compared to that of PEG-CD/AD and SF physical mixtures, indicating stronger inhibitory effect against HepG2 cells by co-loading these two drugs. In summary, this novel supramolecular nanosystem provided a simple strategy to co-deliver doxorubicin and sorafenib toward hepatoma cells, which showed promising potential for treatment of HCC.

Keywords: reduction-responsive, supramolecular nanoassemblies, doxorubicin, sorafenib, hepatocellular carcinoma

INTRODUCTION

Hepatocellular carcinoma (HCC) is the second leading cause of cancer-related death (International Agency for Research on Cancer. GLOBOCAN, 2012), characterized by its insidious onset, poor diagnosis, and intrinsic resistance to chemotherapy agents. Doxorubicin (DOX), a widely used chemotherapeutic drug, plays an undisputed key role in transcatheter arterial chemoembolization

(TACE) for HCC (Vilaseca et al., 1978). However, the therapeutic efficacy of DOX for HCC is often limited because of the emergence of drug resistance (Deng et al., 2015; Galun et al., 2017) and its irreversible cardiotoxicity (Singal and Iliskovic, 1998). Sorafenib (SF), an oral multiple kinase inhibitor, is successful to prolong the survival of advanced HCC patients and has been approved by FDA for the standard treatment of patients with unresectable HCC (Llovet et al., 2015). However, during the clinical application, it was found that SF was only beneficial to about 33% HCC patients while showed low tumor response to other majority of patients (Cheng et al., 2009). It has been reported that combining two or more drugs of different molecular mechanisms might be a promising alternative option for long-term application of a single drug and would exert better therapeutic effects on HCC (Lin et al., 2016; Sun et al., 2017; Zhao et al., 2017). Moreover, clinical trial studies have demonstrated that combination of DOX with SF exhibited remarkable improvement in the overall survival of HCC patients (Hutchinson, 2011; Pazo Cid et al., 2011).

However, due to the hydrophobic properties and varied pharmacokinetic profiles of these two drugs, the co-delivery of both drugs toward HCC is still a major challenge. With the development of nanotechnology in biomedical fields, nanoparticles provide a valid platform to achieve co-loading of multiple drugs and deliver them toward tumor cells simultaneously (Hu et al., 2016). Among these nanoparticles, supramolecular nanosystems, especially formed by host-guest interaction, have attracted researchers' great attention in drug delivery (Feng et al., 2017; Ping et al., 2017). Cyclodextrins (CDs), a series of natural cyclic oligosaccharides composed of D-glucose units, are the most commonly used macrocyclic hosts to construct supramolecular nanosystems in virtue of their low toxicity and low immunogenicity (Zhang et al., 2013; Feng et al., 2017; Xiong et al., 2017). The most prominent structural feature of CDs is their hydrophobic cavities, which can accommodate a variety of guest molecules such as adamantine (Luo et al., 2012) and trans-azobenzene (Li et al., 2013) *via* host-gust interaction. During the past few decades, CDs and their derivatives have been extensively utilized in the construction of drug delivery system. Zhang and coworkers established a supramolecular photosensitizer delivery system through the self-assembly of supramolecular amphiphiles constructed by the host–guest interaction between poly (ethylene glycol)-β-cyclodextrin and adamantane-terminated porphyrin derivatives (Liu et al., 2015). In our previous study, a series of well-defined cyclodextrin-based polymers were synthesized by atom transfer radical polymerization and then further used for drug delivery (Xiong et al., 2014; Zhang M. et al., 2014).

Recently, stimuli-responsive nanoparticles have drawn a lot of attentions due to their responsiveness to tumor or intracellular micro-environmental stimuli, such as low pH-values (Chen et al., 2016), high concentration of certain enzymes (Zhang et al., 2017), and more reductive environment (Wang et al., 2013), and thus releasing their payloads in a controlled manner. According to the previous studies (Wang et al., 2012; Yin et al., 2013), the cytosolic glutathione (GSH) concentration is around 2–10 mM, which is substantially higher than that in the extracellular fluids and blood (2–10 μM). Disulfide bond, which is stable in blood circulation but can be cleaved under reducing intracellular microenvironment, has been widely used as a linker in the design of reduction-responsive drug delivery system. In Sun's work, they reported a prodrug-based nanoplatform self-assembled by the disulfide bond linked conjugates of paclitaxel (PTX) and oleic acid, achieving the rapid and differential release of PTX in tumor cells (Luo et al., 2016). Moreover, the prodrug strategy provides several advantages such as enhanced *in vivo* stability, the prolonged half-life in blood, the improved water solubility, etc. (Yang et al., 2015; Li D. et al., 2016; Li W. et al., 2016).

In this paper, we prepared a novel reduction-responsive supramolecular nanosystem by a facile method for co-delivery of DOX and SF toward hepatoma cells (**Figure 1**). A reduction-responsive prodrug of doxorubicin (Ada-ss-DOX) was first synthesized by conjugation of doxorubicin with amantadine through disulfide bond, and then complexed with poly (ethylene glycol)-β-cyclodextrin (PEG-CD) *via* host-guest interaction between CD cavity and Ada moiety to form PEG-CD/AD supramolecular amphiphiles (I). Using a modified nanoprecipitation method, PEG-CD/AD amphiphiles could self-assemble into spherical nanoparticles in aqueous medium (II). The reduction-responsive disassembly of PEG-CD/AD nanoparticles triggered by dithiothreitol (DTT) was then investigated (III). Moreover, SF could also be incorporated into the hydrophobic cores of the nanoparticles by hydrophobic interaction and π-π stacking interaction with DOX (IV), and thus achieved the co-loading of DOX and SF. The size and morphology of these nanoparticles were respectively characterized by dynamic light scattering (DLS) and transmission electron microscopy (TEM). The cellular uptake and intracellular locations of PEG-CD/AD nanoparticles were investigated by flow cytometry analysis and confocal laser scanning microscopy (CLSM). In addition, the cytotoxicity of PEG-CD/AD/SF nanoparticles against hepatoma HepG2 cells were evaluated by CCK-8 assay in detail.

MATERIALS AND METHODS

Materials

Amantadine hydrochloride (Ada), and dithiodiglycolic acid (DTGA, ≥98%) 4′,6-diamidino-2-phenylindole (DAPI) were obtained from Sigma-Aldrich (St. Louis, MO, USA) and used without further purification. Doxorubicin hydrochloride (DOX·HCl) and sorafenib (SF) base was purchased from Dalian Meilun Biotech Co., Ltd. (Dalian, China). 1-(3-Dimethylaminopropyl)-3-ethylcarbodiimide hydrochloride (EDC·HCl), 1-hydroxybenzotriazole hydrate (HOBt, 99%), O-(7-azabenzotriazol-1-yl)-N,N,N′,N′-tetramethyluronium hexafluorophosphate (HATU, 99%), and N,N-diisopropylethylamine (DIPEA, 99%) was purchased from J&K Scientific (Beijing, China). Methoxypoly(ethylene glycol) succinimidyl succinate (PEG-NHS, $M_n = 2000$) was purchased from JenKem Technology Co., Ltd (Beijing, China). Other chemical reagents in the study were analytical grade and obtained from commercial sources. PEG-CD was synthesized according to the previous study (Peng et al., 2014) and the synthetic route was described in the supplementary data (Figure S1A). The ^1H NMR spectrum of PEG-CD was displayed in Figure S1B.

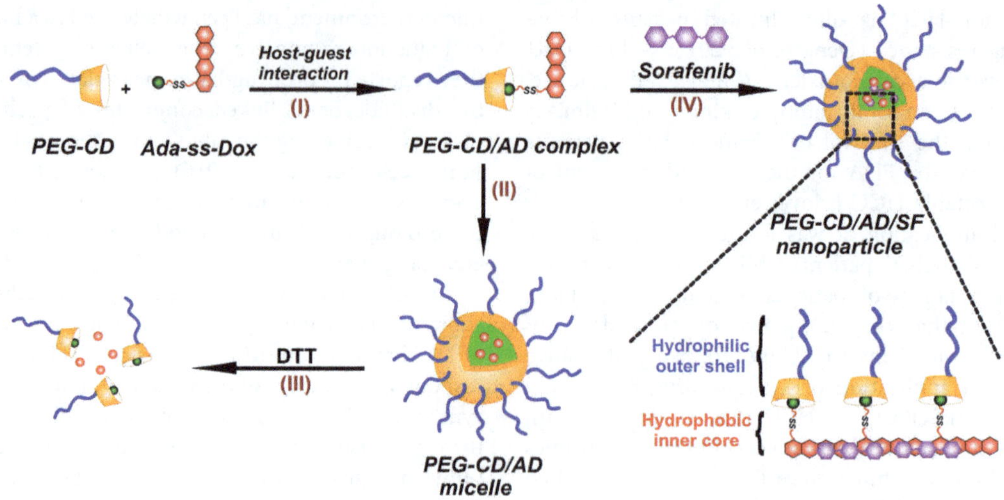

FIGURE 1 | Illustration for the preparation of PEG-CD/AD/SF nanoparticles. (I) PEG-CD/AD supramolecular amphiphile was formed *via* the host-gust interaction between CD cavity and Ada moiety; (II) PEG-CD/AD nanoparticles were prepared by self-assembly of PEG-CD/AD amphiphile in aqueous medium; (III) PEG-CD/AD nanoparticles disassemble after incubation with DTT; (IV) PEG-CD/AD/SF nanoparticles were prepared by incorporating SF in the self-assembly process of PEG-CD/AD amphiphile.

Synthesis of Amantadine-Terminated Doxorubicin Prodrug (Ada-ss-DOX)

Ada-ss-DOX was synthesized by the following two steps. DTGA (5 mmol, 0.9110 g) was dissolved 15 mL of dichloromethane. Subsequently, HOBt (4.5 mmol, 0.6070 g), EDC·HCl (4.5 mmol, 0.8612 g) and triethylamine (15 mmol, 1.5178 g) were added. After the mixture was stirred at 20°C for 1 h, Ada (3 mmol, 0.4549 g) was added. The resulting mixture was stirred at 20°C for another 3 h and filtered to give the filtrate. The filtrate was concentrated to give the crude product and then purified by prep-HPLC system (Instrument: GILSON 281, Column: ASB C18 150*25 mm. Mobile phase: A: deionized water containing 0.1% HCl; B: acetonitrile, Gradient: B from 40 to 70% in 10 min. Flow rate: 25 mL/min) to obtain Ada-ss-COOH as a brown solid (Yield 6.8%).

Subsequently, the synthesized Ada-ss-COOH (3.17 mmol, 1.00 g) and DOX·HCl (2.85 mmol, 1.65 g) were co-dissolved in 20 mL dimethyl formamide (DMF) and then HATU (4.76 mmol, 1.81 g) and DIPEA (9.51 mmol, 1.23 g) were added. The mixture was stirred at 20°C for 2 h and then diluted by 20 mL of water. The resulting mixture was extracted with ethyl acetate. The organic phases were collected, washed with brine and dried with anhydrous Na_2SO_4, filtered and finally concentrated under vacuum to give Ada-ss-DOX (hereafter "AD") as a red solid powder (Yield 45.5%).

Preparation of PEG-CD/AD and PEG-CD/AD/SF Nanoparticles

PEG-CD/AD nanoparticles were prepared by a modified nanoprecipitation and dialysis method. PEG-CD and AD were dissolved in DMF respectively to obtain solutions with a concentration of 1 mg/mL. Then, PEG-CD solution and Ada-ss-DOX solution with molar ratio of 1:1 was mixed and stirred overnight to obtain PEG-CD/AD supramolecular amphiphiles. Afterwards, an equal volume of water was slowly dropped into the above mixed solution under stirring at 400 rpm. The solution was stirred for another 4 h, followed by dialyzed against deionized water for 24 h to remove DMF (MWCO 3500). The dialysate was further concentrated by ultra-filtration membrane (MWCO 5000).

PEG-CD/AD/SF nanoparticles were prepared by a similar method. A determined volume of SF solution in DMF was stirred with PEG-CD/AD mixed solution for 4 h and then water was added. The solution was stirred, dialyzed and concentrated as described above to obtain PEG-CD/AD/SF nanoparticles.

Characterization

^1H NMR analysis was carried out on a AVANCE III HD nuclear magnetic resonance spectrometer at 400 MHz (Bruker, Germany). The molecular weight of AD was analyzed by mass spectrometry (Agilent, 6510 Q-TOF LC/MS, USA). The size, size distribution, and zeta potential of the nanoparticles in aqueous solution were determined by a Zetasizer Nano ZS instrument (Malvern, England) at 25°C. The nanoparticle morphology was visualized using Tecnai G2 20STwin transmission electron microscope (FEI, USA).

Reduction-Triggered Disassembly of PEG-CD/AD Nanoparticles

PEG-CD/AD nanoparticles were added into DTT solutions with different concentrations and then treated for determined periods. The fluorescence intensities of the mixed solutions were measured on a F-4500 fluorescence spectrometer (Hitachi, Japan) at an excitation wavelength of 485 nm. Meanwhile, the size and morphology changes of PEG-CD/AD nanoparticles were monitored by DLS and TEM.

Cellular Uptake and Intracellular Distributions of PEG-CD/AD Nanoparticles

Flow cytometry was employed to determine the cellular uptake of PEG-CD/AD nanoparticles in HepG2 cells. Briefly, the cells were seeded on a 12-well plate and cultured for 24 h. Then the cultural media were replaced with fresh media containing free DOX or PEG-CD/AD nanoparticles at a DOX concentration of 2 μg/mL. After incubation for determined periods, the cells were collected and analyzed on a BD FACSVerse™ flow cytometer (BD Biosciences, USA).

For confocal laser scanning microscope (CLSM) study, the cells were placed onto 12-well glass plates. After incubation for 24 h, the cells were treated as the same as flow cytometry analysis. Then the cells were washed with PBS, fixed with 4% formaldehyde and the cell nuclei were stained by DAPI. Thereafter, the cells were observed under FV 1000 CLSM (Olympus, Japan).

In vitro Drug Releases of DOX and SF from PEG-CD/AD/SF Nanoparticles

The *in vitro* releases of DOX and SF from PEG-CD/AD/SF nanoparticles were evaluated using dynamic dialysis method in four kinds of release media (I: pH 7.4 PBS; II: pH 7.4 PBS with 10 mM DTT; III: pH 5.0 PBS; IV: pH 5.0 PBS with 10 mM DTT). Briefly, PEG-CD/AD/SF nanoparticle solutions (1 mL) were placed into dialysis bags (MWCO 7000) and dialyzed against above media at 37°C in the air bath shaking with 100 rpm. At designated time points, 0.5 mL of release media was withdrawn and replaced with an equal volume of fresh release media. The amounts of DOX and SF in the release media were determined by UV/Vis spectrophotometer (Beckman DU-640, USA) at a wavelength of 490 and 267 nm, respectively (Malarvizhi et al., 2014). The release tests were repeated for three times and the accumulative releases of drug were calculated.

In vitro Cytotoxicity Analysis

The cytotoxicities of PEG-CD/AD and PEG-CD/AD/SF nanoparticles compared with free DOX, free SF, and PEG-CD/AD nanoparticles and SF physical mixtures were evaluated in HepG2 cells using CCK-8 regents. Briefly, the cells were seeded onto 96-well plate and cultured for 24 h, and then the media were replaced with fresh media containing free DOX, free SF, PEG-CD/AD nanoparticles, PEG-CD/AD and free SF physical mixtures, and PEG-CD/AD/SF nanoparticles followed by further incubation for 48, 72, and 96 h, respectively. Next, the media were removed and 10 μL of CCK-8 regents and 90 μL of fresh media were added into each well. After incubated for 2 h, the plates were gently shaken for 2 min and the absorbance was measured at 450 nm using an Epoch 2 microplate spectrophotometer (BioTek, Winooski, USA). The cell viabilities were calculated as the ratio of the absorbance values of treated cells to those of untreated cells. The inhibitory effect of PEG-CD on HepG2 cell growth for 48 h was also assessed as the similar method.

Statistical Analysis

Each experiment was repeated for three times. All data were presented as mean ± standard deviation and compared using one-way ANOVA. The differences were significant when $p < 0.05$.

RESULTS AND DISCUSSION

Synthesis and Characterization of Ada-ss-DOX

DTGA, with two active carboxyl groups, was chosen as the disulfide reagent to produce Ada-ss-DOX prodrug. The synthesis route is displayed in **Figure 2A**. Firstly, Ada-ss-COOH was synthesized *via* the condensation reaction between Ada and DTGA. To ensure that the product with only one of the carboxyl groups of DTGA conjugated with Ada was collected, excess DTGA was added during the reaction process and the product was further purified by prep-HPLC. From the ^{1}H NMR spectrum of Ada-ss-COOH in **Figure 2B**, the integration ratio of the peaks at 3.66 and 3.38 ppm, corresponding to the methylene protons of DTGA (*signal a and b*), to the peaks at 1.75 ppm, originating from the methylene protons of Ada (*signal d*), was calculated to be 1:3, which indicated that the molar ratio of Ada and DTPA is 1:1. Moreover, the molecular weight of Ada-ss-COOH ($C_{14}H_{22}NO_3S_2^+$) determined by ESI-MS in **Figure 2C** was found to be 315.9 g/mol (calcd 316.5 g/mol), further indicating the success synthesis of Ada-ss-COOH.

Subsequently, Ada-ss-DOX was obtained by the reaction between the end carboxyl group of Ada-ss-COOH and the reactive amine group of DOX. The characteristic peaks of hydroxyl protons of DOX (*signal a' and b'*) located at 13.93 and 13.20 ppm were obviously observed in the ^{1}H NMR spectrum of Ada-ss-DOX (**Figure 2B**). Due to the steric-hindrance effect after conjugation of DOX, the signals attributed to the methylene protons of DTGA (*signal a and b*) significantly decreased in the^{1}H NMR spectrum of Ads-ss-DOX. The ESI-MS result showed that the molecular weight of Ada-ss-DOX ($C_{41}H_{49}N_2O_{13}S_2^+$) was 841.3 g/mol, which was consistence with calculated 841.9 g/mol (**Figure 2C**). Altogether, the above results demonstrated that Ada-ss-DOX was successfully prepared.

Preparation and Characterization of PEG-CD/AD Nanoparticles

To our knowledge, the formation of nanoparticles was often due to the self-assembly process of amphiphilic block copolymers driven by hydrophobic interaction among the hydrophobic segments (Zhao et al., 2012). In this study, PEG-CD/AD nanoparticles were self-assembled from PEG-CD/AD supramolecular amphiphiles with hydrophilic segment PEG-CD and hydrophobic segment DOX (**Figure 1**). The DMF solution of PEG-CD and AD was stirred overnight to obtain the supramolecular amphiphiles *via* host-guest interaction between CD cavities and Ada moieties, and then the deionized water was slowly added to induce the self-assembly of PEG-CD/AD nanoparticles. Finally, the solution

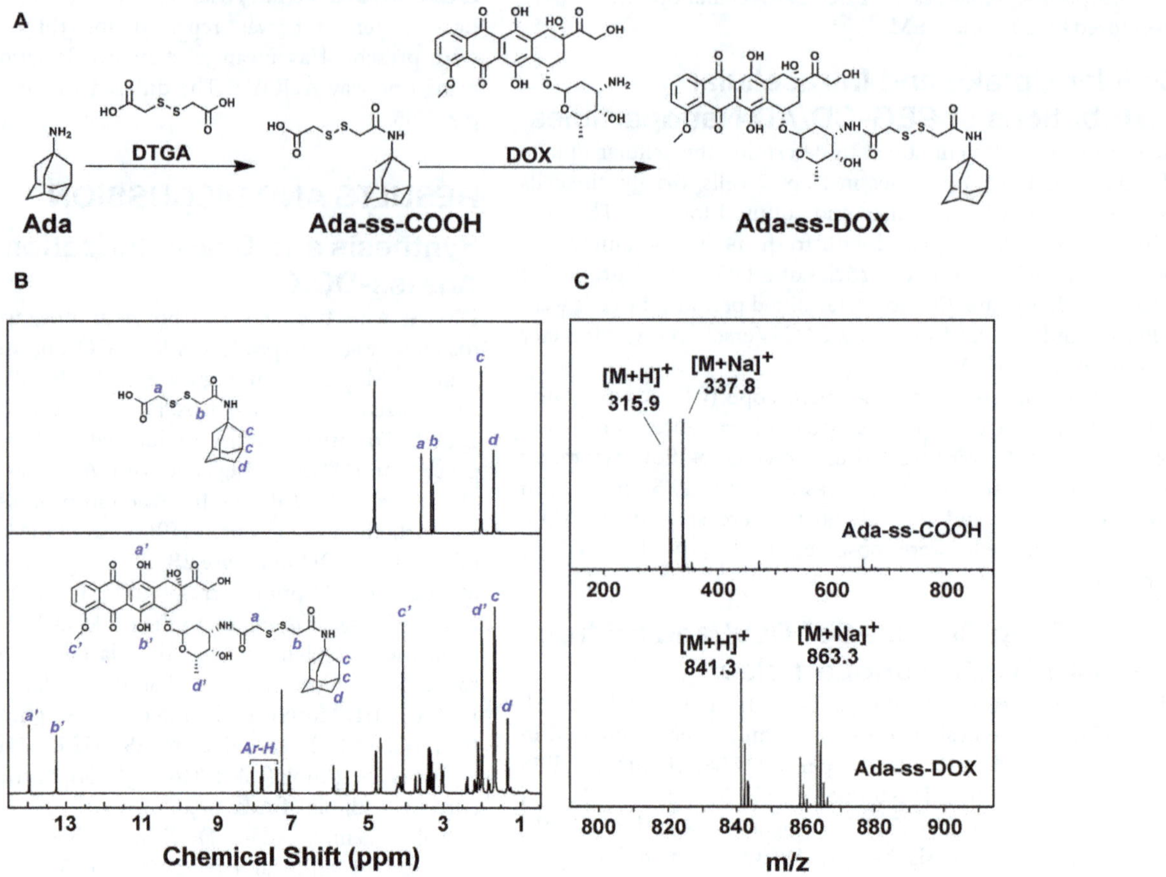

FIGURE 2 | Synthetic route **(A)**, ^{1}H NMR spectra **(B)** and mass spectra **(C)** of Ada-ss-DOX.

was dialyzed against deionized water to remove DMF. The DOX content was calculated to be 13.5% as the molar ratio of PEG-CD and AD was 1:1. The hydrodynamic diameter and morphology of PEG-CD/AD nanoparticles was determined by DLS and TEM. As shown in **Figure 3B**, the average size of PEG-CD/AD nanoparticles was 166.4 nm and polydispersity (PDI) of 0.089. TEM image in **Figure 3Ca** showed that PEG-CD/AD nanoparticles had spherical shape and the average particle size was about 100 nm, which was significantly smaller that measured by DLS. It was perhaps because that the PEG chains in the outer surface of PEG-CD/AD nanoparticles were extended in aqueous solution while collapsed in dry samples.

Reduction-Responsive Disassembly of PEG-CD/AD Nanoparticles

DTT was used to mimic the reductive environment as it was a prevailing GSH stimulant (Dai et al., 2011; Zhang B. et al., 2014). As shown in **Figure 3A**, the fluorescence intensity of the PEG-CD/AD solution containing 10 mM DTT gradually increased as time prolonged. By contrast, almost no change in the emission spectra of the PEG-CD/AD solution was observed for 48 h in the absence of DTT (Figure S2). Moreover, the emission spectra of the nanoparticles were also detected after incubation with DTT of different concentrations for 2 h. It was obviously found that the fluorescence intensity increased with the DTT concentration increasing from 1 to 50 mM (Figure S3). The above results suggested that the disulfide bond could be cleaved under the stimulation of DTT, resulting in the disassembly of PEG-CD/AD nanoparticles and release of DOX.

The hydrodynamic diameters of PEG-CD/AD nanoparticles were also measured after incubation with DTT for 4 h and 24 h (**Figure 3B**). After 4 h, the average size of the nanoparticles increased to 683.6 nm with a corresponding increase of PDI to 0.29. The nanoparticles changed to be larger than 1 µm with PDI of 0.89 after 24 h incubation. TEM images in **Figures 3Cb,c** showed that the morphology of the nanoparticles was irregular and large aggregated particles could be observed, which further confirmed that the disassembly due to reductive cleavage of the disulfide bonds. To be noticed, the hydrodynamic diameters of PEG-CD/AD nanoparticles after incubation with DTT seemed larger than the sizes of nanoparticles displayed in TEM images. This might be attributed that the average size measured by DLS was determined by intensity, and in this case, the size would be larger than the actual size when very large aggregated particles existed.

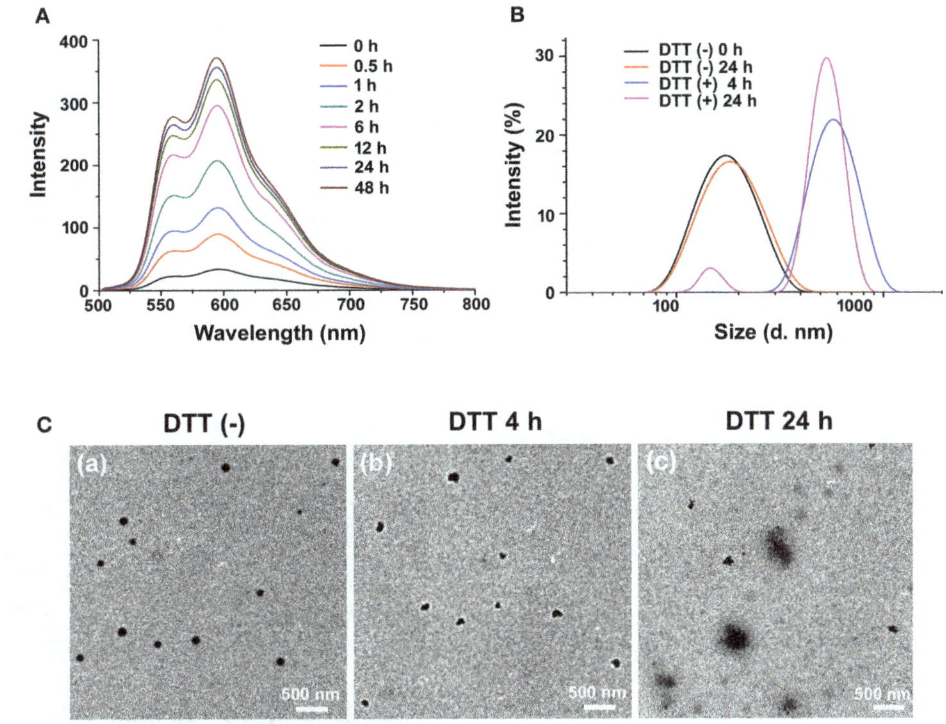

FIGURE 3 | Reduction-responsive disassembly of PEG-CD/AD nanoparticles triggered by DTT. **(A)** Emission spectra of DOX in PEG-CD/AD solutions containing DTT at different time with an excitation wavelength of 485 nm. [PEG-CD/AD = 40 μg/mL] **(B)** Hydrodynamic diameter distribution change of PEG-CD/AD nanoparticles treated with 10 mM DTT for 24 h; **(C)** TEM images of PEG-CD/AD nanoparticles treated without DTT **(a)** and with 10 mM DTT for 4 h **(b)** or 24 h **(c)**.

Cellular Uptake and Intracellular Locations of PEG-CD/AD Nanoparticles

The cellular uptake of PEG-CD/AD nanoparticles was investigated in HepG2 cells by flow cytometry and CLSM. HepG2 cells were incubated with PEG-CD/AD nanoparticles or free DOX for 2 h at DOX concentration of 2.0 μg/mL and then collected for flow cytometry analysis. As shown in **Figure 4A**, PEG-CD/AD nanoparticles exhibited much stronger fluorescence intensity than the control, which indicated that the nanoparticles could be effectively internalized into HepG2 cells. However, PEG-CD/AD nanoparticles showed slightly lower intracellular fluorescence intensity than that of free DOX. It was probably because DOX could not be completely released from the nanoparticles in 2 h.

Next, CLSM was employed to track the intracellular locations of PEG-CD/AD nanoparticles after internalization. HepG2 cells were treated with PEG-CD/AD nanoparticles for predetermined time and the nuclei were stained by DAPI (blue). As shown in **Figure 4B**, the fluorescence signals of DOX (red) in the cells exhibited time-dependent manner. Weak fluorescence signals were observed in the cytoplasm after 0.5 h of incubation and the signals tended to be stronger after 2 h of incubation. Minor red fluorescence signals could be observed in the nuclei after 8 h of incubation, suggesting that DOX was released from the nanoparticles and began to accumulate in the nuclei. After 24 h, the red fluorescence signals were almost overlapped with the shrunken nuclei, which indicated that most of DOX entered the nuclei and exerted an evident cytotoxic effect. Besides, the dynamic intracellular process of free DOX was also investigated and the results are shown in Figure S4. Unlike PEG-CD/AD nanoparticles, free DOX could rapidly enter the nuclei since the red fluorescence signals were obviously observed in the nuclei after 0.5 h. The drug release from free DOX was much faster than that from DOX-loaded nanoparticles (Figure S5), thus, this difference might be attributed to the fact that free DOX can quickly transport into the cells *via* passive diffusion, while PEG-CD/AD nanoparticles entered the cells through endocytosis and then released DOX into the nuclei, thus showing a lagged effect. According to the above results, we might draw the conclusion that, after PEG-CD/AD nanoparticles were taken up, the disulfide bond could be cleaved by the high GSH environment in the cytoplasm and PEG-CD/AD nanoparticles disassembled to release free DOX (**Figure 4C**).

In vitro Cytotoxicity of PEG-CD/AD Nanoparticles against HepG2 Cells

The *in vitro* cytotoxicity of PEG-CD/AD nanoparticles against HepG2 cells was evaluated by CCK-8 agents. Firstly, we determined the inhibitory effect of PEG-CD on the growth of the cells and no significant cytotoxicity was detected since the cell viabilities were larger than 95% at the concentration range of 5–50 μM (**Figure 5A**). By comparison, PEG-CD/AD nanoparticles exhibited obvious inhibition on cell growth in time- and dose-dependent manners (**Figure 5B**). The half maximal inhibitory concentrations (IC_{50} values), denoted as the concentration of DOX causing 50% of cell growth, were calculated to be 19.47, 9.31, and 6.64 μM for 48, 72, and 96 h, respectively. In addition, PEG-CD/AD nanoparticles showed weaker cytotoxicity in HepG2 cells than that of free DOX (Figure S6). According to other disulfide linked DOX-prodrug reported previously (Song et al., 2016), we deduced that it was because PEG-CD/AD showed a sustained release of DOX and thus exhibited delayed therapeutic effects, while free DOX entered the cell nuclei directly and exerted their therapeutic effects instantly.

Physicochemical Characterization of PEG-CD/AD/SF Nanoparticles

Sorafenib (SF) was further integrated into the nanosystem *via* hydrophobic interaction and π-π stacking interaction (Zhao et al., 2015) between DOX and SF. The core of the nanosystem was composed of DOX and SF, while the shell was a layer of PEG-CD. According to a previous study (Zhang et al., 2016), the CI values (combination index determined by IC_{50}) in DOX-based combinations (DOX/SF molar ratio: 1/0.1, 1/0.2, 1/0.5) were much lower than that of SF-based combinations (DOX/SF molar ratio: 0.1/1, 0.2/1), indicated that DOX-based combinations present better cytotoxic effect. In our work, the hydrodynamic

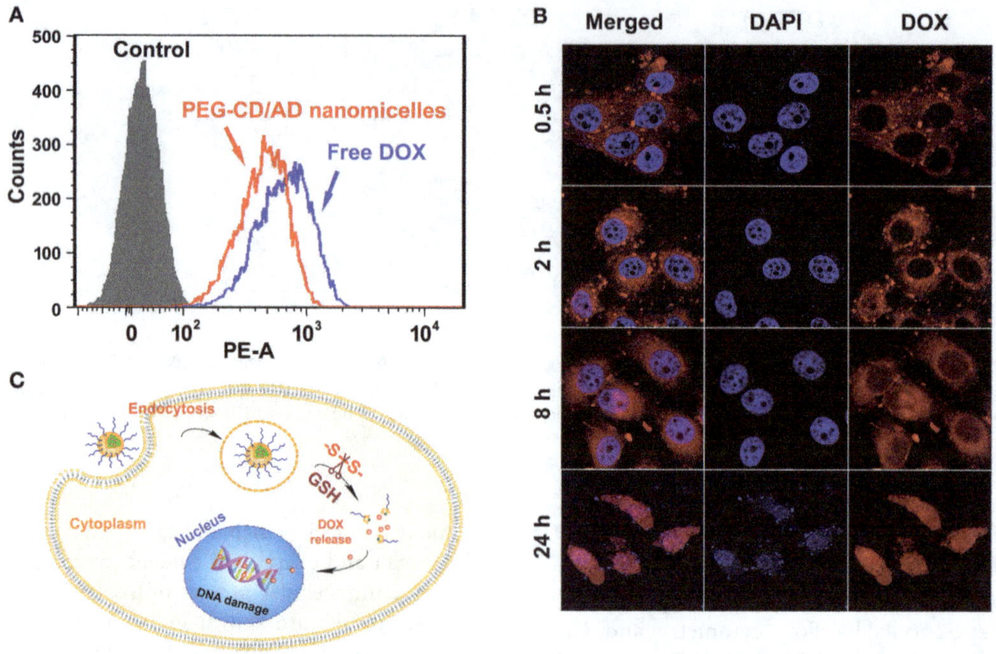

FIGURE 4 | Cellular uptake and intracellular locations of PEG-CD/AD nanoparticles in HepG2 cells. **(A)** Flow cytometry analysis of the cells with the treatments of PEG-CD/AD nanoparticles for different time. **(B)** Confocal images of the cells. **(C)** Schematic illustration of cell internalization of PEG-CD/AD nanoparticles and intracellular release of DOX.

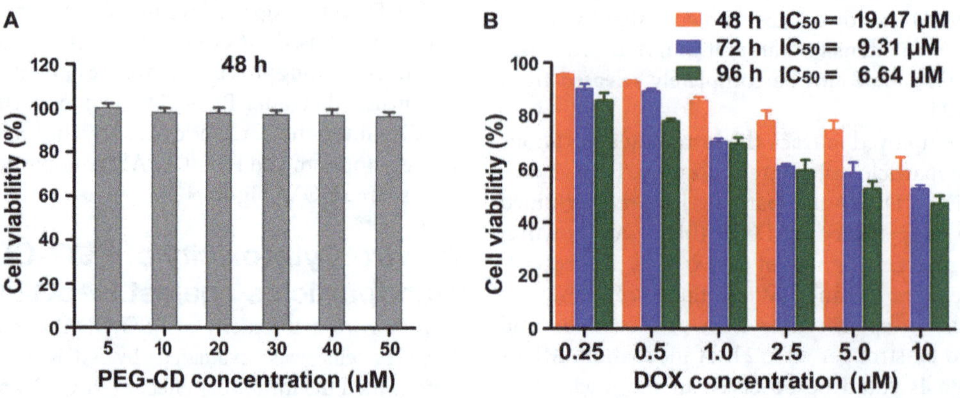

FIGURE 5 | *In vitro* cytotoxicities of PEG-CD **(A)** and PEG-CD/AD nanoparticles **(B)** against HepG2 cells at different concentrations. Data are means ± standard deviation for three separate experiments.

diameters of PEG-CD/AD/SF nanoparticles at different molar ratios were evaluated and the results are displayed in **Table 1**. The average size of PEG-CD/AD/SF nanoparticles increased as the molar ratio of PEG-CD: AD: SF changed from 1/1/0.1 to 1/1/2. Meanwhile, the PDI of PEG-CD/AD/SF nanoparticles tended to be large when more SF was added, indicating that excess SF had a negative effect on the stability of PEG-CD/AD/SF nanoparticles. Taken a comprehensive consideration of CI values and sizes, 1/1/0.2 was believed as the optimal ratio to prepare PEG-CD/AD/SF nanoparticles. As shown in **Figure 6A**, PEG-CD/AD/SF nanoparticles prepared at this ratio had an average size of 186.2 nm with a relatively narrow size distribution (PDI = 0.114). TEM images showed that PEG-CD/AD/SF nanoparticles displayed uniform spherical structure (**Figure 6B**).

The *in vitro* releases of DOX and SF from PEG-CD/AD/SF nanoparticles were investigated in different media and the release profiles are displayed in **Figures 6C,D**. Obviously, DOX releases from PEG-CD/AD/SF nanoparticles in the media containing DTT were significantly faster than that in the media without DTT. DOX release amounts reached up to 20.2 and 33.0% in 84 h with the presence of DTT at pH 7.4 and pH 5.0, respectively, whereas were less than 10% in the media without DTT at both pH. We believed that the higher DOX release rates in pH 5.0 PBS with DTT was attributed to the reduction sensitive properties of disulfide bond as well as better DOX solubility in slightly acid media. The same trend was also observed in the releases profiles of SF from PEG-CD/AD/SF nanoparticles in different media. However, the overall release rates of SF were much higher than that of DOX at the same condition. For example, SF release amounts were 76.3 and 92.8% in 84 h with the presence of DTT at pH 7.4 and pH 5.0, respectively. This difference could be attributed to their distinct drug-loading modes. SF was incorporated into the nanoparticles by physical π-π stacking interaction and hydrophobic interaction, while DOX was loaded by chemical bond and thus exhibited sustained release property.

TABLE 1 | Characterization of PEG-CD/AD/SF nanoparticles by DLS.

PEG-CD/AD/SF (molar ratio)	1/1/0.1	1/1/0.2	1/1/0.5	1/1/1	1/1/2
Size (nm)	176.1	186.2	202.3	246.4	560.2
PDI	0.096	0.114	0.218	0.306	0.572

In vitro Cytotoxicity of PEG-CD/AD/SF Nanoparticles against HepG2 Cells

The cytotoxicity of free SF, PEG-CD/AD+SF physical mixtures and PEG-CD/AD/SF nanoparticles against HepG2 cells were investigated for different time (**Figure 7**). Compared to PEG-CD/AD nanoparticles (**Figure 5B**) and free SF, PEG-CD/AD+SF

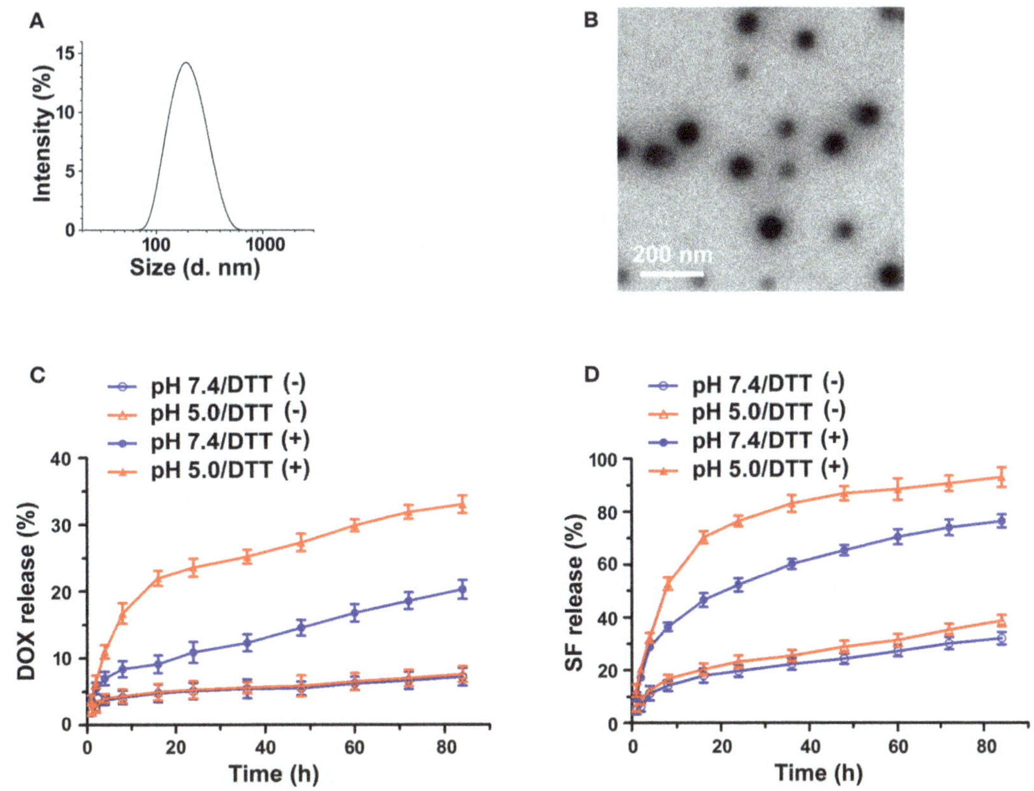

FIGURE 6 | Characterization of PEG-CD/AD/SF nanoparticles. Hydrodynamic diameter distribution **(A)** and TEM image **(B)** of PEG-CD/AD/SF nanoparticles; *in vitro* releases of DOX **(C)**, and SF **(D)** from PEG-CD/AD/SF nanoparticles in different release media. Data are means ± standard deviation for three separate experiments.

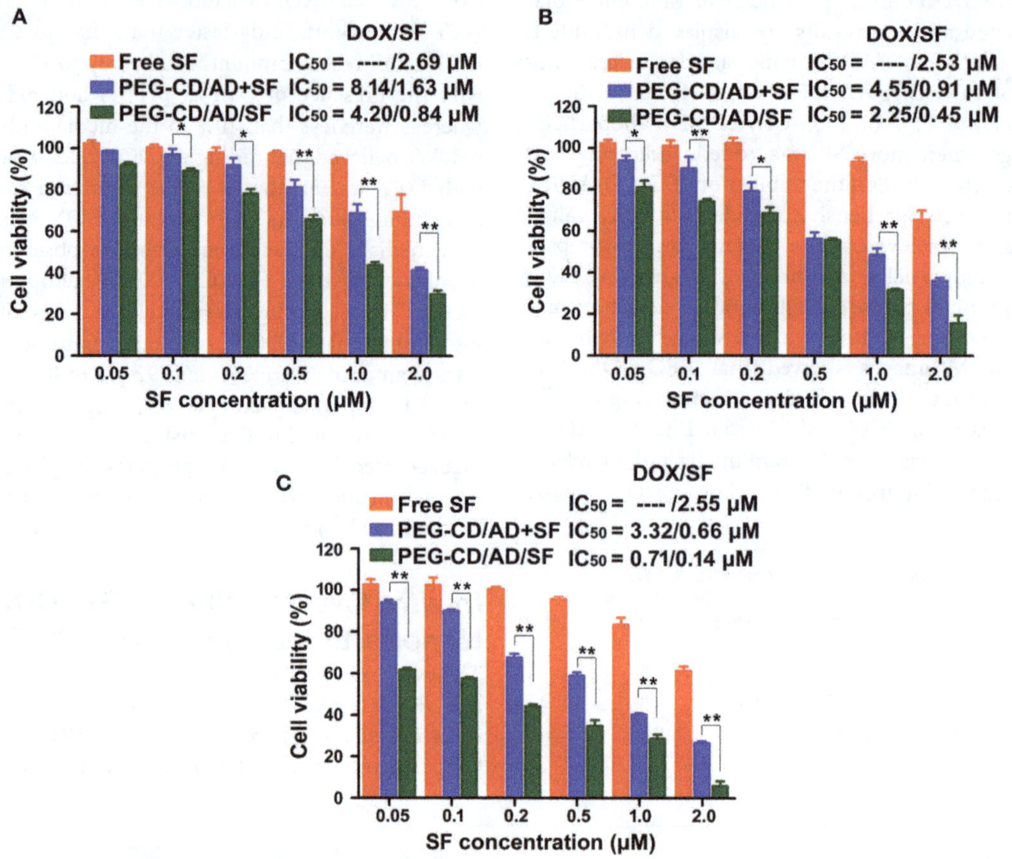

FIGURE 7 | *In vitro* cytotoxicity of HepG2 cells with the treatments of free SF, PEG-CD/AD, and SF physical mixture, PEG-CD/AD/SF nanoparticles for 48 h **(A)**, 72 h **(B)**, and 96 h **(C)**. Data are means ± standard deviation for three separate experiments. $^*p < 0.05$, $^{**}p < 0.01$.

physical mixtures showed an additive cytotoxicity toward HepG2 cells. PEG-CD/AD/SF nanoparticles exhibited higher cytotoxicity than PEG-CD/AD+SF physical mixtures ($p < 0.05$) and the IC_{50} values of PEG-CD/AD/SF nanoparticles were approximately 1.9-, 2.0-, and 4.7-fold decrease compared to that of PEG-CD/AD+ SF physical mixtures after treating HepG2 cells for 48, 72, and 96 h, respectively. The results suggested that PEG-CD/AD/SF nanoparticles exert stronger inhibitory effect against HepG2 cells by co-loading DOX and SF into the same nanosystem. This might perhaps because the solubility of sorafenib greatly improved after loading into the PEG-CD/AD/SF nanoparticles. Moreover, by comparing the IC_{50} values of PEG-CD/AD/SF nanoparticles at different time, we could easily found that the cytotoxicity of PEG-CD/AD/SF nanoparticles increased remarkably as the time increased. This sustained cytotoxicity would be beneficial for treatment of HCC *in vivo*.

CONCLUSION

In this study, we successfully synthesized a disulfide linked prodrug of DOX, which could complex with PEG-CD to form supramolecular amphiphiles. PEG-CD/AD amphiphiles could then self-assemble into nanostructures in aqueous solution with a uniform size of 166.4 nm and meanwhile load SF to form PEG-CD/AD/SF nanoparticles with a size of 186.2 nm. PEG-CD/AD nanoparticles possessed reduction-responsive property and could be effectively uptaken by HepG2 cells. The *in vitro* release of DOX and SF from PEG-CD/AD/SF nanoparticles exhibited reduction-responsive manners. Finally, the *in vitro* cytotoxicity assay illustrated that PEG/AD/SF nanoparticles showed two- to five-fold increased cytotoxicity toward HepG2 cells than PEG-CD/AD+SF physical mixtures. Altogether, this reduction-responsive nanoparticle system showed great potential for HCC treatment.

AUTHOR CONTRIBUTIONS

QX and TS: designed the experiments and wrote the manuscript; MC, JW, and GY: carried out the research and analysis of data and contributed to manuscript writing.

ACKNOWLEDGMENTS

This work was financially supported by National Natural Science Foundation of China (Grant No. 81501575 and 81602569), Key research Project of Tianjin health industry (Grant No. 14KG142) and The Science & Technology Development Fund of Tianjin Education Commission for Higher Education (Grant No. 2017KJ197).

REFERENCES

Chen, J. X., Shi, Y., Zhang, Y. R., Teng, L. P., and Chen, J. H. (2016). One-pot construction of boronate ester based pH-responsive micelle for combined cancer therapy. *Colloids Surfaces B* 143, 285–292. doi: 10.1016/j.colsurfb.2016.03.053

Cheng, A. L., Kang, Y. K., Chen, Z., Tsao, C. J., Qin, S., Kim, J. S., et al. (2009). Efficacy and safety of sorafenib in patients in the Asia-Pacific region with advanced hepatocellular carcinoma: a phase III randomised, double-blind, placebo-controlled trial. *Lancet Oncol.* 10, 25–34. doi: 10.1016/S1470-2045(08)70285-7

Dai, J., Lin, S., Cheng, D., Zou, S., and Shuai, X. (2011). Interlayer-crosslinked micelle with partially hydrated core showing reduction and pH dual sensitivity for pinpointed intracellular drug release. *Angew. Chem. Int. Ed Engl.* 50, 9404–9408. doi: 10.1002/anie.201103806

Deng, G. L., Zeng, S., and Shen, H. (2015). Chemotherapy and target therapy for hepatocellular carcinoma: new advances and challenges. *World J. Hepatol.* 7, 787–798. doi: 10.4254/wjh.v7.i5.787

Feng, X., Ding, J., Gref, R., and Chen, X.-S. (2017). Poly(β-cyclodextrin)-mediated polylactide-cholesterol stereocomplex micelles for controlled drug delivery. *Chin. J. Polym. Sci.* 35, 693–699. doi: 10.1007/s10118-017-1932-7

Galun, D., Srdic-Rajic, T., Bogdanovic, A., Loncar, Z., and Zuvela, M. (2017). Targeted therapy and personalized medicine in hepatocellular carcinoma: drug resistance, mechanisms, and treatment strategies. *J. Hepatocell. Carcinoma* 4, 93–103. doi: 10.2147/JHC.S106529

Hu, Q., Sun, W., Wang, C., and Gu, Z. (2016). Recent advances of cocktail chemotherapy by combination drug delivery systems. *Adv. Drug Deliv. Rev.* 98, 19–34. doi: 10.1016/j.addr.2015.10.022

Hutchinson, L. (2011). Targeted therapies: doxorubicin and sorafenib improves survival in patients with advanced hepatocellular carcinoma. *Nat. Rev. Clin. Oncol.* 8:61. doi: 10.1038/nrclinonc.2010.208

International Agency for Research on Cancer. GLOBOCAN (2012). *Estimated Cancer Incidence, Mortality and Prevalence Worldwide in 2012.* Accessed (July 11, 2017). Available online at: http://globocan.iarc.fr/Pages/fact_sheets_population.aspx

Li, D., Xu, W., Li, P., Ding, J., Cheng, Z., Chen, L., et al. (2016). Self-targeted polysaccharide prodrug suppresses orthotopic hepatoma. *Mol. Pharm.* 13, 4231–4235. doi: 10.1021/acs.molpharmaceut.6b00747

Li, W., Jiang, M., Cao, Y., Yan, L., Qi, R., Li, Y., et al. (2016). Turning ineffective transplatin into highly potent anticancer drug via a prodrug strategy for drug delivery and inhibiting cisplatin drug resistance. *Bioconjug. Chem.* 27, 1802–1806. doi: 10.1021/acs.bioconjchem.6b00302

Li, Z. Q., Zhang, Y. M., Chen, H. Z., Chen, H. Z., Zhao, J., and Liu, Y. (2013). Hierarchical organization of spherical assembly with reversibly photocontrollable cross-links. *J. Org. Chem.* 78, 5110–5114. doi: 10.1021/jo400772j

Lin, J., Wu, L., Bai, X., Xie, Y., Wang, A., Zhang, H., et al. (2016). Combination treatment including targeted therapy for advanced hepatocellular carcinoma. *Oncotarget* 7, 71036–71051. doi: 10.18632/oncotarget.11954

Liu, F., Ma, Y., Xu, L., Liu, L., and Zhang, W. (2015). Redox-responsive supramolecular amphiphiles constructed via host-guest interactions for photodynamic therapy. *Biomater. Sci.* 3, 1218–1227. doi: 10.1039/C5BM00045A

Llovet, J. M., Villanueva, A., Lachenmayer, A., and Finn, R. S. (2015). Advances in targeted therapies for hepatocellular carcinoma in the genomic era. *Nat. Rev. Clin. Oncol.* 12, 408–424. doi: 10.1038/nrclinonc.2015.103

Luo, C., Sun, J., Sun, B., Liu, D., Miao, L., Goodwin, T. J., et al. (2016). Facile fabrication of tumor redox-sensitive nanoassemblies of small-molecule oleate prodrug as potent chemotherapeutic nanomedicine. *Small* 12, 6353–6362. doi: 10.1002/smll.201601597

Luo, G. F., Xu, X. D., Zhang, J., Yang, J., Gong, Y. H., Lei, Q., et al. (2012). Encapsulation of an adamantane-doxorubicin prodrug in pH-responsive polysaccharide capsules for controlled release. *ACS Appl. Mater. Interfaces* 4, 5317–5324. doi: 10.1021/am301258a

Malarvizhi, G. L., Retnakumari, A. P., Nair, S., and Koyakutty, M. (2014). Transferrin targeted core-shell nanomedicine for combinatorial delivery of doxorubicin and sorafenib against hepatocellular carcinoma. *Nanomed. Nanotechnol. Biol. Med.* 10, 1649–1659. doi: 10.1016/j.nano.2014.05.011

Pazo Cid, R. A., Lao, J., and Lanzuela, M. (2011). Doxorubicin plus sorafenib in treatment of advanced hepatocellular carcinoma. *JAMA* 305, 781–781. doi: 10.1001/jama.2011.159

Peng, L., Feng, A., Zhang, H., Wang, H., Jian,C., Liu, B., et al. (2014). Voltage-responsive micelles based on the assembly of two biocompatible homopolymers. *Polym Chem.* 5, 1751–1759. doi: 10.1039/C3PY01204B

Ping, Y., Ding, D., Ramos, R. A. N. S., Mohanram, H., Deepankumar, K., Gao, J., et al. (2017). Supramolecular β-sheets stabilized protein nanocarriers for drug delivery and gene transfection. *ACS Nano* 11, 4528–4541. doi: 10.1021/acsnano.6b08393

Singal, P. K., and Iliskovic, N. (1998). Doxorubicin-Induced Cardiomyopathy. *New Engl. J. Med.* 339, 900–905. doi: 10.1056/NEJM199809243391307

Song, Q., Wang, X., Wang, Y., Liang, Y., Zhou, Y., Song, X., et al. (2016). Reduction responsive self-assembled nanoparticles based on disulfide-linked drug-drug conjugate with high drug loading and antitumor efficacy. *Mol. Pharm.* 13, 190–201. doi: 10.1021/acs.molpharmaceut.5b00631

Sun, W., Wang, Y., Cai, M., Lin, L., Chen, X., Cao, Z., et al. (2017). Codelivery of sorafenib and GPC3 siRNA with PEI-modified liposomes for hepatoma therapy. *Biomater. Sci.* 5, 2468–2479. doi: 10.1039/C7BM00866J

Vilaseca, J., Guardia, J., Bacardí, R., and Monné, J. (1978). Doxorubicin for liver cancer. *Lancet* 311:1367. doi: 10.1016/S0140-6736(78)92448-0

Wang, J., Sun, X., Mao, W., Sun, W., Tang, J., Sui, M., et al. (2013). Tumor redox heterogeneity-responsive prodrug nanocapsules for cancer chemotherapy. *Adv. Mat.* 25, 3670–3676. doi: 10.1002/adma.201300929

Wang, W., Sun, H., Meng, F., Ma, S., Liu, H., and Zhong, Z. (2012). Precise control of intracellular drug release and anti-tumor activity of biodegradable micellar drugs via reduction-sensitive shell-shedding. *Soft Matter* 8, 3949–3956. doi: 10.1039/c2sm07461c

Xiong, Q., Cui, M., Bai, Y., Liu, Y., Liu, D., and Song, T. (2017). A supramolecular nanoparticle system based on β-cyclodextrin-conjugated poly-l-lysine and hyaluronic acid for co-delivery of gene and chemotherapy agent targeting hepatocellular carcinoma. *Colloids Surf. B* 155, 93–103. doi: 10.1016/j.colsurfb.2017.04.008

Xiong, Q., Zhang, M., Zhang, Z., Shen, W., Liu, L., and Zhang, Q. (2014). Anti-tumor drug delivery system based on cyclodextrin-containing pH-responsive star polymer: *In vitro* and *in vivo* evaluation. *Int. J. Pharm.* 474, 232–240. doi: 10.1016/j.ijpharm.2014.08.018

Yang, Q., Qi, R., Cai, J., Kang, X., Sun, S., and Xiao, H. (2015). Biodegradable polymer-platinum drug conjugates to overcome platinum drug resistance. *RSC Adv.* 5, 83343–83349. doi: 10.1039/C5RA11297D

Yin, Q., Shen, J., Zhang, Z., Yu, H., and Li, Y. (2013). Reversal of multidrug resistance by stimuli-responsive drug delivery systems for therapy of tumor. *Adv. Drug Deliv. Rev.* 65, 1699–1715. doi: 10.1016/j.addr.2013.04.011

Zhang, B., Luo, Z., Liu, J., Ding, X., Li, J., and Cai, K. (2014). Cytochrome c end-capped mesoporous silica nanoparticles as redox-responsive drug delivery vehicles for liver tumor-targeted triplex therapy *in vitro* and *in vivo*. *J. Control. Release* 192, 192–201. doi: 10.1016/j.jconrel.2014.06.037

Zhang, C., Pan, D., Li, J., Hu, J., Bains, A., Guys, N., et al. (2017). Enzyme-responsive peptide dendrimer-gemcitabine conjugate as a controlled-release drug delivery vehicle with enhanced antitumor efficacy. *Acta Biomater.* 55, 153–162. doi: 10.1016/j.actbio.2017.02.047

Zhang, J., Hu, J., Chan, H. F., Skibba, M., Liang, G., and Chen, M. (2016). iRGD decorated lipid-polymer hybrid nanoparticles for targeted co-delivery of doxorubicin and sorafenib to enhance anti-hepatocellular carcinoma efficacy. *Nanomed. Nanotechnol. Biol. Med.* 12, 1303–1311. doi: 10.1016/j.nano.2016.01.017

Zhang, M., Xiong, Q., Wang, Y., Zhang, Z., Shen, W., and Liu, L. (2014). A well-defined coil–comb polycationic brush with "star polymers" as side chains for gene delivery. *Polym. Chem.* 5, 4670–4678. doi: 10.1039/C4PY00311J

Zhang, Y., Ren, K., He, Z., Li, H., Chen, T., Lei, Y., et al. (2013). Development of inclusion complex of brinzolamide with hydroxypropyl-β-cyclodextrin. *Carbohyd. Polym.* 98, 638–643. doi: 10.1016/j.carbpol.2013.06.052

Zhao, R., Li, T., Zheng, G., Jiang, K., Fan, L., and Shao, J. (2017). Simultaneous inhibition of growth and metastasis of hepatocellular carcinoma by co-delivery of ursolic acid and sorafenib using lactobionic acid modified and pH-sensitive chitosan-conjugated mesoporous silica nanocomplex. *Biomaterials* 143, 1–16. doi: 10.1016/j.biomaterials.2017.07.030

Zhao, X., Poon, Z., and Engler, A. C. (2012). Enhanced stability of polymeric nanoparticles based on postfunctionalized poly(ethylene glycol)-b-poly(γ-propargyl l-glutamate): the substituent effect. *Biomacromolecules* 13, 1315–1322. doi: 10.1021/bm201873u

Zhao, Y., Chen, F., Pan, Y., Li, Z., Xue, X., Okeke, C. I., et al. (2015). Nanodrug formed by coassembly of dual anticancer drugs to inhibit cancer cell drug resistance. *ACS Appl. Mater. Interfaces* 7, 19295–19305. doi: 10.1021/acsami.5b05347

6

Controlled Drug Delivery by Polylactide Stereocomplex Micelle for Cervical Cancer Chemotherapy

Kai Niu[1†], Yunming Yao[2†], Ming Xiu[3†], Chunjie Guo[4], Yuanyuan Ge[5] and Jianmeng Wang[5]*

[1] *Department of Otorhinolaryngology Head and Neck Surgery, The First Hospital of Jilin University, Changchun, China,* [2] *Department of Abdominal Ultrasound, The First Hospital of Jilin University, Changchun, China,* [3] *Department of Intensive Care Unit, The First Hospital of Jilin University, Changchun, China,* [4] *Department of Radiology, The First Hospital of Jilin University, Changchun, China,* [5] *Department of Geriatrics, The First Hospital of Jilin University, Changchun, China*

***Correspondence:**
Jianmeng Wang
jmwang1981@126.com

† These authors have contributed equally to this work

A stable doxorubicin (DOX)-loaded stereocomplex micelle drug delivery system was developed via the stereocomplex interaction between enantiomeric 4-armed poly(ethylene glycol)–poly(D-lactide) and poly(ethylene glycol)–poly(L-lactide) to realize control drug release and improve tumor cell uptake for efficient cervical carcinoma therapy. All these DOX-loaded micelles including poly(D-lactide)-based micelle (PDM/DOX), poly(L-lactide)-based micelle (PLM/DOX), and stereocomplex micelle (SCM/DOX) exhibited appropriate sizes of ~100 nm for the enhanced permeability and retention (EPR) effect. In addition, compared to PDM/DOX and PLM/DOX, SCM/DOX exhibited the slowest DOX releaser, highest tumor cell uptake and the most efficient tumor cell suppression *in vitro*. Moreover, the excellent tumor inhibiting rates of the DOX-loaded micelles, especially SCM/DOX, were verified in the U14 cervical carcinoma mouse model. Increased tumorous apoptosis and necrosis areas were observed in the DOX-loaded micelles treatment groups, especially the SCM/DOX group. In addition, all these DOX-loaded micelles obviously alleviated the systemic toxicity of DOX. As a result, SCM can be a promising drug delivery system for the future therapy of cervical carcinoma.

Keywords: controlled drug delivery, chemotherapy, cervical carcinoma, enhanced stability, stereocomplex polylactide micelle

INTRODUCTION

Cervical carcinoma is still one of the main causes of cancer-related deaths of female patients' worldwide (Ferlay et al., 2015). In clinic, even though the use of neoadjuvant radio and chemotherapy have decreased the incidence and mortality rates of cervical carcinoma, lots of patients have suffered from intrinsic and acquired resistance to the therapy (Walch-Rückheim et al., 2016). In addition, the substantial severe side effect, low bioavailability, and poor delivery efficiency of the chemotherapeutic agent are still the major clinical challenges for the therapy. To solve these deficiencies, lots of nanodrug delivery systems including micelles (Tan et al., 2017; Wang et al., 2018), liposomes (de Jong et al., 2007; Chuang et al., 2017), nanogels (Ding et al., 2013; Li S. et al., 2018; Zhang et al., 2018), quantum dots (Tao et al., 2017a), nanosheet (Tao et al., 2017b; Zhu et al., 2018), modified nanoparticles (Tao et al., 2014, 2015, 2016; Ding et al., 2017), and nanospheres (Wang et al., 2016; El-Boubbou et al., 2017) have been developed to achieve the spatiotemporally controlled drug release in the tumor sites, increase the drug accumulation in the tumor cells and alleviate the systemic toxicity (Tao et al., 2013; Rosenblum et al., 2018).

Among these nanodrug delivery systems, micelles are generally the perfect choice due to the special core–shell structures, which can make them load a wide variety of drugs with a high drug loading capacity (Ma et al., 2015; Sun et al., 2017; Zhao et al., 2017; Li D. et al., 2018). In addition, due to the appropriate volumes, micelles are very suitable as nanodrug carriers to selectively accumulate at the tumor sites through the enhanced permeation and retention effect (EPR) (Wang et al., 2015c; Chen et al., 2017a,b; Khan et al., 2017; Xu et al., 2017). However, one remaining challenge for micelles-based delivery systems is the instability of them, which often leads to premature release of payloads during the circulation in the body. Chemical cross-linking of either the core or shell is one of the traditional strategies to improve the stability of micelles. However, the application of chemical cross-linkers may unfavorably affect the bioactivity of the loaded agents and the biodegradability of the delivery system (Chen et al., 2011). As an alternative, numerous non-covalent interactions including electrostatic interactions, host-guest, hydrogen bonding and stereocomplexation have been adopted as efficient strategies to improve the stability of micelles (Kim et al., 2008; Pounder et al., 2011; Shen et al., 2017).

Stereocomplexes can be considered as physical crosslinking, which are formed by the interaction between stereoregular chains of enantiomeric polymers (Feng et al., 2017). Poly(lactide) (PLA), as a biodegradable and biocompatible aliphatic polyester, has been verified to be a typical example used for stereocomplexation. PLA has a multitude of primary structures, such as isotactic poly(L-lactic acid) (PLLA) and poly(D-lactic acid) (PDLA) and syndiotactic and atactic/heterotactic PDLLA (Li et al., 2016). It has been reported that the equimolar mixture of PDLA/PLLA could form stereocomplexes with distinctive physical and chemical stability, such as improved mechanical properties, enhanced thermal resistance, and hydrolytic stability, due to the interactions between the L-lactyl and D-lactyl unit sequences (Ikada et al., 1987; Fukushima and Kimura, 2006). Concerning the advantages of PLA stereocomplexed materials in drug delivery, various PLA-based stereocomplexed formations have been developed for the transportation and delivery of different treatment agents. For instance, Ma et al. used sequential ring-opening polymerization to successfully fabricate poly(ethylene glycol)-b-poly(L-lactic acid)-bpoly(D-lactic acid) (PEG-b-PLLA-b-PDLA) stereoblock copolymers (Ma et al., 2015). The stereoblock copolymer micelles showed higher drug loading content (DLC), slower degradation, and drug release rate. In another report, Zhao and co-workers fabricated a biodegradable stereocomplex micelles (SCMs) based on amphiphilic dextran-block-polylactide (Dex-b-PLA) for efficient intracellular drug deliveries (Zhao et al., 2013). This doxorubicin (DOX) loaded SCMs exhibited high stability and sustained release profiles *in vitro*. Wang et al. previously fabricated a DOX-loaded stereocomplex micelle (SCM/DOX) via the equimolar enantiomeric 4-armed poly(ethylene glycol)–polylactide copolymers (Wang et al., 2015a). All the DOX-loaded micelles, especially the SCM/DOX displayed proper sizes for EPR, controlled DOX release, and enhanced antitumor efficacy *in vitro*. However, the *in vivo* antitumor efficacy of these DOX-loaded micelles and whether they can alleviate the systemic toxicity of DOX are not verified.

In order to further confirm the *in vivo* antitumor efficacy and systemic toxicity of DOX-loaded micelles, especially the SCM/DOX toward cervical carcinoma, in the present study, an *in vivo* tumor inhibition test was evaluated on the U14 cells-bearing BALB/c mouse models (**Scheme 1**). Our results indicated that all of these DOX-loaded micelles, especially the SCM/DOX, showed satisfactory tumor suppression efficacy and a higher level of safety in comparison to free DOX·HCl. These DOX-loaded micelles, especially the SCM/DOX, can serve as an excellent nanoplatform for the chemotherapy of cervical carcinoma.

MATERIALS AND METHODS

Materials

4-Armed PEG (number-average molecular weight (M_n) = 10,000 Da) was purchased from Shanghai Seebio Biotech, Inc. (Shanghai, China). DLA and LLA were obtained from Changchun SinoBiomaterials Co., Ltd. (Changchun, China) and recrystallized from ethyl acetate under argon atmosphere before use. The stereocomplex micelle (SCM) was fabricated by the equimolar mixture of the enantiomeric 4-armed poly(ethylene glycol)–polylactide copolymers. Doxorubicin hydrochloride (DOX·HCl) was purchased from Beijing Huafeng United Technology Co., Ltd. (Beijing, China). 4′,6-Diamidino-2-phenylindole (DAPI), Alexa Fluor 488 phalloidin (Alexa 488), and 3-(4,5-dimethylthiazol-2-yl)-2,5-diphenyltetrazolium bromide (MTT) were purchased from Sigma-Aldrich (Shanghai, China). Human cervical cancer HeLa cells and mouse cervical cancer U14 cells were purchased from the American Type Culture Collection (ATCC). Clear 6-well and 96-well tissue culture polystyrene (TCP) plates were purchased from Corning Costar Co. (Cambridge, MA, United States). The deionized water used in this study was prepared through a Milli-Q water purification equipment (Millipore Co., MA, United States).

Preparation of DOX-Loaded Micelles

DOX-loaded micelles were prepared through a nanoprecipitation method.(Benival and Devarajan, 2012). In briefly, DOX·HCl (20.9 mg) were dissolved in 6.0 mL of Milli-Q water, and then were slowly added into 10.0 mL of PEG–PLLA copolymer solution in *N*,*N*-dimethylformamide (DMF) (10.0 mg mL^{-1}). After that, 2.0 mL of phosphate-buffered saline (PBS) was dropwise added into the above solution. The final solution was continuous stirring at room temperature for 12 h and subsequently dialyzed against Milli-Q water for 12 h (molecular weight cut-off (MWCO) = 3500 Da). At last, the PLM/DOX was obtained by lyophilisation. PDM/DOX and SCM/DOX were also fabricated by the same protocol.

In vitro Cellular Uptake

Confocal laser scanning microscopy (CLSM) and flow cytometry (FCM) were used for quantitative analysis of cell uptake *in vitro*.

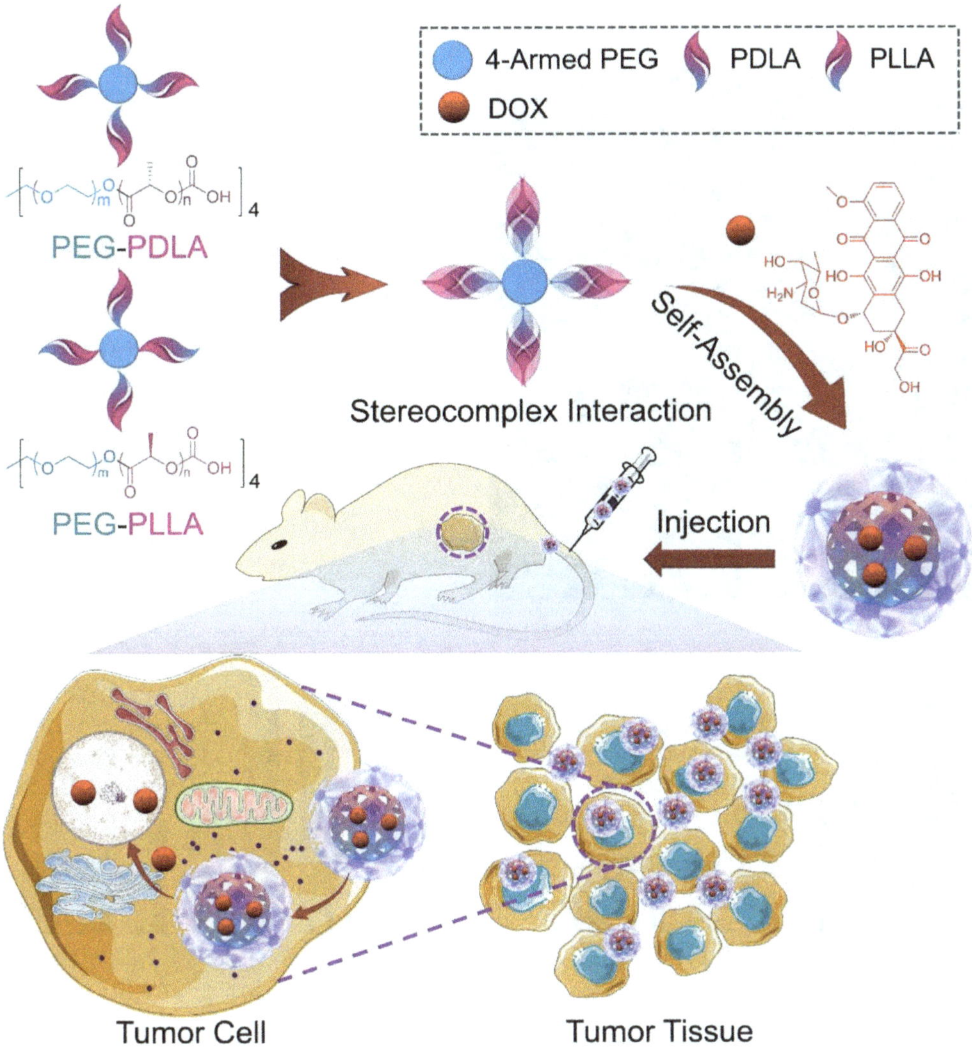

SCHEME 1 | Illustration of the preparation of SCM/DOX and its passive targeting recognition (EPR effect) of the tumor cells.

CLSM. 2.0 × 10^5 of HeLa cells were seeded on glass coverslips per well in 2.0 mL of complete high glucose Dulbecco's modified Eagle's medium (HG-DMEM) in 6-well plates for 24 h. PDM/DOX, PLM/DOX, SCM/DOX, or free DOX·HCl at a final DOX concentration of 10.0 μg mL^{-1} was added to each well. After coincubation for 2 h, the medium was removed, and the cells on glass coverslips were washed with PBS five times and fixed with 4% (W/V) PBS-buffered paraformaldehyde for 20 min at room temperature. And then, the cells were washed for five times by PBS and reacted with 0.1% (V/V) Triton X-100 in PBS for 12 min at room temperature. And then, the nuclei were then stained with DAPI for 3 min at 37 °C, after which the cells were washed with PBS five times. At last, the filamentous actin was stained with Alexa 488 for 30 min at 37°C, and washed with PBS five times. The CLSM micro-images were taken by a CLSM (LSM 780, Carl Zeiss, Jena, Germany). FCM. 2.0 × 10^5 of HeLa cells were seeded in each well of 6-well plates and cultured for 24 h. And then, PDM/DOX, PLM/DOX, SCM/DOX, or free DOX·HCl at a final DOX concentration of 10.0 μg mL^{-1} was added to each well. The cells without any treatment were set as control. After a 2 h co-incubation, the medium was removed, and the cells were washed with PBS five times and then digested by trypsin. Subsequently, 1.0 mL of PBS was added and collected in centrifuge tubes. The harvested cells were centrifuged at 3000 rpm for 5 min. After removing the supernatants, the bottom cells were resuspended in 0.3 mL of PBS and examined by a flow cytometer (λ_{ex} = 488 nm; Beckman, CA, United States).

Cytotoxicity Assays

The cytotoxicities of DOX-loaded micelles and free DOX·HCl with a DOX·HCl concentration of 0.16–10.0 μg mL^{-1} were conducted toward HeLa cells and U14 cells by an MTT assay. In brief, 8.0 × 10^3 cells in 180.0 μL complete HG-DMEM was planted into 96-well plates and incubated at 37°C for 24 h. And then, 20.0 μL of PBS containing various DOX formulations were added to each well and cultured for another 48 h. Subsequently,

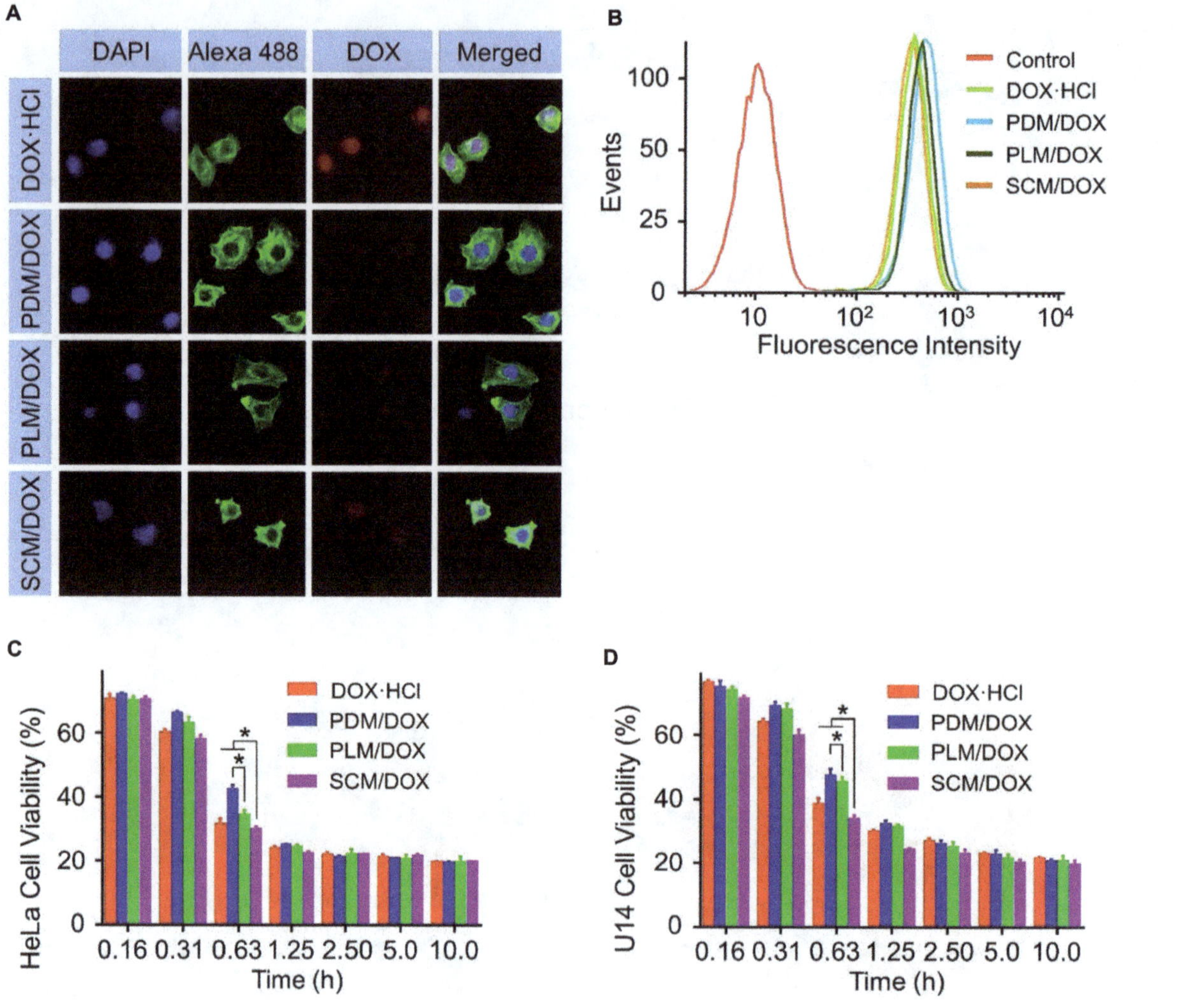

FIGURE 1 | *In vitro* cellular internalization and cytotoxicity of DOX-loaded micelles on HeLa cells. **(A)** CLSM study of HeLa cells after 2 h incubation with DOX·HCl and DOX-loaded micelles (Scale bar = 10 μm). **(B)** FCM study of HeLa cells after 2 h incubation with DOX·HCl and DOX-loaded micelles. **(C)** HeLa cell viability and **(D)** U14 cell viability after treatment with DOX·HCl and DOX-loaded micelles for 48 h. Data are presented as mean ± SD (n = 8; *P < 0.001).

20.0 μL of MTT at a concentration of 5.0 mg mL^{-1} was added and incubated for another 4 h. After that, the medium was carefully removed, and 150.0 μL of dimethyl sulfoxide (DMSO) was added to each well to dissolve the MTT formazan generated by the live cells. The plates were shocked for 5 min before detection. The absorbance of medium was measured at 490 nm using a Bio-Rad 680 microplate reader. The cell viability was calculated as Equation (1).

$$\text{Cell viability (\%)} = \frac{\text{A sample}}{\text{A control}} \times 100 \quad (1)$$

In Equation (1), the A_{sample} and $A_{control}$ represented the absorbances of sample and control wells, respectively.

In vivo Antitumor Efficacy Assay

Female BALB/c mice (~4 weeks) were obtained from Vital River Laboratory Animal Center (Beijing, China). All animals were carefully treated under the guidelines approved by the Institutional Animal Care and Use Committee of Jilin University. The antitumor efficacy of DOX-loaded micelles and free DOX·HCl was evaluated using subcutaneous U14 cells bearing female BALB/c mouse models. Mice treated with NS (normal saline) were used as control. When the tumor volume reached about 100 mm^3, the mice were randomly divided into 6 groups (n = 8 for each group) and treated with NS, free DOX·HCl at a DOX·HCl concentration of 3.0 mg [kg Body Weight (BW)]$^{-1}$ or 6.0 mg (kg BW)$^{-1}$, or DOX-loaded micelles at a DOX·HCl concentration of 3.0 mg (kg BW)$^{-1}$ via tail vein injection every 3 days for a total of 6 doses. The groups were noted as DOX-3 and DOX-6, PDM/DOX, PLM/DOX, and SCM/DOX, respectively. The tumor sizes and body weights were monitored once-every-other-day. Tumor volume was calculated according to the following formula: tumor volume (mm^3) = 0.5 × a × b^2, where a and b are the largest and smallest diameter of tumor, respectively. The tumor inhibition ratio was calculated using the following formula: Tumor inhibition rate (%) = $(V_{control} - V_{sample})/V_{control}$

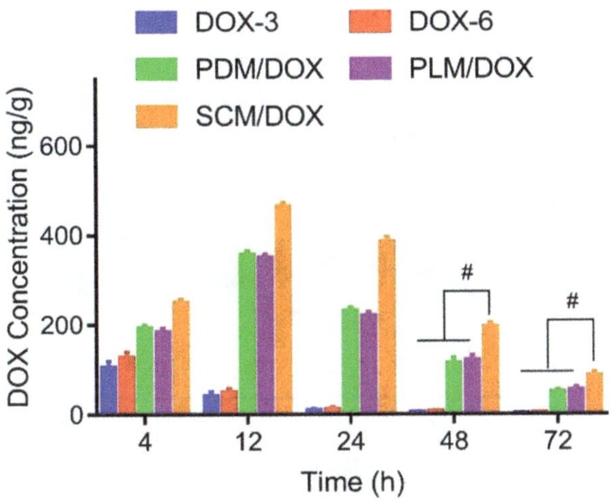

FIGURE 2 | *In vivo* biodistribution of DOX·HCl, or DOX-loaded micelles at 4, 12, 24, 48, and 72 h after injection, respectively. Data were presented as mean ± SD (n = 6), $^{\#}P < 0.01$.

X100, where $V_{control}$ and V_{sample} represented the tumor volumes of control and sample groups, respectively. In addition, the weights of the major organs were recorded. The organ indices of all the organs of mice were calculated according to the following formula: organ index (%) = ($w_{control} - w_{sample}$) × 100.

In vivo DOX Biodistribution of Dox-Loaded Micelles at Tumor Sites

To investigate the *in vivo* DOX biodistribution of DOX-loaded micelles, female BALB/c mice bearing U14 cells (tumor volumes were about 200 mm^3) were randomly assigned to five groups and intravenously injected with free DOX·HCl at a DOX·HCl concentration of 3.0 mg (kg BW)$^{-1}$ or 6.0 mg (kg BW)$^{-1}$), or DOX-loaded micelles at a DOX·HCl concentration of 3.0 mg (kg BW)$^{-1}$. At 4, 12, 24, 48, and 72 h after administration, mice were sacrificed and tumors were collected, rinsed with cold PBS. Methanol was added to each tumor to extract the content of DOX. The mixture was homogenized, centrifuged, and the supernatants were collected. The amount of DOX in each tumor was determined by HPLC. The data were normalized to the tissue weight.

Histopathological and Biochemical Analyses of Organs

The mice were sacrificed 4 days after the last treatment. After that, tumors and major organs (*i.e.*, heart, liver, spleen, lung, kidney, and sternum) were isolated, collected, were fixed in 4% (*W*/*V*) PBS-buffered paraformaldehyde overnight except sternum, and then embedded in paraffin. The organs from healthy mice were also isolated and treated as a normal control. The paraffin-embedded tumor and organ tissues were cut at a thickness of 5 μm, and prepared for hematoxylin and eosin (H&E) staining. The histopathological sections were assessed by a microscope (Nikon Eclipse *Ti*, Optical Apparatus Co., Ardmore, PA, United States). For the tumor tissues, three observation fields were evaluated to get an average value of relative necrosis area with the total area of observation field as "100%." These data were analyzed by ImageJ software (National Institutes of Health, Bethesda, MD, United States). The relative necrotic area (%) of tumor tissues was calculated by Equation (2):

$$\text{Relative necrotic area } (\%) = \frac{\text{Necrotic area in tumor section}}{\text{Total area of observed tumor section}} \times 100 \quad (2)$$

For the histopathological assays of sternums, the isolated sternums were handled as described previously. Four paraffin sections of each sternum were performed for H&E staining.

The damages of tissues and organs were confirmed by testing the corresponding functional enzymes in blood and organs, which were detected with commercial enzyme-linked immunosorbent assay (ELISA) kits (Shanghai Lichen Biotechnology Co., Ltd., Shanghai, China). The heart indices contained creatine kinase-MB (CK-MB), creatine kinase (CK), and lactate dehydrogenase (LDH), liver-related aspartate aminotransferase (AST) and alanine aminotransferase (ALT), and kidney-associated blood urea nitrogen (BUN) and creatinine (Cr), both in serum and organs were detected by the corresponding ELISA kits according to the standard protocols provided by the suppliers.

Detections of Marrow Micronucleus Cell Rates and White Blood Cell Count

The marrow micronucleus cell rate (MMCR) of each group was evaluated from H&E section. For white blood cell count, 20.0 μL of anticoagulated blood from each mouse was employed to count white blood cells (WBCs).

Immunohistochemical Analysis

Immunohistochemistry was carried out to detect the expression of Bax, Bcl-2, caspase-3, and survivin *in ex vivo* tumor tissues, which were performed as described previously (Dai et al., 2011; Dolka et al., 2016).

Statistical Analysis

All experiments were carried out at least three times. All data are presented as mean ± standard deviation (SD) and analyzed for statistical significance using SPSS (Version 13.0, SPSS Inc., Chicago, IL, United States). $^{\&}P < 0.05$ was considered statistically significant, $^{\#}P < 0.01$ and $^{*}P < 0.001$ were considered highly significant, respectively.

RESULTS AND DISCUSSION

Preparation and Characterization of DOX-Loaded Micelles

The unsatisfactory stability of micelles is still an obvious challenge for their extensive application in controlled drug delivery. Herein,

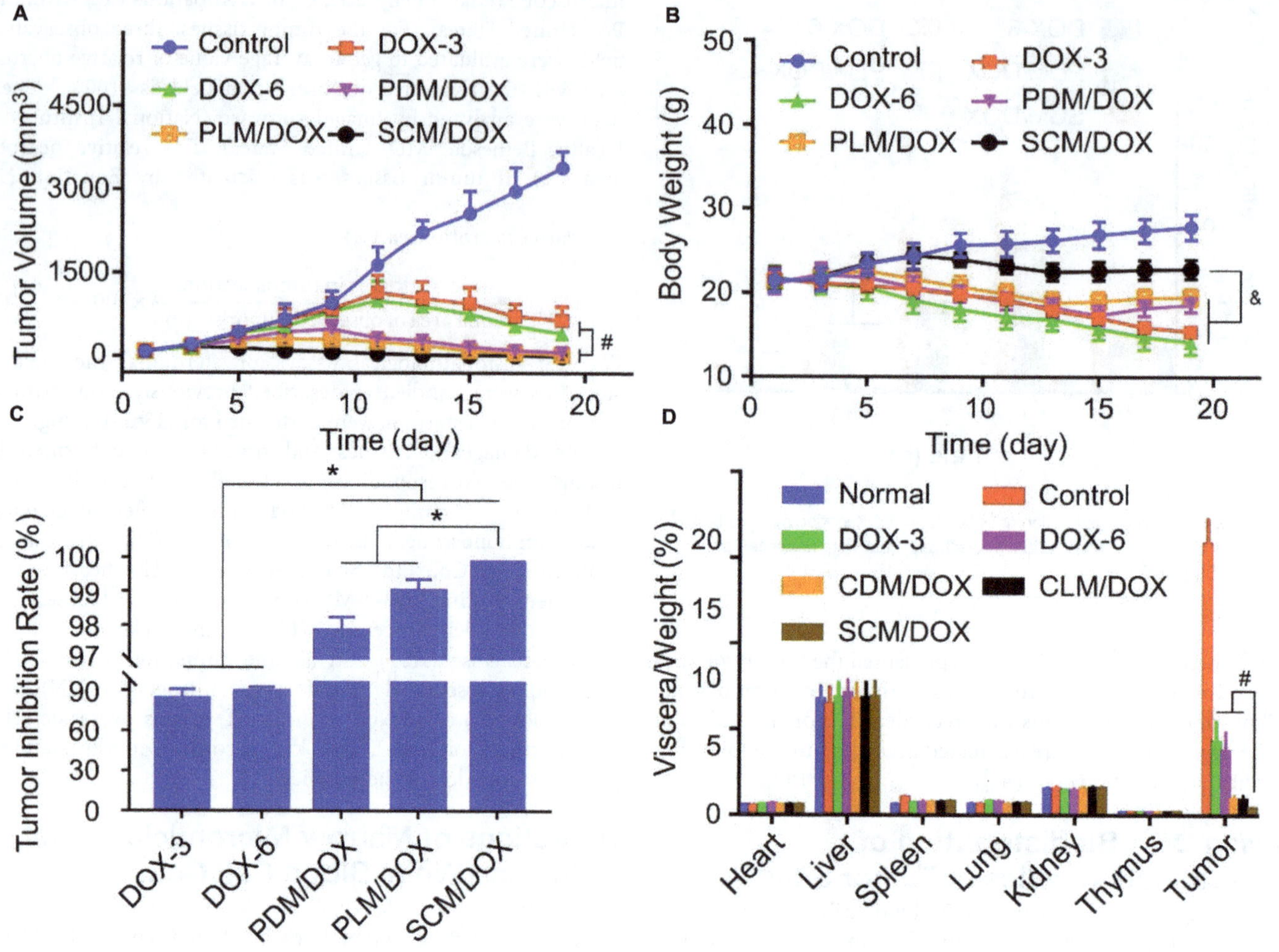

FIGURE 3 | *In vivo* antitumor effect of DOX-loaded micelles in the U14 tumor-bearing BALB/c mice. **(A)** Tumor growth profles, **(B)** body weight changes, **(C)** quantitative analysis of the tumor inhibition rates, and **(D)** organ indices of U14 cervical cancer-allografted mice after injected with NS, DOX·HCl, or DOX-loaded micelles. Each set of data is represented as mean ± SD (n = 8; $^{\&}P < 0.05$, $^{\#}P < 0.01$, $^{*}P < 0.001$).

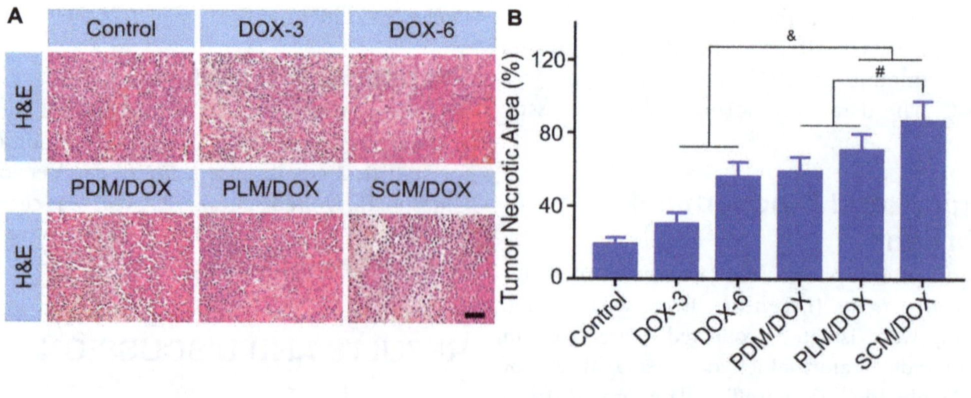

FIGURE 4 | Histopathological analysis of tumor tissues. **(A)** H&E staining (Scale bar = 50 μm) of the tumor tissues from the mice. **(B)** Quantitative analysis of the tumor necrotic area of each group. Each set of data is represented as mean ± SD (n = 3; $^{\&}P < 0.05$, $^{\#}P < 0.01$).

pairs of enantiomeric copolymers of PEG–PDLA and PEG–PLLA were employed as matrices to enhance the stability of micelles via stereocomplex interaction. In aqueous solution, PEG–PDLA, PEG–PLLA and an equimolar mixture of them could self-assemble into micelles due to their amphiphilic nature. They were noted as PDM, PLM, and SCM, respectively. As depicted in **Scheme 1**, DOX was encapsulated by PDM, PLM, or SCM by nanoprecipitation. In the previous work, all of these DOX-loaded micelles showed clear spherical morphologies and the average diameters of the micelles were about 100, 90, and 80 nm, respectively. The appropriate sizes of these micelles made them suitable candidates to selectively accumulate at tumor sites by the EPR effect.(Kobayashi et al., 2014; Liu et al., 2014) Moreover, all the loaded micelles exhibited excellent stability both in PBS and bovine serum albumin (BSA) solutions.(Wang et al., 2015a). In addition, critical micellization concentration (CMC) is one of the key parameters to describe the physical properties of micelles. The CMCs of PDM, PLM, and SCM were 0.063, 0.052, and 0.045 g/L, respectively (Liu et al., 2014). The CMC value of SCM was lower than that of PDM and PLM, induced by the stereocomplex interaction, which played an important role in the stability of the micelle.

Intracellular DOX Release and Cell Viability Assays

The cell uptake and intracellular release behaviors of DOX-loaded micelles were employed through CLSM and FCM. As shown in **Figure 1A**, after 2 h of incubation, the intracellular DOX fluorescences of the groups treated with DOX-loaded micelles were weaker than those cultured with free DOX·HCl. The different intracellular cell uptake behavior of DOX-loaded micelles and free DOX·HCl. was most likely due to the manner of free DOX·HCl enters cells was diffusion, which was faster than the endocytosis of DOX-loaded micelles (Li et al., 2014). Furthermore, the SCM/DOX group showed higher DOX fluorescences than PDM/DOX and PLM/DOX groups. This might be related to the slower extracellular DOX release and more efficient intracellular DOX release of SCM/DOX induced by stereocomplex interaction (Liu et al., 2014). These results were further confirmed by FCM analyses. In **Figure 1B**, the intracellular DOX fluorescence intensity of SCM/DOX group was higher than that in PDM/DOX and PLM/DOX group, while lower than free DOX·HCl. Both the CLSM and FCM verified the effective internalization of DOX-loaded micelles by HeLa cells, especially the SCM/DOX.

MTT assays in HeLa cells and U14 cells revealed that the SCM/DOX displayed significant cell killing activity after 48 h incubation (**Figures 1C,D**). It should be noted that the half maximal inhibitory concentrations (IC_{50}) values for SCM/DOX against HeLa, and U14 cells were 0.47 and 0.50 $\mu g\ mL^{-1}$, respectively, which were lower than those obtained with the PDM/DOX, PLM/DOX, and free DOX·HCl [(IC_{50} = 0.60, 0.52, and 0.49 $\mu g\ mL^{-1}$, HeLa cells) and (IC_{50} = 0.65, 0.73, and 0.68 $\mu g\ mL^{-1}$, U14 cells)]. This higher cell killing activity of SCM/DOX was attributed to the enhanced cellular uptake via stereocomplex interaction and the improved intracellular DOX release.

In vivo Biodistribution of DOX-Loaded Micelles at Tumor Sites

The *in vivo* DOX biodistribution at tumor sites was explored by treating tumor-bearing mice with free DOX·HCl and DOX-loaded micelles, respectively. As shown in **Figure 2**, free DOX·HCl was rapidly distributed in tumors at 4 h and rapidly eliminated at 12 h. The signal of DOX in tumors was negligible after 24 h. In contrast, DOX in the DOX-loaded micelles groups showed a much slower elimination. The concentrations of DOX in the primary tumors gradually reached to the maximum contents at 12 h post injection and was significantly increased compared to the free DOX·HCl groups (both the D0X-3 and DOX-6 groups). Until 72 h later, the DOX-loaded micelles groups still showed high DOX concentrations in tumor than free DOX·HCl groups ($P < 0.01$). Furthermore, compared to PDM/DOX and PLM/DOX, SCM/DOX exhibited the highest DOX concentration in tumor sites, which further verified the enhanced cellular uptake via stereocomplex interaction. This long-lasting delivery of DOX-loaded micelles was beneficial to the treatment of the tumor. These results could be due to the improved EPR effect and the decreased reticulo-endothelia system (RES) elimination by the PEG coating.

In vivo Antitumor Efficacy Measurement

The *in vivo* antitumor efficacy of DOX-loaded micelles was evaluated using a U14 subcutaneous cervical carcinoma model in BALB/c mice. As shown in **Figure 3A**, in comparison to free DOX·HCl, DOX-loaded micelles showed a stronger tumor inhibition effect, probably due to the enhanced accumulation at tumor site through EPR effect.(Wang et al., 2015a,b) Importantly, SCM/DOX group exhibited better antitumor efficacy than PDM/DOX and PLM/DOX, which might be related to the improved stability of SCM/DOX, suggesting less extracellular DOX release and greater internalized in the tumor cells. Moreover, the tumor inhibition rates of PDM/DOX, PLM/DOX, and SCM/DOX were 97.8 ± 0.40, 99.0 ± 0.35, and 99.8% ± 0.02%, which were higher than that of DOX-3 and DOX-6 groups (*i.e.*, 83.7 ± 7.01 and 89.2 ± 3.21%; $P < 0.001$) (**Figure 3C**). Although free DOX·HCl also showed some tumor inhibition effect, severe body weight loss was observed during therapy (**Figure 3B**), indicating its serious systemic toxicity to mice. In contrast, the DOX-loaded micelles-treated groups did not exhibit significant body weight loss, indicating satisfactory tolerance of mice to DOX-loaded micelles. In addition, organ indices were calculated by the weight ratios between organs (mg) and the whole body (g) to provide a general impression of toxicity. As shown in **Figure 3D**, no obvious difference was observed in the heart, liver, spleen, lung, kidney, and thymus indices among all the groups, indicating the DOX-loaded micelles would not lead to severe systemic toxicities when they were used *in vivo*. Conversely, the tumor indices of the DOX-loaded micelles groups, especially the SCM/DOX, were much lower than that of free DOX·HCl groups. These indices were consistent with

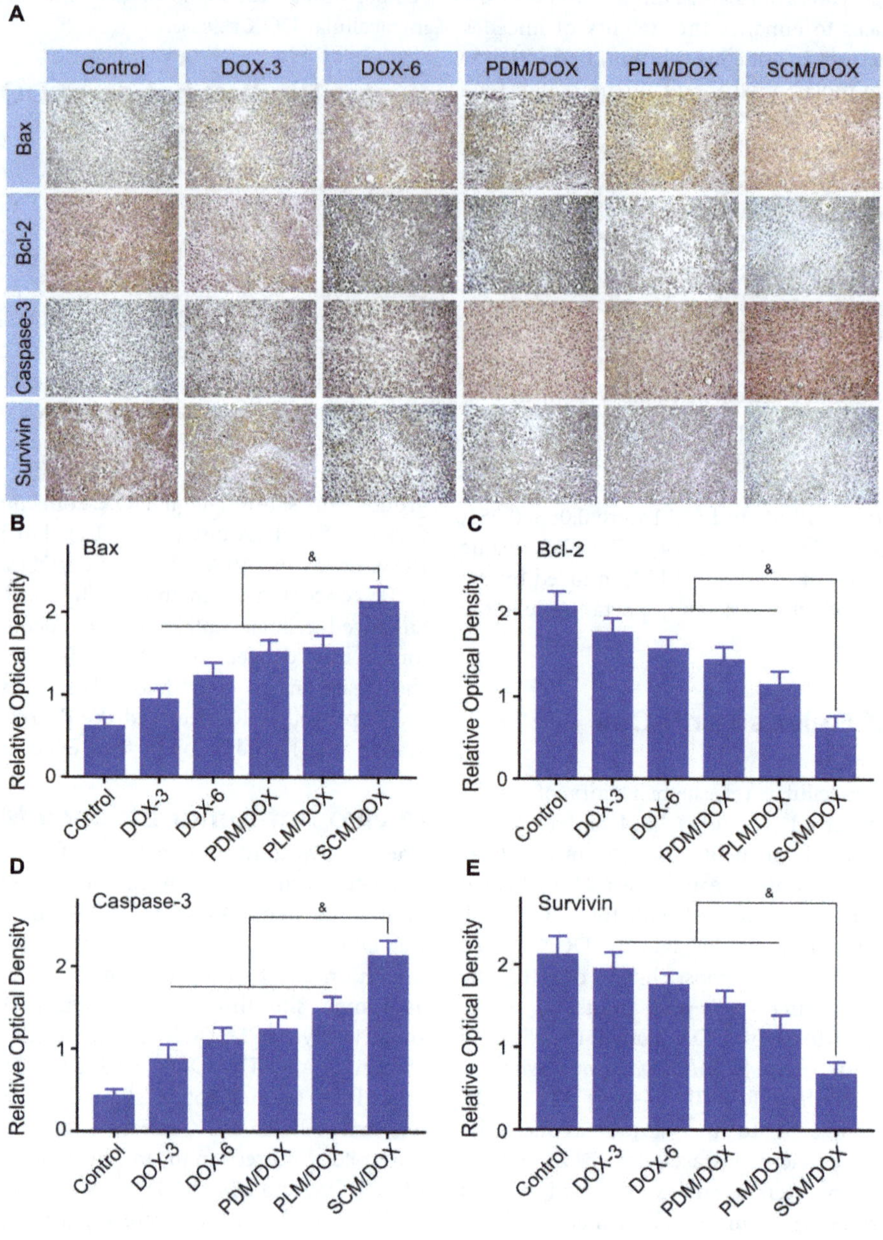

FIGURE 5 | Immunohistochemical analysis of tumor tissues. **(A)** Immunohistochemical (*i.e.*, Bax, caspase-3, survivin, and Bcl-2) analyses (Scale bar = 50 μm) of tumor tissues sections. Relative positive area of tumor sections from Bax **(B)**, Bcl-2 **(C)**, caspase-3 **(D)**, and survivin **(E)** after all treatments. Each set of data is represented as mean ± SD (n = 3; $^{\&}P$ < 0.05).

the tumor inhibition rates. H&E staining of tumor sections was performed to investigate the fate of tumor cells after experiencing treatment in the four groups (**Figure 4A**). As shown, tumor tissues from mice in control group showed no obvious necrosis or apoptosis and the tumor cells retained their normal morphology and nuclear structure, indicating that the tumor cells in control group proliferated quickly. In contrast, tumor tissues showed various degrees of necrosis in the free DOX·HCl and DOX-loaded micelles-treated groups. Furthermore, DOX-loaded micelles-treated groups showed larger necrosis area than free DOX·HCl-treated groups. In detail, the quantitative necrosis area of PDM/DOX, PLM/DOX, and SCM/DOX-treated groups were 58.6, 70.3, and 86.2% (**Figure 4B**), respectively, which were higher than that in DOX-3-treated group (30.1%) and DOX-6-treated group (55.7%) (P < 0.05). This observation indicated the effective antitumor efficacy of DOX-loaded micelles, especially the SCM/DOX.

Immunohistochemical staining analysis was performed to further verify the antitumor efficacy of DOX-loaded micelles. As shown in **Figure 5A**, the pro-apoptotic protein Bax (brown) and caspase-3 (brown) signals of from the tumor cells that received the treatment of DOX-loaded micelles, especially the

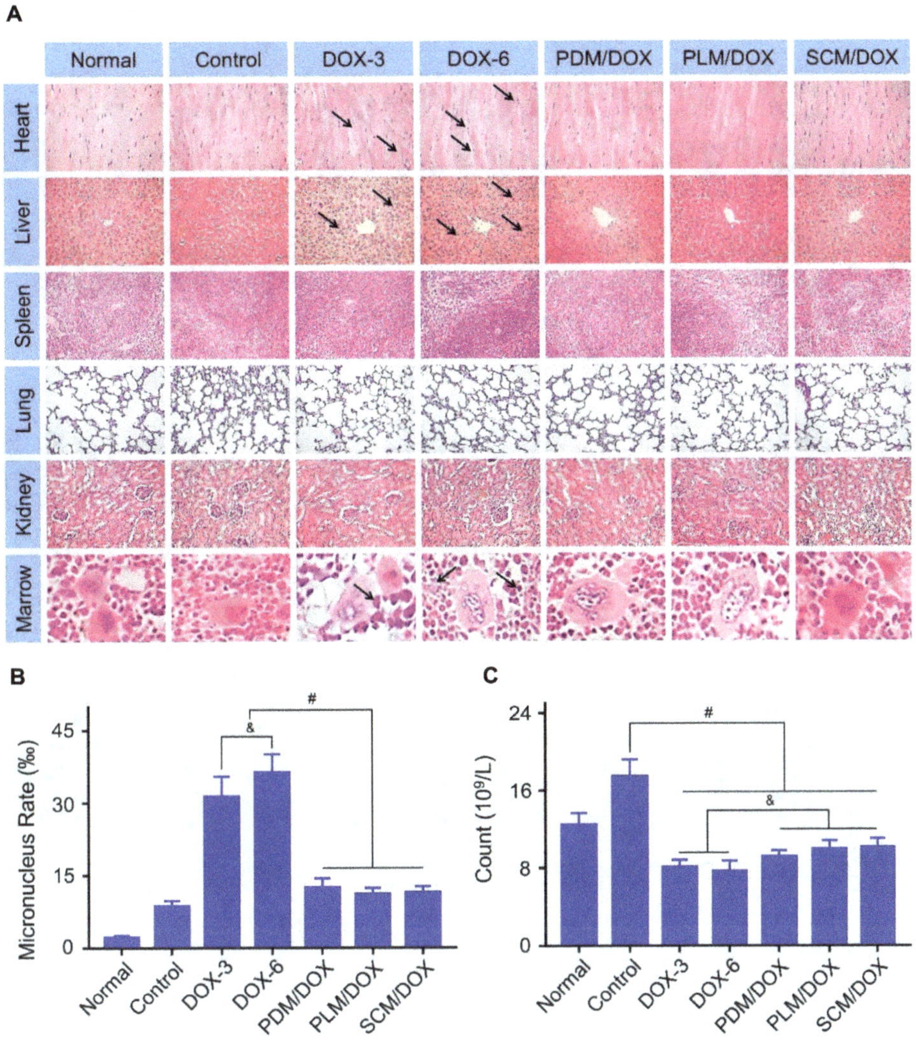

FIGURE 6 | Histopathological examination of visceral tissues. **(A)** Histopathological analyses (Scale bar = 50 μm) of internal tissues from normal mouse, or U14 cervical cancer-allografted BALB/c mice after treatment with NS, DOX·HCl, or DOX-loaded micelles. Black arrows indicated the occurrence of pathological changes. **(B)** Micronucleus rate and **(C)** WBC count of normal mouse or U14 cervical cancer-allografted BALB/c mice after all treatments. Each set of data is represented as mean ± SD (n = 3; $^{\&}P < 0.05$, $^{\#}P < 0.01$).

SCM/DOX, were much higher than free DOX·HCl groups. In detail, the SCM/DOX-treated group showed 2.3, 1.7, 1.4, and 1.4 times Bax signal (**Figure 5B**) ($P < 0.05$) and 2.5, 2.0, 1.7, and 1.4 times caspase-3 signal than DOX-3, DOX-6, PDM/DOX, and PLM/DOX (**Figure 5D**) ($P < 0.05$), respectively. In contrast, the expression of antiapoptotic protein Bcl-2 (brown) decreased significantly in the DOX-loaded micelles-treated groups, especially the SCM/DOX group. The Bcl-2 signal of SCM/DOX group was 0.7, 0.6, 0.6, and 0.5-fold decrease compared with DOX-3, DOX-6, PDM/DOX, and PLM/DOX ($P < 0.05$), respectively (**Figure 5C**). In addition, survivin, which can improve the survival of tumor cells primarily, was also used to evaluate cell survival. As shown in **Figure 5E**, the expressions of survivin (brown) decreased in the DOX-loaded micelles-treated groups, especially the SCM/DOX group. The SCM/DOX group showed a 0.7, 0.6, 0.6, and 0.4-fold decrease of survival signal compared with DOX-3, DOX-6, PDM/DOX, and PLM/DOX ($P < 0.05$), respectively. These data clearly demonstrated that our DOX-loaded micelles, especially SCM/DOX, could serve as highly effective nano therapeutic agents.

In vivo Security Evaluation

The *in vivo* toxicity of DOX was detected by the histopathological analysis. As shown in **Figure 6A**, the obvious accumulation of neutrophils and myocardial fiber breakage were detected in the heart of free DOX·HC-treated groups, especially the DOX-6 group, indicating the evident cardiotoxicity of free DOX·HCl. All of these damages were pointed out by black arrows in **Figure 6A**. In contrast, DOX-loaded micelles-treated groups did not show neutrophils accumulation and the myocardial cells lined in order and their sarcolemma-maintained integrity, which could be due to the decreased distribution of DOX in heart.

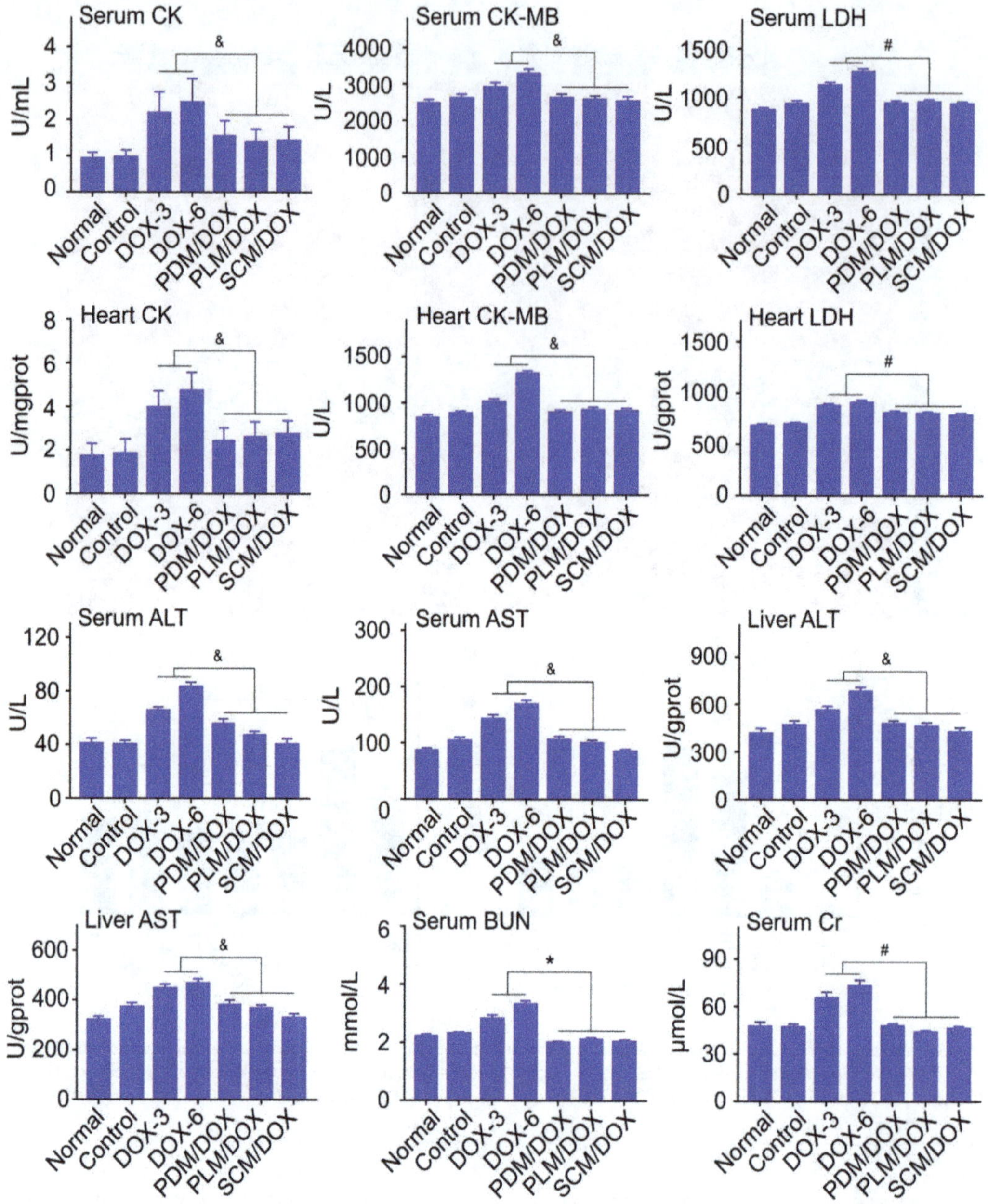

FIGURE 7 | Biochemical parameter assays for safety evaluation. Examinations of CK, CK-MB, LDH, ALT, AST, BUN, and Cr in serum and corresponding internal organs of normal mice or U14 cervical cancer-allografted BALB/c mice after treatment with NS, DOX·HCl, or DOX-loaded micelles. Each set of data is represented as mean ± SD ($n = 3$; $^{\&}P < 0.05$, $^{\#}P < 0.01$, $^{*}P < 0.001$).

Besides, free DOX·HCl-treated group showed hepatotoxicity, which was revealed in the microregional necrosis of hepatocytes. In contrast, less structural disturbance was showed in the DOX-loaded micelles-treated groups. In addition, free DOX·HCl-treated group also showed nephrotoxicity, as judged through the shriveled glomerular and unclear cell morphology. On the contrary, the structure of the kidney in the DOX-loaded micelles-treated groups was intact. All the data demonstrated the decreased systematic toxicity of DOX-loaded micelles, which could be due to the decreased DOX release from the micelles during blood circulation and less DOX accumulated at normal tissues and organs. No obvious pathological change was found in the spleens and lungs of the DOX-loaded micelles groups, indicating the good biocompatibility of them.

The damages of small molecular chemotherapeutic drugs to chromosomes can be reflected in the increase of MMCR.(Chen et al., 1994) As shown in **Figure 6A**, various quantities of bone marrow mononuclear cells were observed in different groups. The specific quantitative proportions of them showed that the MMCRs in DOX-3 and DOX-6 groups were ascendant, while the MMCRs of DOX-loaded micelles-treated groups were slightly ascendant ($P < 0.01$) (**Figure 6B**). The results were in accordance with the histopathological analysis of tissues and organs, which further demonstrated the detoxification of DOX-loaded micelles.

It is reported that the count of WBC can reflect the influence of chemotherapy on the immune status.(Homma et al., 2014) In **Figure 6C**, the WBC count of the control group significantly raised in comparison to other groups, indicating that the treatments with free DOX·HCl and DOX-loaded micelles could effectively eliminate the inflammation caused by tumor ($P < 0.01$). In addition, the DOX-loaded micelles showed a more efficient anti-inflammatory efficacy than free DOX·HCl ($P < 0.05$). All the data further verified the advantages of DOX-loaded micelles in the application of anti-cervical carcinoma than free DOX·HCl.

Clinical chemical parameters, including CK, CK-MB, LDH, ALT, AST, BUN, and Cr were tested to further demonstrate the security of DOX-loaded micelles *in vivo*. As shown in **Figure 7**, the relevant parameters for both serum and organs were obviously raised in free DOX·HCl-treated groups, especially the DOX-6 group, which indicated that free DOX·HCl caused obvious damage to heart, liver, and kidney ($P < 0.05$). In contrast, all the DOX-loaded micelles-treated groups, especially the SCM/DOX group, showed negligible changes of relevant parameters, which were almost the same with normal group. The data verified that all the DOX-loaded micelles, especially the SCM/DOX could minimize the damage of DOX to the body. All of the up-mentioned results were consistent with the body weight changes and immunohistochemistry results of tissues and organs. All these results demonstrated that all of the DOX-loaded micelles, especially the SCM/DOX, were relatively safe and could be potentially applied in clinical studies in the future.

CONCLUSION

In this study, DOX-loaded polylactide based micelles (PDM/DOX and PLM/DOX) and stereocomplex micelle (SCM/DOX) were fabricated. *In vitro* studies showed that SCM/DOX increased the cellular uptake compared to PDM/DOX and PLM/DOX and exhibited the strongest cytotoxicity against HeLa cells, which was even stronger than free DOX·HCl. Furthermore, in a mouse U14 cervical carcinoma model, SCM/DOX also exhibited the most efficient antitumor efficacy compared to either PDM/DOX, PLM/DOX or free DOX·HCl. Importantly, all the DOX-loaded micelles, especially the SCM/DOX could obviously alleviate the systemic toxicity of DOX. Therefore, the stereocomplex micelle could serve as a promising nanodrug delivery system with high systemic safety for the future cervical carcinoma therapy.

AUTHOR CONTRIBUTIONS

These studies were conceived of and designed by all authors. Experiments were performed by KN and YY. Data analysis, data interpretation, manuscript preparations were done by MX, CG, YG, and JW.

REFERENCES

Benival, D. M., and Devarajan, P. V. (2012). Lipomer of doxorubicin hydrochloride for enhanced oral bioavailability. *Int. J. Pharm.* 423, 554–561. doi: 10.1016/j.ijpharm.2011.11.035

Chen, H., Rupa, D. S., Tomar, R., and Eastmond, D. A. (1994). Chromosomal loss and breakage in mouse bone marrow and spleen cells exposed to benzene in vivo. *Cancer Res.* 54, 3533–3539.

Chen, J., Ding, J., Wang, Y., Cheng, J., Ji, S., Zhuang, X., et al. (2017a). Sequentially responsive shell-stacked nanoparticles for deep penetration into solid tumors. *Adv. Mater.* 29. doi: 10.1002/adma.201701170

Chen, J., Ding, J., Xu, W., Sun, T., Xiao, H., Zhuang, X., et al. (2017b). Receptor and microenvironment dual-recognizable nanogel for targeted chemotherapy of highly metastatic malignancy. *Nano Lett.* 17, 4526–4533. doi: 10.1021/acs.nanolett.7b02129

Chen, S., Cheng, S. X., and Zhuo, R. X. (2011). Self-assembly strategy for the preparation of polymer-based nanoparticles for drug and gene delivery. *Macromol. Biosci.* 11, 576–589. doi: 10.1002/mabi.201000427

Chuang, C.-H., Wu, P.-C., Tsai, T.-H., Fang, Y.-P., Tsai, Y.-H., Cheng, T.-C., et al. (2017). Development of pH-sensitive cationic pegylated solid lipid nanoparticles for selective cancer-targeted therapy. *J. Biomed. Nanotechnol.* 13, 192–203. doi: 10.1166/jbn.2017.2338

Dai, J., Lin, S., Cheng, D., Zou, S., and Shuai, X. (2011). Interlayer-crosslinked micelle with partially hydrated core showing reduction and ph dual sensitivity for pinpointed intracellular drug release. *Angew. Chem. Int. Ed.* 50, 9404–9408. doi: 10.1002/anie.201103806

de Jong, S., Chikh, G., Sekirov, L., Raney, S., Semple, S., Klimuk, S., et al. (2007). Encapsulation in liposomal nanoparticles enhances the immunostimulatory, adjuvant and anti-tumor activity of subcutaneously administered CpG ODN. *Cancer Immunol. Immunother.* 56, 1251–1264. doi: 10.1007/s00262-006-0276-x

Ding, J., Xu, W., Zhang, Y., Sun, D., Xiao, C., Liu, D., et al. (2013). Self-reinforced endocytoses of smart polypeptide nanogels for "on-demand" drug delivery. *J. Control. Release* 172, 444–455. doi: 10.1016/j.jconrel.2013.05.029

Ding, L., Zhu, X., Wang, Y., Shi, B., Ling, X., Chen, H., et al. (2017). Intracellular fate of nanoparticles with polydopamine surface engineering and a novel strategy for exocytosis-inhibiting, lysosome impairment-based cancer therapy. *Nano Lett.* 17, 6790–6801. doi: 10.1021/acs.nanolett.7b03021

Dolka, I., Król, M., and Sapierzyński, R. (2016). Evaluation of apoptosis-associated protein (Bcl-2, Bax, cleaved caspase-3 and p53) expression in canine mammary tumors: an immunohistochemical and prognostic study. *Res. Vet. Sci.* 105, 124–133. doi: 10.1016/j.rvsc.2016.02.004

El-Boubbou, K., Azar, D., Bekdash, A., and Abi-Habib, R. J. (2017). Doxironide magnetic nanoparticles for selective drug delivery to human acute myeloid leukemia. *J. Biomed. Nanotechnol.* 13, 500–512. doi: 10.1166/jbn.2017.2365

Feng, X.-R., Ding, J.-X., Gref, R., and Chen, X.-S. (2017). Poly(β-*cyclodextrin*)-mediated polylactide-cholesterol stereocomplex micelles for controlled drug delivery. *Chinese J. Polym. Sci.* 35, 693–699. doi: 10.1007/s10118-017-1932-7

Ferlay, J., Soerjomataram, I., Dikshit, R., Eser, S., Mathers, C., Rebelo, M., et al. (2015). Cancer incidence and mortality worldwide: sources, methods and major patterns in GLOBOCAN 2012. *Int. J. Cancer* 136, E359–E386. doi: 10.1002/ijc.29210

Fukushima, K., and Kimura, Y. (2006). Stereocomplexed polylactides (Neo-PLA) as high-performance bio-based polymers: their formation, properties, and application. *Polym. Int.* 55, 626–642. doi: 10.1002/pi.2010

Homma, Y., Taniguchi, K., Nakazawa, M., Matsuyama, R., Mori, R., Takeda, K., et al. (2014). Changes in the immune cell population and cell proliferation in peripheral blood after gemcitabine-based chemotherapy for pancreatic cancer. *Clin. Transl. Oncol.* 16, 330–335. doi: 10.1007/s12094-013-1079-0

Ikada, Y., Jamshidi, K., Tsuji, H., and Hyon, S. H. (1987). Stereocomplex formation between enantiomeric poly (lactides). *Macromolecules* 20, 904–906. doi: 10.1021/bm400228x

Khan, S., Chen, Z., Nadimidla, K., and Kanapathipillai, M. (2017). Inhibition of glioblastoma cell proliferation by hyaluronan synthesis inhibiting nanoparticles. *J. Biomed. Nanotechnol.* 13, 815–821. doi: 10.1166/jbn.2017.2391

Kim, S. H., Tan, J. P., Nederberg, F., Fukushima, K., Yang, Y. Y., Waymouth, R. M., et al. (2008). Mixed micelle formation through stereocomplexation between enantiomeric poly (lactide) block copolymers. *Macromolecules* 42, 25–29. doi: 10.1016/j.msec.2018.06.006

Kobayashi, H., Watanabe, R., and Choyke, P. L. (2014). Improving conventional enhanced permeability and retention (EPR) effects; what is the appropriate target? *Theranostics* 4, 81–89. doi: 10.7150/thno.7193

Li, D., Feng, X., Chen, L., Ding, J., and Chen, X. (2018). One-step synthesis of targeted acid-labile polysaccharide prodrug for efficiently intracellular drug delivery. *ACS Biomater. Sci. Eng.* 4, 539–546. doi: 10.1021/acsbiomaterials.7b00856

Li, S., Zhang, T., Xu, W., Ding, J., Yin, F., Xu, J., et al. (2018). Sarcoma-targeting peptide-decorated polypeptide nanogel intracellularly delivers shikonin for upregulated osteosarcoma necroptosis and diminished pulmonary metastasis. *Theranostics* 8, 1361–1375. doi: 10.7150/thno.18299

Li, M., Tang, Z., Lv, S., Song, W., Hong, H., Jing, X., et al. (2014). Cisplatin crosslinked pH-sensitive nanoparticles for efficient delivery of doxorubicin. *Biomaterials* 35, 3851–3864. doi: 10.1016/j.biomaterials.2014.01.018

Li, Z., Yuan, D., Jin, G., Tan, B. H., and He, C. (2016). Facile layer-by-layer self-assembly toward enantiomeric poly (lactide) stereocomplex coated magnetite nanocarrier for highly tunable drug deliveries. *ACS Appl. Mater. Interfaces* 8, 1842–1853. doi: 10.1021/acsami.5b09822

Liu, D.-H., Ding, J.-X., Xu, W.-G., Song, X.-F., Zhuang, X.-L., and Chen, X.-S. (2014). Stereocomplex micelles based on 4-armed poly (ethylene glycol)-polylactide enantiomeric copolymers for drug delivery. *Acta Polym. Sin.* 9, 1265–1273. doi: 10.3390/ma8010216

Ma, C., Pan, P., Shan, G., Bao, Y., Fujita, M., and Maeda, M. (2015). Core–shell structure, biodegradation, and drug release behavior of poly (lactic acid)/poly (ethylene glycol) block copolymer micelles tuned by macromolecular stereostructure. *Langmuir* 31, 1527–1536. doi: 10.1021/la503869d

Pounder, R. J., Willcock, H., Ieong, N. S., Rachel, K., and Dove, A. P. (2011). Stereocomplexation in novel degradable amphiphilic block copolymer micelles of poly (ethylene oxide) and poly (benzyl α-malate). *Soft Matter* 7, 10987–10993. doi: 10.1039/c1sm06164j

Rosenblum, D., Joshi, N., Tao, W., Karp, J. M., and Peer, D. (2018). Progress and challenges towards targeted delivery of cancer therapeutics. *Nat. Commun.* 9:1410. doi: 10.1038/s41467-018-03705-y

Shen, K., Li, D., Guan, J., Ding, J., Wang, Z., Gu, J., et al. (2017). Targeted sustained delivery of antineoplastic agent with multicomponent polylactide stereocomplex micelle. *Nanomedicine* 13, 1279–1288. doi: 10.1016/j.nano.2016.12.022

Sun, C., Liang, Y., Zhao, M., Hao, N., Xu, L., Cheng, F., et al. (2017). Multi-activated polymeric micelles with charge-conversion and ros-controlled drug release for efficient cancer therapy. *J. Biomed. Nanotechnol.* 13, 946–959. doi: 10.1166/jbn.2017.2411

Tan, L., Ma, B., Zhao, Q., Zhang, L., Chen, L., Peng, J., et al. (2017). Toxicity evaluation and anti-tumor study of docetaxel loaded mpeg-polyester micelles for breast cancer therapy. *J. Biomed. Nanotechnol.* 13, 393–408. doi: 10.1166/jbn.2017.2356

Tao, W., Ji, X., Xu, X., Islam, M. A., Li, Z., Chen, S., et al. (2017a). Antimonene quantum dots: synthesis and application as near-infrared photothermal agents for effective cancer therapy. *Angew. Chem.* 129, 12058–12062. doi: 10.1002/anie.201703657

Tao, W., Zhu, X., Yu, X., Zeng, X., Xiao, Q., Zhang, X., et al. (2017b). Black phosphorus nanosheets as a robust delivery platform for cancer theranostics. *Adv. Mater.* 29. doi: 10.1002/adma.201603276

Tao, W., Zeng, X., Liu, T., Wang, Z., Xiong, Q., Ouyang, C., et al. (2013). Docetaxel-loaded nanoparticles based on star-shaped mannitol-core PLGA-TPGS diblock copolymer for breast cancer therapy. *Acta Biomater.* 9, 8910–8920. doi: 10.1016/j.actbio.2013.06.034

Tao, W., Zeng, X., Wu, J., Zhu, X., Yu, X., Zhang, X., et al. (2016). Polydopamine-based surface modification of novel nanoparticle-aptamer bioconjugates for in vivo breast cancer targeting and enhanced therapeutic effects. *Theranostics* 6, 470–484. doi: 10.7150/thno.14184

Tao, W., Zeng, X., Zhang, J., Zhu, H., Chang, D., Zhang, X., et al. (2014). Synthesis of cholic acid-core poly (ε-caprolactone-ran-lactide)-b-poly (ethylene glycol) 1000 random copolymer as a chemotherapeutic nanocarrier for liver cancer treatment. *Biomater. Sci.* 2, 1262–1274. doi: 10.1039/C4BM00134F

Tao, W., Zhang, J., Zeng, X., Liu, D., Liu, G., Zhu, X., et al. (2015). Blended nanoparticle system based on miscible structurally similar polymers: a safe, simple, targeted, and surprisingly high efficiency vehicle for cancer therapy. *Adv. Healthc. Mater.* 4, 1203–1214. doi: 10.1002/adhm.201400751

Walch-Rückheim, B., Pahne-Zeppenfeld, J., Fischbach, J., Wickenhauser, C., Horn, L. C., Tharun, L., et al. (2016). STAT3/IRF1 pathway activation sensitizes cervical cancer cells to chemotherapeutic drugs. *Cancer Res.* 76, 3872–3883. doi: 10.1158/0008-5472.CAN-14-1306

Wang, J., Li, S., Han, Y., Guan, J., Chung, S., Wang, C., et al. (2018). Poly (Ethylene Glycol)–polylactide micelles for cancer therapy. *Front. Pharmacol.* 9:202. doi: 10.3389/fphar.2018.00202

Wang, J., Shen, K., Xu, W., Ding, J., Wang, X., Liu, T., et al. (2015a). Stereocomplex micelle from nonlinear enantiomeric copolymers efficiently transports antineoplastic drug. *Nanoscale Res. Lett.* 10:907. doi: 10.1186/s11671-015-0907-2

Wang, X., Shan, H., Wang, J., Hou, Y., Ding, J., Chen, Q., et al. (2015b). Characterization of nanostructured ureteral stent with gradient degradation in a porcine model. *Int. J. Nanomed.* 10, 3055–3064. doi: 10.2147/IJN.S80810

Wang, X., Zhang, L., Chen, Q., Hou, Y., Hao, Y., Wang, C., et al. (2015c). A nanostructured degradable ureteral stent fabricated by electrospinning for upper urinary tract reconstruction. *J. Nanosci. Nanotechnol.* 15, 9899–9904.

Wang, X., Li, X., Ito, A., Watanabe, Y., Sogo, Y., Tsuji, N. M., et al. (2016). Stimulation of in vivo antitumor immunity with hollow mesoporous silica nanospheres. *Angew. Chem. Int. Ed.* 55, 1899–1903. doi: 10.1002/anie.201506179

Xu, W., Ding, J., and Chen, X. (2017). Reduction-responsive polypeptide micelles for intracellular delivery of antineoplastic agent. *Biomacromolecules* 18, 3291–3301. doi: 10.1021/acs.biomac.7b00950

Zhang, Y., Wang, F., Li, M., Yu, Z., Qi, R., Ding, J., et al. (2018). Self-stabilized hyaluronate nanogel for intracellular codelivery of doxorubicin and cisplatin to osteosarcoma. *Adv. Sci.* 5:1700821. doi: 10.1002/advs.201800811

Zhao, K., Li, D., Xu, W., Ding, J., Jiang, W., Li, M., et al. (2017). Targeted hydroxyethyl starch prodrug for inhibiting the growth and metastasis of prostate cancer. *Biomaterials* 116, 82–94. doi: 10.1016/j.biomaterials.2016.11.030

Zhao, Z., Zhang, Z., Chen, L., Cao, Y., He, C., and Chen, X. (2013). Biodegradable stereocomplex micelles based on dextran-block-polylactide as efficient drug deliveries. *Langmuir* 29, 13072–13080. doi: 10.1021/la402890k

Zhu, X., Ji, X., Kong, N., Chen, Y., Mahmoudi, M., Xu, X., et al. (2018). Intracellular mechanistic understanding of 2D MoS2 nanosheets for anti-exocytosis-enhanced synergistic cancer therapy. *ACS Nano* 12, 2922–2938. doi: 10.1021/acsnano.8b00516

7

Effects of Chitosan Oligosaccharides on Human Blood Components

Xi Guo[1,2]*, Tong Sun*[1,2]*, Rui Zhong*[3]*, Lu Ma*[2]*, Chao You*[1,2,4]*, Meng Tian*[1,2,4*]*, Hao Li*[2*] *and Chengwei Wang*[5*]

[1] *Department of Neurosurgery, West China Hospital, Sichuan University, Chengdu, China,* [2] *Neurosurgery Research Laboratory, West China Hospital, Sichuan University, Chengdu, China,* [3] *Institute of Blood Transfusion, Chinese Academy of Medical Sciences & Peking Union Medical College, Chengdu, China,* [4] *West China Brain Research Centre, West China Hospital, Sichuan University, Chengdu, China,* [5] *Department of Integrated Traditional and Western Medicine, West China Hospital, Sichuan University, Chengdu, China*

***Correspondence:**
Meng Tian
6744710@qq.com;
tianmong007@gmail.com
Hao Li
coscolh@126.com
Chengwei Wang
21270526@qq.com

Chitosan oligosaccharide (COS) is known for its unique biological activities such as anti-tumor, anti-inflammatory, anti-oxidant, anti-bacterial activity, biological recognition, and immune enhancing effects, and thus continuous attracting many research interests in drug, food, cosmetics, biomaterials and tissue engineering fields. In comparison to its corresponding polymer, COS has much higher absorption profiles at the intestinal level, which results in permitting its quick access to the blood flow and potential contacting with blood components. However, the effects of COS on blood components remain unclear to date. Herein, two COS with different molecular weight (MW) were characterized by FTIR and ^{1}H NMR, and then their effects on human blood components, including red blood cells (RBCs) (hemolysis, deformability, and aggregation), coagulation system [activated partial thromboplastin time (APTT), prothrombin time (PT), thrombin time (TT), and the concentration of fibrinogen (Fib)], complement (C3a and C5a activation), and platelet (activation and aggregation), were comprehensively studied. In the case of RBCs, COS exhibited a low risk of hemolysis in a dose and molecular weight dependent manner and the irreversible aggregation was observed in their high concentration. For coagulation system, COS has a mild anticoagulation activity through blocking the intrinsic coagulation pathway. In addition, COS showed no effect on complement activation in C3a and C5a and on platelet activation while inhibition of platelet aggregation was evident. Finally, the mechanism that effects of COS on blood components was discussed and proposed.

Keywords: chitosan oligosaccharide (COS), red blood cells (RBC), coagulation, complement, platelet

INTRODUCTION

Chitosan oligosaccharide (COS) is an oligomer of chitosan with an average molecular weight (MW) < 5,000 Da, and its chemical structure, like chitosan, is a linear binary copolymer consisting of β-1, 4-linked 2-acetamido-2-deoxy-β-D-glucopyranose (GlcNAc) and 2-amino-2-deoxy-β-D-glucopyranose (GlcN) (Kumar et al., 2004; Muanprasat and Chatsudthipong, 2017). The great research interest on this oligomer results not only from its physical-chemical properties such as better water solubility and cationic nature at neutral pH, but also from its biological activities, e.g., anti-tumor, anti-inflammatory, anti-oxidant, anti-bacterial activity, biological recognition, and immune enhancing effects (Liu et al., 2009; Lu et al., 2014, 2015; Zhang et al., 2014, 2018; Huang et al., 2016; Kunanusornchai et al., 2016; Mattaveewong et al., 2016; Ding et al., 2017; Kalagatur et al., 2018). These unique properties and activities continuously attract many research interests in drug, food, cosmetics, biomaterials and tissue engineering fields (Swiatkiewicz et al., 2015; Lee et al., 2017; Bai et al., 2018; El-Sayed et al., 2018; Nan et al., 2018).

Although the use of COS has been broadened in many research and applied areas, there are some dilemmas that need to be elucidated. For example, it is well-known that oral administration of COS has much higher absorption profiles at the intestinal level than that of its corresponding polymer, chitosan, which results in permitting its quick access to the blood flow and potential contacting with blood components (Chae et al., 2005). This is also applicable to chitosan based tissue-engineering scaffolds, because the degraded fragments that mainly composed of COS would finally enter into the blood circulation. For these reasons, the effect of COS on the blood such as its main components, including red blood cells (RBCs), coagulation, protein adsorption, complement, and platelets, has to be taken into account, since the hemocompatibility of the COS has not been reported to date. In general, chitosan formed a coagulum in contact with whole blood where platelets showed distinct adhesion to its surface within a short time, and the clotting time was reported to reduce by 40% compared to whole blood alone (Rao and Sharma, 1997; Chen et al., 2017). As a result, chitosan is normally used as a hemostatic dressing for wound healing in clinic instead of a blood-contact medical device (Muzzarelli et al., 2005). The hemostatic property was attributed to the polycationic characteristic of chitosan and its non-specific binding to cell membranes resulting from the positively charged amino groups along the molecular chains (Benesch and Tengvall, 2002). In the case of COS, however, some different phenomena were observed. Lin et al. compared the whole blood clotting time of COS and chitosan and found that the former showed no hemostatic effect (Lin and Lin, 2003). Similarly, Fernandes et al. studied the interactions of COS with human RBCs and the results showed that no significant hemolysis was evident and the damage of COS on the RBCs was dependent on the concentration and MW of the used samples (Fernandes et al., 2008). The above reports indicated that COS appears to be better hemocompatiblility than chitosan. Besides the positively charged amino groups, there are numerous hydroxyl groups along the molecular chains of the COS. Previous studies on the effect of functional groups such as hydroxyl, carboxyl, and amino groups on the blood components have suggested that hydroxyl groups resulted in a mild anticoagulation as well as complement activation in spite of no report on COS (Sperling et al., 2005). In this regard, it can be expected that the hydroxyl groups along the molecular chains of COS probably also have some specific effects on the blood components.

Herein, we hypothesize that COS would affect the blood components in a different manner comparable to chitosan, which might be related with its MW and functional groups along the molecular chains. To address this hypothesis, the effects of COS with two different MW on the human blood components were comprehensively investigated in this work (**Figure 1**). Specifically, the effect of COS on RBCs included hemolysis, deformability and aggregation; the blood coagulation was evaluated by coagulation time, including prothrombin time (PT), activated partial thromboplastin time (APTT) and thrombin time (TT), and the concentration of fibrinogen (Fib); for complement system, complement 3a (C3a) and 5a (C5a) using ELISA method were considered; and in terms of platelet, platelet activation, and aggregation were determined. Based on above results, the mechanism of action was discussed and proposed.

MATERIALS AND METHODS

Materials Preparation

Two COS samples with distinct MW, 3 (COS-3K) and 5 (COS-5K) kDa, were purchased from Zhejiang Aoxing Biotechnology Co., Ltd. (Zhejiang, China). Both samples were obtained by enzymatic hydrolysis of chitosan derived from crab shells. PEI and Heparin sodium were purchased from Aladdin Co., Ltd. (Chengdu, China). Coagulation-related kits were purchased from Union Bio-tech Co., Ltd. (Chengdu, China). The ELISA Kit II was purchased from Becton-Dickinson Co., Ltd, (USA). Flow cytometry-related agents, anti-CD61-fluorecein isothiocyanate (FITC) and anti-CD62p-phycoerythrin (PE) were purchased from BD Pharmingen, BD Bioscience Co., Ltd. Adenosine-diphosphate and epinephrine, which were platelet aggregation-inducers, were purchased from Kelong Co., Ltd. (Chengdu, China). COS-3K/5K were mixed with normal saline to get the COS stock solution.

Structure Characterization

The structure of the two COS was characterized by Fourier transform infrared spectra (FTIR) and ^{1}H nuclear magnetic resonance spectroscopy (NMR). FTIR analyses of the COSs were recorded with KBr compressed pellets on a Nicolet 670 FT-IR Spectrometer. ^{1}H NMR analyses were recorded on a Bruker AV II-400MHz spectrometer. The DD was calculated by ^{1}H NMR according to equation (1), where "A_{CH3}" and "$A_{GlcNH-2}$," respectively correspond to the integral of the N-acetyl proton signal and H-2 proton signal of GlcN units.

$$DD(\%) = 1 - \frac{\frac{1}{3}A_{CH_3}}{\frac{1}{3}A_{CH_3} + A_{GlcNH-2}} \times 100 \qquad (1)$$

Blood Collection

The study was approved by Ethical Committee of Institute of Blood Transfusion, Chinese Academy of Medical Sciences & Peking Union Medical College. Anticoagulated whole blood samples (3.8% sodium citrate/blood 1:9) and fresh frozen plasma (FFP) anticoagulated with citrate-phosphate-adenine used in this study were obtained from Chengdu Blood Center. For RBC tests, RBC suspension was gained by washing anticoagulated whole blood with normal saline for three times and then adjusting hematocrit (HCT) to 10%. The whole blood samples were centrifuged at 1,200 g for 20 min under 4°C to obtain platelet-poor plasma (PPP) and at 150 g for 10 min under 4°C to acquire platelet-rich plasm (PRP).

Red Blood Cells

Hemolysis

Washed RBC suspension with 10% HCT (270 μl) was mixed with COS-3K/5K solution (30 μl) to obtain a final COS concentration

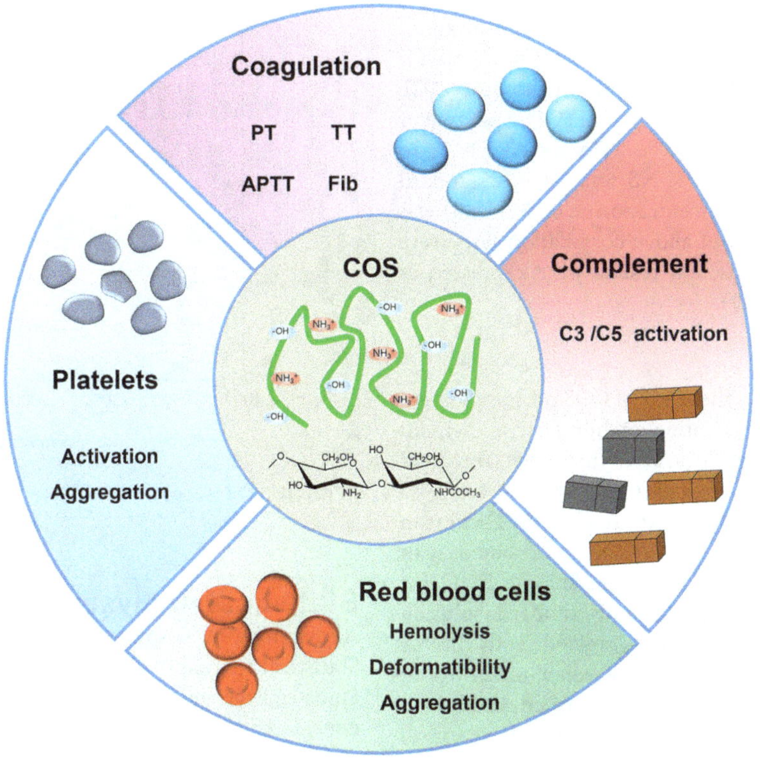

FIGURE 1 | Schematic presentation of COS and blood components.

of 0.01, 0.1, 0.5, 1 mg/ml. The mixtures then were gently centrifuged at 1,500 g for 5 min after 1 h incubation under 37°C. Supernatant (0.02 ml) obtained after centrifuge was added to ortho-tolidine solution (1 ml; 0.2 g in 60 ml acetic acid) and hydrogen peroxide (1 ml; 1 g/L). After incubation for 10 min, the reaction was stopped by mixed with acetic acid (10 ml; 10%). The spectrophotometer was used to measure absorbance at a wavelength of 435 nm. A standard hemoglobin solution with concentration of 100 mg/L was used as a standard control and diluted water (DW) was used as a hemolysis control. To figure out the extent of hemolysis, the following equation was used (Lewis, 1965).

$$Hemolysis(\%) = \left(\frac{A_1}{A_S} \times 100\right) \times \frac{100 - Hct(\%)}{C_{Hb}(g/L) \times 1000} \quad (2)$$

A_1 means the absorbance (435 nm) of sample; A_S means the absorbance of standard sample (100 mg/L); Hct (%) means hematocrit; C_{Hb} means concentration of hemoglobin.

Deformability

To measure RBC deformability, the washed RBC suspension (270 μl) were incubated with COS stock solution (30 μl) to attain the final concentration of 0.01, 0.1, 0.5, and 1 mg/ml. After 1 h incubation, the suspension was centrifuged at 1,500 g for 4 min and then the precipitate was gently mixed with 1 ml of polyvinylpyrrolidone solution (15% in PBS). A laser-diffraction Ektacytometer system (LBY-BX, Beijing Pencil Instrument Co., Ltd, China) was used. About 0.5 ml of the mixture was added to the system and the sheared between two concentric cylinders of the machine, in which size of gap was 0.5 mm, under four different shear stresses of 0.39, 0.77, 1.54, and 7.7 Pa (corresponding to shear rates of 50, 100, 200, and 1,000) at 37°C. Then the parameter was presented as elongation index (EI) by the system through measuring the diffraction of passing laser. Normal saline and diluted water mixed with RBC suspension were used as standard and positive control, respectively.

Aggregation

To determine whether COS can lead to RBC aggregation, anti-coagulated whole blood samples (270 μl) was mixed with COS stock solution (30 μl) to attain the final concentration of 1 and 5 mg/ml for 1 h incubation. The mixtures then were centrifuged at 1,000 g for 3 min. The precipitate (3 μl) and supernatant (40 μl) were gently mixed and mixtures (4 μl) were made into slides. Images of slides were captured by a digital microscope camera. Polyetherimide (PEI), which can lead to obvious erythrocytes aggregation, was used as positive control and normal saline was used as standard control.

Coagulation

Activated partial thrombin time (APTT), prothrombin time (PT), thrombin time (TT) and the concentration of fibrinogen (Fib) were measured to determine the effect of COS on coagulation system by a modified strategy according to previous study (Nikitina et al., 2018). Briefly, COS stock solution (60 μl) were mixed with FFP (540 μl) to attain a final concentration of 0.01, 0.1, and 0.5 mg/ml and then was incubated at 37°C for 3 min. A coagulation analyzer (Instrumentation Laboratory ACL ELITE, USA) was used to test the incubated FFP. The parameter range available for the machine is 6 s to 245 s for APTT, 5 s to 165 s for PT, and 3 s to 169 s for TT. NS was used as standard control and heparin (HP, final concentration of 0.75 IU/ml) was used as positive control. Values of above coagulation tests were mean from three measurements and results were expressed as mean ± standard deviation (SD).

Complement

Complement activation reflects the effect of COS on complement system. We focused on the activation of human complement C3 and C5 in circulation and measured their cleft fragment C3a and C5a. The method of measurement was followed by the standard protocol of ELISA Kit II (Becton-Dickinson Co., Ltd, USA). Briefly, serum (90 μl) was incubated with COS (final concentration of 0.1 and 1 mg/ml) at 37°C for 1 h. Then incubated serum (100 μl) and standard solution (100 μl) of the kit were, respectively, mixed with ELISA dilution (50 μl) in antibody coated well-sealed under room temperature for 2 h. After that, wells were washed and added detection antibody and enzyme concentrate of the kit for 1-h incubation. Finally, the wells were read and absorbance of 450 nm was measured by spectrophotometer (EON, Bio-Tech CO., Ltd, USA). The concentration of C3a and C5a was calculated according to the standard curve of standard samples of kit.

Platelet

Activation

CD61, a specific marker of platelet surface, and CD62p, the marker of activated platelet, were involved in this test. Platelet-rich plasm (PRP) (90 μl) was incubated with COS stock solution (10 μl) at 37°C for 1 h to obtain a final concentration of 0.1 and 0.5 mg/ml. Incubated PRP (5 μl) was mixed with anti-CD61-fluorecein isothiocyanate (5 μl), anti-CD62p-phycoerythrin (5 μl), and PBS buffer (10 mM, 40 μl) in dark for 15 min and then added 400 μl of PBS buffer. The flow cytometry (Becton-Dickinson, San Jose', CA, USA) were used to measure the number of CD62p-expressing platelets. Normal saline and thrombin (10 U/ml) were used as normal control and positive control, respectively (Zhong et al., 2013).

Aggregation

To investigate whether platelet aggregation was affected by COS, PRP (270 μl) was incubated with COS stock solution (30 μl) at 37°C for 1 h. After incubation, we added adenosine diphosphate (0.1 mM, 12.5 μl) and epinephrine (0.15 mM, 12.5 μl) to the incubated PRP to induce platelet aggregation. And the aggregometry (MODEL700, CHRONO-LOG CO. LTD, USA) was used to measure extent of aggregation. PRP incubated with normal saline and thrombin (10 U/ml) were used as control groups.

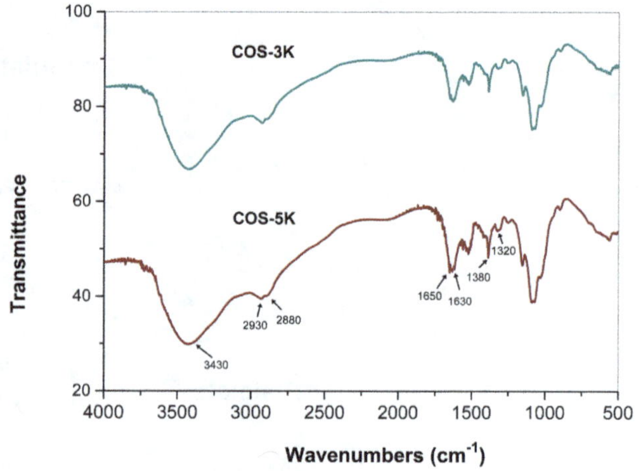

FIGURE 2 | FTIR spectra of two COS.

Statistical Analysis

All results were described as means ± standard deviation (SD). Statistical analysis of all data was performed using SPSS 19 (IBM, Statistic Package for Social Science). A value of $p < 0.05$ was considered as being statistically significant.

RESULTS AND DISCUSSIONS

Structure Characterization of COS

The FTIR spectra of the two COS are shown in **Figure 2**, both of which displayed characteristic absorptions that are similar to that of chitosans with high DD as reported previously. The absorption band at around 3,430 cm^{-1} is attributed to the N-H and O-H stretching vibrations (Chen et al., 2016; Wu et al., 2017). The peaks at 2,880 and 2,930 cm^{-1} are assigned to C-H stretching vibrations, and the peaks at 1,650, 1,630, and 1,320 cm^{-1} are, respectively, assigned to amide I, II, and III. The band at 1,380 is corresponds to C-H bending and C-H stretching vibrations, and the band in the range 1,150–890 are assigned to the characteristics of its polysaccharide structure. As previous literature reported, the COS prepared by chemical degradation approaches such as oxidative degradation with peroxide hydrogen shown a weakened amide Iband due to the H-abstraction at C-1 and C-2 during degradation that both led to the partly deamination. However, the two COS samples in this study obtained by enzymatic hydrolysis remain exhibited a strong amide Iband, which indicated that the two COS samples are both degradation products with high DD.

The chemical structure of the two COS samples was further studied by ^1H NMR. As shown in **Figure 3**, the two samples exhibited similar ^1H NMR spectrum. According to previous literatures, signals at 2.0 and 3.1 ppm are assigned to protons of CH3 and H-2 of GlcN, respectively. In the low field, the signals at 3.5–4.0 ppm are assigned to H-3, 4, 5, 6 of GlcN and H-2, 3, 4, 5, 6 of GlcNAc, and the signals at 4.5 ppm are attributed to H-1 of GlcN (Trombotto et al., 2008). Compared to ^1H NMR spectrum of the chitosan as previous reported, there is no significant

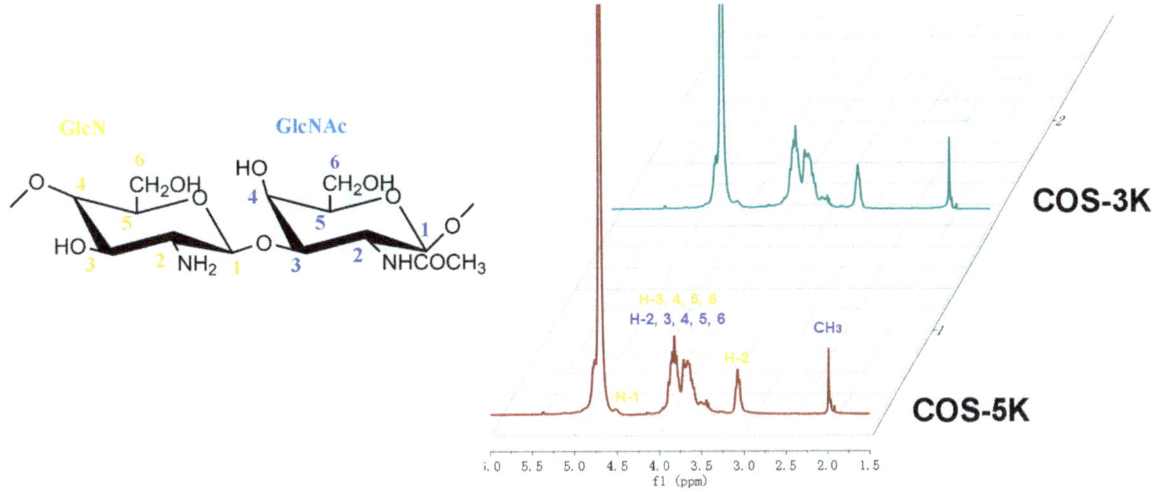

FIGURE 3 | ^{1}H NMR spectra of two COS.

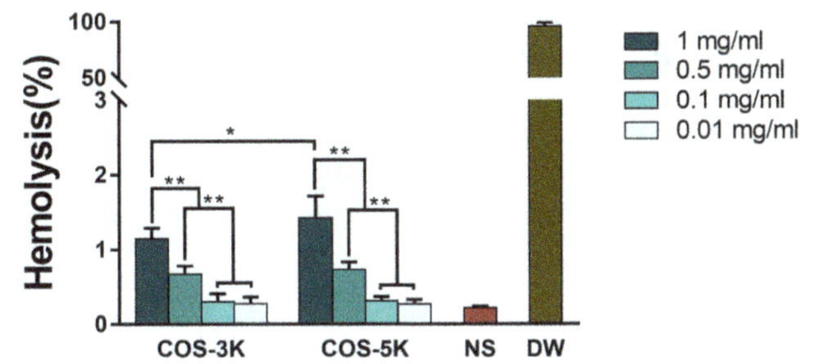

FIGURE 4 | Hemolysis percentage of RBC suspension induced by COS. NS, normal saline; DW, diluted water. $^{*}p < 0.05$; $^{**}p < 0.01$.

difference for the two samples. In addition, the DD values for the two samples were calculated by ^{1}H NMR spectrum according to equation (1). The calculated DD were 88.4 and 87.4% for COS-5K and COS-3K, respectively, which is consistent with the results of the FTIR.

Red Blood Cells

In order to investigate the effect of two COS on RBCs, three main parameters of RBCs including hemolysis, deformability and aggregation were studied. Hemolysis is a crucial and direct parameter evaluating the safety of biomaterials and defined as the percentage of RBCs lysis when the biomaterial interacting with RBCs suspension (Fernandes et al., 2008). According to ISO10993-5, percentage of hemolysis induced by exogenous materials under 5% was considered as a low risk (Weber et al., 2018). As shown in **Figure 4**, percentages of hemolysis presented in a dose-dependent manner. As the concentration increasing from 0.1 to 1 mg/ml, the hemolysis increased from 0.30 ± 0.10 to 1.15 ± 0.14% (p < 0.01) in COS-3K group and from 0.30 ± 0.06 to 1.42 ± 0.30% (p <0.01) in COS-5K group. When the concentration below 0.1 mg/ml, the hemolysis in both COS groups had no significant difference with that in NS group. We also observed that hemolysis in COS-5K group was significantly higher than that in COS-3K group when the concentration was above 0.1 mg/ml, indicating that the hemolysis of COS also presented as a MW-dependent manner.

As for deformability of RBCs, an index representing the ability of RBCs to change their biconcave disk shape against the exogenous force from vascular walls, we used four different sheer forces in the tests (Zhao et al., 2010). As shown in **Figures 5A–D**, as sheer force increasing from 0.39 to 7.7 Pa (corresponding sheer rate 50 to 1,000), elongation index was generally increased except in DW group with a stable and lowest EI due to containing no intact RBCs. Under sheer rate of 50 and 100, EI presented a dose dependent manner where EI was significant higher at 0.5 and 1 mg/ml than 0.01 and 0.1 mg/ml. Though under sheer rate of 200, there was no statistical difference on EI between 0.5, 1, and 0.01, 0.1 mg/ml in COS-3K group, EI in COS-5K group had the same trend as under 50 and 100 sheer rate.

Results of erythrocytes aggregation was in accordance with hemolysis. As shown in **Figure 6**, at the concentration of 1 mg/ml, RBCs displayed biconcave shape and some erythrocytes rouleaux defined as reversible aggregation were observed compared to normal distribution of RBCs in NS group. However, with the concentration increasing to 5 mg/ml, RBCs all aggregated forming erythrocytes clusters which are irreversible aggregation and the normal shape of erythrocytes was absent. As previous report, amidocyanogen of chitosan could neutralize the negatively charged neuraminic acid residues located on the surface of RBCs (Fernandes et al., 2008). Likely, the positive charge of COS can change the distribution of charge and break the electrokinetic balance on erythrocyte surface leading to aggregation in a dose-dependent manner.

Coagulation

Effect on coagulation is an essential property of biomaterial due to both anti-coagulation and pro-coagulation can cause fetal

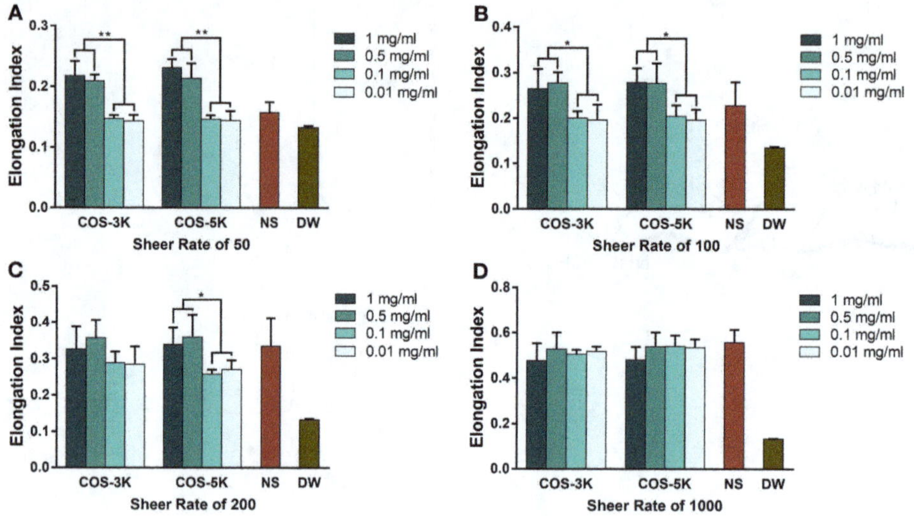

FIGURE 5 | Deformability of RBC detected by a laser-diffraction Ektacytometer system under shear rate of 50 **(A)**, 100 **(B)**, 200 **(C)**, 1,000 **(D)** with the presence of COS with different concentration. NS, normal saline; DW, diluted water. $^*p < 0.05$; $^{**}p < 0.01$.

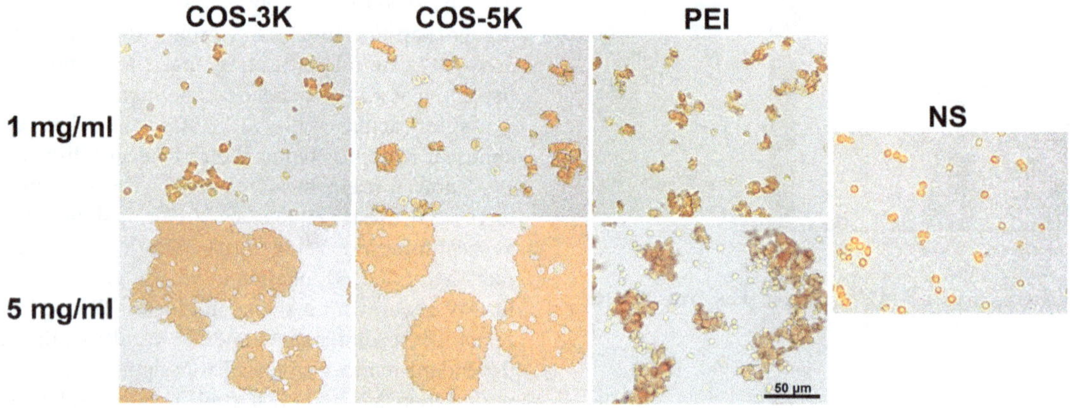

FIGURE 6 | Pictures of RBC aggregation induced by COS under an optical microscope. RBC incubated with PEI was positive control. PEI, polyetherimide; NS, normal saline.

complications or side effects on human such as bleeding and thrombosis formation (Zhang et al., 2013). In order to study effect on coagulation, APTT, PT, TT, and Fib were involved in the tests. It is defined as disordered hemostatic property of human blood when APTT changes more than 10 s or PT/TT changes more than 3 s (Yang et al., 2008). In our study, as shown in **Figure 7A**, high concentration (0.5 and 0.1 mg/ml) COS prolonged APTT compared to NS group ($p < 0.01$) in a dose-dependent manner and the maximum APTT even exceeded the machine available value (>245 s). In contrast, TT was normal in all COS group (**Figure 7B**). For PT showing in **Figure 7C**, though it was slightly longer at 0.1 and 0.5 mg/ml group, all the PT values were in normal range when considering 3 s mobility scale. Similar to TT, concentration of Fib in COS groups was equal to that in NS group (**Figure 7D**). Within our expectation, heparin (0.75 IU/ml) group (TT positive control) showed a prolonged TT value which exceeded 169 s.

APTT and PT, respectively, reflect the status of intrinsic and extrinsic blood coagulation, while TT is used to check the effect on the conversion from fibrinogen to insoluble fibrin induced by thrombin or whether there exist an anticoagulant when APTT and PT are prolonged. Our study indicated COS influenced intrinsic coagulation pathway due to prolonging APTT while PT, TT, and Fib were in normal range. To the best of our knowledge, it is the first time to report that COS has anticoagulation activity through blocking the intrinsic coagulation pathway, which is different from chitosan with pro-coagulant activity. On the other hand, it should be noted that the anticoagulation activity of the COS is mild compared to other anticoagulants such as alginate sulfates, whose APTT was prolonged by 180 s in the

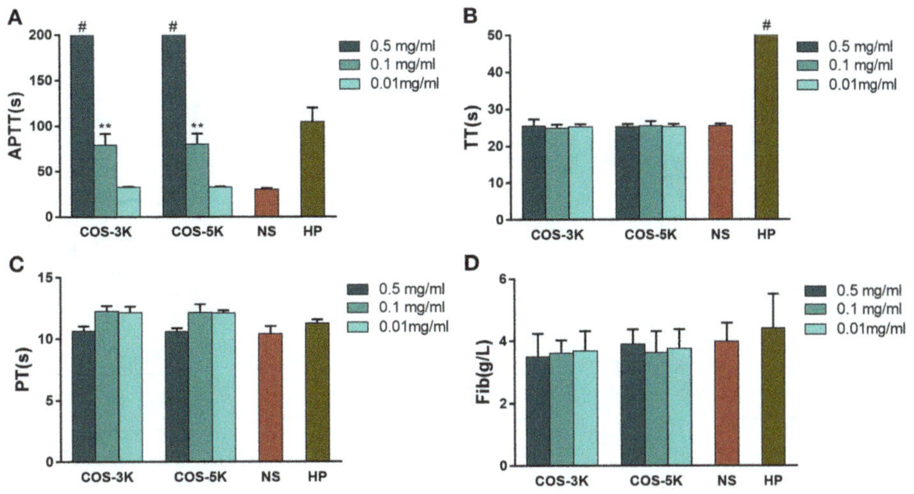

FIGURE 7 | Analysis of influence on coagulation caused by COSs. **(A)** APTT of COSs and heparin. **(B)** TT of COSs and heparin. **(C)** PT of COSs and heparin. **(D)** Concentration of Fib. $^{**}p < 0.01$ vs. NS group; # means the parameter exceeded machine available. NS, normal saline; HP, heparin.

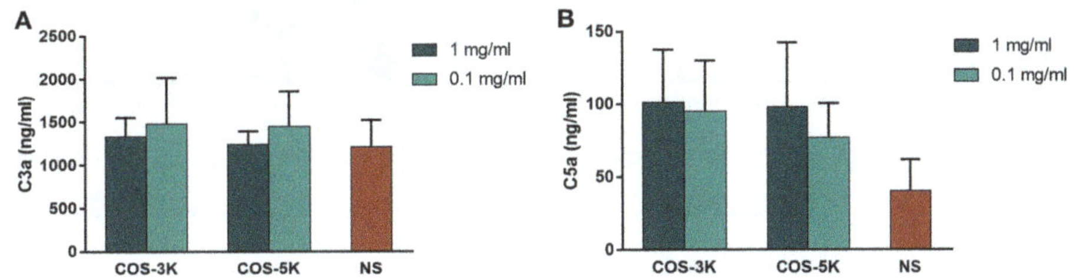

FIGURE 8 | Effects of COS on complement system. **(A)** Concentration of C3a in serum. **(B)** Concentration of C5a in serum. NS, normal saline.

concentration of 80 μg/ml, while the APTT of the COS was around 80 s in the concentration of 0.1 mg/ml.

Complement

Complement activation is an important indicator of hemocompatibility of biomaterials. Complement system is an innate part of immune system and can be activated via three pathways, classical pathway, alternative pathway and lectin pathway (Coulthard and Woodruff, 2015). Once complement system activated, C3 cleaves to fragments C3a and C3b, and leads to its downstream generation of C5a. As shown in **Figure 8**, at low concentration, COS seemed to induce more C3a than NS group than that at high concentration. However, the difference has no statistical significance.

Chitosan is suggested to activated complement system by deplete or absorb C3 and C5 proteins from serum (Benesch and Tengvall, 2002). Interestingly, in our study, COS demonstrated relative complement compatibility that C3a and C5a in all groups was in a normal range. Similar to our findings, Marchand et al. reported that chitosan with 80% and 95% DD do not activate complement system for that C3 and C5 bind to chitosan as intact proteins (Marchand et al., 2010). Hence, DD might be a significant factor that determined whether the chitosan induced complement activation.

Platelet

CD62P, a platelet activation marker, was used to investigate the effect of COS on platelet. As shown in **Figures 9A,B**, with presence of COS at 0.1 and 0.5 mg/ml, expression of CD62P was in normal range ($p > 0.05$) indicating platelet was not activated by COS. Heparin demonstrated a strong ability to stimulate platelet that CD62P was remarkable high in heparin group. In terms of platelet aggregation, reduced aggregation was observed in all COS groups ($p < 0.05$ for all COS) compared to normal saline (**Figure 9C**). Moreover, there was no statistical significant difference between two concentrations or two COSs.

Platelet was a vital component in blood participating in coagulation cascade and provided large scale of coagulation factors, such as platelet factor 3 and factor Va, when activated leading to generate platelet micro particles (Gorbet and Sefton, 2004). In coagulation process, induced platelet micro particles promote platelet adherence to fibrin resulting in congregation of platelet and anti-bleeding function. In accordance to coagulation results, COS did not activate platelet and inhibited platelet aggregation indicating it played as an anti-coagulant. Under such

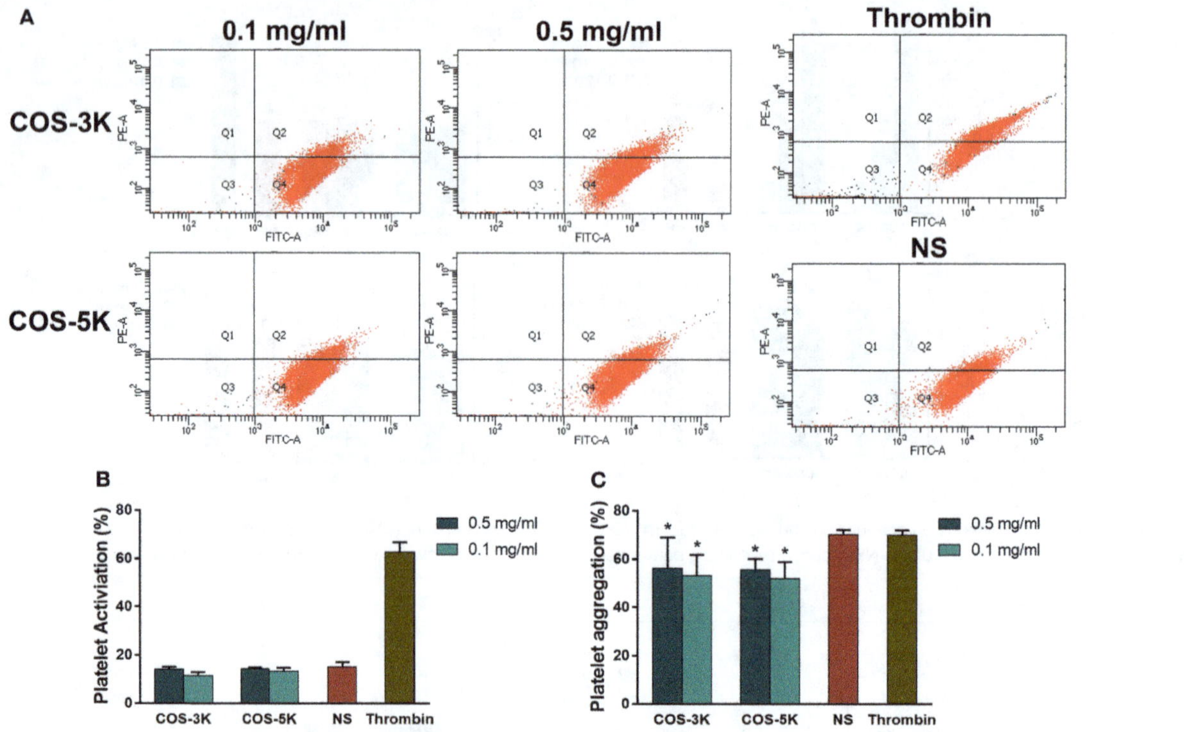

FIGURE 9 | Analysis of influence on platelet caused by COSs: **(A)** Flow cytometry of activated platelets. **(B)** Percentage of platelet activation. **(C)** Effects on Platelet aggregation. NS, normal saline. $^{*}p < 0.05$.

concentrations of 0.5 and 0.1 mg/ml, COS with two MW has no difference in ability of inhibiting platelet.

DISCUSSION OF MECHANISM

Chitosan derived from chitin is a cationic polysaccharide that is widely used as a hemostasis, wound dressing, or anti-bacterial material in clinic (Kumar et al., 2004; Muzzarelli et al., 2005). However, application in blood-contacting is occluded by its inferior compatibility with blood components such as procoagulant function and complement activation. Interesting, here it was found that COS exhibited quite different effects on human blood components comparable to chitosan (**Figure 10**). To explain this phenomenon, a mechanism was proposed as follows based on literatures and our results.

The procoagulant function of chitosan is due to its cationic nature that induced by positively charged amino groups, in which these groups induction of fibrinogen adsorption, activation of platelets, releasing of coagulation factors, and then trigger extrinsic coagulation pathway (Benesch and Tengvall, 2002; Zhang et al., 2013). However, when chitosan was degraded into COS, the decreased MW resulted in decreasing of local positive charge density and thus weakened the electrostatistic interactions between the positively charged amino groups and the blood components in comparison to that of chitosan. In the case of RBCs, the electrostatic interactions results in membrane damage, hemolysis as well as aggregation, while low risk of hemolysis, deformability and aggragation were observed for COS-3k and 5k resulting from the decreased MW and positive charge density. Similarly, the decreased positive charge density may reduce the procoagulant function of chitosan as well. However, our results shown that the both two COS exhibited a mild anticoagulation activity in a dose-dependent manner. The anticoagulation activity probably related with the hydroxyl groups along the molecular chains, since it has been demonstrated that hydroxyl groups are capable of anticoagulation as previously reported (Sperling et al., 2005).

CONCLUSION

In summary, the molecular structure of the two COS with different MW was characterized by FTIR and ^{1}H NMR, and then the effects of the COS on the human blood components, including RBCs, coagulation system, complement, and platelet, were studied in this work. The results indicated that: (i) COS exhibited a low risk of hemolysis in a dose and MW dependent manner and the irreversible aggregation was observed in their high concentration; (ii) COS has a mild anticoagulation activity through blocking the intrinsic coagulation pathway; (iii) COS has no effect on complement activation in C3a and C5a; (iv) COS has no effect on platelet activation while inhibition of platelet aggregation was evident. Finally, the mechanism of action was discussed and proposed.

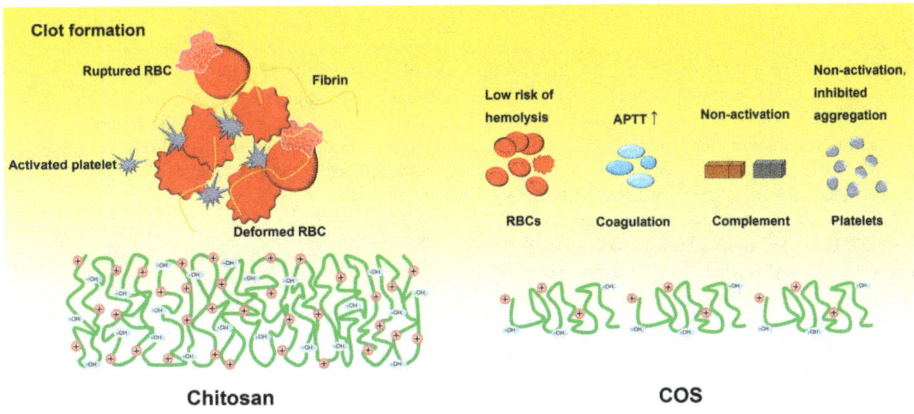

FIGURE 10 | Schematic presentation of the effects of chitosan and COS on blood components.

AUTHOR CONTRIBUTIONS

XG: results discussion, writing the article, and hemocompatibility evaluation. TS: results discussion, hemocompatibility evaluation. RZ: hemocompatibility evaluation, statistic analysis. LM: results discussion. CY: evaluating the results of study. MT: article design, NMR spectroscopy, and FTIR characterization. HL and CW: results discussion, statistic analysis.

ACKNOWLEDGMENTS

This work is supported by National Natural Science Foundation of China (No. 81401528, 51403238), The National Key Research and Development Program of China (No. YS2018YFA010082), Sichuan Province Science and Technology Key R&D Project (No. 2018SZ0029, 2018SZ0100, 2015SZ0051), and 1.3.5 project for disciplines of excellence, West China Hospital, Sichuan University (No. ZY2016102, and ZY2016203).

REFERENCES

Bai, M. Y., Tang, S. L., Chuang, M. H., Wang, T. Y., and Hong, P. D. (2018). Evaluation of chitosan derivative microparticles encapsulating superparamagnetic Iron oxide and doxorubicin as a pH-sensitive delivery carrier in hepatic carcinoma treatment: an *in vitro* comparison study. *Front. Pharmacol.* 9:1025. doi: 10.3389/fphar.2018.01025

Benesch, J., and Tengvall, P. (2002). Blood protein adsorption onto chitosan. *Biomaterials* 23, 2561–2568. doi: 10.1016/S0142-9612(01)00391-X

Chae, S. Y., Jang, M. K., and Nah, J. W. (2005). Influence of molecular weight on oral absorption of water soluble chitosans. *J. Control. Release* 102, 383–394. doi: 10.1016/j.jconrel.2004.10.012

Chen, Y., Li, J., Li, Q., Shen, Y., Ge, Z., Zhang, W., et al. (2016). Enhanced water-solubility, antibacterial activity and biocompatibility upon introducing sulfobetaine and quaternary ammonium to chitosan. *Carbohydr. Polym.* 143, 246–253. doi: 10.1016/j.carbpol.2016.01.073

Chen, Z., Yao, X., Liu, L., Guan, J., Liu, M., Li, Z., et al. (2017). Blood coagulation evaluation of N-alkylated chitosan. *Carbohydr. Polym.* 173, 259–268. doi: 10.1016/j.carbpol.2017.05.085

Coulthard, L. G., and Woodruff, T. M. (2015). Is the complement activation product C3a a proinflammatory molecule? Re-evaluating the evidence and the myth. *J. Immunol.* 194, 3542–3548. doi: 10.4049/jimmunol.1403068

Ding, B., Yu, C., Li, C., Deng, X., Ding, J., Cheng, Z., et al. (2017). cis-Platinum pro-drug-attached CuFeS2 nanoplates for *in vivo* photothermal/photoacoustic imaging and chemotherapy/photothermal therapy of cancer. *Nanoscale* 9, 16937–16949. doi: 10.1039/C7NR04166G

El-Sayed, N. S., Sharma, M., Aliabadi, H. M., El-Meligy, M. G., El-Zaity, A. K., Nageib, Z. A., et al. (2018). Synthesis, characterization, and *in vitro* cytotoxicity of fatty acyl-CGKRK-chitosan oligosaccharides conjugates for siRNA delivery. *Int. J. Biol. Macromol.* 112, 694–702. doi: 10.1016/j.ijbiomac.2018.01.213

Fernandes, J. C., Eaton, P., Nascimento, H., Belo, L., Rocha, S., Vitorino, R., et al. (2008). Effects of chitooligosaccharides on human red blood cell morphology and membrane protein structure. *Biomacromolecules* 9, 3346–3352. doi: 10.1021/bm800622f

Gorbet, M. B., and Sefton, M. V. (2004). Biomaterial-associated thrombosis: roles of coagulation factors, complement, platelets and leukocytes. *Biomaterials* 25, 5681–5703. doi: 10.1016/j.biomaterials.2004.01.023

Huang, B., Xiao, D., Tan, B., Xiao, H., Wang, J., Yin, J., et al. (2016). Chitosan oligosaccharide reduces intestinal inflammation that involves Calcium-Sensing Receptor (CaSR) activation in Lipopolysaccharide (LPS)-challenged piglets. *J. Agric. Food Chem.* 64, 245–252. doi: 10.1021/acs.jafc.5b05195

Kalagatur, N. K., Nirmal Ghosh, O. S., Sundararaj, N., and Mudili, V. (2018). Antifungal activity of chitosan nanoparticles encapsulated with cymbopogon martinii essential oil on plant pathogenic fungi *Fusarium graminearum*. *Front. Pharmacol.* 9:610. doi: 10.3389/fphar.2018.00610

Kumar, M. N., Muzzarelli, R. A., Muzzarelli, C., Sashiwa, H., and Domb, A. J. (2004). Chitosan chemistry and pharmaceutical perspectives. *Chem. Rev.* 104, 6017–6084. doi: 10.1021/cr030441b

Kunanusornchai, W., Witoonpanich, B., Tawonsawatruk, T., Pichyangkura, R., Chatsudthipong, V., and Muanprasat, C. (2016). Chitosan oligosaccharide suppresses synovial inflammation via AMPK activation: an *in vitro* and *in vivo* study. *Pharmacol. Res.* 113, 458–467. doi: 10.1016/j.phrs.2016.09.016

Lee, J. Y., Termsarasab, U., Lee, M. Y., Kim, D. H., Lee, S. Y., Kim, J. S., et al. (2017). Chemosensitizing indomethacin-conjugated chitosan oligosaccharide nanoparticles for tumor-targeted drug delivery. *Acta Biomater.* 57, 262–273. doi: 10.1016/j.actbio.2017.05.012

Lewis, G. P. (1965). Method using ortho-tolidine for the quantitative determination of haemoglobin in serum and urine. *J. Clin. Pathol.* 18, 235–239. doi: 10.1136/jcp.18.2.235

Lin, C. W., and Lin, J. C. (2003). Characterization and blood coagulation evaluation of the water-soluble chitooligosaccharides prepared by a facile fractionation method. *Biomacromolecules* 4, 1691–1697. doi: 10.1021/bm034129n

Liu, H. T., Li, W. M., Xu, G., Li, X. Y., Bai, X. F., Wei, P., et al. (2009). Chitosan oligosaccharides attenuate hydrogen peroxide-induced stress injury in human umbilical vein endothelial cells. *Pharmacol. Res.* 59, 167–175. doi: 10.1016/j.phrs.2008.12.001

Lu, Y., Shah, A., Hunter, R. A., Soto, R. J., and Schoenfisch, M. H. (2015). S-Nitrosothiol-modified nitric oxide-releasing chitosan oligosaccharides as antibacterial agents. *Acta Biomater.* 12, 62–69. doi: 10.1016/j.actbio.2014.10.028

Lu, Y., Slomberg, D. L., and Schoenfisch, M. H. (2014). Nitric oxide-releasing chitosan oligosaccharides as antibacterial agents. *Biomaterials* 35, 1716–1724. doi: 10.1016/j.biomaterials.2013.11.015

Marchand, C., Bachand, J., Périnêt, J., Baraghis, E., Lamarre, M., Rivard, G. E., et al. (2010). C3, C5, and factor B bind to chitosan without complement activation. *J. Biomed. Mater. Res. A* 93, 1429–1441. doi: 10.1002/jbm.a.32638

Mattaveewong, T., Wongkrasant, P., Chanchai, S., Pichyangkura, R., Chatsudthipong, V., and Muanprasat, C. (2016). Chitosan oligosaccharide suppresses tumor progression in a mouse model of colitis-associated colorectal cancer through AMPK activation and suppression of NF-kappaB and mTOR signaling. *Carbohydr. Polym.* 145, 30–36. doi: 10.1016/j.carbpol.2016.02.077

Muanprasat, C., and Chatsudthipong, V. (2017). Chitosan oligosaccharide: biological activities and potential therapeutic applications. *Pharmacol. Ther.* 170, 80–97. doi: 10.1016/j.pharmthera.2016.10.013

Muzzarelli, R. A., Guerrieri, M., Goteri, G., Muzzarelli, C., Armeni, T., Ghiselli, R., et al. (2005). The biocompatibility of dibutyryl chitin in the context of wound dressings. *Biomaterials* 26, 5844–5854. doi: 10.1016/j.biomaterials.2005.03.006

Nan, W., Ding, L., Chen, H., Khan, F. U., Yu, L., Sui, X., et al. (2018). Topical use of quercetin-loaded chitosan nanoparticles against ultraviolet B radiation. *Front. Pharmacol.* 9:826. doi: 10.3389/fphar.2018.00826

Nikitina, L. E., Kiselev, S. V., Startseva, V. A., Bodrov, A. V., Azizova, Z. R., Shipina, O. T., et al. (2018). Sulfur-containing monoterpenoids as potential antithrombotic drugs: research in the molecular mechanism of coagulation activity using Pinanyl Sulfoxide as an example. *Front. Pharmacol.* 9:116. doi: 10.3389/fphar.2018.00116

Rao, S. B., and Sharma, C. P. (1997). Use of chitosan as a biomaterial: studies on its safety and hemostatic potential. *J. Biomed. Mater. Res.* 34, 21–28. doi: 10.1002/(SICI)1097-4636(199701)34:1<21::AID-JBM4>3.0.CO;2-P

Sperling, C., Schweiss, R. B., Streller, U., and Werner, C. (2005). *In vitro* hemocompatibility of self-assembled monolayers displaying various functional groups. *Biomaterials* 26, 6547–6557. doi: 10.1016/j.biomaterials.2005.04.042

Swiatkiewicz, S., Swiatkiewicz, M., Arczewska-Wlosek, A., and Jozefiak, D. (2015). Chitosan and its oligosaccharide derivatives (chito-oligosaccharides) as feed supplements in poultry and swine nutrition. *J. Anim. Physiol. Anim. Nutr.* 99, 1–12. doi: 10.1111/jpn.12222

Trombotto, S., Ladavière, C., Delolme, F., and Domard, A. (2008). Chemical preparation and structural characterization of a homogeneous series of chitin/chitosan oligomers. *Biomacromolecules* 9, 1731–1738. doi: 10.1021/bm800157x

Weber, M., Steinle, H., Golombek, S., Hann, L., Schlensak, C., Wendel, H., et al. (2018). Blood-contacting biomaterials: evaluation of the hemocompatibility. *Front. Bioeng. Biotechnol.* 6:99. doi: 10.3389/fbioe.2018.00099

Wu, T., Wu, C., Fu, S., Wang, L., Yuan, C., Chen, S., et al. (2017). Integration of lysozyme into chitosan nanoparticles for improving antibacterial activity. *Carbohydr. Polym.* 155, 192–200. doi: 10.1016/j.carbpol.2016.08.076

Yang, J., Tian, F., Wang, Z., Wang, Q., Zeng, Y. J., and Chen, S. Q. (2008). Effect of chitosan molecular weight and deacetylation degree on hemostasis. *J. Biomed. Mater. Res. Part B Appl. Biomater.* 84, 131–137. doi: 10.1002/jbm.b.30853

Zhang, G., Jia, P., Liu, H., Hu, T., and Du, Y. (2018). Conjugation of chitosan oligosaccharides enhances immune response to porcine circovirus vaccine by activating macrophages. *Immunobiology* 223, 663–670. doi: 10.1016/j.imbio.2018.07.012

Zhang, P., Liu, W., Peng, Y., Han, B., and Yang, Y. (2014). Toll like receptor 4 (TLR4) mediates the stimulating activities of chitosan oligosaccharide on macrophages. *Int. Immunopharmacol.* 23, 254–261. doi: 10.1016/j.intimp.2014.09.007

Zhang, W., Zhong, D., Liu, Q., Zhang, Y., Li, N., Wang, Q., et al. (2013). Effect of chitosan and carboxymethyl chitosan on fibrinogen structure and blood coagulation. *J. Biomater. Sci. Polym. Ed.* 24, 1549–1563. doi: 10.1080/09205063.2013.777229

Zhao, L., You, G., Liao, F., Kan, X., Wang, B., Sun, Q., et al. (2010). Sodium alginate as viscosity modifier may induce aggregation of red blood cells. *Artif. Cells Blood Substit. Immobil. Biotechnol.* 38, 267–276. doi: 10.3109/10731191003776736

Zhong, R., Wang, H., Wu, X., Cao, Y., He, Z., He, Y., et al. (2013). *In vitro* investigation of the effect of plasticizers on the blood compatibility of medical grade plasticized poly (vinyl chloride). *J. Mater. Sci. Mater. Med.* 24, 1985–1992. doi: 10.1007/s10856-013-4950-1

8

Enhanced Anti-Tumor of Pep-1 Modified Superparamagnetic Iron Oxide/PTX Loaded Polymer Nanoparticles

Baoyan Wang[1†], Weijun Wu[1†], Hongjin Lu[2], Zhi Wang[3] and Hongliang Xin[2]*

[1] Nanjing Drum Tower Hospital, The Affiliated Hospital of Nanjing University Medical School, Nanjing, China, [2] Department of Pharmaceutics, School of Pharmacy, Nanjing Medical University, Nanjing, China, [3] Department of Pharmacy, The Second Affiliated Hospital of Nanjing Medical University, Nanjing, China

***Correspondence:**
Hongliang Xin
xhl@njmu.edu.cn

† These authors have contributed equally to this work

Superparamagnetic iron-oxide nanoparticle (SPION) has gained tremendous attention for drug delivery applications due to their unique properties. In this study, we developed a dual targeted delivery system with paclitaxel (PTX) and SPION co-loaded PLGA nanoparticles, modified with Pep-1 peptide (Pep-NP-SPION/PTX), to achieve magnetic targeting and active targeting for tumor treatment. SPION was synthesized by a co-precipitation method and was then encapsulated with PTX simultaneously into PLGA nanoparticles. After that, the non-complex was conjugated with Pep-1 through chemical modification. The resulting Pep-NP-SPION/PTX showed a spherical morphology and an average size of 100 nm. The enhancement cellular uptake of Pep-NP-SPION was demonstrated in *in vitro* through cell experiments. The IC_{50} value of Pep-NP-SPION/PTX and NP-SPION/PTX was determined to be 10.2 and 19.4 μg/mL, respectively. A biodistribution study showed that obvious higher accumulations of Pep-NP-SPION was observed in tumors, compared with that of non-targeting nanocomposites. Moreover, under the condition of a magnetic field, both NP-SPION and Pep-NP-SPION exhibited much higher tumor distribution. Furthermore, Pep-NP-SPION/PTX presented desirable *in vivo* anti-tumor effects based on active targeting and magnetic targeting characteristics. Altogether, Pep-NP-SPION/PTX can offer magnetic targeting and receptor mediated targeting to enhance the anti-tumor outcome.

Keywords: tumor, drug delivery system, superparamagnetic iron oxide nanoparticle, interleukin-13 receptor α2, dual targeting nanocarrier

INTRODUCTION

Current tumor chemotherapy still faces a major problem with the of lack of selectivity of drugs on tumor cells, which leads to a narrow therapeutic index of most anti-tumor drugs (Wong et al., 2016). As a result, the achievement of an adequate therapeutic effect requires a high concentration of anti-tumor drugs, which in turn enhances the systematic toxicity. Thus, in order to reduce the toxicity of a chemotherapy drug at its minimum dose, specific nanoparticulate drug delivery systems, such as nanoparticle, liposome and polymeric micelle, could provide a non-invasive treatment strategy due to its passive targeting properties (Huang et al., 2016; Muralidharan et al., 2017;

Roberts et al., 2017). However, these conventional drug delivery systems lack the capability of active targeting for tumor section.

Recently, superparamagnetic iron-oxide nanoparticles (SPION) consisting of cores made of iron oxides, have been considered to be attractive in cancer theranostic applications, since they can be delivered to the required tissue through an external magnetic field (Hachani et al., 2016). Due to the superparamagnetism, a high saturation field and a high field irreversibility, SPION has been widely used for various biological applications (Li et al., 2016). Moreover, SPIONs could lose their magnetization and become highly dispersed even after the removal of the magnetic field (Nagesh et al., 2016). However, biological application of SPION was limited because of the high surface hydrophobicity, making them susceptible to being ingested and eliminated by mononuclear phagocyte systems (MPS). In order to prolong the circulation time, it is necessary to modify the surface of SPION by amphiphilic copolymer coating to convert hydrophobic SPION into hydrophilic ones (Mirsadeghi et al., 2016; Silva et al., 2016).

Under an external magnetic field, SPION-encapsulated polymer nanoparticles could easily reach around the tumor section. In order to increase the active targeting of nanoparticles and uptake by tumor cells, receptor-mediated endocytosis could serve as a versatile targeting strategy *via* linking nanoparticles with multifunctional ligands to construct a potentially multiple targeting drug nanocarrier (Zhao et al., 2015; Rabiej et al., 2016; Shen et al., 2018). It is reported that various receptors are over-expressed on tumor cells, including folate receptor, neuropilin-1 receptor and transferrin receptor (Wang et al., 2011; Du et al., 2015; Song et al., 2015). Based on these receptors, drug delivery systems have been modified with corresponding targeting ligands and explored to deliver drugs through receptor-mediated endocytosis. The interleukin 13 receptor α2 (IL-13Rα2) is a subtype of the interleukin-13 receptor family, which is over-expressed on tumor cells (Mintz et al., 2002; Balyasnikova et al., 2012). It has been reported that IL-13Rα2, acting as a decoy receptor, has an intimate relationship with the progression of a tumor and can undergo internalization after binding to ligands (Kawakami et al., 2001). This property indicates that IL-13Rα2 could serve as a promising targeted moiety for anti-tumor drug delivery.

Pep-1 peptide (CGEMGWVRC) that was screened by the phage display library, could bind to IL-13Rα2 with high affinity and specificity and could be exploited to target ligand to tumor cells (Pandya et al., 2012). In our previous study, we demonstrated that Pep-1 conjugated paclitaxel (PTX) loaded nanoparticles, could be internalized into tumor cells *via* IL-13Rα2 mediated endocytosis (Wang et al., 2014). However, the accumulation of the targeted drug delivery system in the tumor tissue was still rather low and could only be by enhanced penetration and retention (EPR) effects (Wilhelm et al., 2016). Therefore, we aimed at developing PTX and SPION co-loaded polymer nanoparticles with Pep-1 peptide modification as a dual targeting nanocarrier (designated as Pep-NP-SPION/PTX) for tumor treatment in this study. SPION was prepared using a co-precipitation method and loaded into PEG-PLGA polymer nanoparticles that were modified with Pep-1 peptide to form Pep-NP-SPION/PTX (**Figure 1A**). As showed in **Figure 1B**, after intravenous (i.v.) injection, Pep-NP-SPION/PTX was expected to accumulate at the tumor tissue in the presence of an external magnetic field and then be internalized into tumor cells through IL-13Rα2 mediated endocytosis, which would reduce the uptake of Pep-NP-SPION/PTX by the MPS and enhance the anti-tumor efficiency of PTX. These physical-chemical properties of the dual targeted nanocarrier were also systematically characterized. Furthermore, the *in vitro* biological targeted capability of Pep-NP-SPION/PTX was investigated. Finally, the *in vitro* and *in vivo* anti-tumor effect of Pep-NP-SPION/PTX was studied using a cell and subcutaneous xenograft tumor mice model, respectively.

MATERIALS AND METHODS

Materials

Qleic acid, Iron(II) chloride, iron(III) chloride and ammonium hydroxide were purchased from Sinopharm Chemical Reagent Co., Ltd. (China). Methoxyl poly(ethylene glycol)-co-poly(D,L-lactic-co-glycolic acid) copolymer(MePEG-PLGA, 40 KDa) and Maleimidyl-poly(ethylene glycol)-co-poly(D,L-lactic- coglycolic acid) copolymer(Male-PEG-PLGA, 41.5 KDa) were purchased from Daigang Biomaterial Co., Ltd. (Jinan, China). PTX was purchased from Zelang Medical Technology Co., Ltd. (Nanjing, China). 3-(4, 5-dimethylthiazol-2-yl)-2, 5-diphenyltetrazolium bromide (MTT) was purchased from Beyotime Biotechnology Co., Ltd. (Nantong, China). Penicillin-streptomycin, RPMI 1640 medium, fetal bovine serum (FBS) and 0.25% (w/v) trypsin solution were obtained from Gibco BRL (Gaithersburg, MD, United States).

Cell Line

The C6 cell line was obtained from the Institute of Biochemistry and Cell Biology, Shanghai Institutes for Biological Sciences, Chinese Academy of Sciences (Shanghai, China). The cell line was cultured in a RPMI 1640 medium, supplemented with 10% FBS, 1% penicillin and 100 mg/mL streptomycin sulfate. Cells were cultured in incubators maintained at 37°C with 5% CO_2. All experiments were performed in the logarithmic phase of cell growth.

Animals

Mice (male, 4–5 weeks, 20–25 g) were supplied by the Department of Experimental Animals, Nanjing Medical University (Nanjing, China) and maintained under standard a housing environment. All animal experiments were performed in accordance with protocols and evaluated and approved by the ethics committee of Nanjing Medical University.

Synthesis of SPION Coated With Oleic Acid (OA-SPION)

Superparamagnetic iron-oxide nanoparticle was prepared by co-precipitating ferrous and ferric salts in an alkaline medium (Schleich et al., 2013). Briefly, 0.10 g of $FeCl_2{\cdot}4H_2O$ and 0.27 g of $FeCl_3{\cdot}6H_2O$ were added into 50 mL PEG600, which was placed

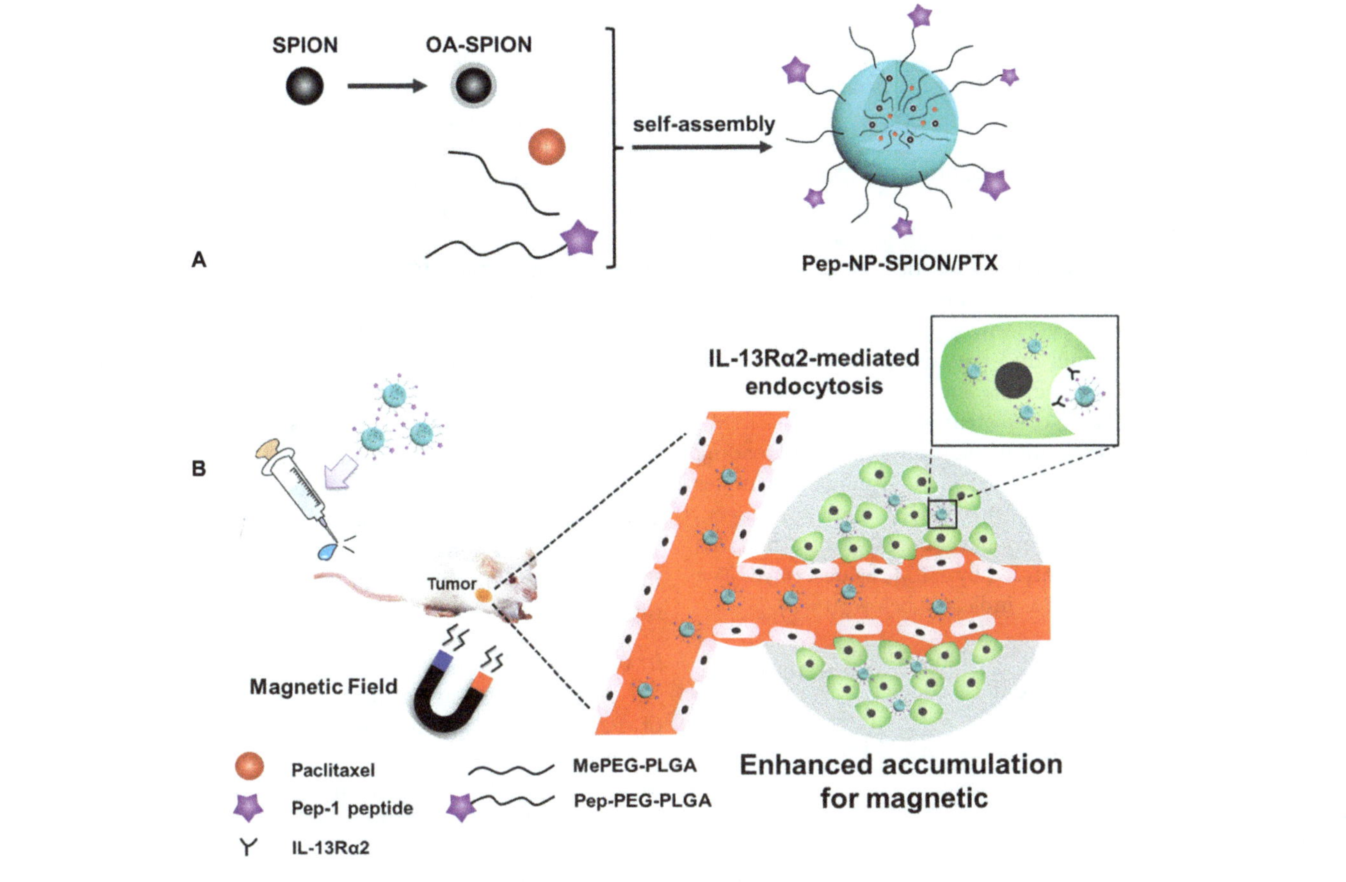

FIGURE 1 | Schematic design of Pep-NP-SPION/PTX. The main components and preparation of the Pep-NP-SPION/PTX **(A)**. After intravenous injection, Pep-NP-SPION/PTX targets to tumor tissue *via* external magnetic field and then is internalized into tumor cells through IL-13Rα2 mediated endocytosis **(B)**.

under a vacuum overnight at 40°C to degas. The mixture was then heated to 125°C under nitrogen protection. Then, 2 mL ammonium hydroxide was added, and the mixture was reheated to 125°C. 5 min later, 20 mL of oleic acid was added into the solution at 125°C and the mixture was kept at this temperature for another 30 min. Finally, the black precipitate was separated by an external magnet and washed three times with absolute ethanol and ultrapure water to remove the unreacted reagent, respectively. Dry SPION coated with oleic acid was prepared through freeze-drying for further use.

Preparation of Pep-NP-SPION/PTX

Paclitaxel and SPION loaded PLGA-based nanoparticles were prepared *via* an emulsion/solvent evaporation method (Wilhelm et al., 2016). Firstly, the conjugation of Pep-1 peptide to PEG-PLGA copolymer *via* the reaction of maleimide with thiol group was carried out as previously reported (Wilhelm et al., 2016). Then, 19 mg MePEG-PLGA and 2 mg Pep-PEG-PLGA polymer were dissolved in 1 mL dichloromethane (DCM) containing PTX (1 mg/mL) and OA-SPION (Fe concentration: 4 mg/mL). Then the mixture was added to a 2 mL 1% (w/v) sodium cholate aqueous solution, which was finally sonicated using a probe sonicator (Xin Zhi Biotechnology Co., Ltd., China) for 5 min at 190 W output. The suspension was added drop-wisely into 10 mL 1% (w/v) sodium cholate solution under moderate stirring. A rotary evaporator was used to evaporate the redundant DCM at 40°C. The solutions were centrifuged at 13500 *g* for 40 min to remove the excess excipient. After being washed three times by water, the Pep-NP-SPION/PTX was collected and re-dispersed in PBS for further use.

Characterization of Pep-NP-SPION/PTX

Morphology, Particle Size and Zeta Potential of Pep-NP-SPION/PTX

The morphology of Pep-NP-SPION/PTX was characterized by the transmission electron microscope (TEM, Philips CM 100) operating at a voltage of 100 kV. The particle size and zeta potential of nanoparticles were assessed by dynamic light scattering (DLS, Zs90, Malvern, United Kingdom).

Determination of SPION Loading Content

The Fe content was measured using the phenanthroline spectrophotometric method. Lyophilized nanoparticles were dissolved in DCM, and then dried under nitrogen. The residue was dissolved with 10% (v/v) HCl solution. The yellow solution was combined with aqueous solutions of hydroxylamine hydrochloride (10%, w/v) and sodium acetate buffer solution (pH = 5, 1 mol/L). Then 0.1% phenanthroline solution was added. After 0.5 h, the absorbance at 510 nm was measured and the Fe content was determined based on a comparison of a standard curve.

Encapsulation Efficiency and Loading Capacity of PTX

The amount of PTX was measured by high performance liquid chromatography (HPLC) with UV detection at 227 nm (LC-10AT, SHIMADZU, Japan). The mobile phase consisted of acetonitrile and water (47:53, v/v) with a gradient elution pumped at a flow rate of 1.0 mL/min and the column was maintained at 30°C. The calibration curve was linear in the range of 0.1–100 μg/mL with a correlation coefficient of $R^2 = 0.9998$.

To determine the encapsulation efficiency (EE%) and loading capacity (LC%) of Pep-NP-SPION/PTX, the lyophilized samples were dissolved in DCM, and then dried under nitrogen. The residue was dissolved in mobile phase solution and the concentration of PTX was analyzed by HPLC as described. The EE% and LC% were calculated as indicated below ($n = 3$).

$$\text{EE\%} = \frac{\text{Amount of PTX in the nanoparticles}}{\text{Total amount of PTX added}} \times 100\%$$

$$\text{LC\%} = \frac{\text{Amount of PTX in the nanoparticles}}{\text{Nanoparticles weight}} \times 100\%$$

In vitro Release

The *in vitro* release kinetics of PTX from Pep-NP-SPION/PTX was measured by a standard dialysis method in PBS (0.04 M, pH 7.4) or HAc-NaAc buffer (0.04 M, pH 5.0) containing 0.1% (w/v) Tween-80 at 37°C. Briefly, nanoparticles were suspended in 1 mL of mediator solution and placed in a dialysis bag (MWCO 3000). The dialysis bag was immersed in 30 mL of the release medium which was shaken at 37°C. At predetermined time intervals, a portion of 0.3 mL dialysate was harvested, and the same volume of fresh mediator solution was added. The PTX concentration of samples was determined by HPLC as described above.

In vitro Evaluation

In vitro Cellular Uptake

C6 cells were seeded into a 24-well plate at the density of 1×10^5 cells per well. After 24 h incubation, the cells were incubated with NP-SPION and Pep-NP-SPION at different concentrations (Fe concentration: 25 and 50 μg/mL) at 37°C for 1 h, respectively. After that, the cells were washed three times with cold PBS and fixed with 4% formaldehyde for 10 min. Then, these cells were stained with Pearls' reagent (2% potassium ferrocyanide/6% HCl: 1/1) for 30 min. Finally, after washing by PBS for three times, the uptake of nanoparticles in the C6 cells was observed using a microscope.

In vitro Cytotoxicity

An MTT assay was used to evaluate the cell cytotoxicity of Pep-NP-SPION/PTX. C6 cells were seeded into 96-well plates at the density of 5000 cells/well and incubated at 37°C in a 5% CO_2 atmosphere, and then incubated with Taxol®, NP-SPION/PTX and Pep-NP-SPION/PTX at different PTX concentration (1, 5, 10, and 20 μg/mL) after 24 h, respectively. All the concentrations of Fe used were based on the corresponding PTX concentrations (Fe concentrations: 3.9, 19.6, 39.2, and

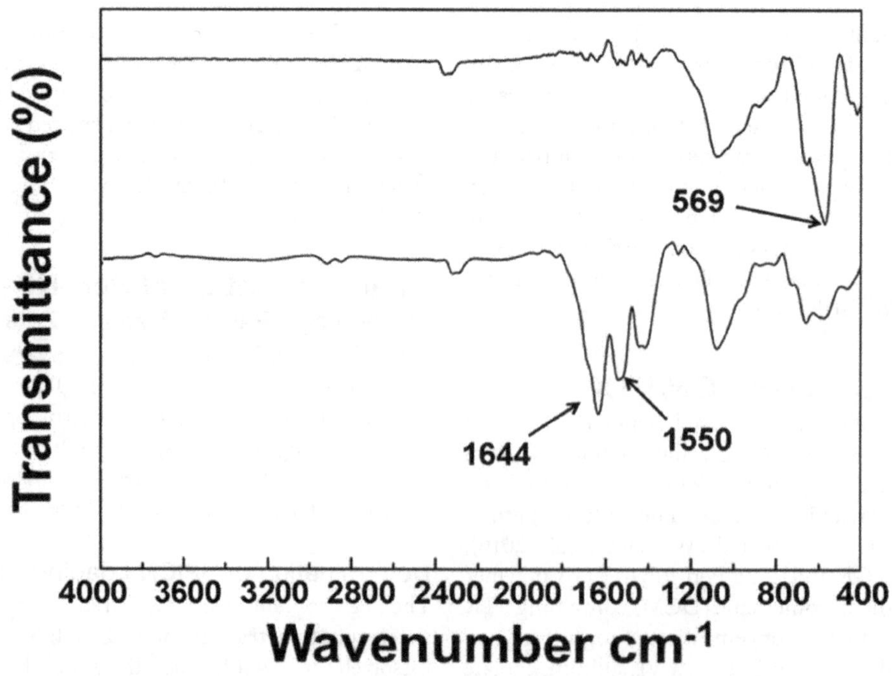

FIGURE 2 | FTIR spectra of SPION and OA-SPION.

78.4 μg/mL). After 48 h, the culture medium was discarded and 20 μL MTT solution was added into each well and incubated for additional 4 h. Then the unreacted dye was removed and 200 μL of DMSO was added to each well. Finally, the optical density was measured by a microplate reader at wavelength of 490 nm.

In vivo Evaluation

Biodistribution of Pep-NP-SPION/PTX in Tumor Tissue

C6 cells (3×10^6 cells suspended in 100 μL PBS) were injected into the armpit of the right anterior limbs of mice subcutaneously. When the tumor volume reached about 300 cm^3, the mice were divided into four groups randomly, then intravenously administrated with NP-SPION/PTX and Pep-NP-SPION/PTX (Fe dose of 15 mg/kg), respectively. The influence of the external magnetic field was also evaluated. 2 h after injection, the mice were sacrificed, and the tumor tissues were harvested and fixed in 4% paraformaldehyde. After paraffin embedding, the tumors were cut into 5 μm and stained with Prussian blue staining.

In vivo Anti-tumor Efficacy

In vivo tumor growth inhibition was carried out to evaluate the anti-tumor efficacy of Pep-NP-SPION/PTX. Subcutaneous xenograft tumor mice model was established as described above. With the tumor volume reached about 100 mm^3, the mice were divided into six groups randomly, and then intravenously administrated with saline, Taxol®, NP-SPION/PTX and Pep-NP-SPION/PTX (PTX dose: 4.5 mg/kg, Fe dose: 15.6 mg/kg), respectively. The influence of external magnetic field was also evaluated. The formulation was given every other day for four injections. 15 days later, the mice were sacrificed with tumor collection and tumor volume was calculated (the formula: $\pi/6 \times$ larger diameter $\times$ smaller diameter^2).

RESULTS

Synthesis of SPION Coated With Oleic Acid

In order to improve the hydrophobicity and dispersibility of SPION, their surfaces were conjugated by oleic acid through physical adsorption. The FTIR spectra of SPION and OA-SPION are shown in **Figure 2**. The absorption peak at 569 cm^{-1} was the characteristic absorption peak of Fe-O bond. The spectrum of OA-SPION showed a sharp absorption peak at 1644 cm^{-1}, which was attributed to the C = O stretching vibrational absorption of oleic acid. However, the characteristic vibrational absorptions were not present in the spectrum of SPION. These results

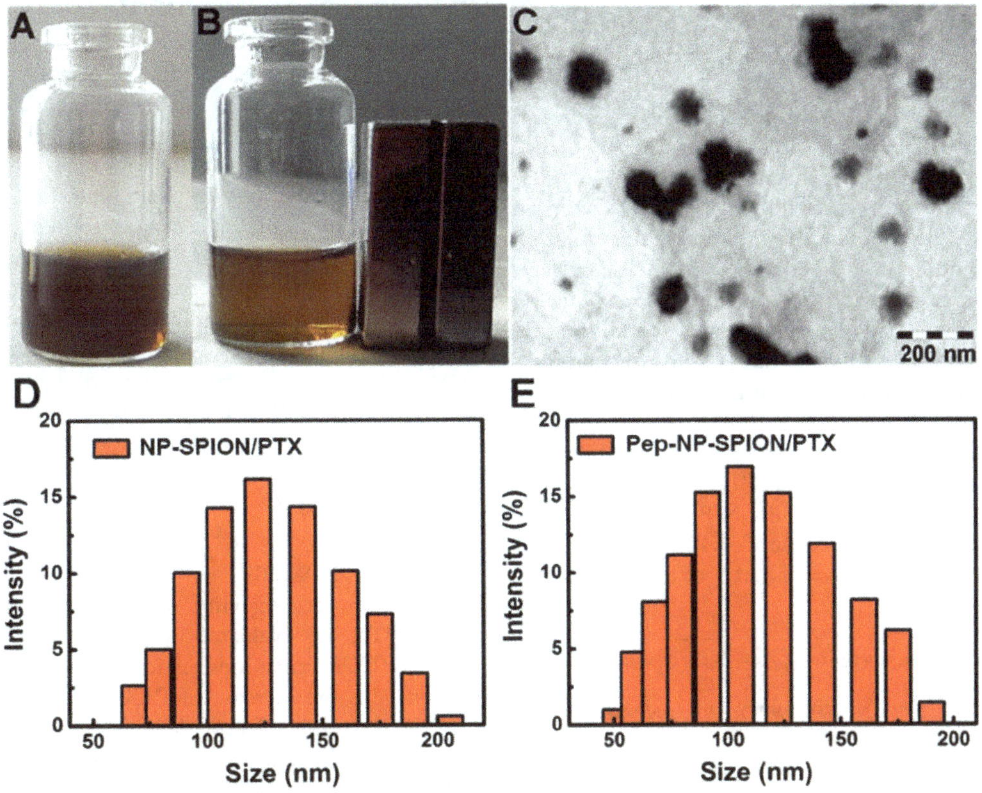

FIGURE 3 | Characterization of Pep-NP-SPION/PTX. Pep-NP-SPION/PTX solution **(A)** or absorption under external magnetic field **(B)**; TEM image of Pep-NP-SPION/PTX **(C)** and size distribution of NP-SPION/PTX **(D)** and Pep-NP-SPION/PTX **(E)**.

demonstrated the successful modification of oleic acid on the surface of SPION.

Characterization of Pep-NP-SPION/PTX

Pep-NP-SPION/PTX was prepared *via* an emulsion/solvent evaporation method. As shown in **Figure 3**, Pep-NP-SPION/PTX was well-dispersed in water and showed a brown color before magnetic separation. When exposed to a magnetic field, the solution become more and more colorless and the nanoparticles were collected near the magnet. Therefore, the magnetic property of SPION was not affected by the encapsulation of PEG-PLGA.

The morphology and size of Pep-NP-SIPION/PTX was characterized by TEM and DLS, respectively. A TEM photograph showed that Pep-NP-SPION/PTX was uniformly spherical and of regular shape with a narrow size distribution. As shown in **Table 1**, the particle size of NP-SPION/PTX and Pep-NP-SPION/PTX were 129.8 ± 1.2 nm and 101.6 ± 1.0 nm, respectively. The particle size difference between NP-SPION/PTX and Pep-NP-SPION/PTX might be due to the modification of hydrophilic Pep-1 peptides, which enhanced the hydrophilicity of polymer nanoparticles. The zeta potential of NP-SPION/PTX and Pep-NP-SPION/PTX were below −20 mV.

The PTX LC% and EE% of Pep-NP-SPION/PTX were 3.54 ± 0.14% and 81.30 ± 3.50%, respectively, compared with 3.22 ± 0.86% and 66.85 ± 1.84% for NP-SPION/PTX. The change of encapsulation efficiency and loading capacity might be attributed to the modification of polymer materials with Pep-1 peptide. The iron loading of NP-SPION/PTX and Pep-NP-SPION/PTX was 12.41 ± 2.75 mg and 13.53 ± 3.38 mg/100 mg polymer, respectively.

In vitro Drug Release

The release profiles of PTX-loaded magnetic nanoparticles under different pH conditions are presented in **Figure 4**. Tween-80 was used to increase the solubility of PTX in a buffer solution and to avoid the binding of PTX to the nanoparticle surface. Herein, the drug release behavior was studied under a simulated physiological environment (pH 7.4) and an acidic condition (pH 5.0) because of the lower pH value in tumor tissues, due to excess lactic acid produced by hypoxia and acidic intracellular organelles (Xu et al., 2012).

Paclitaxel-loaded magnetic nanoparticles all exhibited an initial burst release profile with total PTX releases of about 60% before 12 h. After 72 h, NP-SPION/PTX and Pep-NP-SPION/PTX showed a total drug release of 63.4 and 65.8% of PTX at pH 7.4, respectively, while 82.3 and 87.1% of the PTX in PBS

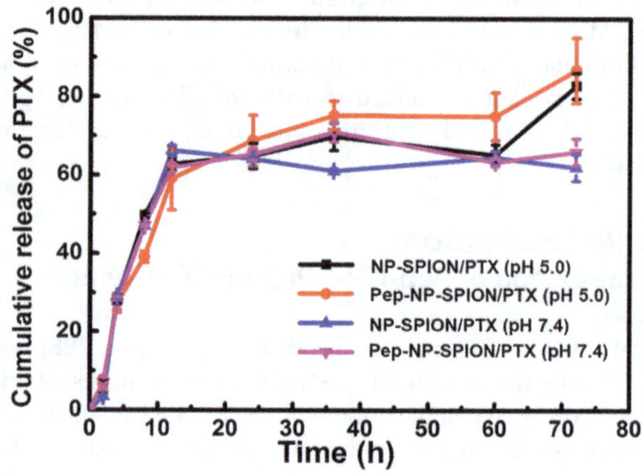

FIGURE 4 | PTX release profiles from NP-SPION/PTX and Pep-NP-SPION/PTX in HAc-NaAc (pH 5.0) and PBS (pH 7.4) buffer solution containing 0.1% (w/v) Tween-80.

(pH 5.0), respectively. These results suggested that solution pH could affect the release pattern of PTX from nanoparticles. The pH responsive release of the dual targeted nanoparticles may be beneficial for enhancing the anti-tumor efficacy of the PTX in the acidic tumor microenvironment.

TABLE 1 | Characterization of NP-SPION/PTX and Pep-NP-SPION/PTX.

	NP-SPION/PTX	Pep-NP-SPION/PTX
Particle size (nm)	129.8 ± 1.2	101.6 ± 1.0
Zeta potential (mV)	−21.9 ± 0.5	−21.2 ± 0.5
Encapsulation efficiency (EE%)	66.85 ± 1.84	81.30 ± 3.50
Loading capacity (LC%)	3.22 ± 0.86	3.54 ± 0.14
Iron loading (mg/100 mg polymer)	12.41 ± 2.75	13.53 ± 3.38

In vitro Cell Experiment

In vitro Cellular Uptake

It has been reported that IL-13Rα2 was upregulated in C6 cell line (Daines et al., 2006), so the C6 cell was used as the cell model to investigate the *in vitro* uptake of Pep-NP-SPION in this study. The cellular uptake of Pep-NP-SPION was studied quantitatively by Prussian blue staining. The number of blue granules within C6 cells was related to the nanoparticle concentration. As shown in **Figure 5**, the blue granules intensity was increased with the increase of iron concentrations ranging from 25 to 50 μg/mL after 1 h incubation, which indicated that the cellular uptake of Pep-NP-SPION exhibited a concentration-dependent mode. Moreover, the cellular uptake of Pep-NP-SPION was obviously higher than that of NP-SPION. These results implied that the modification of Pep-1 peptide could enhance the cellular uptake of nanoparticles through receptor-mediated endocytosis.

In vitro Cytotoxicity

The *in vitro* cell viability of NP-SPION/PTX and Pep-NP-SPION/PTX was evaluated by MTT assay. The cytotoxicity of various PTX formulations exhibited a concentration-dependent pattern with the increase of PTX concentration ranging from 1 to 20 μg/mL. Different degrees of cytotoxicity were found in all the PTX formulations. As shown in **Figure 6**, the cell viability of Pep-NP-SPION/PTX was even lower than 50% at PTX concentration of 10 μg/ml. The IC_{50} value of Pep-NP-SPION/PTX and NP-SPION/PTX is 10.2 and 19.4 μg/mL, respectively.

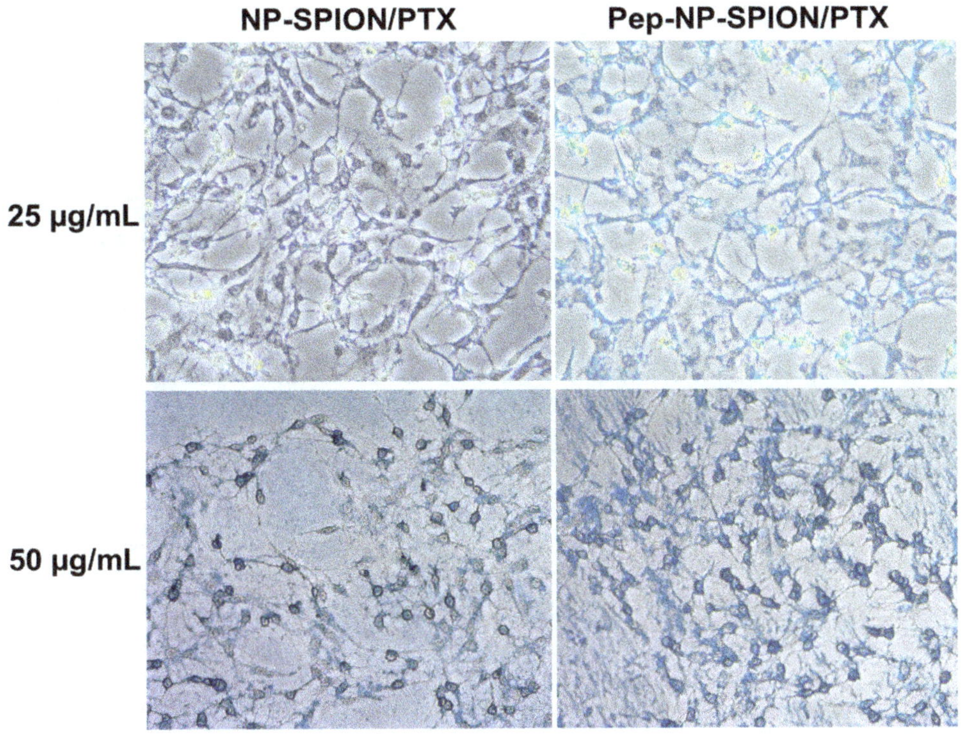

FIGURE 5 | Prussian blue staining images of C6 cells after 1 h incubation with NP-SPION/PTX and Pep-NP-SPION/PTX with Fe concentration at 25 and 50 μg/mL. Original magnification: 200×.

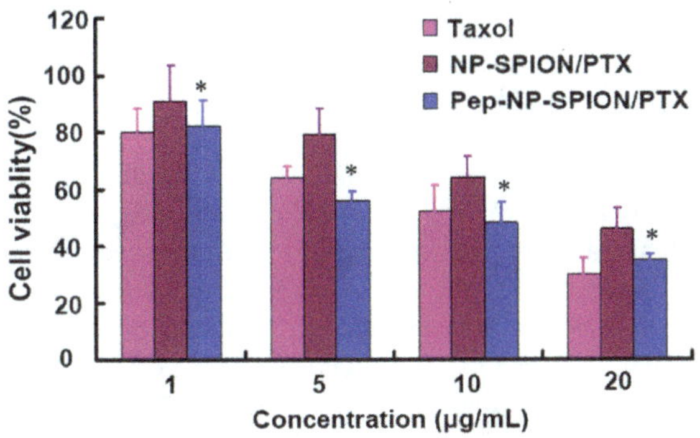

FIGURE 6 | *In vitro* cytotoxicity of Taxol®, NP-SPION/PTX and Pep-NP-SPION/PTX at various concentrations at 48 h. Data represented mean ± SD ($n = 3$). *$p < 0.05$ significantly lower than that of NP-PTX.

Biodistribution of Pep-NP-SPION/PTX in Tumor Tissue

The *in vivo* tumor targeting capability of magnetic nanoparticles was studied qualitatively by Prussian blue staining. Iron oxide was indicated as blue and cell nucleus as red. As shown in **Figure 7**, in the presence of an external magnetic field, both NP-SPION/PTX and Pep-NP-SPION/PTX exhibited much higher tumor distribution than those without magnetic field intervention, which indicated that the constructed nanoparticles had an attractive magnetic targeting character for improving tumor distribution. Moreover, compared with the NP-SPION/PTX group, Pep-NP-SPION/PTX showed an obvious higher distribution no matter whether an external magnetic field was added, which revealed that the modification of Pep-1 peptide could accelerate the accumulation of nanoparticles into the tumor section *via* IL-13Rα2 mediated endocytosis. Altogether, based on the active targeting and magnetic targeting, Pep-NP-SPION/PTX can be used as a potential dual targeting nanocarrier for the treatment of tumors.

In vivo Anti-tumor Efficacy

In this study, mice bearing subcutaneous tumor xenograft were used to evaluate the *in vivo* anti-tumor efficacy of Pep-NP-SPION/PTX. The mice were intravenously injected with Taxol, NP-SPION/PTX and Pep-NP-SPION/PTX (PTX dose: 4.5 mg/kg, Fe dose: 15.6 mg/kg) every other day for four consecutive administrations with tumor sizes recorded every 3 days, respectively. As shown in **Figure 8**, the tumor size of the saline group was obviously all larger than that of the PTX formulations. In the initial days, there was no significant difference in tumor size among these groups. At the experimental terminal, the tumor size of all PTX formulations followed the order: Pep-NP-SPION/PTX with magnetic field < Pep-NP-SPION/PTX < NP-SPION/PTX with magnetic field < NP-SPION/PTX < Taxol < Saline. These results showed that the modification of Pep-1 peptide could improve the anti-tumor efficacy of nanoparticles through IL-13Rα2-mediated

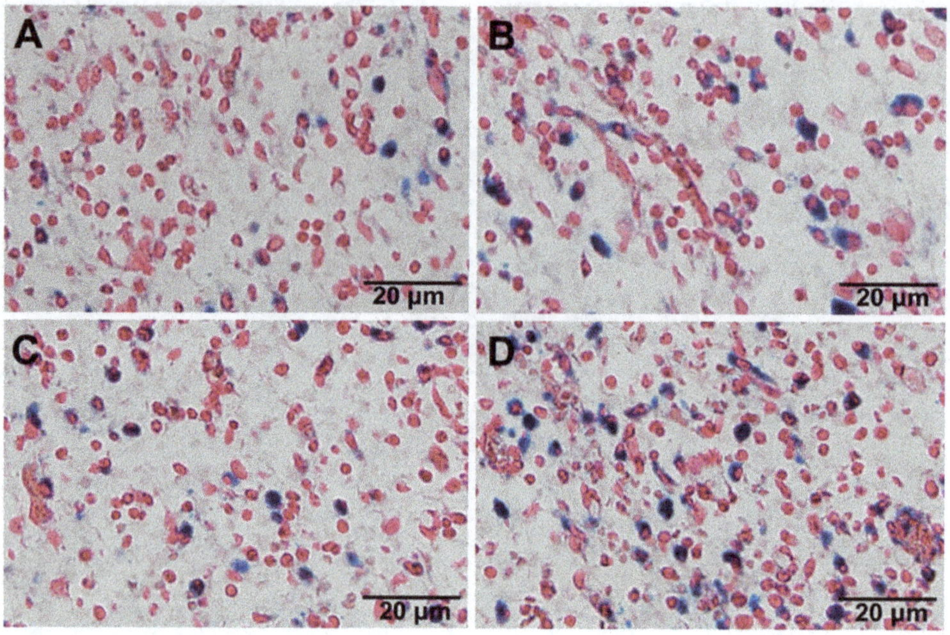

FIGURE 7 | The distribution of nanoparticles in tumor section visualized by Prussian blue staining. Histological sections were extracted at 2 h after intravenous injection of NP-SPION/PTX **(A)**, NP-SPION/PTX with magnetic field **(B)**, Pep-NP-SPION/PTX **(C)**, and Pep- NP-SPION/PTX with external magnetic field **(D)**.

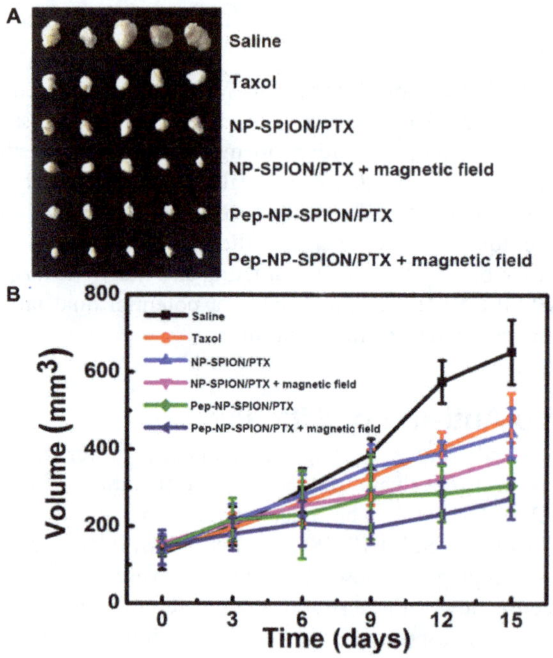

FIGURE 8 | Anti-tumor efficacy of Taxol®, NP-SPION/PTX and Pep-NP-SPION/PTX on tumor xenograft mice. Tumor xenografts alignment of each group taken out from the sacrificed mice at the end point **(A)** and tumor growth volume vs. time **(B)**. (n = 5).

endocytosis, consistent with our previous study. Moreover, the encapsulation of SPION endowed nanoparticles with the magnetic targeting property and enhanced the anti-tumor efficacy with the magnetic field. Together, Pep-NP-SPION/PTX constructed in this study could offer a potential magnetic targeting and receptor mediated targeting to enhance the anti-tumor efficacy for tumor treatment.

CONCLUSION

In this study, we successfully constructed PTX and SPION co-loaded polymer nanoparticles with Pep-1 peptide modification as a dual targeted nanocarrier for tumor treatment. The cellular uptake of Pep-NP-SPION/PTX showed a concentration-dependent manner and significantly enhanced than that of unmodified NP-SPION/PTX. Pep-NP-SPION/PTX exhibited cytotoxicity comparable to Taxol at the PTX concentrations ranging from 1 to 20 μg/mL *in vitro* cell experiments. Furthermore, Pep-NP-SPION/PTX showed a satisfactory tumor accumulation and the magnetic field significantly enhanced the bio-distribution of nanoparticles in the tumor section. More importantly, the *in vivo* anti-tumor efficacy showed that Pep-NP-SPION/PTX exhibited desirable anti-tumor efficacy and the magnetic field could also enhance the anti-tumor efficacy. Altogether, these results indicate that the modification of Pep-1 peptide could enhance the active targeting property through receptor-mediated endocytosis and the encapsulation of SPION which obviously improves the physical targeting property of nanoparticles under an external magnetic field. The physical magnetic targeting and IL-13Rα2 mediated active targeting characteristics could synergistically increase the targeted efficiency for a tumor. Therefore, Pep-NP-SPION/PTX could serve as a potential dual targeting nanocarrier for tumor therapy.

AUTHOR CONTRIBUTIONS

HX designed the experiments. BW and WW performed the experiments. BW and HX wrote the main manuscript. HL and ZW prepared the figures and tables. All authors reviewed the manuscript.

FUNDING

This work was supported by the grants from the National Natural Science Foundation of China (31671018), the Natural Science Foundation of Jiangsu Province-Excellent Young Scientist Fund (BK20160096), the 2016 Qing Lan Program of Jiangsu Province, and the 2017 Six Talent Peaks Project of Jiangsu Province.

ACKNOWLEDGMENTS

The authors acknowledge the support from the School of Pharmacy, Fudan University and the Open Project Program of Key Lab of Smart Drug Delivery (Fudan University), Ministry of Education, China (SDD2012-4).

REFERENCES

Balyasnikova, I. V., Wainwright, D. A., Solomaha, E., Lee, G., Han, Y., Thaci, B., et al. (2012). Characterization and immunotherapeutic implications for a novel antibody targeting interleukin (IL)-13 receptor α2. *J. Biol. Chem.* 287, 30215–30227. doi: 10.1074/jbc.M112.370015

Daines, M. O., Tabata, Y., Walker, B. A., Chen, W., Warrier, M. R., Basu, S., et al. (2006). Level of expression of IL-13Rα2 impacts receptor distribution and IL-13 signaling. *J. Immunol.* 176, 7495–7501. doi: 10.4049/jimmunol.176.12.7495

Du, W. W., Fan, Y. C., He, B., Zheng, N., Yuan, L., Dai, W. B., et al. (2015). Bionano interactions of MCF-7 breast tumor cells with a transferrin receptor targeted nanoparticle. *Mol. Pharmacol.* 12, 1467–1476. doi: 10.1021/mp500796d

Hachani, R., Lowdell, M., Birchall, M., Hervault, A., Mertz, D., Begin-Colin, S., et al. (2016). Correction: polyol synthesis, functionalisation, and biocompatibility studies of superparamagnetic iron oxide nanoparticles as potential MRI contrast agents. *Nanoscale* 8, 3278–3287. doi: 10.1039/c5nr03867g

Huang, W. C., Chen, S. H., Chiang, W. H., Huang, C. W., Lo, C. L., Chern, C. S., et al. (2016). Tumor microenvironment-responsive nanoparticle delivery of chemotherapy for enhanced selective cellular uptake and transportation within tumor. *Biomacromolecules* 17, 3883–3892. doi: 10.1021/acs.biomac.6b00956

Kawakami, K., Taguchi, J., Murata, T., and Puri, R. K. (2001). The interleukin-13 receptor α2 chain: an essential component for binding and internalization but not for interleukin-13-induced signal transduction through the STAT6 pathway. *Blood* 97, 2673–2679. doi: 10.1182/blood.V97.9.2673

Li, L., Gao, F. M., Jiang, W. W., Wu, X. L., Cai, Y. Y., Tang, J. T., et al. (2016). Folic acid-conjugated superparamagnetic iron oxide nanoparticles for tumor-targeting MR imaging. *Drug Deliv.* 23, 1726–1733. doi: 10.3109/10717544.2015.1006404

Mintz, A., Gibo, D. M., Slagle-Webb, B., Christensen, N. D., and Debinski, W. (2002). IL-13Ralpha2 is a glioma-restricted receptor for interleukin-13. *Neoplasia* 4, 388–399. doi: 10.1038/sj.neo.7900234

Mirsadeghi, S., Shanehsazzadeh, S., Atyabi, F., and Dinarvand, R. (2016). Effect of PEGylated superparamagnetic iron oxide nanoparticles (SPIONs) under magnetic field on amyloid beta fibrillation process. *Mater. Sci. Eng. C Mater. Biol. Appl.* 59, 390–397. doi: 10.1016/j.msec.2015.10.026

Muralidharan, R., Babu, A., Amreddy, N., Srivastava, A., Chen, A., Zhao, Y. D., et al. (2017). Tumor-targeted nanoparticle delivery of HuR siRNA inhibits lung tumor growth *In Vitro* and *In Vivo* by disrupting the oncogenic activity of the RNA-binding protein HuR. *Mol. Cancer Ther.* 16, 1470–1486. doi: 10.1158/1535-7163.MCT-17-0134

Nagesh, P. K. B., Johnson, N. R., Boya, V. K. N., Chowdhury, P., Othman, S. F., Khalilzad-Sharghi, V., et al. (2016). PSMA targeted docetaxel-loaded superparamagnetic iron oxide nanoparticles for prostate cancer. *Colloids Surf. B Biointerfaces* 144, 8–20. doi: 10.1016/j.colsurfb.2016.03.071

Pandya, H., Gibo, D. M., Garg, S., Kridel, S., and Debinski, W. (2012). An interleukin 13 receptor α2-specific peptide homes to human Glioblastoma multiforme xenografts. *Neuro Oncol.* 14, 6–18. doi: 10.1093/neuonc/nor141

Rabiej, V. K., Pflanzner, T., Wagner, T., Goetze, K., Storck, S. E., Eble, J. A., et al. (2016). Low density lipoprotein receptor-related protein 1 mediated endocytosis of β1-integrin influences cell adhesion and cell migration. *Exp. Cell Res.* 340, 102–115. doi: 10.1016/j.yexcr.2015.11.020

Roberts, C. M., Shahin, S. A., Wen, W., Finlay, J. B., Dong, J., Wang, R., et al. (2017). Nanoparticle delivery of siRNA against TWIST to reduce drug resistance and tumor growth in ovarian cancer models. *Nanomedicine* 13, 965–976. doi: 10.1016/j.nano.2016.11.010

Schleich, N., Sibret, P., Danhier, P., Ucakar, B., Laurent, S., Muller, R. N., et al. (2013). Dual anticancer drug/superparamagnetic iron oxide-loaded PLGA-based nanoparticles for cancer therapy and magnetic resonance imaging. *Int. J. Pharm.* 447, 94–101. doi: 10.1016/j.ijpharm.2013.02.042

Shen, Z. Q., Ye, H. L., Kröger, M., and Li, Y. (2018). Aggregation of polyethylene glycol polymers suppresses receptor-mediated endocytosis of PEgylated liposomes. *Nanoscale* 10, 4545–4560. doi: 10.1039/c7nr09011k

Silva, A. H., Lima, E. Jr., Mansilla, M. V., Zysler, R. D., Troiani, H., Pisciotti, M. L. M., et al. (2016). Superparamagnetic iron-oxide nanoparticles mPEG350- and mPEG2000-coated: cell uptake and biocompatibility evaluation. *Nanomedicine* 12, 909–919. doi: 10.1016/j.nano.2015.12.371

Song, H. J., Zhang, J., Wang, W. W., Huang, P. S., Zhang, Y. M., Liu, J. F., et al. (2015). Acid-responsive PEGylated doxorubicin prodrug nanoparticles for neuropilin-1 receptor-mediated targeted drug delivery. *Colloids Surf. B Biointerfaces* 136, 365–374. doi: 10.1016/j.colsurfb.2015.09.030

Wang, B. Y., Lv, L. Y., Wang, Z. Y., Zhao, Y., Wu, L., Fang, X. L., et al. (2014). Nanoparticles functionalized with Pep-1 as potential glioma targeting delivery system *via* interleukin 13 receptor α2-mediated endocytosis. *Biomaterials* 35, 5897–5907. doi: 10.1016/j.biomaterials.2014.03.068

Wang, X., Li, J., Wang, Y. X., Koenig, L., Gjyrezi, A., Giannakakou, P., et al. (2011). A folate receptor-targeting nanoparticle minimizes drug resistance in a human cancer model. *ACS Nano* 5, 6184–6194. doi: 10.1021/nn200739q

Wilhelm, S., Tavares, A. J., Dai, Q., Ohta, S., Audet, J., Dvorak, H. F., et al. (2016). Analysis of nanoparticle delivery to tumours. *Nat. Rev. Mater.* 1:16014. doi: 10.1038/natrevmats.2016.14

Wong, M. H., Chan, D. L., Lee, A., Li, B. T., Lumba, S., Clarke, S. J., et al. (2016). Systematic review and meta-analysis on the role of chemotherapy in advanced and Metastatic Neuroendocrine Tumor (NET). *PLoS One* 11:e0158140. doi: 10.1371/journal.pone.0158140

Xu, Q., Liu, Y. X., Su, S. S., Li, W., Chen, C. Y., and Wu, Y. (2012). Anti-tumor activity of paclitaxel through dual-targeting carrier of cyclic RGD and transferrin conjugated hyperbranched copolymer nanoparticles. *Biomaterials* 33, 1627–1639. doi: 10.1016/j.biomaterials.2011.11.012

Zhao, R. B., Visentin, M., and Goldman, I. D. (2015). Determinants of the activities of antifolates delivered into cells by folate-receptor-mediated endocytosis. *Cancer Chemother. Pharmacol.* 75, 1163–1173. doi: 10.1007/s00280-015-2733-8

9

Nanoliposome-Encapsulated Brinzolamide-Hydropropyl-β-Cyclodextrin Inclusion Complex: A Potential Therapeutic Ocular Drug-Delivery System

Fazhan Wang[1†], Xingting Bao[1†], Aiping Fang[1,2†], Huili Li[1], Yang Zhou[1], Yongmei Liu[1], Chunling Jiang[1], Jinhui Wu[1] and Xiangrong Song[1*]*

[1] State Key Laboratory of Biotherapy, Geriatrics and Cancer Center, West China Hospital and Collaborative Innovation Center for Biotherapy, Sichuan University, Chengdu, China, [2] West China School of Public Health, Sichuan University, Chengdu, China

***Correspondence:**
Xiangrong Song
songxr@scu.edu.cn
Jinhui Wu
wujinhui@scu.edu.cn

† These authors have contributed equally to this work.

Novel ocular drug delivery systems (NODDSs) remain to be explored to overcome the anatomical and physiological barriers of the eyes. This study was to encapsulate brinzolamide (BRZ)-hydropropyl-β-cyclodextrin (HP-β-CD) inclusion complex (HP-β-CD/BRZ) into nanoliposomes and investigate its potential as one of NODDS to improve BRZ local glaucomatous therapeutic effect. HP-β-CD/BRZ was firstly prepared to enhance the solubility of poorly water-soluble BRZ. The HP-β-CD/BRZ loaded nanoliposomes (BCL) were subsequently constructed by thin-film dispersion method. After the optimization of the ratio of BRZ to HP-β-CD, the optimal BCL showed an average size of 82.29 ± 6.20 nm, ζ potential of −3.57 ± 0.46 mV and entrapment efficiency (EE) of 92.50 ± 2.10% with nearly spherical in shape. The X-ray diffraction (XRD) confirmed the formation of HP-β-CD/BRZ and BCL. The *in vitro* release study of BCL was evaluated using the dialysis technique, and BCL showed moderate sustained release. BCL (1 mg/mL BRZ) showed a 9.36-fold increase in the apparent permeability coefficient and had a sustained and enhanced intraocular pressure reduction efficacy when compared with the commercially available formulation (BRZ-Sus) (10 mg/mL BRZ). In conclusion, BCL might have a promising future as a NODDS for glaucoma treatment.

Keywords: brinzolamide, cyclodextrin, inclusion complex, nanoliposomes, intraocular pressure, ocular drug delivery

INTRODUCTION

Despite easy accessibility for topical drug administration, overcoming the anatomical and physiological barriers of the eye remains one of the greatest challenges for ocular drug delivery (Bucolo et al., 2012; Zhang et al., 2015). Drug retention is impeded by tear reflex, blinking, and nasolacrimal drainage (Morrison et al., 2013). Cornea barrier protects the eye from the passage of any foreign molecules including drugs into the eye, and thus only a small fraction of the topically applied drug penetrates the cornea and reaches intraocular tissues (Mun et al., 2014). As a result, repeated dosing is needed, which increases the patient discomfort and other adverse effects (Luo et al., 2011). A system which behaves like a solution and at the same time can lead to retention of drug in the eye and increase corneal permeability is of great urgency.

Nanoliposomes, as biodegradable, biocompatible and non-immunogenic drug delivery system, have been widely applied (van Rooijen and van Nieuwmegen, 1980; Mugabe et al., 2006; Arias, 2013; Sercombe et al., 2015; Ji et al., 2017). They can encapsulate hydrophilic drugs into the inner aqueous phase, whereas entrap hydrophobic drugs into the hydrophobic lipid phase (Allen and Cullis, 2004; Chen et al., 2009). However, it is difficult to obtain high drug-loading capacity in the lipid phase because of the limited space offered by the lipid phase, and a large amount of hydrophobic drugs can destabilize the structural integrity of the liposomal layers (Song et al., 2012). Inclusion complexes are one of the most useful strategies in the pharmaceutical field, which can solubilize a wide range of hydrophobic drugs (Morrison et al., 2013; Zhang et al., 2013; Alomrani et al., 2014; Ji et al., 2016; Maria et al., 2017; Soliman et al., 2017). The binding force between the guest drug molecule and the cyclodextrin host molecule is usually weak, possibly leading to rapid dissociation of the inclusion complexes due to dilution by plasma or extracellular fluids (Chen et al., 2014). Encapsulation of hydrophobic drugs in the form of inclusion complexes into nanoliposomes has been investigated as a new strategy to combine the advantages of inclusion complexes and nanoliposomes, namely the drug-in-cyclodextrin-in-nanoliposome (DCL) system (Piel et al., 2006; Hatzi et al., 2007; Zhang et al., 2015). The presence of cyclodextrin in the aqueous compartment of nanoliposomes would not affect the characteristics of conventional liposomes but prolong drug release compared to conventional liposomes (Maestrelli et al., 2010; Zhang et al., 2015). Although a number of studies on DCL systems have been reported (Dhule et al., 2012; Rahman et al., 2012; Lapenda et al., 2013; Alomrani et al., 2014), to date, the therapeutic application of DCL systems as an ocular delivery system remains to be explored.

Nanoliposome systems are applicable in ocular delivery, which have the potential of increasing corneal permeability and improving retention time (de Sa et al., 2015; Li et al., 2016). Moreover, some functional liposomes have been constructed (Eriksen et al., 2017; Huang et al., 2017; Tan et al., 2017). Cyclodextrin, with a hydrophilic outer surface and a cavity at its center and low renal toxicity, has the ability to form hydrophilic inclusion complexes by a molecular complexation with a lot of hydrophobic drugs (Ji et al., 2016; Maria et al., 2016, 2017; Abd El-Gawad et al., 2017). Hydropropyl-β-cyclodextrin (HP-β-CD), a type of cyclodextrin, is commonly used for ocular drug delivery and has been approved by the FDA (Bozkir et al., 2012). Many *in vitro* and *in vivo* studies also showed that the inclusion complex of poor water-soluble drugs by HP-β-CD could increase drug solubility, corneal permeability, and ophthalmic bioavailability (Ito et al., 2013; Morrison et al., 2013). Encouraged by these previous results, we postulated that DCL might have the potential to enhance ocular permeation of the hydrophobic model drug brinzolamide (BRZ) and enhance its therapeutic efficacy for glaucoma.

Previously, we have used inclusion complex and nanoliposomes to encapsulate the low water-soluble drug BRZ, respectively. Both formulations improved the corneal permeation and therapeutic efficacy of BRZ to some extent (Zhang et al., 2013; Li et al., 2016). Here, we further combined HP-β-CD and nanoliposomes to prepare BRZ-HP-β-CD inclusion complex (HP-β-CD/BRZ)-loaded nanoliposomes (BCL) as shown in **Figure 1**. The pharmaceutical properties including UV/vis spectra, particle size, surface charge, entrapment efficiency (EE) of BRZ, X-ray diffraction (XRD), and *in vitro* release profile were then characterized systemically. The *ex vivo* corneal permeability, *in vivo* intraocular pressure (IOP) reduction efficiency and preliminary safety of BCL were finally evaluated.

MATERIALS AND METHODS

Materials

BRZ (purity > 99%) was obtained from Dalian Meilun Biology Technology Company (Dalian, China). HP-β-CD (purity > 99%, DS = 7) was supplied by Xi'an Deli Chemicals Corporation (Xi'an, China). Soybean phosphatidylcholine (SPC) was provided by Shanghai A.V.T. Pharmaceutical, Co., Ltd. (Shanghai, China). Cholesterol was purchased from Shanghai Yuanju Biology Technology Company (Shanghai, China). The commercial formulation AZOPT® (BRZ-Sus) was supplied by Alcon Laboratories (Puurs, Belgium). All the other reagents were of analytical grade unless otherwise stated.

Animals

White New Zealand rabbits (male, 2.0–2.5 kg) were used for each formulation ($n = 6$). Animals were housed individually and allowed free access to food and water with a 12:12 h cyclic lighting schedule. After a week of adaptation, animals were admitted to experiments. All animal experiments were approved and supervised by the State Key Laboratory of Biotherapy Animal Care and Use Committee (Sichuan University, Chengdu, Sichuan, China).

Preparation of H-β-CD/BRZ Inclusion Complex

According to previously described methods by Zhang et al. (2013), the inclusion complex was prepared with some

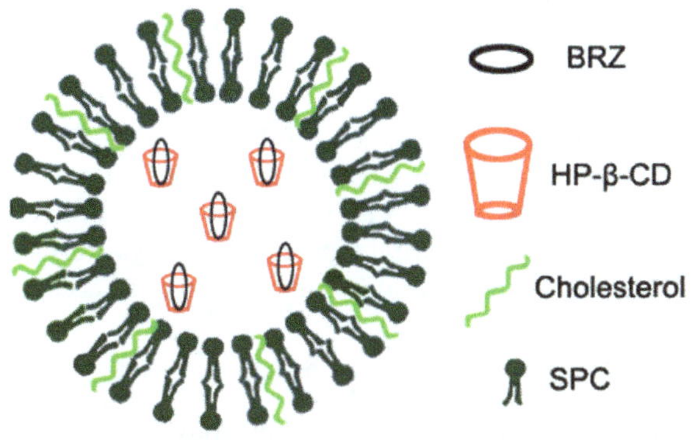

FIGURE 1 | Schematic structure of HP-β-CD/BRZ-inclusion complex loaded nanoliposomes.

modifications. Briefly, BRZ and HP-β-CD at different molar ratio (2:1, 1:1, 1:2, and 1:3) were dissolved by ethanol in a round-bottomed flask. After 1 h of ultrasound at 37°C, the ethanol was removed using a rotary evaporator in vacuum. To dissolve the inclusion complex, PBS was added to the flask followed by filtering through a 0.22 μm membrane. The content of BRZ in the inclusion complex was analyzed by high-performance liquid chromatography (HPLC, Waters, Milford, MA, United States) at 252 nm. The mobile phase, at 1 mL/min flow rate, was composed of acetonitrile and water at a volume ratio of 40:60.

Preparation of BCL

BCL was prepared using a modified thin-film dispersion method (Lapenda et al., 2013; Li et al., 2016). Briefly, SPC and cholesterol were dissolved in a mixture solvent of chloroform/methanol (4:1, v/v). The organic solvents were evaporated using a rotary evaporator at 37°C, and then the formed thin film was further dried under high vacuum for 1 h. The lipid film was hydrated with HP-β-CD/BRZ inclusion complexes at 60°C for 1 h to obtain a suspension. To obtain BCL, the above suspension was sonicated for 3 min at 100 W in an ice bath and filtered through a 0.22-μm membrane filter.

The BRZ-loaded nanoliposomes (LP/BRZ) were obtained using the similar procedure with the addition of BRZ into the chloroform/methanol (4:1 v/v) solvent mixture and hydrating lipid film with sterile PBS. The blank liposomes (Blank LP) were also prepared using the similar preparation process of LP/BRZ without adding BRZ.

Characterization of BCL

Ultraviolet-Visible (UV/vis) Spectroscopy

The UV/vis absorption spectra of BRZ, HP-β-CD, Blank LP, inclusion complex, LP/BRZ, and BCL were recorded using a SHIMADZU UV-2600 UV/vis spectrophotometer in the range of 200–600 nm.

Particle Size and ζ Potential

The average particle size, size distribution [polydispersity index (PDI)], and ζ potential of diluted BCL were recorded by Zetasizer Nano ZS90 (Malvern Instruments, Malvern, United Kingdom). All measurements were carried out at 25°C after 3 min of equilibration and were conducted in triplicate. All the data were presented as mean ± standard deviation (SD).

Morphology

The morphological examination of BCL was performed by transmission electron microscopy (TEM, H-600, Hitachi, Japan). Briefly, a drop of liposomal suspension was placed onto copper electron microscopy grids, and then they were negatively stained with 2% phosphotungstic acid for observation at an acceleration voltage of 100 kV.

Drug Entrapment Efficiency

According to previously described methods (Rahman et al., 2012), the drug content of BCL was determined by separating BCL from the unentrapped drug using cooling centrifugation at 50,000 rpm for 30 min at a temperature of 4°C. Following the removal of the supernatant, 1 ml of acetonitrile was added into the BCL sediment and sonicated for 20 min to extract BRZ from BCL. After centrifugation at 13,000 rpm for 10 min, the content of BRZ in the supernatant diluted with acetonitrile was quantified by HPLC as described previously. Analysis was performed in triplicate and the values were expressed as mean ± SD. EE was calculated by the following calculation equation:

$$EE = (\text{amount of BRZ in BCL}/\text{initial BRZ amount}) \times 100\%.$$

Stability of BCL

The optimized formulation was stored at 4°C for 2 weeks in order to investigate the preliminary stability. In the test, the physicochemical characteristics such as particle size and EE were recorded and changes over time were evaluated.

XRD Analysis

X-ray diffraction was performed to investigate the crystal structure according to the former study (Tao et al., 2017). Different samples (pure BRZ, HP-β-CD, HP-β-CD/BRZ, and BCL) were examined using an X-ray diffractometer (X'Pert Pro Philips, Netherlands) at a voltage of 40 kV and a current of 40 mA. The scans were carried out at a scanning rate of 10°C/min in the 2θ range from 0 to 50°C.

In Vitro BRZ Release from BCL

In vitro release studies were carried out using the dynamic dialysis technique in sink conditions. Briefly, 2 mL of different formulations containing the drug were placed into different dialysis bags (molecular weight cut-off = 3,500 Da) and immersed in 40 mL of simulated tear fluid (STF) and continuously agitated in an orbital shaker maintained at 37°C. At given time intervals, 1 mL of receptor phase was removed and replaced with an equal volume of STF. The drug concentration was quantified by the HPLC method as described above. All data were presented as mean ± SD of three independent measurements.

Corneal Permeability

The transcorneal permeability of BCL was evaluated using a Franz diffusion chamber which consisted of a donor and a receiver compartment (with a volume of 1.0 and 2.0 mL, respectively). The diffusion chamber was maintained at a constant temperature (37 ± 0.2°C) by a thermostatic water bath, under mixing conditions using a magnetic stirrer. The cornea together with a 2-mm ring of sclera was excised immediately after the rabbits (n = 3) were sacrificed and stored in glutathione bicarbonate ringer (GBR) buffer after rinsing with cold saline before use. One mL of the GBR solution was added to the endothelial (receptor) side of the cornea, while 0.5 mL of different formulations was added to the epithelial (donor) side of the cornea. Different samples from the receptor chamber were withdrawn at 0, 0.5, 1, 1.5, 2, 3, 4, 5 and 6 h and replaced with fresh GBR buffer-receptor solution. The content of drug permeation across the cornea was determined by the HPLC method as described above. The experiment was done in triplicate.

The apparent permeation coefficient (P_{app}, cm/s) of each formulation was calculated using the following equation

(Goskonda et al., 2000):

$$P_{app} = (1/AC_0) * (dM/dt)$$

where A is the available corneal surface area for diffusion (cm^2), C_0 is the initial drug concentration (μg/mL) in the donor compartment, and dM/dt is the flux across the cornea (μg/cm^2h).

Corneal Hydration Level

According to the literature (Vega et al., 2008), the corneal hydration level (HL) was evaluated by measuring total water content by the gravimetric method. At the end of the corneal permeability study (n = 3), the wet weight of each cornea (W_1) and dry corneal weight (W_2) after a desiccation at 100°C for 6 h were obtained, respectively. The corneal HL was calculated using the following equation: HL% = $(W_1\text{-}W_2)/W_1 \times 100\%$.

In Vivo IOP Measurement

IOP was recorded in mmHg with a Tono-pen XL® tonometer (Reichert, NY, United States) calibrated according to the manufacturer's instructions. IOP was recorded until the animals (n = 6) were accustomed to the experimental procedure. Each formulation (50 μL) was instilled topically into the right eye, while the left eye received no treatment to minimize the diurnal and individual variations. The IOP was measured at 0.5, 1, 2, 3, 4, 5, 6, 8, 10, 12 and 24 h after instilled.

Statistical Analysis

The data were expressed as mean ± SD. Statistical significance was assessed by a two-way analysis of variance using SPSS 16.0 (SPSS, Inc., Chicago, IL, United States). The p-values < 0.05 were considered statistically significant difference.

RESULTS

UV/vis Spectroscopy

The influence of the BCL on the absorption of BRZ was evaluated by UV/vis spectroscopy. The absorption spectra of BRZ, HP-β-CD, Blank LP, HP-β-CD/BRZ inclusion complex, LP/BRZ and BCL in acetonitrile were determined (**Figure 2**). The spectrum of BCL exhibited a characteristics absorption peak at 252 nm, which was similar to the peak of BRZ. These results suggested that the HPLC method developed for BRZ measurement with a detection wavelength of 252 nm could also be applied to determine the BRZ concentration in BCL.

Preparation of BCL

Different ratios of BRZ and HP-β-CD were used to establish the optimal preparation conditions in which BCL are formed. The drug content of BCL ranged between 84.38 and 92.50% and the size of BCL ranged between 82.29 ± 6.20 nm and 90.62 ± 11.30 nm depending on the BRZ/ HP-β-CD molar ratio (**Figure 3A**).

Characterization of BCL

Particle Size, ζ Potential, and EE

The physicochemical properties of optimal BCL were evaluated. The particle size of the optimal BCL was 82.29 ± 6.20 nm with a narrow size distribution (PDI = 0.21 ± 0.01) (**Figure 3C**). The ζ potential of BCL was −3.57 ± 0.46 mV (**Figure 3D**). The appearance and morphological studies of BCL were also conducted. LP/BRZ and BCL colloidal solution were observed as a slightly blue opalescence with obvious Tyndall effect compared with water (**Figures 3E,F**). BCL were seen to be distinct lipid membrane structure with a particle size diameter of about 70 nm (**Figure 3G**).

Storage Stability

The particle size and EE of BCL were determined at a predetermined time of storage at 4°C. BCL displayed good stability with no detectable changes in particle size and EE for at least 3 days (**Figure 3B**).

XRD Analysis

X-ray diffractograms were obtained from different samples of BRZ, HP-β-CD, HP-β-CD/BRZ and BCL to evaluate the crystal structure and entrapment of BRZ in BCL. The X-ray spectrum of BRZ showed several sharp and narrow peaks between 5 and 50°C (2θ) with a maximal peak at 2θ = 24.97°C, indicating their crystalline nature. HP-β-CD displayed a specific broad peak at 2θ = 20°C in its X-ray diffractogram. Neither HP-β-CD/BRZ nor BCL showed the peak at 2θ = 24.97°C (**Figure 4**).

In Vitro Release Profile

The *in vitro* release experiments were performed to investigate the successful inclusion and the sustained release characteristic of BCL. A sustained release phase was observed in BCL within a period of 9 h (1–10 h) as presented in **Figure 5**. BRZ release from the inclusion complex was slightly slower than free drug but faster than LP/BRZ. Moreover, BCL displayed a slower release compared to LP/BRZ.

Corneal Permeation and Corneal Hydration

The corneal penetration study was performed to evaluate the effect of BCL on transcorneal transportation. The corneal permeation characteristics of BRZ-Sus (10 mg/mL), LP/BRZ (1 mg/mL), and BCL (1 mg/mL) were shown in **Figure 6**. There was no significant difference in the cumulative permeation amount at 0–2 h among the three groups. At 3–6 h, BRZ-Sus and BCL showed a significant increase of BRZ cumulative permeation compared with LP/BRZ. A linear relationship was observed for all preparations over the time period from 0.5 to 6 h, indicating that the corneal integrity was maintained throughout the experiment. Moreover, the permeation coefficient of BCL was much larger than those of BRZ-Sus and LP/BRZ (**Table 1**, p < 0.001). BCL showed a 9.36- and 0.40-fold increase in P_{app} when compared with Brz-Sus and LP/BRZ, respectively.

Corneal HL was used to evaluate the safety of BCL (Vega et al., 2008). Its normal value is often from 75 to 80% (Vega et al., 2008). The corneal HL of BRZ-Sus, LP/BRZ, and BCL were

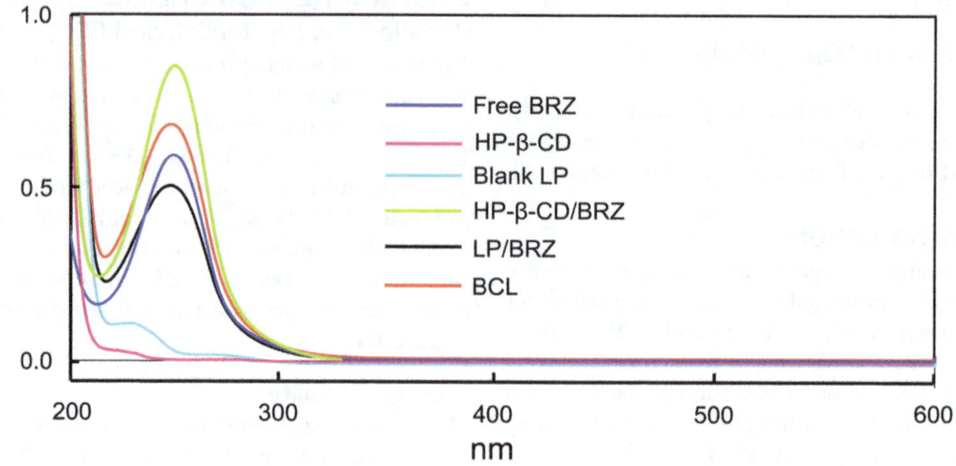

FIGURE 2 | The UV/vis spectra of free BRZ, HP-β-CD, Blank LP, HP-β-CD/BRZ inclusion complex, LP/BRZ, and BCL in acetonitrile.

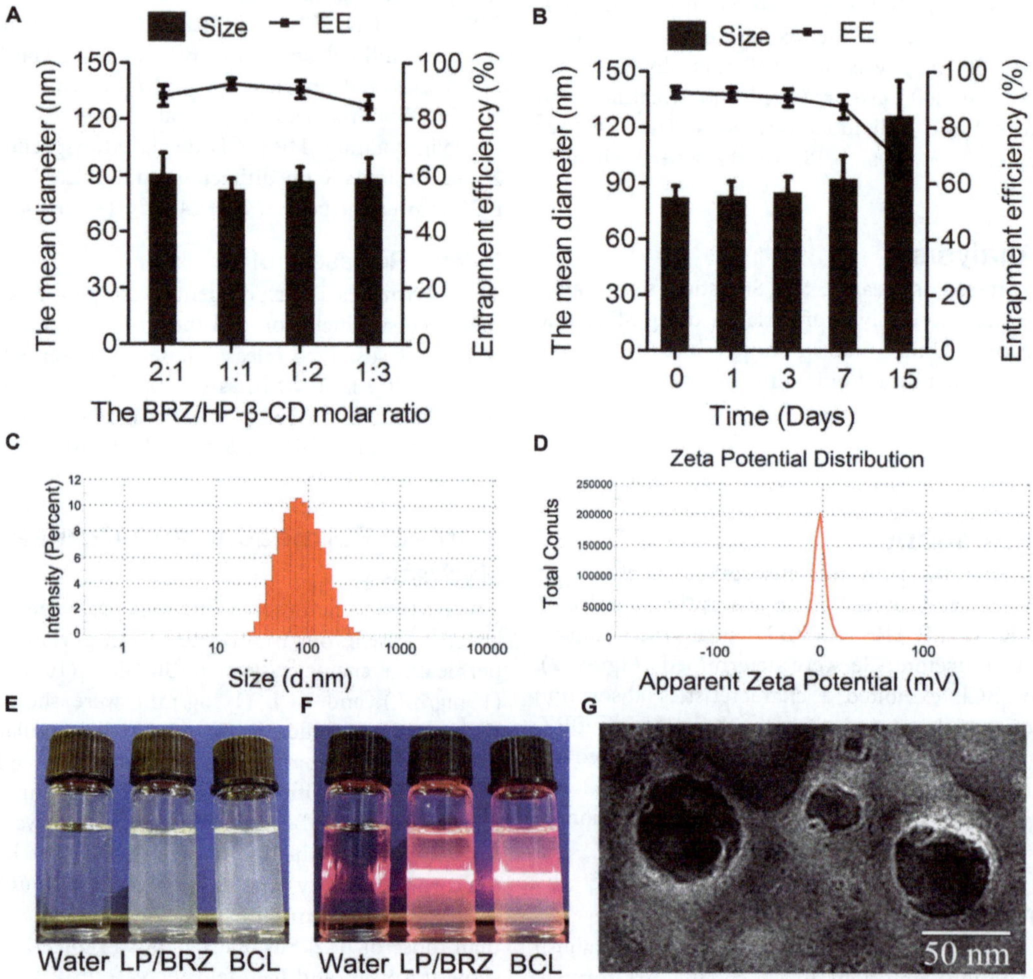

FIGURE 3 | Effects of various HP-β-CD/BRZ ratios on diameter and drug entrapment efficiency of BCL **(A)** (n = 3). Change in size and entrapment efficiency of BCL at various time points stored at 4°C **(B)** (n = 3). Size distribution **(C)**, ζ potential **(D)**, appearance **(E)**, and tyndall effect **(F)** of BCL. TEM images of BCL **(G)**.

80.12 ± 2.43%, 79.37 ± 2.19%, and 78.56 ± 3.04%, respectively. No statistical difference in HL % was found ($p > 0.05$), indicating BCL might be safe for topical ocular use.

In Vivo IOP-Lowering Effect

As shown in **Figure 7**, BCL (1 mg/mL BRZ) presented more effective IOP reduction with a longer term role than BRZ-Sus (10 mg/mL Brz) and LP/BRZ (1 mg/mL Brz). The novel formulation of BRZ had an onset of less than 1 h, achieved a maximum IOP reduction of 32.3% at 2 h, and sustained an effective IOP reduction until the 12th hour, while Brz-Sus began to result in an effective IOP reduction at 0.5 h and quickly reached its peak effect at 1 h (an average reduction of 16.12% from baseline). Furthermore, IOP was significantly lower in the BCL group at any time point from 2 to 12 h than Brz-Sus group. Even though the dosage of BRZ was just 10% in BCL compared with BRZ-Sus, the IOP reduction efficacy was much higher.

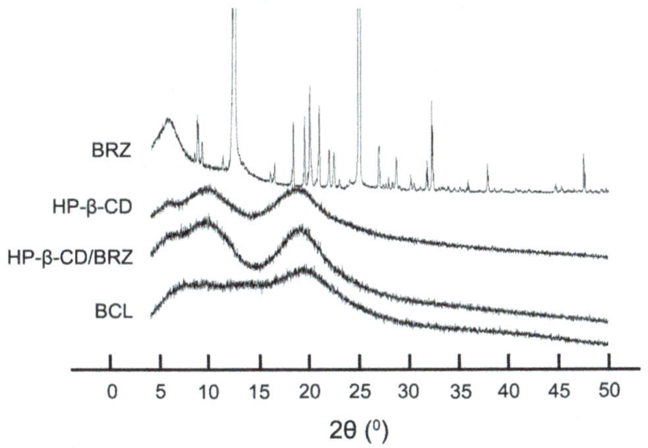

FIGURE 4 | X-ray diffractograms of BRZ, HP-β-CD, HP-β-CD/BRZ, and BCL.

DISCUSSION

In this work, we aimed to construct a novel ocular delivery system DCL loaded with BRZ (BCL) and investigate its potential to improve BRZ local glaucomatous therapeutic effect. BCL was prepared by hydrating lipid film with inclusion complex (Lapenda et al., 2013), and HP-β-CD was selected to enhance the solubility of poorly soluble drug BRZ (Zhang et al., 2013). According to the literature, the content of HP-β-CD was critical for the physicochemical properties of DCL (Chen et al., 2014; Cutrignelli et al., 2014). Cyclodextrins would interact with the lipid membrane and influence the formation of DCL (Cutrignelli et al., 2014). Thus, the amount of HP-β-CD was optimized based on the particle size and EE of BCL in this study. As seen in **Figure 3A**, EE first increased and then reached a plateau with the decrease of the BRZ/HP-β-CD molar ratio while the average diameter of BCL first decreased and then increased. Further increase in the HP-β-CD content (when the BRZ/HP-β-CD molar ratio was set at 1:3) cannot correspondingly enhance the BRZ entrapment into BCL but reduced EE. The cholesterol in the lipid bilayer of nanoliposomes might enter the excessive HP-β-CD cavity (Morrison et al., 2013; Chen et al., 2014), thereby forming unstable nanoliposomes which cannot incorporate enough HP-β-CD/BRZ-inclusion complex. The highest EE and the smallest particle size of BCL were achieved when BRZ and HP-β-CD was fed at a 1:1 molar ratio, and thus BCL containing 1:1 BRZ/H-β-CD were chosen for the subsequent investigations.

The optimal BCL were nano-sized (less than 100 nm) with negative surface charge probably resulting from the phosphatidylcholine head group in the outer nanoliposomes surface (Ascenso et al., 2013). Interestingly, BCL colloidal suspension had a similar appearance, average size, and surface charge to LP/BRZ despite the introduction of HP-β-CD (Maestrelli et al., 2010). This phenomenon indicated that HP-β-CD might mainly distribute in the inner aqueous core of the nanoliposomes, which was consistent with the literature (Cavalcanti et al., 2011; Lapenda et al., 2013; Chen et al., 2014). Moreover, it was clear that the peaks of BRZ disappeared from

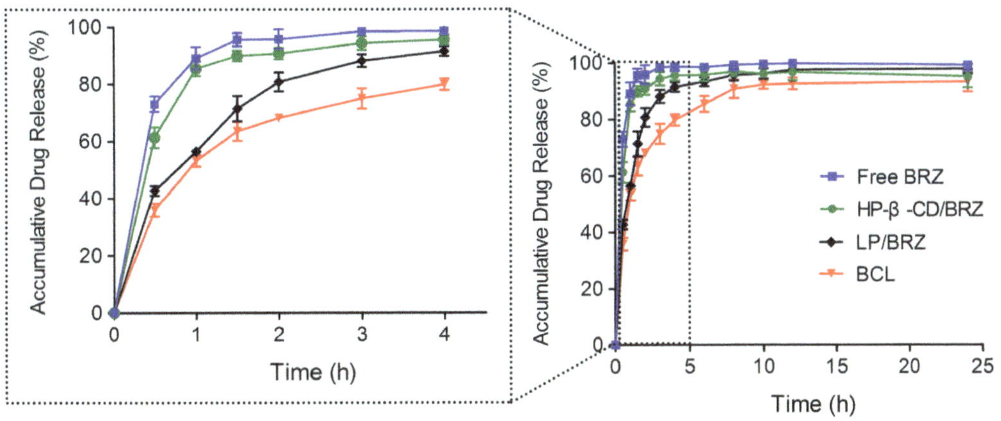

FIGURE 5 | *In vitro* release profiles of BRZ from BRZ solution (free drug), HP-β-CD/BRZ, LP/BRZ, and BCL at 37°C in simulated tear fluid. Data are expressed as mean ± SD ($n = 3$).

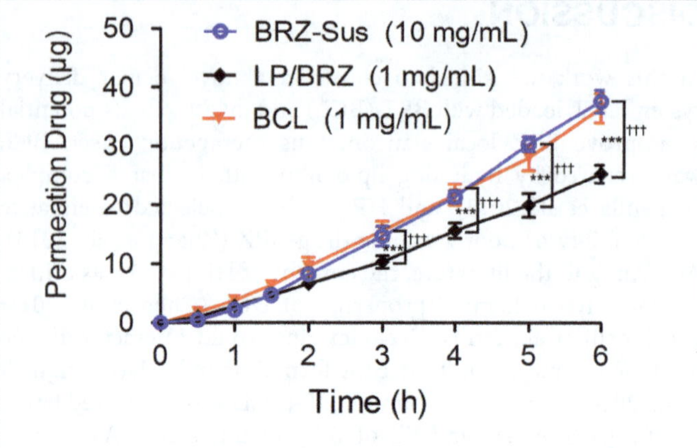

FIGURE 6 | *In vitro* transcorneal permeation profiles of BRZ-Sus, LP/BRZ, and BCL versus time. Data are expressed as mean ± SD (n = 3) (***p < 0.001 vs. BRZ-Sus; †††p < 0.001 vs. BCL).

TABLE 1 | Corneal hydration level and P_{app} of different formulations containing brinzolamide. Data are expressed as mean ± SD (n = 3).

Formulation	HL%	P_{app} ($\times 10^6$ cm/s)
BRZ-Sus	80.12 ± 2.43	0.36 ± 0.02
LP/BRZ	79.37 ± 2.19	2.59 ± 0.07
BCL	78.56 ± 3.04	3.73 ± 0.13

the diffraction pattern of BCL, demonstrating that BRZ was completely and successfully encapsulated into BCL.

BCL could be stable for about 7 days at 4°C, which might benefit from the negatively charged surface. However, EE sharply declined when BCL were kept for 15 days. The cholesterol in BCL might go into the hydrophobic cavity of HP-β-CD to compete with BRZ (Lapenda et al., 2013; Morrison et al., 2013), hence partially contributing to partial leakage of BRZ from the inclusion complex and the instability of nanoliposomes. HP-β-CD has previously been reported to extract cholesterol from cell membranes (Morrison et al., 2013) and decrease the integrity of liposomes composed of cholesterol and saturated phospholipids (Hatzi et al., 2007). The phenomenon found in this study was in line with these former studies. The free BRZ would easily pass through the lipid bilayer of the unstable BCL, which led to the reduced EE after relatively long-term storage. Generally, this kind of destructive role of HP-β-CD on DCL basically depends on the HP-β-CD affinity balance between the guest drug molecules and lipid components of nanoliposomes (Piel et al., 2006; Chen et al., 2014). According to the preliminary stability results, BCL would be further developed to be a freeze-drying formulation for long-term storage.

BCL performed a slower release than HP-β-CD/BRZ inclusion complex and LP/BRZ. It seems that the slower release profile of BCL was partially attributed to the fact that there were more barriers to the diffusion of BRZ from the BCL than LP/BRZ. As for BCL, two definitely different routes may account for the BRZ release (Chen et al., 2014). The whole HP-β-CD/BRZ inclusion complex might release from the destructive BCL or transport to lipid phase and then release. For the other way, BRZ might release from the dissociated HP-β-CD/BRZ inclusion complex inside BCL followed by diffusion out of the nanoliposomes and dispersion through the dialysis bag (Chen et al., 2014). To date, there still remains a lot of work to do to clarify the relative contributions of the two definitely different routes in release of BCL.

BCL exhibited enhanced and sustained IOP reduction effect as shown in **Figure 7**. This promising efficacy of BCL on glaucoma treatment may be mainly explained by the combinatorial advantages of BCL with HP-β-CD and nanoliposomes. Neutral liposome with a size of about 100 nm were reported to be safe for ocular applications without ocular irritability (Taniguchi et al., 1988). Moreover, particle size < 10 μm was recommended and considered optimal for ophthalmic preparation to minimize eye irritation (Kassem et al., 2007; Yuan et al., 2009). Accordingly, BCL colloidal solution with small size rather than BRZ-Sus might attenuate ocular irritation, thereby reducing the loss of BRZ by tear flushing. In addition, BCL with higher corneal binding affinity (Natarajan et al., 2012) can increase the retention on the surface of cornea, probably extending the absorption of BRZ. BCL displayed significant improvement in corneal permeation in contrast to the conventionally prepared LP/BRZ. This was thought to be the cause of the more efficient IOP lowering effect of BCL. Moreover, the intact HP-β-CD/BRZ inclusion complex

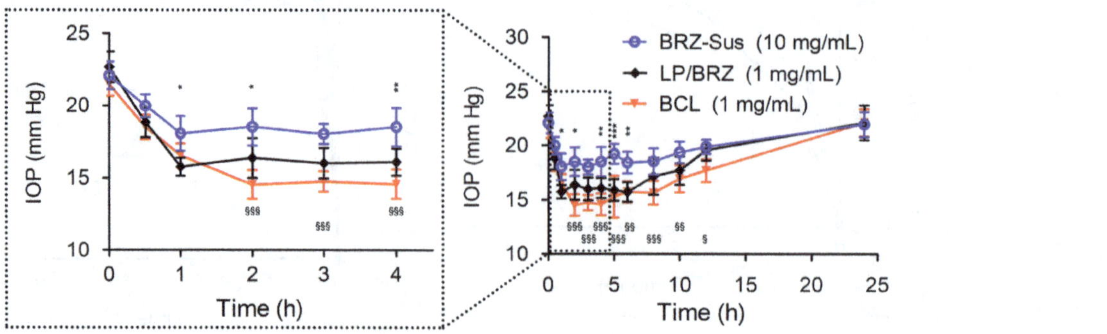

FIGURE 7 | *In vivo* intraocular pressure (IOP) profiles of white New Zealand rabbits treated with BRZ-Sus, LP/BRZ, and BCL. Data are expressed as mean ± SD (n = 6) (*p < 0.05, **p < 0.01, and ***p < 0.001 vs. LP/BRZ; §p < 0.05, §§p < 0.01, and §§§p < 0.001 vs. BCL).

released from BCL might lead to the enhanced penetration according to our previous study (Zhang et al., 2013). Of note, the sustained release profile of BCL as shown in the *in vitro* release study might be linked to the prolonged therapeutic efficacy of BCL.

CONCLUSION

In this study, a novel drug-in-cyclodextrin-in-nanoliposome system containing BRZ was successfully prepared and its potential application in glaucomatous treatment was investigated. The optimized ratio of BRZ and HP-β-CD was set at 1:1 to prepare BCL with small size and high drug content. BCL incorporated BRZ very well and showed a sustained release profile and enhanced corneal permeation. Moreover, this new formulation of BRZ achieved an improved and prolonged effect of IOP reduction with similar safety to the commercially available formulation on white New Zealand rabbits. However, further studies are still required to investigate the *in vitro* release properties of BCL and elucidate how the release profile affects the therapeutic efficacy of BCL. In sum, all the data indicated that DCL might be one of the potential ocular delivery systems for hydrophobic drugs and BCL were worthy of further investigation as a novel anti-glaucoma formulation candidate of BRZ.

AUTHOR CONTRIBUTIONS

XS conceived of the study. JW designed the experiments. XS and FW wrote the manuscript. FW and XB conducted most of the experiments. AF performed the statistical analysis and drafted the manuscript. HL and YZ performed all the preliminary experiments. YL and CJ participated in literature research and manuscript editing. All authors reviewed and approved the manuscript.

ACKNOWLEDGMENTS

This work was financially supported by the Sichuan Province Science and Technology Support Program (Grant Nos. 2015SZ0234 and 2017GZ0413) and the National Natural Science Foundation of China (Grant No. 81600006).

REFERENCES

Abd El-Gawad, A. E. H., Soliman, O. A., El-Dahan, M. S., and Al-Zuhairy, S. A. S. (2017). Improvement of the ocular bioavailability of econazole nitrate upon complexation with cyclodextrins. *AAPS PharmSciTech* 18, 1795–1809. doi: 10.1208/s12249-016-0609-9

Allen, T. M., and Cullis, P. R. (2004). Drug delivery systems: entering the mainstream. *Science* 303, 1818–1822. doi: 10.1126/science.1095833

Alomrani, A. H., Shazly, G. A., Amara, A. A., and Badran, M. M. (2014). Itraconazole-hydroxypropyl-beta-cyclodextrin loaded deformable liposomes: *in vitro* skin penetration studies and antifungal efficacy using *Candida albicans* as model. *Colloids Surf. B Biointerfaces* 121, 74–81. doi: 10.1016/j.colsurfb.2014.05.030

Arias, J. L. (2013). Liposomes in drug delivery: a patent review (2007 – present). *Expert Opin. Ther. Pat.* 23, 1399–1414. doi: 10.1517/13543776.2013.828035

Ascenso, A., Cruz, M., Euleterio, C., Carvalho, F. A., Santos, N. C., Marques, H. C., et al. (2013). Novel tretinoin formulations: a drug-in-cyclodextrin-in-liposome approach. *J. Liposome Res.* 23, 211–219. doi: 10.3109/08982104.2013.788026

Bozkir, A., Denli, Z. F., and Basaran, B. (2012). Effect of hydroxypropyl-beta-cyclodextrin on the solubility, stability and in-vitro release of ciprofloxacin for ocular drug delivery. *Acta Pol. Pharm.* 69, 719–724.

Bucolo, C., Drago, F., and Salomone, S. (2012). Ocular drug delivery: a clue from nanotechnology. *Front. Pharmacol.* 3:188. doi: 10.3389/fphar.2012.00188

Cavalcanti, I. M., Mendonca, E. A., Lira, M. C., Honrato, S. B., Camara, C. A., Amorim, R. V., et al. (2011). The encapsulation of beta-lapachone in 2-hydroxypropyl-beta-cyclodextrin inclusion complex into liposomes: a physicochemical evaluation and molecular modeling approach. *Euro. J. Pharm. Sci.* 44, 332–340. doi: 10.1016/j.ejps.2011.08.011

Chen, J., Lu, W. L., Gu, W., Lu, S. S., Chen, Z. P., Cai, B. C., et al. (2014). Drug-in-cyclodextrin-in-liposomes: a promising delivery system for hydrophobic drugs. *Expert Opin. Drug Deliv.* 11, 565–577. doi: 10.1517/17425247.2014.884557

Chen, Y., Lu, Y., Chen, J., Lai, J., Sun, J., Hu, F., et al. (2009). Enhanced bioavailability of the poorly water-soluble drug fenofibrate by using liposomes containing a bile salt. *Int. J. Pharm.* 376, 153–160. doi: 10.1016/j.ijpharm.2009.04.022

Cutrignelli, A., Lopedota, A., Denora, N., Laquintana, V., Tongiani, S., and Franco, M. (2014). Characterization and release studies of liposomal gels containing glutathione/cyclodextrins complexes potentially useful for cutaneous administration. *J. Pharm. Sci.* 103, 1246–1254. doi: 10.1002/jps.23900

de Sa, F. A., Taveira, S. F., Gelfuso, G. M., Lima, E. M., and Gratieri, T. (2015). Liposomal voriconazole (VOR) formulation for improved ocular delivery. *Colloids Surf. B Biointerfaces.* 133, 331–338. doi: 10.1016/j.colsurfb.2015.06.036

Dhule, S. S., Penfornis, P., Frazier, T., Walker, R., Feldman, J., Tan, G., et al. (2012). Curcumin-loaded gamma-cyclodextrin liposomal nanoparticles as delivery vehicles for osteosarcoma. *Nanomedicine* 8, 440–451. doi: 10.1016/j.nano.2011.07.011

Eriksen, A. Z., Brewer, J., Andresen, T. L., and Urquhart, A. J. (2017). The diffusion dynamics of PEGylated liposomes in the intact vitreous of the *ex vivo* porcine eye: a fluorescence correlation spectroscopy and biodistribution study. *Int. J. Pharm.* 522, 90–97. doi: 10.1016/j.ijpharm.2017.03.003

Goskonda, V. R., Hill, R. A., Khan, M. A., and Reddy, I. K. (2000). Permeability of chemical delivery systems across rabbit corneal (SIRC) cell line and isolated corneas: a comparative study. *Pharm. Dev. Technol.* 5, 409–416. doi: 10.1081/PDT-100100557

Hatzi, P., Mourtas, S., Klepetsanis, P. G., and Antimisiaris, S. G. (2007). Integrity of liposomes in presence of cyclodextrins: effect of liposome type and lipid composition. *Int. J. Pharm.* 333, 167–176. doi: 10.1016/j.ijpharm.2006.09.059

Huang, Y., Tao, Q., Hou, D., Hu, S., Tian, S., Chen, Y., et al. (2017). A novel ion-exchange carrier based upon liposome-encapsulated montmorillonite for ophthalmic delivery of betaxolol hydrochloride. *Int. J. Nanomed.* 12, 1731–1745. doi: 10.2147/IJN.S122747

Ito, Y., Nagai, N., Okamoto, N., Shimomura, Y., Nakanishi, K., and Tanaka, R. (2013). Reduction of enhanced rabbit intraocular pressure by instillation of pyroglutamic acid eye drops. *Biol. Pharm. Bull.* 36, 1017–1023. doi: 10.1248/bpb.b13-00159

Ji, T., Lang, J., Wang, J., Cai, R., Zhang, Y., Qi, F., et al. (2017). Designing liposomes to suppress extracellular matrix expression to enhance drug penetration and pancreatic tumor therapy. *ACS Nano* 11, 8668–8678. doi: 10.1021/acsnano.7b01026

Ji, T., Li, S., Zhang, Y., Lang, J., Ding, Y., Zhao, X., et al. (2016). An MMP-2 responsive liposome integrating antifibrosis and chemotherapeutic drugs for enhanced drug perfusion and efficacy in pancreatic cancer. *ACS Appl. Mater. Interfaces* 8, 3438–3445. doi: 10.1021/acsami.5b11619

Kassem, M. A., Abdel Rahman, A. A., Ghorab, M. M., Ahmed, M. B., and Khalil, R. M. (2007). Nanosuspension as an ophthalmic delivery system for certain glucocorticoid drugs. *Int. J. Pharm.* 340, 126–133. doi: 10.1016/j.ijpharm.2007.03.011

Lapenda, T. L., Morais, W. A., Almeida, F. J., Ferraz, M. S., Lira, M. C., Santos, N. P., et al. (2013). Encapsulation of trans-dehydrocrotonin in liposomes: an enhancement of the antitumor activity. *J. Biomed. Nanotechnol.* 9, 499–510. doi: 10.1166/jbn.2013.1554

Li, H., Liu, Y., Zhang, Y., Fang, D., Xu, B., Zhang, L., et al. (2016). Liposomes as a novel ocular delivery system for brinzolamide: *in vitro* and *in vivo* studies. *AAPS PharmSciTech* 17, 710–717. doi: 10.1208/s12249-015-0382-1

Luo, Q., Zhao, J., Zhang, X., and Pan, W. (2011). Nanostructured lipid carrier (NLC) coated with Chitosan Oligosaccharides and its potential use in ocular drug delivery system. *Int. J. Pharm.* 403, 185–191. doi: 10.1016/j.ijpharm.2010.10.013

Maestrelli, F., Gonzalez-Rodriguez, M. L., Rabasco, A. M., Ghelardini, C., and Mura, P. (2010). New "drug-in cyclodextrin-in deformable liposomes" formulations to improve the therapeutic efficacy of local anaesthetics. *Int. J. Pharm.* 395, 222–231. doi: 10.1016/j.ijpharm.2010.05.046

Maria, D. N., Abd-Elgawad, A. H., Soliman, O. A., El-Dahan, M. S., and Jablonski, M. M. (2017). Nimodipine ophthalmic formulations for management of glaucoma. *Pharm. Res.* 34, 809–824. doi: 10.1007/s11095-017-2110-x

Maria, D. N., Mishra, S. R., Wang, L., Abd-Elgawad, A. H., Soliman, O. A., El-Dahan, M. S., et al. (2016). Water-soluble complex of curcumin with cyclodextrins: enhanced physical properties for ocular drug delivery. *Curr. Drug Deliv.* 14, 875–886.

Morrison, P. W., Connon, C. J., and Khutoryanskiy, V. V. (2013). Cyclodextrin-mediated enhancement of riboflavin solubility and corneal permeability. *Mol. Pharm.* 10, 756–762. doi: 10.1021/mp3005963

Mugabe, C., Azghani, A. O., and Omri, A. (2006). Preparation and characterization of dehydration-rehydration vesicles loaded with aminoglycoside and macrolide antibiotics. *Int. J. Pharm.* 307, 244–250. doi: 10.1016/j.ijpharm.2005.10.005

Mun, E. A., Morrison, P. W., Williams, A. C., and Khutoryanskiy, V. V. (2014). On the barrier properties of the cornea: a microscopy study of the penetration of fluorescently labeled nanoparticles, polymers, and sodium fluorescein. *Mol. Pharm.* 11, 3556–3564. doi: 10.1021/mp500332m

Natarajan, J. V., Ang, M., Darwitan, A., Chattopadhyay, S., Wong, T. T., and Venkatraman, S. S. (2012). Nanomedicine for glaucoma: liposomes provide sustained release of latanoprost in the eye. *Int. J. Nanomedicine* 7, 123–131. doi: 10.2147/IJN.S25468

Piel, G., Piette, M., Barillaro, V., Castagne, D., Evrard, B., and Delattre, L. (2006). Betamethasone-in-cyclodextrin-in-liposome: the effect of cyclodextrins on encapsulation efficiency and release kinetics. *Int. J. Pharm.* 312, 75–82. doi: 10.1016/j.ijpharm.2005.12.044

Rahman, S., Cao, S., Steadman, K. J., Wei, M., and Parekh, H. S. (2012). Native and beta-cyclodextrin-enclosed curcumin: entrapment within liposomes and their in vitro cytotoxicity in lung and colon cancer. *Drug Deliv.* 19, 346–353. doi: 10.3109/10717544.2012.721143

Sercombe, L., Veerati, T., Moheimani, F., Wu, S. Y., Sood, A. K., and Hua, S. (2015). Advances and challenges of liposome assisted drug delivery. *Front. Pharm.* 6:286. doi: 10.3389/fphar.2015.00286

Soliman, O. A. E., Mohamed, E. A. M., El-Dahan, M. S., and Khatera, N. A. A. (2017). Potential use of cyclodextrin complexes for enhanced stability, anti-inflammatory efficacy, and ocular bioavailability of loteprednol etabonate. *AAPS PharmSciTech* 18, 1228–1241. doi: 10.1208/s12249-016-0589-9

Song, C. K., Balakrishnan, P., Shim, C. K., Chung, S. J., Chong, S., and Kim, D. D. (2012). A novel vesicular carrier, transethosome, for enhanced skin delivery of voriconazole: characterization and *in vitro/in vivo* evaluation. *Colloids Surf. B Biointerfaces* 92, 299–304. doi: 10.1016/j.colsurfb.2011.12.004

Tan, G., Yu, S., Pan, H., Li, J., Liu, D., Yuan, K., et al. (2017). Bioadhesive chitosan-loaded liposomes: a more efficient and higher permeable ocular delivery platform for timolol maleate. *Int. J. Biol. Macromol.* 94, 355–363. doi: 10.1016/j.ijbiomac.2016.10.035

Taniguchi, K., Yamamoto, Y., Itakura, K., Miichi, H., and Hayashi, S. (1988). Assessment of ocular irritability of liposome preparations. *J. Pharmacobiodyn.* 11, 607–611. doi: 10.1248/bpb1978.11.607

Tao, W., Zhu, X., Yu, X., Zeng, X., Xiao, Q., Zhang, X., et al. (2017). Black phosphorus nanosheets as a robust delivery platform for cancer theranostics. *Adv. Mater.* 29:1603276. doi: 10.1002/adma.201603276

van Rooijen, N., and van Nieuwmegen, R. (1980). Liposomes in immunology: multilamellar phosphatidylcholine liposomes as a simple, biodegradable and harmless adjuvant without any immunogenic activity of its own. *Immunol. Commun.* 9, 243–256. doi: 10.3109/08820138009065997

Vega, E., Gamisans, F., Garcia, M. L., Chauvet, A., Lacoulonche, F., and Egea, M. A. (2008). PLGA nanospheres for the ocular delivery of flurbiprofen: drug release and interactions. *J. Pharm. Sci.* 97, 5306–5317. doi: 10.1002/jps.21383

Yuan, J., Zhai, J. J., Chen, J. Q., Ye, C. T., and Zhou, S. Y. (2009). Preparation of 0.05% FK506 suspension eyedrops and its pharmacokinetics after topical ocular administration. *J. Ocul. Pharmacol. Ther.* 25, 345–350. doi: 10.1089/jop.2008.0125

Zhang, L., Zhang, Q., Wang, X., Zhang, W., Lin, C., Chen, F., et al. (2015). Drug-in-cyclodextrin-in-liposomes: a novel drug delivery system for flurbiprofen. *Int. J. Pharm.* 492, 40–45. doi: 10.1016/j.ijpharm.2015.07.011

Zhang, Y., Ren, K., He, Z., Li, H., Chen, T., Lei, Y., et al. (2013). Development of inclusion complex of brinzolamide with hydroxypropyl-beta-cyclodextrin. *Carbohydr. Polym.* 98, 638–643. doi: 10.1016/j.carbpol.2013.06.052

10

A Robust Nanoparticle Platform for RNA Interference in Macrophages to Suppress Tumor Cell Migration

Shi Liang[1,2,3], Junmeng Zheng[1,2], Wei Wu[1,2,3], Quan Li[1,2,3], Phei Er Saw[1,2], Jianing Chen[1,2,3], Xiaoding Xu[1,2], Herui Yao[1,2,3]* and Yandan Yao[1,2,3]**

[1] Guangdong Provincial Key Laboratory of Malignant Tumor Epigenetics and Gene Regulation, Medical Research Center, Sun Yat-sen Memorial Hospital, Sun Yat-sen University, Guangzhou, China, [2] RNA Biomedical Institute, Sun Yat-sen Memorial Hospital, Sun Yat-sen University, Guangzhou, China, [3] Breast Tumor Center, Sun Yat-sen Memorial Hospital, Sun Yat-sen University, Guangzhou, China

***Correspondence:**
Xiaoding Xu
xuxiaod5@mail.sysu.edu.cn
Herui Yao
yaoherui@126.com
Yandan Yao
yaoyand@mail.sysu.edu.cn

Macrophages are one of the most abundant immune cells in the solid tumor and their increased density is associated with the specific pathological features of cancers, including invasiveness, metastasis, immunosuppression, neovascularization, and poor response to therapy. Therefore, reprogramming macrophage behavior is emerging as a promising therapeutic modality for cancer treatment. RNA interference (RNAi) technology is one of the powerful strategies for the regulation of macrophage activities by silencing specific genes. However, as polyanionic biomacromolecules, RNAi therapeutics such as small interfering RNA (siRNA) cannot readily cross cell membrane and thus specific delivery vehicles are required to facilitate the cytosolic siRNA delivery. Herein, we developed a robust nanoparticle (NP) platform for efficient siRNA delivery and gene silencing in macrophages. This NP platform is composed of biodegradable poly (ethylene glycol)-*b*-poly (ε-caprolactone) (PEG-*b*-PCL), poly (ε-caprolactone)-*b*-poly (2-aminoethyl ethylene phosphate) (PCL-*b*-PPEEA), and PCL homopolymer. We chose CC-chemokine ligand 18 (CCL-18) as a proof of concept therapeutic target and our results demonstrate that the CCL-18 silencing in macrophages can significantly inhibit the migration of breast cancer cells. The successful regulation of the macrophage behavior demonstrated herein shows great potential as an effective strategy for cancer therapy.

Keywords: macrophages, RNAi, nanoparticle, cancer therapy, siRNA delivery

INTRODUCTION

Macrophages are important cells of immune system with two major phenotypes, i.e., pro-inflammatory phenotype (M1) and anti-inflammatory phenotype (M2) (Mantovani et al., 2008; Noy and Pollard, 2014; Ostuni et al., 2015). In solid tumors, tumor-associated macrophages (TAMs) are one of the most abundant cell types (up to 50% of the tumor mass) and are present at all stages of tumor progression (Caillou et al., 2011; Ginhoux et al., 2015; Parayath et al., 2018). Numerous clinical and epidemiological studies have demonstrated that TAMs are primary M2-like macrophages (Gordon and Martinez, 2010; Sica and Mantovani, 2012; Bronte and Murray, 2015) and their increased density is associated with the specific pathological features of cancers, including invasiveness, metastasis, immunosuppression, neovascularization, and poor response to therapy (Qian and Pollard, 2010; McAllister and Weinberg, 2014; Bronte and Murray, 2015). Therefore, macrophages represent an important therapeutic target and strategies that can effectively regulate undesirable macrophage activities are always pursued for future cancer therapy.

One of the promising strategies for the regulation of macrophage activities is using RNA interference (RNAi) technology to silence specific genes (Aouadi et al., 2009; Kortylewski et al., 2009; Yu et al., 2013). Since its discovery in 1998, RNAi technology has demonstrated significant potential for disease treatment by silencing the expression of target gene(s), especially those encoding "undruggable" proteins (Melnikova, 2007; Burnett and Rossi, 2012; Kanasty et al., 2013; Zuckerman and Davis, 2015). The key challenge is the safe and effective delivery of RNAi therapeutics such as small interfering RNA (siRNA) to aberrant macrophages (e.g., TAMs). Due to its polyanionic and macromolecular characteristics, naked siRNA cannot readily cross the cell membrane and thus requires specific delivery vehicles to facilitate its intracellular uptake and cytosolic delivery for bioactivity (Whitehead et al., 2009; Zhang et al., 2012; Shi et al., 2017; Xu et al., 2017b). Over the past decade, nanoparticles (NPs), which present the advantage of preferential and selective accumulation at tumor sites via the enhanced permeation and retention (EPR) effect, have been widely used for cancer treatment (Chen et al., 2017; Zeng et al., 2017; Liu et al., 2018; Xiao et al., 2018). Up to now, numerous innovative NPs have been developed to enhance the siRNA delivery efficacy (Tseng et al., 2009; Xu et al., 2016, 2017a; Cheng et al., 2017; Saw et al., 2018). However, a substantial number of these NPs are designed to directly target tumor cells. At present, modest effort has been made to develop RNAi NPs for the modulation of undesirable macrophage activities.

Herein, we developed a robust RNAi NP platform for the efficient regulation of macrophage activities. This NP platform is composed of biodegradable poly (ε-caprolactone)-*b*-poly (2-aminoethyl ethylene phosphate) (PCL-*b*-PPEEA), poly (ethylene glycol)-*b*-poly (ε-caprolactone) (PEG-*b*-PCL), and PCL homopolymer (**Figure 1**). Through optimizing the NP size by adjusting the formulation, we demonstrated that larger size NPs can deliver siRNA and silence target gene in macrophages with higher efficacy. As a proof-of-concept, we chose CC-chemokine ligand 18 (CCL-18) as a therapeutic target and evaluated the influence of CCL-18 silencing on the macrophage activities. CCL-18 is a key factor secreted by TAMs to induce cancer cell epithelial-mesenchymal transition (EMT), enhance breast cancer metastasis, and reduce patient survival (Chen et al., 2011; Su et al., 2014; Nie et al., 2017). Our results show that the optimal NP platform can efficiently silence the CCL-18 expression in macrophages, leading to significant inhibition of breast cancer cell migration (**Figure 1**).

MATERIALS AND METHODS

Materials

Methoxyl-poly (ethylene glycol) (Meo-PEG_{114}-OH, M_n = 5000), phorbol myristate acetate (PMA), *N*-2-hydroxyethylpiperazine-*N*′-2-ethanesulfonic acid buffered saline (HEPES), stannous octoate [Sn $(Oct)_2$], RNase A, and heparin sulfate were acquired from Sigma-Aldrich and used directly. ε-Caprolactone (CL) was provided by Sigma-Aldrich and distilled before use. The poly (ε-caprolactone) homopolymer with 34 repeating units (PCL_{34}) and polydispersity of 1.21 was synthesized according to the previous report (Wang et al., 2006). The block copolymers, methoxyl-poly (ethylene glycol)-*block*-poly (ε-caprolactone) ($mPEG_{114}$-*b*-PCL_{41}) and poly (ε-caprolactone)-*block*-poly (2-aminoethyl ethylene phosphate) (PCL_{25}-*b*-$PPEEA_{17}$), were synthesized according to our previous reports (Wang et al., 2013; Liang et al., 2015). The degree of polymerization of each repeating unit was calculated based on proton nuclear magnetic resonance (^{1}HNMR) analysis. Dulbecco's modified Eagle's medium (DMEM), 3-[4,5-dimethylthiazol-2-yl]-2,5-diphenyltetrazoliumbromide (MTT), fetal bovine serum (FBS), and trypsin were purchased from Gibco BRL. Lipofectamine 2000 (Lipo) RNAi MAX transfection kit and DAPI were provided by Invitrogen Corp. Fluorescent dye (Cy5) labeled CCL-18 siRNA (Cy5-si*CCL-18*) and negative control siRNA (si*NC*) were acquired from Suzhou Ribo Life Science Co., The siRNA sequences are as follows: si*NC*, 5′-TTG GGA AAA TGA GTG GTT dTdT-3′ (sense) and 5′-AAC CAC TCA ACT TTT TCC CAA dTdT-3′ (antisense); si*CCL-18*, 5′-ACA AGU UGG UAC CAA CAA ATT-3′ (sense) and 5′-UUU GUU GGU ACC AAC UUG UGC -3′ (antisense). The fluorescent dye was labeled at the 5′-end of the sense strand of si*CCL-18*. All other organic solvents or reagents were analytical grade and used without further purification.

Methods

Preparation and Characterizations of Nanoparticles (NPs)

The NPs with different sizes were prepared by using the classic nanoprecipitation method. The polymers, mPEG-*b*-PCL (10 mg), PCL-*b*-PPEEA (10 mg), and PCL (50 mg) were, respectively, dissolved in 1 mL of acetonitrile and methyl alcohol (v/v, 1:1). Subsequently, mPEG-*b*-PCL and PCL-*b*-PPEEA were mixed in a molar ratio of 1.5:1 and then added dropwise to 10-fold volume of deionized water which was under vigorously stirring. After stirring for another 20 min, the NP suspension was transferred into a rotary evaporator to remove the organic solvent. The final NP suspension was dispersed in deionized water at a concentration of 1 mg/mL. To adjust the NP size, different amount of PCL was mixed with the mixture of mPEG-*b*-PCL and PCL-*b*-PPEEA (molar ratio, 1.5:1) and the resulting NPs were

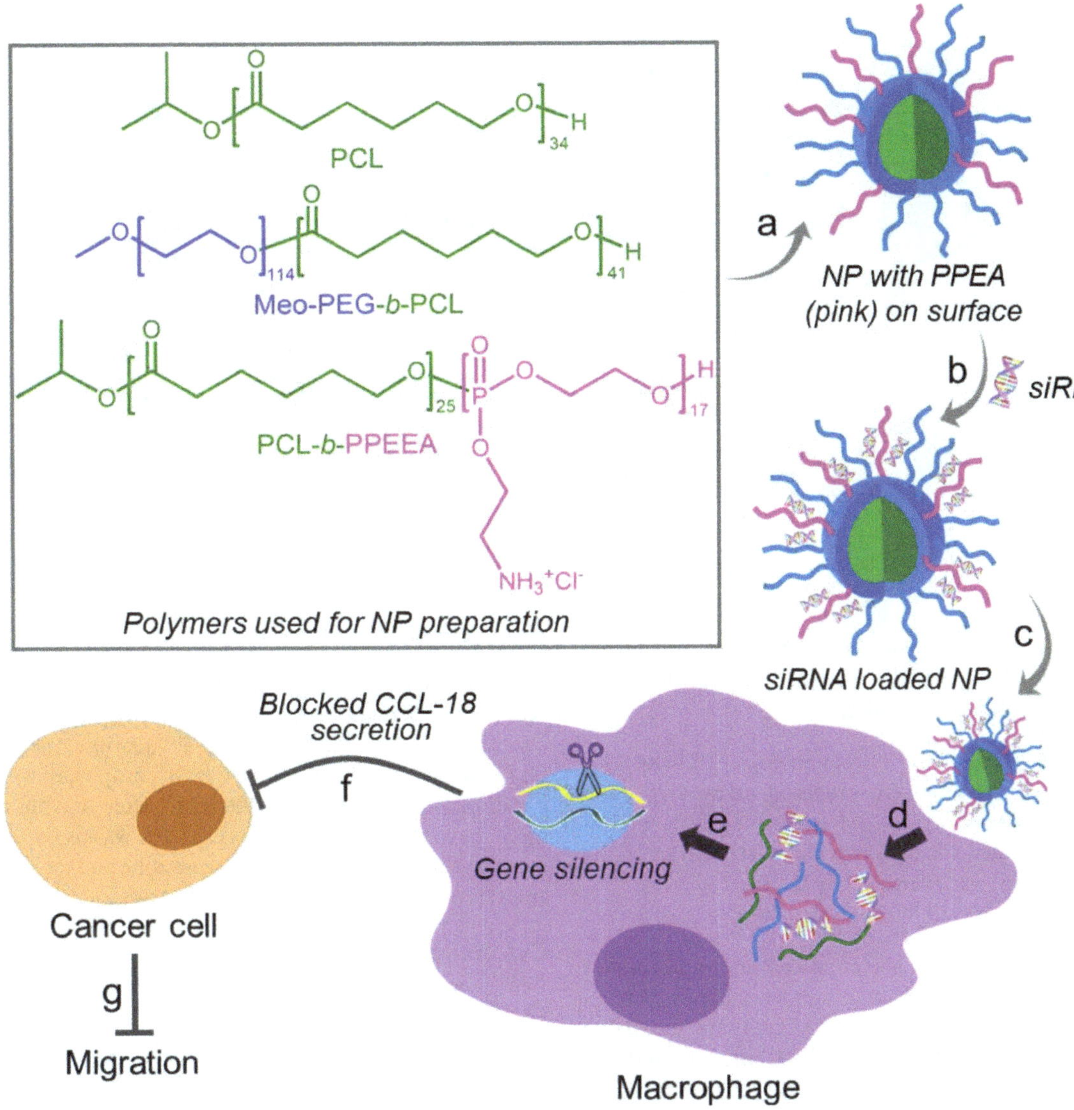

FIGURE 1 | Chemical structures of the polymers (PCL, Meo-PEG-*b*-PCL, and PCL-*b*-PPEEA) and schematic illustration of the self-assembly of the polymers into nanoparticles (NPs) for small interfering RNA (siRNA) delivery and CCL-18 silencing in macrophages to inhibit breast cancer migration. The amphiphilic Meo-PEG-*b*-PCL and PCL-*b*-PPEEA can spontaneously self-assemble into NPs with hydrophobic PCL chains embedded in the cores and hydrophilic PEG and PPEEA chains positioned on the surface **(a)**. After siCCL-18 loading via the electrostatic interaction **(b)** and then internalized by macrophages **(c,d)**, the siCCL-18 can knock down CCL-18 expression **(e)** and thus CCL-18 secretion from the macrophages would be blocked **(f)**, leading to the inhibition of tumor migration **(g)**.

prepared according to the same method described above. The size distribution and zeta potential of the NPs were examined by dynamic light scattering (DLS, Malvern Instruments Corporation). The morphology of the NPs was observed by transmission electron microscopy (TEM, Tecnai G^2 Spirit BioTWIN).

Gel Retardation Assay

The NPs prepared above were mixed with the si*CCL-18* aqueous solution (20 mM) at different N/P ratios. After incubating at room temperature for 20 min, the formed NP/si*CCL-18* complexes were electrophoresed on a 1% agarose gel at 120 mV for 10 min in pH 8.3 Tris/borate/EDTA buffer (89 mM Tris, 89 mM boric acid, 2 mMEDTA). The siRNA bands were visualized with ethidium bromide staining under a UV transilluminator at a wavelength of 365 nm. Naked si*CCL-18* was used as control.

In vitro siRNA Release

The NP/Cy5-si*CCL-18* complexes at an N/P ratio of 10:1 were prepared according the same method described above and then suspended in pH 7.4 PBS solution at a siRNA concentration of 200 nM. Subsequently, the siRNA loaded NP suspension was transferred to a dialysis device (MWCO 100 kDa) that was immersed in pH 7.4 PBS solution at 37°C. At a predetermined

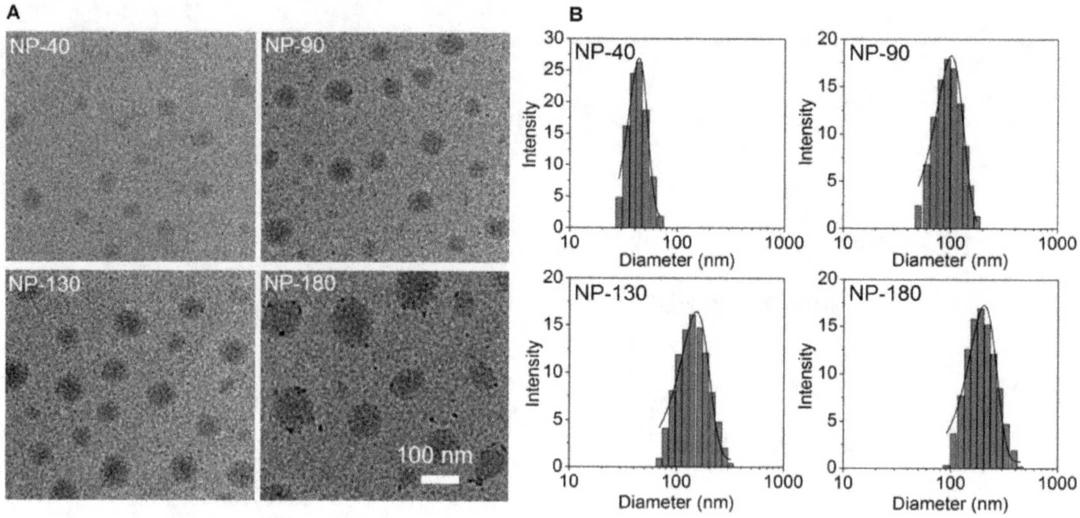

FIGURE 2 | (A) Transmission electron microscopic (TEM) images and **(B)** size distribution of the NP-40, NP-90, NP-130, and NP-180.

interval, 5 μL of the NP suspension was withdrawn and mixed with 20-fold DMSO. The fluorescence intensity of Cy5-si*CCL-18* was determined by a microplate reader.

Evaluation of the Stability of NP/siRNA Complexes

The NP/si*CCL-18* complexes were prepared at an N/P ratio of 10:1 and then dispersed in DMEM containing 10% FBS at 37°C. At a predetermined interval, the size distribution of the NP/si*CCL-18* complexes was examined by DLS.

Cell Culture

THP-1 cells (human monocytic leukemia cell line) and human breast cancer cells (MDA-MB-231 cell line) were obtained from the American Type Culture Collection (ATCC) and incubated in DMEM medium with 10% FBS at 37°C in a humidified atmosphere containing 5% CO_2.

Construction of M2-Like Macrophages

THP-1 cells were incubated in DMEM medium containing 10% FBS and PMA (10 ng/mL) at for 8 h. Subsequently, the medium was replaced by fresh DMEM medium containing interleukin-4 (IL-4, 20 ng/mL). After 48 h incubation, the cells will differentiate into M2-like macrophages and the mRNA level of CCL-18 was examined using quantitative reverse transcription real-time PCR (qRT-PCR).

Confocal Laser-Scanning Microscope (CLSM)

After successful construction of the M2-like macrophages, the cells (50,000 cells) were seeded in round disks and incubated in 2 mL of DMEM medium containing 10% FBS. After 24 h incubation, the medium was replaced and the NP/Cy5-si*CCL-18* complexes were added to the disks at a siRNA concentration of 200 nM. After 4 h incubation, the medium was removed and the cells were washed with pH 7.4 PBS solution thrice. Finally, the nuclei were stained with DAPI and the cells were viewed under a Carl Zeiss LSM 710 CLSM.

Flow Cytometry

The M2-like macrophages were seeded in six-well plate (50,000 cells per well) and incubated in 2 mL of DMEM medium containing 10% FBS. After 24 h incubation, the medium was replaced and the NP/Cy5-si*CCL-18* complexes were added at a siRNA concentration of 200 nM. After 4 h incubation, the medium was removed and the cells were washed with pH 7.4 PBS solution thrice. Finally, the cells were collected for flow cytometry analysis using a BD FACSCalibur flow cytometer.

Cytotoxicity

The cytotoxicity of the NPs was evaluated by using MTT assay. The M2-like macrophages were seeded in 96-well plates at 5,000 cells per well and incubated in 100 μL of DMEM medium containing 10% FBS. After 24 h incubation, the medium was removed and different amounts of the NPs suspended in the culture medium were added. After 48 h incubation, the medium was removed and the cell viability was examined using the MTT assay according to the manufacturer's protocol.

CCL-18 Silencing

The M2-like macrophages were seeded in six-well plate (50,000 cells per well) and incubated in 2 mL of DMEM medium containing 10% FBS. After 24 h incubation, the medium was replaced and the NP/si*CCL-18* complexes were added at different siRNA concentrations. After 48 h incubation, the medium was removed and the cells were washed with pH 7.4 PBS solution thrice. The intracellular mRNA was isolated and the mRNA level of CCL-18 was examined using qRT-PCR.

Inhibition of Migration

MDA-MB-231 cells (50,000 cells) were seeded in round disks and incubated in 2 mL of DMEM medium containing 10% FBS. After 24 h incubation, the cells in the predesigned area of the disks were removed using tips. After washing the cells with PBS thrice,

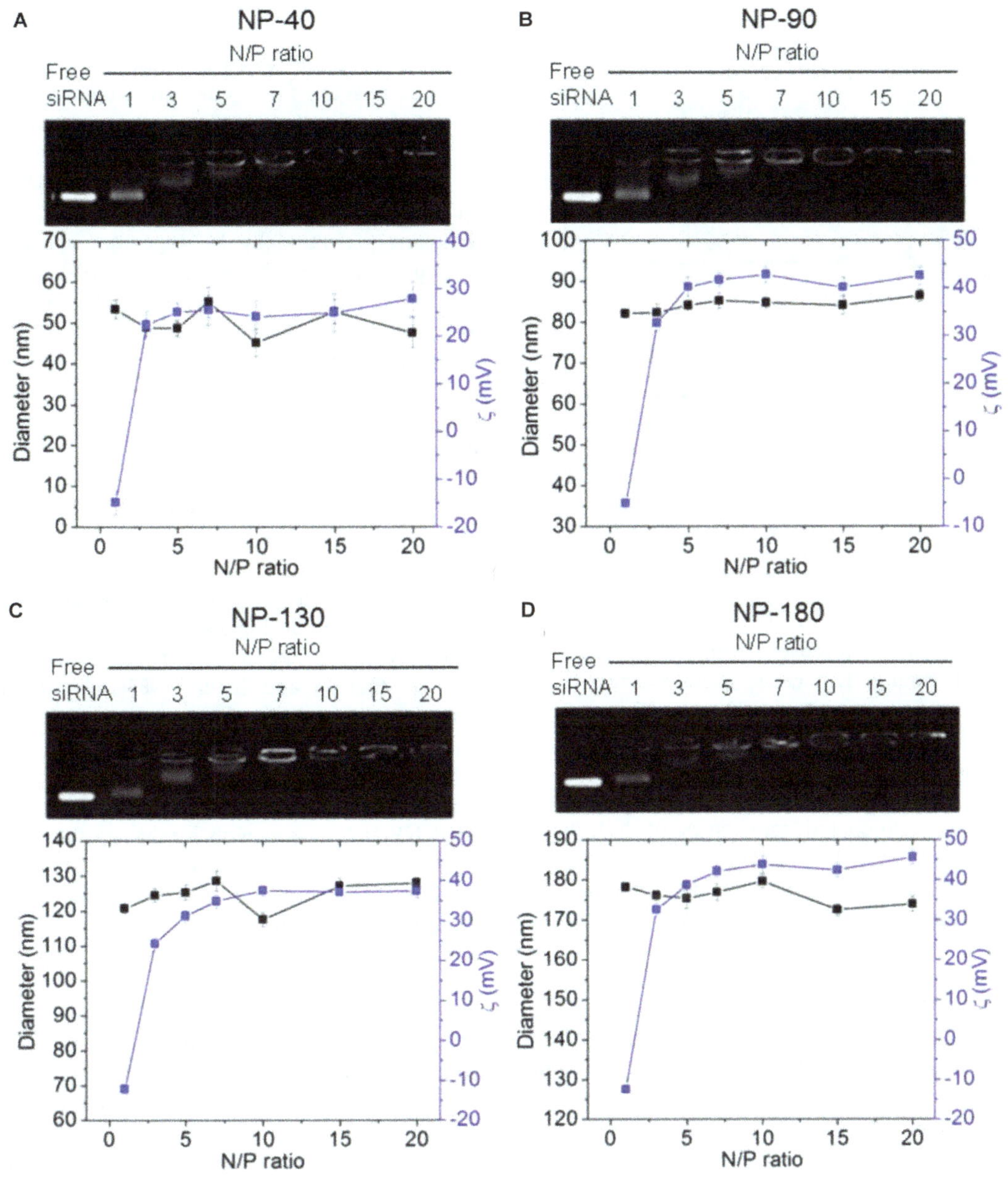

FIGURE 3 | Gel retardation analysis, size, and zeta potential of the complexes formed between si*CCL-18* and the NP-40 **(A)**, NP-90 **(B)**, NP-130 **(C)**, or NP-180 **(D)**.

the cells were incubated with the conditioned medium from the macrophages, in which the CCL-18 has been silenced by the NP-180/si*CCL-18* at a siRNA concentration of 400 nM. After 48 h incubation, the medium was removed and the cells were viewed under optical microscope after washing with PBS thrice.

RESULTS AND DISCUSSION

Preparation and Characterizations of Nanoplatform

Starting from the commercial available mPEG-OH and ε-CL, we employed ring-opening polymerization (ROP) to synthesize the mPEG-*b*-PCL and PCL homopolymer (Sun et al., 2008). The amphiphilic polymer PCL-*b*-PPEEA was also prepared by ROP method (Sun et al., 2008), in which the cationic PPEEA segment was used to complex siRNA via electrostatic interaction. By mixing these three polymers in acetonitrile and methyl alcohol (v/v, 50:50) followed by the addition to deionized water, well-defined NPs can be formed with spherical morphology (**Figure 2A**). In this self-assembly system, the amphiphilic PEG-*b*-PCL and PCL-*b*-PPEEA can spontaneously self-assemble into NPs with hydrophobic PCL chains embedded in the cores and hydrophilic PEG and PPEEA chains positioned on the surface that can, respectively, stabilize the NPs and complex

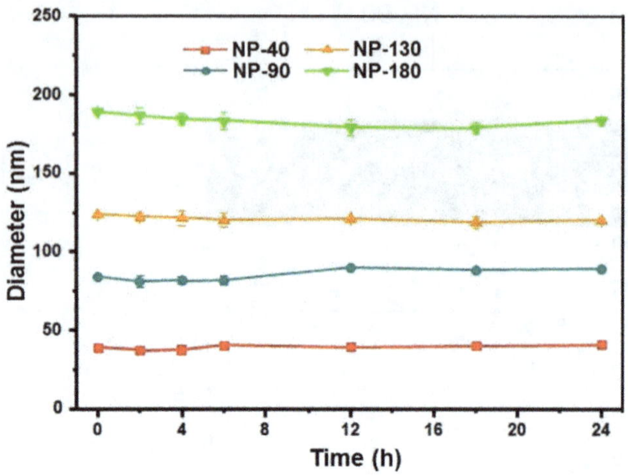

FIGURE 4 | Size of the complexes formed between si*CCL-18* and NP-40, NP-90, NP-130, or NP-180 incubated in DMEM medium containing 10% FBS for different times.

negatively charged siRNA. Moreover, with the increasing feed amount of PCL homopolymer, the average size of the resulting NPs increases from ~40 to 180 nm (**Figure 2B**). The possible reason is that the increased percentage of PCL homopolymer in the NPs induces the size increase of their hydrophobic inner cores (Mao et al., 2014; Liang et al., 2015). In this work, we prepared four types of NPs with the size of 40, 90, 130, and 180 nm (respectively, denoted NP-40, NP-90, NP-130, and NP-180) to evaluate their ability to deliver CCL-18 siRNA (si*CCL-18*) for gene silencing in macrophages.

We next used gel retardation assay to evaluate the siRNA loading capacity of the NPs. As shown in **Figure 3**, due to the presence of cationic PPEEA segment on the surface, all the NPs can effectively load si*CCL18* at an N/P ratio of 10:1, without apparent size change after si*CCL18* loading. Furthermore, all the si*CCL18* loaded NPs show good stability in 10% FBS-containing cell culture medium (**Figure 4**). More importantly, in comparison with the naked *siCCL18*, the use of the NPs can protect the si*CCL18* from degradation by RNase. As shown in **Figure 5A**, with the protection by the NPs, the addition of RNase does not induce the siRNA degradation and the loaded siRNA can still bind with the NPs even under electric field. In contrast, without the NP protection, the naked siRNA has been degraded by the RNase and thus no siRNA band can be observed in the gel retardation assay experiment. All these results demonstrate the NP platform developed in this work shows a strong ability to load and protect the si*CCL-18*, which would thus ensure its bioactivity when used for regulation of macrophage activities. Notably, since we only varied the feed amount of hydrophobic PCL homopolymer to adjust the NP size, while the other two polymers (Meo-PEG-*b*-PCL and PCL-*b*-PPEEA) remain constant in the NP formulations, all the NPs showed the similar ability to load and release the siRNA (**Figure 5B**).

Evaluation of CCL-18 Silencing

After validation of the siRNA loading ability of the NPs, we next examined whether these NPs can deliver siRNA to macrophages for gene silencing. THP-1, a human monocytic leukemic cell line, was used to construct M2-type macrophage-like cells through treatment with PMA and interleukin-4 (IL-4) (Liang et al., 2015). As shown in **Figure 6A**, the high expression of CCL-18, a well-known chemokine generated by M2-type macrophages (Chen et al., 2011), demonstrated the success of THP-1 cells differentiation from monocytes to M2-type macrophages (denoted THP-1-originated macrophages). With this encouraging result, we subsequently encapsulated dye-labeled si*CCL-18* (Cy5-si*CCL-18*) into the NPs and investigated their cellular uptake by the differentiated THP-1 macrophages obtained above. From the flow cytometry (FACS) analysis shown in **Figure 6B**, the THP-1-originated macrophages show higher uptake of the Cy5-si*CCL18* loaded NPs compared to the naked siRNA. The intracellular mean fluorescence intensity (MFI) is at least 1.3-fold stronger than that of the macrophages treated with the naked siRNA. Among these NP formulations, the uptake of NP-180 is highest and the possible reason is that macrophages are apt to internalize foreign materials with large size (Tabata and Ikada, 1988; Champion et al., 2008). **Figure 6C** shows the fluorescent images of macrophages incubated with the Cy5-si*CCL-18* loaded NP-180. Similar as the results of FACS analysis, the THP-1-originated macrophages show strong ability to internalize the siRNA loaded NP-180 as seen with bright red fluorescence and these NPs are mainly dispersed in the cytoplasm where siRNA functions (Whitehead et al., 2009). Although the THP-1-originated macrophages show higher cellular uptake of the NP-180, these NPs do not induce apparent cytotoxicity (**Figure 7A**).

Based on the results of FACS analysis and toxicity assay, the NP-180 shows higher uptake by the THP-1-originated macrophages with negligible toxicity. Therefore, we chose this NP platform as si*CCL-18* delivery tool to examine its gene silencing efficacy in macrophages. As shown in **Figure 7B**, the NP-180 can indeed transport si*CCL-18* into the THP-1-originated macrophages and thereby down-regulate CCL-18 expression. Compared to the macrophages without any treatment (Control), the mRNA level of CCL-18 is down-regulated by 20% at a si*CCL-18* concentration of 100 nM and more than 70% of CCL-18 is suppressed at a si*CCL-18* concentration of 400 nM.

Evaluation of the Inhibition of Migration

It is known that CCL-18 is an important factor secreted by TAMs that can enhance breast cancer metastasis and therefore reduce patient survival (Chen et al., 2011; Su et al., 2014). Previous reports demonstrate that CCL-18 released by TAMs in breast cancer promotes the invasiveness of cancer cells by triggering integrin clustering and enhancing their adherence to extracellular matrix and silencing the CCL-18 expression can inhibit the consistent activation

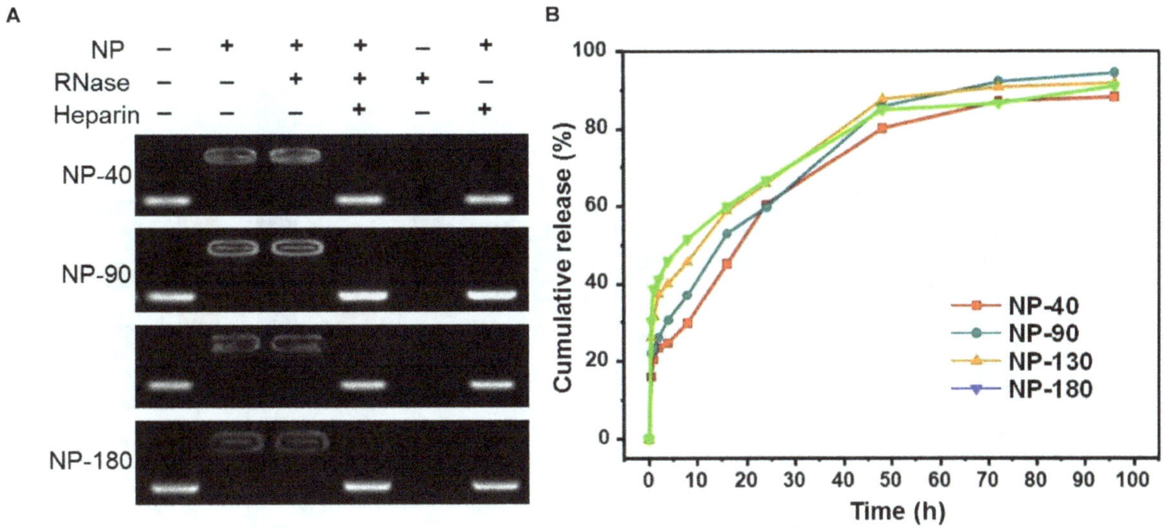

FIGURE 5 | (A) Gel retardation assay of the siRNA loading capacity of the NP-40, NP-90, NP-130, and NP-180; **(B)** Cumulative siRNA release profile of the complexes formed between Cy5-si*CCL-18* and the NP-40, NP-90, NP-130, or NP-180.

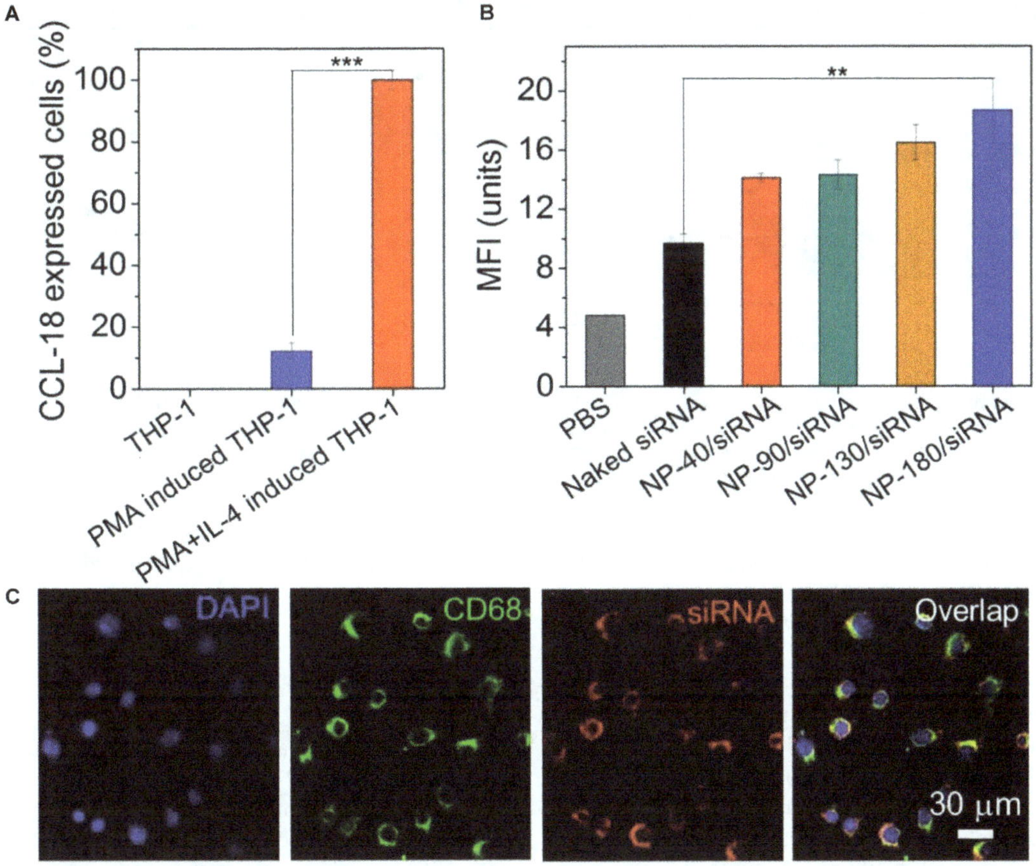

FIGURE 6 | (A) The mRNA level of CCL-18 in the THP-1 cells treated with PMA and IL-4. **(B)** MFI determined by FACS analysis of the THP-1-originated macrophages incubated with the Cy5-si*CCL-18* loaded NPs for 4 h at a siRNA concentration of 200 nM. **(C)** Fluorescent images of the macrophages incubated with the Cy5-si*CCL-18* loaded NP-180 for 4 h at a siRNA concentration of 200 nM. The nuclei and macrophages were staining with DAPI as blue fluorescence and anti-CD68 as green fluorescence, respectively. $^{**}P < 0.01$; $^{***}P < 0.001$.

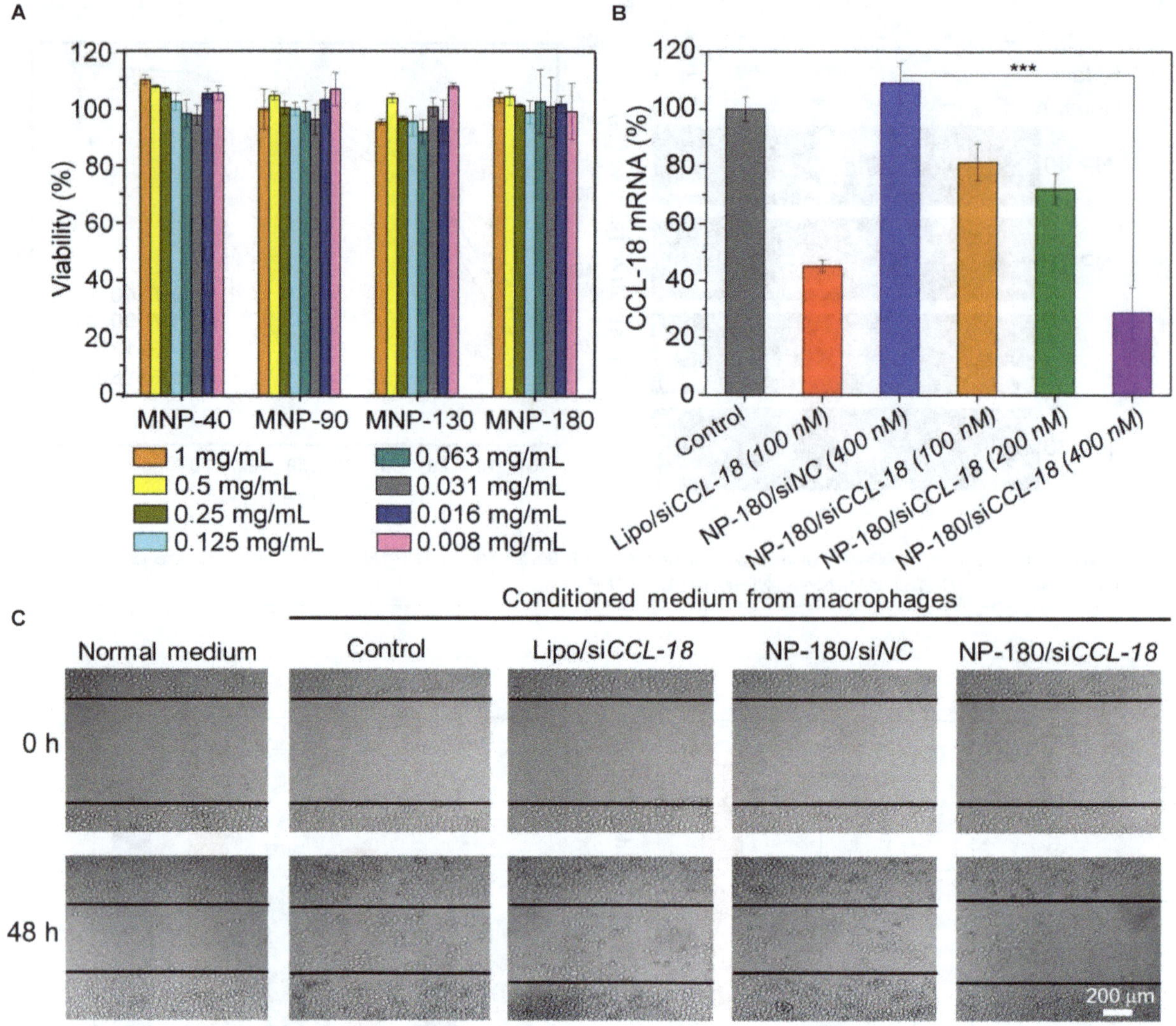

FIGURE 7 | (A) Cell viability of the macrophages incubated with the si*CCL-18* loaded NPs at various concentrations for 48 h. **(B)** The mRNA level of CCL-18 in the macrophages treated by Lipo/si*CCL-18* complexes (Lipo/si*CCL-18*), negative control siRNA loaded NP-180 (NP-180/si*NC*), and si*CCL-18* loaded NP-180 (NP-180/si*CCL-18*). **(C)** Optical images of MDA-MB-231 cells incubated with the conditioned medium from the macrophages that treated with Lipo/si*CCL-18*, NP-180/si*NC*, and NP-180/si*CCL-18* at a siRNA concentration of 400 nM. ****P* < 0.001.

of downstream signal pathways to prevent the migration of breast cancer (Chen et al., 2011). Therefore, we finally simulated tumor microenvironment *in vitro* by incubating breast cancer cell line (MDA-MB-231) with the medium that was obtained from THP-1-originated macrophage (denoted conditioned medium), and examined the influence of CCL-18 silencing on the behavior of MDA-MB-231 cells. As shown **Figure 7C**, due to presence of secreted CCL-18 by macrophages, the addition of conditioned medium to MDA-MB-231 cells can enhance their migration compared to the cells incubated in normal medium. In contrast, after using si*CCL-18* loaded NP-180 to suppress CCL-18 expression in macrophages, the migration of MDA-MB-231 cells is significantly inhibited when incubated with the conditioned medium. This result is consistent with our previous reports (Chen et al., 2011; Su et al., 2014; Nie et al., 2017), and highlights the importance of CCL-18 to the breast cancer cell migration.

CONCLUSION

We have developed a robust RNAi NP platform for efficient gene silencing in M2-type macrophages. Through varying the percentage of hydrophobic PCL homopolymer in the NP formulation, we successfully constructed four types of NPs with different sizes and systemically evaluated their siRNA loading ability and gene silencing efficacy. Experimental results demonstrate that the NP platform with larger size (NP-180) shows higher cellular uptake and efficient CCL-18 silencing in macrophages, leading to efficient inhibition of the breast cancer cell migration. Notably, this NP platform may passively target the tumor tissues via the EPR effect. However, the NP size is very large (~180 nm) and will affect the therapeutic effect if used for *in vivo* regulation of macrophage behaviors. We are currently optimizing the NP formulation and small size NPs will be developed in the future for *in vivo* regulation of macrophage behaviors and cancer treatment.

AUTHOR CONTRIBUTIONS

SL, HY, YY, and XX conceived and designed the experiments. SL, JZ, WW, QL, and JC performed the experiments. SL, PS, XX, HY, and YY analyzed the data and co-wrote the paper.

FUNDING

This work was supported by grants from the Natural Science Foundation of China (81874226, 81272897, 81772837, 81372819, and 81702618), the Thousand Talents Program for Distinguished Young Scholars, the National Key Research and Development Program of China (2017YFA0106300 and 2016YFC1302300), the Guangdong Science and Technology Department (2014A050503029, 2015B050501004, and 2016B030229004), the Natural Science Foundation of Guangdong Province (2017A030313828), and the funding from Guangzhou Science and Technology Bureau (201704020131).

REFERENCES

Aouadi, M., Tesz, G. J., Nicoloro, S. M., Wang, M., Chouinard, M., Soto, E., et al. (2009). Orally delivered siRNA targeting macrophage Map4k4 suppresses systemic inflammation. *Nature* 458, 1180–1184. doi: 10.1038/nature07774

Bronte, V., and Murray, P. J. (2015). Understanding local macrophage phenotypes in disease: modulating macrophage function to treat cancer. *Nat. Med.* 21, 117–119. doi: 10.1038/nm.3794

Burnett, J. C., and Rossi, J. J. (2012). RNA-based therapeutics: current progress and future prospects. *Chem. Biol.* 19, 60–71. doi: 10.1016/j.chembiol.2011.12.008

Caillou, B., Talbot, M., Weyemi, U., Pioche-Durieu, C., Al Ghuzlan, A., Bidart, J. M., et al. (2011). Tumor-associated macrophages (TAMs) form an interconnected cellular supportive network in anaplastic thyroid carcinoma. *PLoS One* 6:e22567. doi: 10.1371/journal.pone.0022567

Champion, J. A., Walker, A., and Mitragotri, S. (2008). Role of particle size in phagocytosis of polymeric microspheres. *Pharm. Res.* 25, 1815–1821. doi: 10.1007/s11095-008-9562-y

Chen, J., Ding, J., Wang, Y., Cheng, J., Ji, S., Zhuang, X., et al. (2017). Sequentially responsive shell-stacked nanoparticles for deep penetration into solid tumors. *Adv. Mater* 29:1701170. doi: 10.1002/adma.201701170

Chen, J., Yao, Y., Gong, C., Yu, F., Su, S., Chen, J., et al. (2011). CCL18 from tumor-associated macrophages promotes breast cancer metastasis via PITPNM3. *Cancer Cell* 19, 541–555. doi: 10.1016/j.ccr.2011.02.006

Cheng, W., Nie, J., Gao, N., Liu, G., Tao, W., Xiao, X., et al. (2017). A Multifunctional nanoplatform against multidrug resistant cancer: merging the best of targeted chemo/gene/photothermal therapy. *Adv. Funct. Mater* 27:1704135. doi: 10.1002/adfm.201704135

Ginhoux, F., Schultze, J. L., Murray, P. J., Ochando, J., and Biswas, S. K. (2015). New insights into the multidimensional concept of macrophage ontogeny, activation and function. *Nat. Immunol.* 17:34. doi: 10.1038/ni.3324

Gordon, S., and Martinez, F. O. (2010). Alternative activation of macrophages: mechanism and functions. *Immunity* 32, 593–604. doi: 10.1016/j.immuni.2010.05.007

Kanasty, R., Dorkin, J. R., Vegas, A., and Anderson, D. (2013). Delivery materials for siRNA therapeutics. *Nat. Mater* 12, 967–977. doi: 10.1038/nmat3765

Kortylewski, M., Swiderski, P., Herrmann, A., Wang, L., Kowolik, C., Kujawski, M., et al. (2009). In vivo delivery of siRNA to immune cells by conjugation to a TLR9 agonist enhances antitumor immune responses. *Nat. Biotechnol.* 27, 925–932. doi: 10.1038/nbt.1564

Liang, S., Yang, X.-Z., Du, X.-J., Wang, H.-X., Li, H.-J., Liu, W.-W., et al. (2015). Optimizing the size of micellar nanoparticles for efficient siRNA delivery. *Adv. Funct. Mater* 25, 4778–4787. doi: 10.1002/adfm.201501548

Liu, S., Pan, J., Liu, J., Ma, Y., Qiu, F., Mei, L., et al. (2018). Dynamically PEGylated and borate-coordination-polymer-coated polydopamine nanoparticles for synergetic tumor-targeted, chemo-photothermal combination therapy. *Small* 14:1703968. doi: 10.1002/smll.201703968

Mantovani, A., Allavena, P., Sica, A., and Balkwill, F. (2008). Cancer-related inflammation. *Nature* 454, 436–444. doi: 10.1038/nature07205

Mao, C. Q., Xiong, M. H., Liu, Y., Shen, S., Du, X. J., Yang, X. Z., et al. (2014). Synthetic lethal therapy for KRAS mutant non-small-cell lung carcinoma with nanoparticle-mediated CDK4 siRNA delivery. *Mol. Ther.* 22, 964–973. doi: 10.1038/mt.2014.18

McAllister, S. S., and Weinberg, R. A. (2014). The tumour-induced systemic environment as a critical regulator of cancer progression and metastasis. *Nat. Cell Biol.* 16, 717–727. doi: 10.1038/ncb3015

Melnikova, I. (2007). RNA-based therapies. *Nat. Rev. Drug Discov.* 6:863. doi: 10.1038/nrd2443

Nie, Y., Chen, J., Huang, D., Yao, Y., Chen, J., Ding, L., et al. (2017). Tumor-associated macrophages promote malignant progression of breast phyllodes tumors by inducing myofibroblast differentiation. *Cancer Res.* 77, 3605–3618. doi: 10.1158/0008-5472.can-16-2709

Noy, R., and Pollard, J. W. (2014). Tumor-associated macrophages: from mechanisms to therapy. *Immunity* 41, 49–61. doi: 10.1016/j.immuni.2014.06.010

Ostuni, R., Kratochvill, F., Murray, P. J., and Natoli, G. (2015). Macrophages and cancer: from mechanisms to therapeutic implications. *Trends Immunol.* 36, 229–239. doi: 10.1016/j.it.2015.02.004

Parayath, N. N., Parikh, A., and Amiji, M. M. (2018). Repolarization of tumor-associated macrophages in a genetically engineered nonsmall cell lung cancer model by intraperitoneal administration of hyaluronic acid-based nanoparticles encapsulating microRNA-125b. *Nano Lett.* 18, 3571–3579. doi: 10.1021/acs.nanolett.8b00689

Qian, B.-Z., and Pollard, J. W. (2010). Macrophage diversity enhances tumor progression and metastasis. *Cell* 141, 39–51. doi: 10.1016/j.cell.2010.03.014

Saw, P. E., Zhang, A., Nie, Y., Zhang, L., Xu, Y., and Xu, X. (2018). Tumor-associated fibronectin targeted liposomal nanoplatform for cyclophilin a siRNA delivery and targeted malignant glioblastoma therapy. *Front. Pharmacol.* 9:1194. doi: 10.3389/fphar.2018.01194

Shi, J., Kantoff, P. W., Wooster, R., and Farokhzad, O. C. (2017). Cancer nanomedicine: progress, challenges and opportunities. *Nat. Rev. Cancer* 17, 20–37. doi: 10.1038/nrc.2016.108

Sica, A., and Mantovani, A. (2012). Macrophage plasticity and polarization: in vivo veritas. *J. Clin. Invest.* 122, 787–795. doi: 10.1172/JCI59643

Su, S., Liu, Q., Chen, J., Chen, J., Chen, F., He, C., et al. (2014). A positive feedback loop between mesenchymal-like cancer cells and macrophages is essential to breast cancer metastasis. *Cancer Cell* 25, 605–620. doi: 10.1016/j.ccr.2014.03.021

Sun, T. M., Du, J. Z., Yan, L. F., Mao, H. Q., and Wang, J. (2008). Self-assembled biodegradable micellar nanoparticles of amphiphilic and cationic block copolymer for siRNA delivery. *Biomaterials* 29, 4348–4355. doi: 10.1016/j.biomaterials.2008.07.036

Tabata, Y., and Ikada, Y. (1988). Effect of the size and surface charge of polymer microspheres on their phagocytosis by macrophage. *Biomaterials* 9, 356–362. doi: 10.1016/0142-9612(88)90033-6

Tseng, Y. C., Mozumdar, S., and Huang, L. (2009). Lipid-based systemic delivery of siRNA. *Adv. Drug Deliv. Rev.* 61, 721–731. doi: 10.1016/j.addr.2009.03.003

Wang, H. X., Xiong, M. H., Wang, Y. C., Zhu, J., and Wang, J. (2013). N-acetylgalactosamine functionalized mixed micellar nanoparticles for targeted delivery of siRNA to liver. *J. Control. Release* 166, 106–114. doi: 10.1016/j.jconrel.2012.12.017

Wang, Y.-C., Shen, S.-Y., Wu, Q.-P., Chen, D.-P., Wang, J., Steinhoff, G., et al. (2006). block copolymerization of ε-caprolactone and 2-methoxyethyl ethylene phosphate initiated by aluminum isopropoxide: synthesis, characterization, and kinetics. *Macromolecules* 39, 8992–8998. doi: 10.1021/ma061821c

Whitehead, K. A., Langer, R., and Anderson, D. G. (2009). Knocking down barriers: advances in siRNA delivery. *Nat. Rev. Drug Discov.* 8, 129–138. doi: 10.1038/nrd2742

Xiao, H., Yan, L., Dempsey, E. M., Song, W., Qi, R., Li, W., et al. (2018). Recent progress in polymer-based platinum drug delivery systems. *Prog. Polym. Sci.* 87, 70–106. doi: 10.1016/j.progpolymsci.2018.07.004

Xu, X., Saw, P. E., Tao, W., Li, Y., Ji, X., Yu, M., et al. (2017a). tumor microenvironment-responsive multistaged nanoplatform for systemic RNAi and cancer therapy. *Nano Lett.* 17, 4427–4435. doi: 10.1021/acs.nanolett.7b01571

Xu, X., Wu, J., Liu, Y., Saw, P. E., Tao, W., Yu, M., et al. (2017b). multifunctional envelope-type siRNA delivery nanoparticle platform for prostate cancer therapy. *ACS Nano* 11, 2618–2627. doi: 10.1021/acsnano.6b07195

Xu, X., Wu, J., Liu, Y., Yu, M., Zhao, L., Zhu, X., et al. (2016). Ultra-pH-responsive and tumor-penetrating nanoplatform for targeted siRNA delivery with robust anti-cancer efficacy. *Angew. Chem. Int. Ed.* 55, 7091–7094. doi: 10.1002/anie.201601273

Yu, S. S., Lau, C. M., Barham, W. J., Onishko, H. M., Nelson, C. E., Li, H., et al. (2013). Macrophage-specific RNA interference targeting via "click", mannosylated polymeric micelles. *Mol. Pharm.* 10, 975–987. doi: 10.1021/mp300434e

Zeng, X., Liu, G., Tao, W., Ma, Y., Zhang, X., He, F., et al. (2017). A drug-self-gated mesoporous antitumor nanoplatform based on pH-sensitive dynamic covalent bond. *Adv. Funct. Mater* 27:1605985. doi: 10.1002/adfm.201605985

Zhang, Y., Satterlee, A., and Huang, L. (2012). In vivo gene delivery by nonviral vectors: overcoming hurdles? *Mol. Ther.* 20, 1298–1304. doi: 10.1038/mt.2012.79

Zuckerman, J. E., and Davis, M. E. (2015). Clinical experiences with systemically administered siRNA-based therapeutics in cancer. *Nat. Rev. Drug Discov.* 14, 843–856. doi: 10.1038/nrd4685

11

Poly(Ethylene Glycol)–Polylactide Micelles for Cancer Therapy

Jixue Wang[1,2], Shengxian Li[1,2], Yuping Han[3], Jingjing Guan[1*], Shirley Chung[4], Chunxi Wang[1] and Di Li[2*]*

[1] Department of Urology, The First Hospital of Jilin University, Changchun, China, [2] Key Laboratory of Polymer Ecomaterials, Changchun Institute of Applied Chemistry, Chinese Academy of Sciences, Changchun, China, [3] Department of Urology, China-Japan Union Hospital of Jilin University, Changchun, China, [4] Department of Biology, University of Waterloo, Waterloo, ON, Canada

***Correspondence:**
Yuping Han
hyp181818@126.com
Jingjing Guan
guanjingjing99@126.com
Di Li
lidi@ciac.ac.cn

For the treatment of malignancy, many therapeutic agents, including small molecules, photosensitizers, immunomodulators, proteins and genes, and so forth, have been loaded into nanocarriers for controllable cancer therapy. Among these nanocarriers, polymeric micelles have been considered as one of the most promising nanocarriers, some of which have already been applied in different stages of clinical trials. The successful advantages of polymeric micelles from bench to bedside are due to their special core/shell structures, which can carry specific drugs in certain disease conditions. Particularly, poly(ethylene glycol)–polylactide (PEG–PLA) micelles have been considered as one of the most promising platforms for drug delivery. The PEG shell effectively prevents the adsorption of proteins and phagocytes, thereby evidently extending the blood circulation period. Meanwhile, the hydrophobic PLA core can effectively encapsulate many therapeutic agents. This review summarizes recent advances in PEG–PLA micelles for the treatment of malignancy. In addition, future perspectives for the development of PEG–PLA micelles as drug delivery systems are also presented.

Keywords: polylactide, poly(ethylene glycol), micelle, nanocarrier, controlled drug release, antitumor treatment

INTRODUCTION

Cancer is one of the major health problems that threaten human life. According to the worldwide statistic, there were 14.1 million new tumor incidences and 8.2 million cancer-related deaths in 2012 (Scsukova et al., 2015). Cancer cells proliferate uncontrollably and rapidly, thus they are characterized by the development of abnormalities and the combination of mutagenic stages. Moreover, they can realize self-sufficiency in growth signals, resistance to growth inhibition and evasion of apoptotic cues (Luo et al., 2009). Furthermore, tumors can induce angiogenesis, evasion from immune surveillance, and metastasis to distant sites through interactions with surrounding stromal cells (Mohme et al., 2017). All of these reasons have led to the refractoriness of cancer. To date, chemotherapy, radiation, surgery, and hormonal therapies are still the major treatment methods for cancer in clinics. Whereas in the research industry, many other treatments, such as photodynamic therapy, photothermal therapy, gene therapy, immunotherapy, and so forth, are being studied. Despite the relatively satisfactory results these therapeutic agents exhibit, they also possess many disadvantages, including poor pharmacokinetics, unspecific bio-distribution, and low targeting ability. The poor solubility and hydrophobicity are considered the major hurdles when therapeutic agents are applied in cancer therapy. Therefore, it is urgent and necessary to overcome these shortcomings to enhance the anti-tumor efficiency.

With the development of nanotechnology, nanomaterials have been widely used in biological application, such as biosensor, tissue engineering as well as drug delivery (Yu et al., 2016a,b,c; Zhang et al., 2017). Nanocarriers have attracted more and more attention in cancer therapy owing to their unique properties, such as nanoscaled size, high surface-to-volume ratio, and favorable physico-chemical characteristics. Various nanocarriers, including liposomes, micelles, and nanocapsules, have been studied in anticancer trials (He et al., 2016; Hofmann et al., 2017; Niu et al., 2017; Tao et al., 2017). They have the capacity to modulate both pharmacokinetic and pharmacodynamic properties, thereby improving their therapeutic index. Among these nanocarriers, polymeric micelles have gained considerably more attention as a multifunctional drug delivery system for poorly water-soluble agents.

Polymeric micelles are the nano-scaled sized particles (5–200 nm) which are self-assembled by amphiphilic polymers. They consist of two parts: the hydrophobic part on the inside (core) and hydrophilic part on the outside (shell). Therefore, the hydrophobic core can serve as a solubilization depot for agents with poor aqueous solubility. The hydrophilic shell provides advantages including longer blood circulation time and increased stability in the blood. In addition, polymeric micelles can be functionalized with targeting ligands to enhance tumor accumulation. As a result, the role of polymeric micelles in delivery of hydrophobic therapeutic agents for anticancer therapy is promising and opportunistic.

Polyethylene glycol (PEG)-polylactide (PLA) is one of the most prominent amphipathic polymers, therefore it is very suitable for constructing micelles. PLA is a form of biodegradable and biocompatible polyester derived from renewable resources and approved by the Food and Drug Administration (FDA) for clinical use. The hydrophobicity of PLA makes it suitable for the hydrophobic portion of micelles. PLA has three types of stereoisomers: poly(L-(-)-*S*-lactide) (PLLA), poly(D-(+)-*R*-lactide) (PDLA), and racemic PDLLA. Interestingly, PLLA and PDLA can form stereocomplexes through physical association of PLLA and PDLA chains (Ikada et al., 1987). PLA can interact with different hydrophilic agents, such as PEG (Danafar et al., 2017), poly(2-methacryloyloxyethyl phosphorylcholine) (PMPC) (Long et al., 2016), poly(ethylene oxide) (PEO) (Fang et al., 2015), and poly(*N*-isopropylacrylamide) (PNIPAAm) (Wei et al., 2009), to form amphiphilic block copolymers and further self-assemble into micelles. Among them, PEG is the most popular hydrophilic agent due to its various advantages, including linearity, lack of charge, immunogenicity, low polydispersity, and easy activation for conjugation. PEG–PLA micelles have been widely used as drug delivery systems for cancer therapy owing to the excellent physicochemical and biological properties, namely nontoxicity, non-protein adsorption, and weakened uptake by the reticulo-endothelial system (RES) after intravenous injection (Wang et al., 2015, 2017). Notably, Genexol®-PM, a paclitaxel formulation based on PEG–PLA copolymer micelles, was approved in Korea in 2007 for the treatment of breast, lung, and ovarian cancers (Luo et al., 2012). Moreover, it is currently under clinical development in the USA (Lee et al., 2008).

In this review paper, an overview of PEG–PLA-based micelles utilized for the effective delivery of therapeutic agents possessing varying mechanisms for cancer treatment is discussed, as shown in **Scheme 1**. Additionally, the applications of different treatment modalities are described in detail. Features of nanocarriers in references are shown in **Table 1**. In particular, the development of stimuli-responsive, targeted-modified, and multifunctional PEG–PLA micelles are also highlighted.

CHEMOTHERAPEUTICS

In clinical settings, surgery and radiotherapy are the most commonly used and effective therapeutic means for local and non-metastatic tumors. However, they are inefficient for metastatic tumors. Currently, application of anti-cancer drugs, such as chemotherapeutic drugs, hormone drugs, and biological drugs, has become the main method of treatment. These anti-cancer drugs are able to reach all parts of the body *via* the bloodstream and primarily inhibit the rapid replication of tumor cells. Unfortunately, they also inhibit the rapid growth of healthy cells which are crucial to maintaining normal function of the organism, such as hair follicles, bone marrow, and gastrointestinal tract cells (Chabner and Roberts, 2005). As a result, serious side effects are apparent in chemotherapeutic drug treatments. Due to the severe toxicity and concomitant multidrug resistance of conventional chemotherapeutic drugs, it is urgent to find new effective drug carriers to solve these problems. PEG–PLA micelles provide significant advantages over standard treatments. Drug-loaded micelles exhibit a huge potential for tumor drug delivery to overcome the limitations of chemotherapeutic agents.

As generally known, many chemotherapeutic drugs are not highly water-soluble. Hydrophobic agents are associated with several problems in therapeutic applications, such as poor absorption, bioavailability, and drug aggregation-related complications. Fortunately, polymeric micelles constructed from amphiphilic copolymers can promisingly increase the water solubility of such hydrophobic chemotherapeutic drugs by 10–5000 folds (Savić et al., 2006). Puntawee et al. improved the aqueous solubility and bioavailability of semi-synthetic andrographolide analog (19-triphenylmethyl ether andrographolide, AG 050) by utilizing the PEG-*b*-PLA micelles. As a result, PEG-*b*-PLA micelle was able to significantly increase the encapsulation efficiency of hydrochloride salt of AG 050 (AG 050-P) in aqueous solution (280-fold) (Puntawee et al., 2016).

It is worth noting that conventional chemotherapeutic drugs are quite small in size. As a result, they are rapidly cleared from the bloodstream, thus leading to decreased concentration within the tumor (Allen and Cullis, 2004). When chemotherapeutic drugs are loaded into PEG–PLA micelles, their circulation time in the bloodstream will be prolonged, therefore allowing adequate amounts of drugs to reach the target site (Jin et al., 2017). Furthermore, compared to other drug carriers, micelles have the advantage of possessing a very small size (10–100 nm). This is critical for passive accumulation through the leaky vasculature and into the tumor site *via* the enhanced

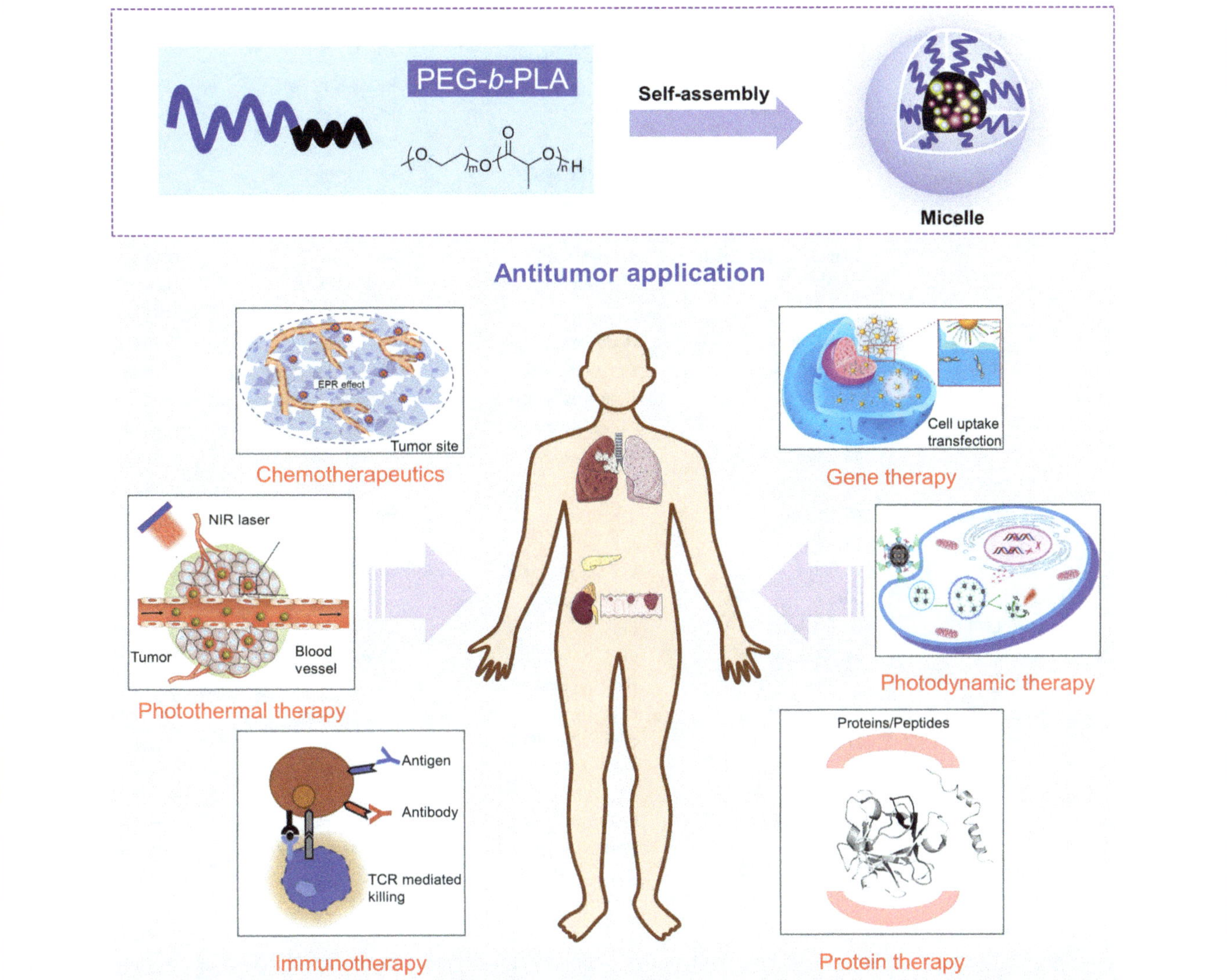

SCHEME 1 | Schematic illustration of PEG-*b*-PLA micelle in application of antitumor. Reproduced with permission from Cho et al. (2016); Peng et al. (2016); Wang et al. (2016); Moy and Tunnell (2017); Yin et al. (2017) and Zhai et al. (2017).

permeability and retention (EPR) effect to solid tumors, particularly to poorly vascularized tumors (Davis and Shin, 2008; Feng et al., 2017). Two main factors are responsible for the EPR effect: (1) the angiogenic vasculature of tumor sites have higher permeability than normal vasculature because of their discontinuous endothelia and (2) the lymphatic drainage is not fully developed in tumors. These conditions result in the exudation of colloidal particles through the "leaky" endothelial layer of tumor vascular and subsequently accumulating in tumor tissues. Majority of vascular pore cutoff size of tumor sites is between 380 and 780 nm (Hobbs et al., 1998). Shi et al. synthesized a docetaxel (DTX)-conjugated mPEG–PLA micelle *via* an ester linkage (DTX-PM). The average size of DTX-PM was 58.2 ± 2.3 nm, which was suitable for passive targeting *via* an EPR effect for anti-cancer drug delivery. More importantly, the DTX-PM significantly induced apoptosis of HSC-3 cancer cells and effectively suppressed the tumor progression in the HSC-3 xenograft model *in vivo* (Shi et al., 2016) (**Figure 1**). Particle size is a critical factor in the efficacy of drug-loaded-micelles. It is of fundamental importance to understand the association between the size of drug-loaded nanocarriers and their fate in biological systems *in vivo* for rational design of drug delivery systems. Yu et al. prepared five different sized (30–230 nm) DTX-loaded methoxy poly(ethylene glycol)-poly(lactide) micelles. They studied the permeation effect of micelles within both multicellular tumor spheroids and tumor xenografts in mice. The results indicated that small micelles could enhance the tissue penetration however, the blood half-life was short. Micelles of 100–200 nm showed prolonged circulation time compared with that of smaller or larger micelles, but the

TABLE 1 | Features of nanocarriers in references.

Treatment methods	Therapeutic agents	Mean size (nm)	Delivery strategy	Cancerous cells	References
Chemotherapeutics	AG 050	10–100 nm	EPR	KKU-M213 cells	Puntawee et al., 2016
	DTX	58.2 ± 2.3 nm	EPR	HSC-3 cells	Shi et al., 2016
		30–230 nm		KB cells	Yu and Qiu, 2016
		111 nm/129 nm	c(RGDfK) targeted	HeLa cells	Li et al., 2016a
		∼ 80 nm	Octreotide targeted	NCI-H446 cells	Zhang et al., 2011
	PTX	80–125 nm	Folate targeted	KB cells	Xiong et al., 2011
		14.6 ± 0.8–104.2 ± 8.1 nm	pH sensitive/EPR	A549 cells	Liang et al., 2016
	DOX	170.87 ± 3.02	Folate targeted /pH sensitive	MCF-7Adr	Li et al., 2015
		150 nm	pH sensitive	MDA-MB231	Wu et al., 2010
		34–107 nm	Redox-responsive	HeLa cells	Yang et al., 2015
Photothermal therapy	TPT–TT NPs	85 nm	Optical excitation	HeLa/HepG2 cells	Sun et al., 2015
Photodynamic therapy	PpIX	80 nm	Optical excitation	C26/B16BL6/ Lewis cells	Ogawara et al., 2016
		30 nm	Optical excitation	H2009 cells	Ding et al., 2011a
		49 ± 6/57 ± 6 nm	Optical excitation	H2009 cells	Ding et al., 2011b
	NEt2Br2BDP	138.4 ± 17.3 nm	Optical excitation/pH sensitive	U87MG cells	Tian et al., 2015
Immune therapy	LD-indolicidin	25 ± 5 nm		EG7 cells	Coumes et al., 2015
	CTLA-4-siRNA	141.6 ± 6.1 nm		B16 melanoma cells	Li et al., 2016b
Protein therapy	Plk1; si*Plk1*	120 nm	$ScFv_{Her2}$ targeted	BT474	Dou et al., 2014
	OX26	50 nm	OX26 targeted		Yue et al., 2012
Gene therapy	TNF cDNA	80 ± 4 nm	EPR	MCF-7 cells	Shukla et al., 2017
	siRNA	54.30 ± 3.48 nm	EPR	MCF-7 cells	Zhao et al., 2012
	TRAIL gene/PTX		RGD targeted	U87 cells	Zhan et al., 2012
Others	curcumin	∼ 33 ± 2.3 nm	EPR	C6/U251 cells	Zheng et al., 2016
		171.0–22.6 nm	pH sensitive/EPR	MCF-7 cells	Yu et al., 2014
		104.6 ± 2.1/169.3 ± 1.52 nm	EPR	B16F10/MDA-MB-231 cells	Kumari et al., 2017
		<100 nm	EPR	HepG2 cells	Yang et al., 2012c
		110 ± 5 nm	EPR	B16F10/MDA-MB-231 cells	Kumari et al., 2016
	DOX/CA4	29.2 ± 2.5 nm	EPR	B16-F10	Wang et al., 2011

penetration was limited. Large micelles (>200 nm) had both short half-life and weak penetration ability, leading to limited tumor accumulation (Yu and Qiu, 2016). Through the EPR effect, drug-loaded PEG–PLA micelles can selectively kill tumor cells and reduce the damage to normal tissues.

Active targeting is another effective method to reduce the damage of chemotherapeutic drugs to normal tissues (Allen, 2002; Szakács et al., 2006). Ligands are modified on the surface of nanocarriers to bind to particular receptors overexpressed by tumor cells or tumor vasculature. Many kinds of targeted ligands have been researched, such as small organic molecules, sugar moieties, peptides, and monoclonal antibodies (Allen, 2002; Brannon-Peppas and Blanchette, 2012). Folate is an example of a small organic molecule that is a cancer targeting ligand because the folate receptor is frequently overexpressed on tumors (Cho et al., 2016). Xiong *et al.* designed folate-conjugated interfacially crosslinked biodegradable micelles consisting of poly(ethylene glycol)-*block*-poly(acryloyl carbonate)-*block*-poly(D,L-lactide) (PEG–PAC–PLA) and folate-PEG–PLA (FA-PEG–PLA) block copolymers for receptor-mediated delivery of paclitaxel (PTX). Remarkably, folate-decorated PTX-loaded crosslinked micelles displayed significantly higher toxicity to KB cells than free PTX. This is most likely due to their much more efficient cellular uptake through FA receptor-mediated endocytosis. Flow cytometry studies also showed that folate-decorated FITC-labeled crosslinked micelles were much more efficiently taken up by KB cells than that of controls without folate ligands. All these results indicated that ligand-conjugated interfacially crosslinked PEG–PLA micelles have great potential in targeted cancer therapy (Xiong et al., 2011). Peptides are another form of actively used ligands in anticancer drug delivery. Li et al. developed DTX-loaded target micelles (c(RGDfK)-PEG–PLA/PEG–PLA/DTX) that were able to targeted delivery DTX to the tumor cells. Cellular uptake and 3-(4,5-dimethylthiazol-2-yl)-2,5-diphenyltetrazolium bromide (MTT) studies revealed that the target micelles were more efficiently taken up by HeLa cells in the presence of c(RGDfK) and significantly improved the cytotoxicity compared to that of non-target micelles (Li et al., 2016a). In another study, researchers constructed somatostatin analog octreotide (OCT)-modified, DTX loaded PEG-*b*-PLA micelles that bind to somatostatin receptors (SSTRs) overexpressed on tumor cells. The results showed that OCT-PM-DTX enhanced intracellular delivery efficiency in cells and exhibited

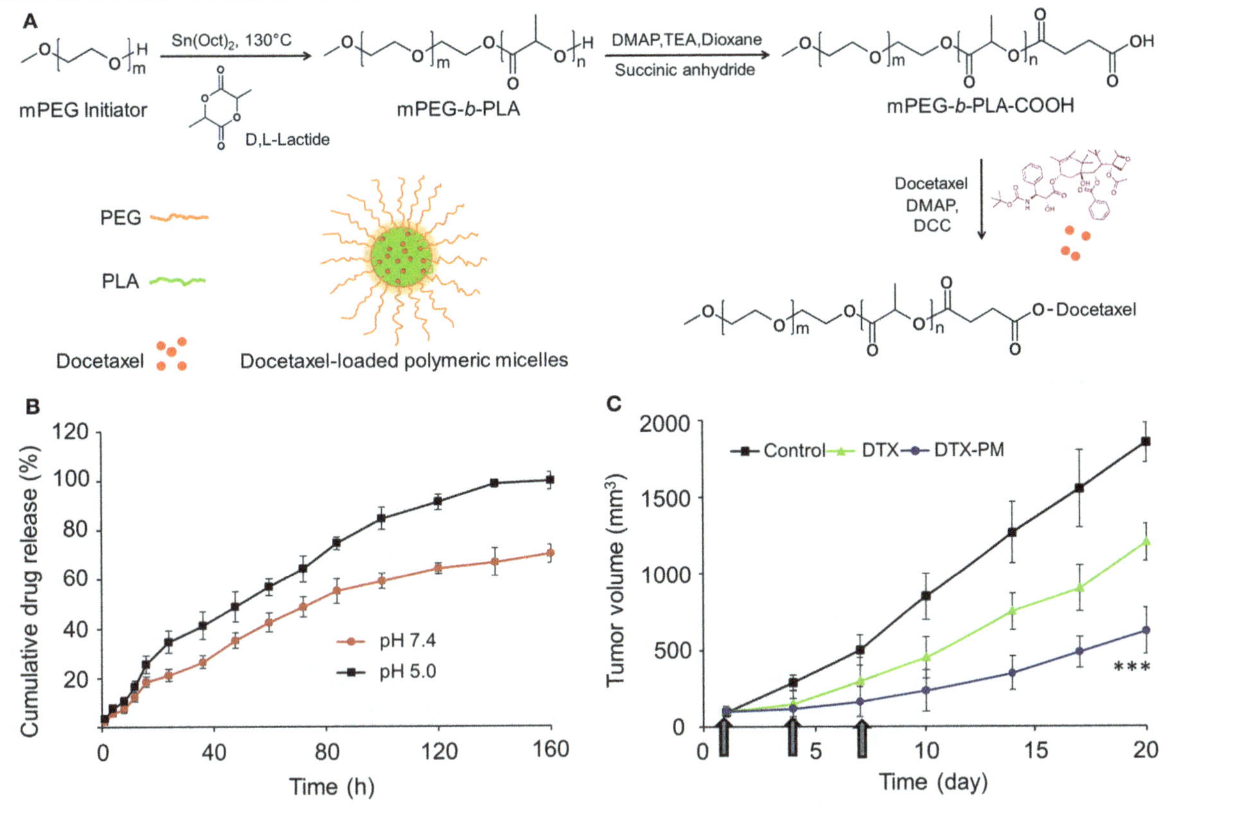

FIGURE 1 | (A) Schematic illustration of synthesis of mPEG–PLA-docetaxel polymer drug conjugate. **(B)** The *in vitro* release of DTX from DTX-PM (PBS, pH 7.4 and pH 5.0, at 37 °C). **(C)** Tumor volume of free DTX and DTX-PM in xenograft tumor model (***$P < 0.0001$). Reproduced with permission from Shi et al. (2016).

higher retardation of tumor growth *in vivo* (Zhang et al., 2011).

In another study, researchers synthesized a folate modified pH sensitive targeted polymeric micelle to reduce the systemic toxicity of doxorubicin (DOX) and to increase the antitumor efficacy in a multi-drug resistant tumor model (Li et al., 2015). A pH sensitive targeted strategy is derived from the pH of the tumor microenvironment which is slightly lower (6.5–7.2) compared to physiological pH (7.4) (Tannock and Rotin, 1989; Gerweck et al., 2006). The triggering mechanisms of most pH sensitive micelles relate to the endosome and release of the loaded drugs into the cytoplasm. This is because the pH significantly drops to 5.0–6.5 in the endosome and to 4.5 in primary and secondary lysosomes (Hubbell, 2003; Schmaljohann, 2006). Therefore, based on the pH of endosomes/lysosomes, pH sensitive PEG–PLA-based micelles loaded with chemotherapeutic drugs have been widely studied to improve the efficiency of cancer therapy. The major strategies used for inducing pH-sensitive behaviors are changing the charges in the micellar system and the dissociating pH-dependent drug binding linkers. Liang *et al.* constructed size shifting micelle nanoclusters (MNC) based on a cross-linked framework interspersed with PEG–PLA micelles. After being internalized into tumor cells, the framework of MNC became swollen and disintegrated within the acidic environment of lysosomes *via* the proton sponge effect of PEI resulting in the release of nanosized micelles for further penetration (Liang et al., 2016). Wu et al. fabricated tumor-targeted and pH-responsive polymeric micelles by mixing AP peptide (CRKRLDRN) conjugated PEG-poly(D,L-lactic acid) block copolymer (AP-PEG–PLA) into the pH-responsive micelles of methyl ether poly(ethylene glycol) (MPEG)-poly(-amino ester) (PAE) block copolymer (MPEG-PAE). This micelle showed a sharp pH-dependent micellization/demicellization transition at the acidic environment of the tumor. When loaded with DOX, the DOX-loaded micelles exhibited excellent anticancer therapeutic efficacy (Wu et al., 2010).

Redox-responsive nanocarriers are another captivating direction of research for effective intracellular anticancer drug release (Meng et al., 2009; Cheng et al., 2011). Unlike pH-sensitive strategies which usually release drugs in the endo/lysosomal compartments, redox-responsive strategies aim to disassemble and release drugs in the cytosol and cell nucleus where many chemotherapeutic drugs, such as DOX and PTX, elicit their therapeutic effects (Zhang et al., 2012; Chuan et al., 2014). Since the amounts of glutathione (GSH) tripeptide in the cytosol and cell nucleus ($\sim$2–10 mM) are confoundedly higher than that of extracellular fluids and circulation ($\sim$2–20 μM), the intracellular redox-response is exceedingly fast and efficient. Yang et al. constructed a type of redox-responsive micelle which could self-assemble from dynamic covalent PEG–PLA block copolymers that contained a double disulfide linkage in the backbone. The *in vitro* drug release analyses indicated that a reductive environment could result in triggered drug release profiles. A cytotoxicity assay of DOX-loaded micelles indicated higher cellular proliferation inhibition against HeLa cells pretreated with 10 mM GSH monoester (GSH-OEt) for 2 h than that of nonpretreated ones (Yang et al., 2015). In order to further improve the anticancer efficiency of chemotherapeutic drug-loaded PEG–PLA micelles, dual or multi-stimuli responsive micelles that respond to a combination of two or more signals mentioned above have also been developed.

PHOTOTHERMAL THERAPY COMPONENTS

Photothermal therapy (PTT) has become an effective alternative in cancer therapy because of the advantages over other treatment methods, such as minimal invasiveness, low toxicity, and high specificity to tumor sites (Geng et al., 2015; Mebrouk et al., 2015). In clinical practice, to maximize the light penetration depth and minimize the influence of biological chromophores, photothermal agents should have strong optical absorbance in the near-infrared (NIR) window (700–900 nm) (Jaque et al., 2014). In recent years, a variety of nanomaterials, such as gold nanostructures (nanoshells, nanorods, nanostars and nanocages) (Chen et al., 2010; Zhang et al., 2012; Ma et al., 2013; Wang et al., 2013), carbon nanomaterials (carbon nanotube and graphene) (Liu et al., 2011; Yang et al., 2012a), and various other inorganic (Tian et al., 2011) and organic nanoparticles (Yang et al., 2012b) have been used for PTT. Although most inorganic nanomaterials have shown effective therapeutic effect for cancers, majority of them are non-biodegradable and will retain in the body for a long time (Sharifi et al., 2012; Zhang et al., 2013). Compared to inorganic nanomaterials, polymeric NIR-absorbing nanomaterials agents have shown great superiority for PTT. Among PTT agents, small molecular organic dyes, such as (ICG) (Fang et al., 2017) and prussian blue (PB) (Hoffman et al., 2014), have been used not only as fluorescent probes in optical imaging, but also as PTT agents. Sun et al. fabricated a new photothermal nano-agent by coprecipitation of 2,5-Bis(2,5-*bis*(2-thienyl)-N-dodecyl pyrrole) thieno[3,4-b][1,2,5] thiadiazole (TPT-TT) and a biodegradable amphiphilic block copolymer, methoxy poly(ethylene glycol)2K-*block*-poly(D,L-lactide)2K (mPEG2K–PDLLA2K). As a result, TPT-NPs showed high photothermal conversion efficiency, excellent photostability, and heating reproducibility. The photostability of TPT-TT NPs was much better than that of ICG. Besides, TPT-TT NPs exhibited significant photothermal therapeutic effects toward human cervical carcinoma (HeLa) and human liver hepatocellular carcinoma HepG2 cells (Sun et al., 2015) (**Figure 2**).

PHOTODYNAMIC THERAPY COMPONENTS

Photodynamic therapy (PDT) is a light triggered method for cancer treatment. Due to the minimal aggressiveness and harmlessness to healthy tissue, PDT can avoid the disadvantages of conventional chemotherapeutic agents, such as serious side

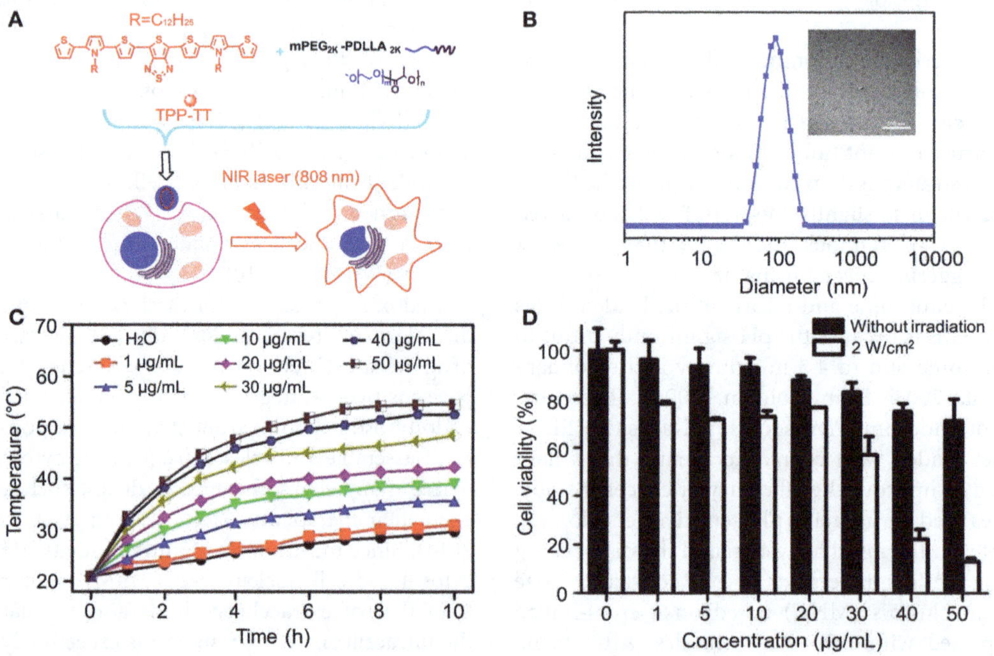

FIGURE 2 | (A) Schematic illustration of the preparation and their cellular action process of TPT-TT NPs. **(B)** TEM image (Scale bar 500 nm) and size distribution determined by DLS of TPT-TT NPs. **(C)** Photothermal conversion behavior of TPT-TT NPs at various concentrations. **(D)** Relative cell viabilities of HepG2 cells incubated with different concentrations of TPT-TT NPs. Reproduced with permission from Sun et al. (2015).

effects or multidrug resistances. PDT can kill tumor cells mainly through the generation of singlet oxygen ($^1O_2$) or free radicals. The reactive oxygen species (ROS) can cause significant cellular damage, destruction of tumor blood vessels, and stimulation of antineoplastic immunity (Juarranz et al., 2008). PDT depends on three factors to perform its anticancer effect: (i) a photosensitizer (PS) agent; (ii) irradiation of the affected region using light of an appropriate wavelength; and (iii) presence of oxygen. During irradiation, highly reactive species, such as ROS, which are capable of causing direct damage to biomolecules and triggering the death of tumor cells, are generated *in situ* (Paszko et al., 2011). Recently, the combination of photodynamic therapeutic agents and nanosystems has proven to be promising. Nanosystems, such as liposomes, micelles, and polymeric nanoparticles, have been widely studied for PDT application, as well as for combination of PDT agents with chemotherapeutic agents or with other forms of therapies. For example, Ogawara et al. encapsulated the photoprotoporphyrin IX dimethyl ester (PppIX-DME) into PEG–PLA nanoparticles (PN-Por). The PN-Por showed significant phototoxicity *in vitro* and effective antitumor effect in C26 tumor-bearing mice *in vivo*. All results exhibited the potency of PN-Por for PDT-based cancer treatments (Ogawara et al., 2016). In another study, in order to increase the solubility and delivery efficiency of PpIX, Ding et al. prepared PpIX loaded polymeric micelles using non-covalent encapsulation and covalent conjugation methods. Micelles with lower PpIX loading density (e.g., 0.2%) showed brighter fluorescence and higher $^1O_2$ yield than higher PpIX loading density (e.g., 4%) in solution. However, 4% PpIX-conjugated micelles demonstrated better antitumor efficiency *in vivo* (Ding et al., 2011a). Moreover, they further studied the effect of carrier microenvironment on photophysical properties of 5,10,15,20-tetrakis(meso-hydroxyphenyl)porphyrin (mTHPP) and its biological efficacy in tumor inhibition. The electron-deficient PEG–PLA micelle was used as a control. Results displayed that the photophysical and photodynamic properties of mTHPP were highly related to the micelle core environment (Ding et al., 2011b).

PDT can also be combined with active targeting strategies to enhance the antitumor efficiency. Cyclic RGD (cRGD) is a type of peptide that can target the $\alpha_v\beta_3$ integrin-rich tumor cells. Tian et al. encapsulated NEt2Br2BDP (a trifunctional photosensitizer) into a cRGD peptide-poly(ethylene glycol)-*block*-poly(lactic acid) (cRGD-PEG–PLA) and methoxyl poly(ethylene glycol)- block-poly(lactic acid) (mPEG–PLA) nanomicelle. Under the acidic tumor environment (pH 4.5–5.0), the nanoprobe could be activated to produce fluorescence for tumor detection and $^1O_2$ for effective tumor therapy (Tian et al., 2015) (**Figure 3**).

Although there are few related studies, the PEG–PLA-micelle-based PDT represents a new kind of therapeutic method, which may be used in clinics in the future.

IMMUNE PREPARATION

Immunotherapy is a method of treatment that utilizes the patients' own immune system to treat their illness. Recent strategies for cancer immunotherapy mainly focus on tumor-associated antigens (TAAs), known as a tumor vaccine, and the induction of antigen-specific T cell-mediated immune responses (Cheever and Higano, 2011; Tefit and Serra, 2011; Ledford, 2014). With the thriving progress of genomics and proteomics, various potential target antigens, such as recombinant proteins, synthetic peptides, and DNA, have been studied (De Gregorio and Rappuoli, 2014). However, when administered alone *in vivo*, they often suffer from short half-life and ineffectively activate the immune system. Hence, adjuvants are required to elicit effective immune responses against tumor cells (Brichard and Lejeune, 2007). Based on the mechanisms of action, vaccine adjuvants can be divided into two categories: immunomodulatory adjuvants and delivery systems (Huang et al., 2011). Coumes et al. synthesized a peptide/polymer conjugate copolymer by conjugation of the amine end-group of LD-indolicidin to the Nhydroxysuccinimide-activated carboxyl end-group of PEG. When the TAA vaccine candidate was formulated with LD-indolicidin-PEG–PLA-stabilized squalene-in-water emulsion, they could effectively elicit a T helper (Th)1-dominant antigen-specific immune response and exhibit satisfactory antitumor activity (Coumes et al., 2015) (**Figure 4**). To induce T cell-mediated immune responses, Li et al. used PEG–PLA based nanoparticles to deliver cytotoxic T lymphocyte-associated molecule-4 (CTLA−4)-siRNA (NPsiCTLA-4). Both the *in vitro* and *in vivo* studies showed that this nanoparticle delivery system could effectively deliver CTLA-4-siRNA into both CD4+ and CD8+ T cells, and could significantly increase the percentage of anti-tumor CD8+ T cells, therefore enhancing the antitumor immune responses (Li et al., 2016b).

PROTEINS

Protein therapeutics, especially applying cytokines and antibodies, have attracted increasing attention in recent clinical cancer treatments. Compared to chemotherapeutic drugs, proteins have many unique advantages including high specificity, incorporation of diversified functions, and minor side effects on normal tissue (Leader et al., 2008). The mechanism of protein therapy for cancer treatment typically depends on the direct induction of apoptosis in tumor cells and indirect tumor inhibition by activating an immune response or targeting the tumor vasculature and stroma. In order to overcome the shortcomings of proteins in cancer treatment, such as rapid *in vivo* degradation, poor pharmacokinetics, and instability, combination of proteins with nano delivery systems has been intensively researched.

Cytokines are a class of secreted or membrane-bound proteins. They play an important role in regulating the growth, differentiation, and activation of immune cells (Dranoff, 2004). Many kinds of cytokines, such as tumor necrosis factors (TNFs), interleukins (ILs), and interferons (INFs), have been widely used in clinical cancer treatment. These cytokines can be targeted through the use of antibodies. Antibodies are one of the most efficient and promising approaches for the treatment of hematological malignant neoplasms and solid

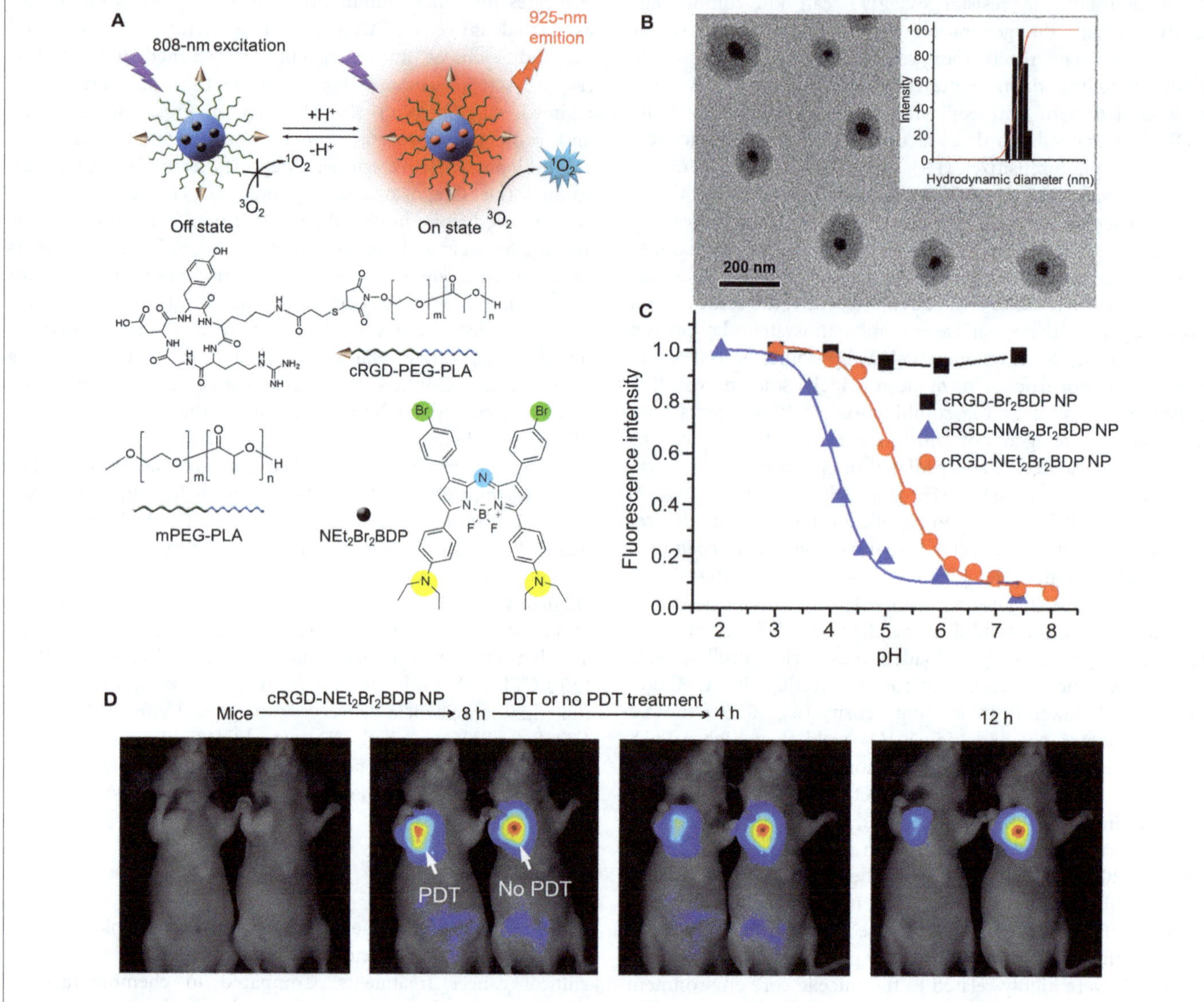

FIGURE 3 | (A) Structure, characterization, and optical properties of cRGD-NEt2Br2BDP. **(B)** NPTEM image of cRGD-NEt_2Br_2BDP NP. Inset: size distribution of cRGD-NEt_2Br_2BDP NP determined with DLS. **(C)** pH titration curves of fluorescence intensity of different NPs. **(D)** *In vivo* PDT and therapeutic monitoring on subcutaneous U87MG tumor-bearing mice with cRGD-NEt_2Br_2BDP NP. Reproduced with permission from Tian et al. (2015).

tumors (Scott et al., 2012). A series of monoclonal antibodies (mAbs) have been approved by the FDA or are being assessed in clinical trials for cancer therapy (Scott et al., 2012). Antibodies can also act as target groups to enhance the uptake of drugs in tumor cells and can be combined with a nano drug delivery system. In order to achieve targeted delivery of si*Plk1* to $Her2^+$ breast cancer, Dou et al. designed an anti-Her2 single-chain variable fragment antibody (ScFv $_{Her2}$)-decorated PEG–PLA-based nanoparticles encapsulated with si*Plk1* (ScFv $_{Her2}$ -NP $_{si}$ *Plk1*). This ScFv $_{Her2}$ -NP $_{siRNA}$ could specifically bind to the Her2 antigen overexpressed on the surface of $Her2^+$ breast cancer cells. Therefore, the antitumor efficiency was evidently improved (Dou et al., 2014). Yue et al. prepared multifunctional hybrid micelles based on amphiphilic mal-PEG-*b*-PLA and mPEG-*b*-P(LA-*co*-DHC/RhB) block copolymers. A specific anti-transferrin receptor antibody, OX26, was then linked onto the surface of the micelles. The results showed that OX26 conjugation visibly increased the uptake efficiency of micelles by target cell lines (C6) and effectively passed through the blood-brain barrier (Yue et al., 2012).

GENE

Nucleic acid (such as plasmid DNA, antisense oligonucleotides, and siRNA)-based gene therapeutics have received an increased amount of attention in the last few decades because of their unique advantages for attacking critical cancer hallmarks (Das and Verma, 2016; Jiang et al., 2017). Even though the use of viral vectors for gene therapy offers highly efficient gene

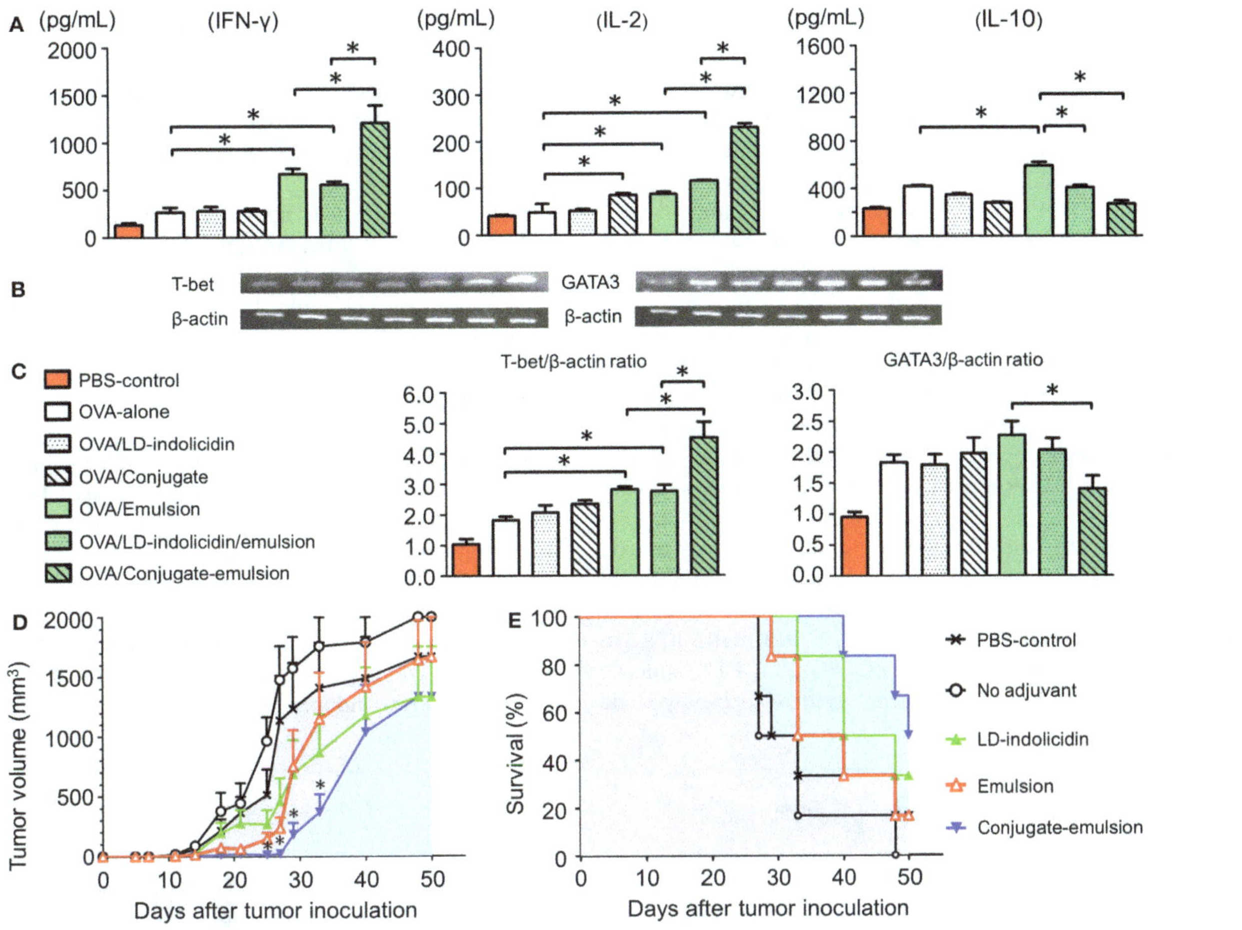

FIGURE 4 | Analysis of T cell immunity. **(A)** Cytokine secretion responses and **(B,C)** mRNA expression levels. Antitumor efficacy of OVA protein formulated with different adjuvants and administered to C57BL/6 mice bearing EG7 tumor cells. Statistical significance was determined by performing ANOVA followed by a Bonferroni post-test. *$p < 0.05$. **(D)** Tumor volume *$p < 0.05$ compared with no adjuvant group and **(E)** survival rate. Reproduced with permission from Coumes et al. (2015).

transfer and has shown satisfactory results in clinical trials (Alton, 2007), they possess various unwanted effects, such as immune stimulation and the potential for mutagenesis. Therefore, it is clear there is still need for further investigation to improve the delivery mechanism (Thomas et al., 2003; Ginn et al., 2013). These unwanted effects have led researchers to turn to non-viral vector solutions with high efficiency, stability, and minimal toxicity (Mykhaylyk et al., 2007; Sun et al., 2008). Among them, cationic polymers have been widely studied due to its unique advantages (Merdan et al., 2002). Polyethyleneimine (PEI), a synthetic polymer which has shown high condensation and superior transfection efficiencies, is one of the most used cationic polymers (Wiseman et al., 2003). In order to achieve high efficiency for either DNA or siRNA loading and transfection efficiency, the molecular weight (MW) of the PEI block must be high (e.g., 25 k Da). However, high MW PEI is known to cause systemic toxicity upon intravenous administration (Moghimi et al., 2005). Moreover, another shortcoming is that polycation/DNA or siRNA complexes have the tendency to aggregate when induced by salt- and serum proteins *in vivo* and can be rapidly cleared by the immune system (Moret et al., 2001). Although PEI can be conjugated with PEG to form block copolymer assemblies and has shown increased stability, reduced toxicity, and lower immunogenicity (Kim et al., 2005; Sato et al., 2007), block copolymers still limit timely release of the internalized gene from the complex due to steric interferences of the associated PEG chains (Grigsby and Leong, 2010; Salcher and Wagner, 2010). Therefore, developing efficient delivery systems based on biomaterials may be an effective means for nucleic acid delivery in therapeutic applications. PEG–PLA micelles are able to resolve parts of the aforementioned problems of gene delivery. In order to systematically deliver DNA expression vectors to tumors, Shukla *et al.* developed a novel dual nanoparticle (DNP) system to deliver DNA expression vectors to tumor cells. The DNP system was consisted of a DNA expression vector–cationic peptide nanocomplex (NC) surrounded by a PEG–PLA nanoparticle. The results showed that the DNP system could effectively induce apoptosis of tumor cells and possess highly anti-tumor efficacy *in vivo* (Shukla et al., 2017).

RNA interference (RNAi) is a post-transcriptional gene silencing phenomenon. The discovery of RNAi was through the mechanism of small interfering RNA (siRNA). The mechanism is that siRNA can be incorporated into the RNA-induced silencing complex (RISC) and specifically degrades the target messenger mRNA through complementary base pairing, thereby prohibiting the translation into target proteins (Amjad et al., 2017). Zhao et al. synthesized a biodegradable amphiphilic tri-block copolymer (mPEG2000-PLA3000-*b*-R15) composed of monomethoxy poly(ethylene glycol), poly(D,L-lactide), and polyarginine. This copolymer can further self-assemble into cationic polymeric nanomicelles for *in vivo* siRNA delivery. The polymeric nanomicelles showed excellent haemocompatibility and higher cell growth inhibition toward EGFR expressed MCF-7 cells. *In vivo* experiments further proved the effective tumor growth inhibition effect of the polymeric nanomicelles (Zhao et al., 2012) (**Figure 5**).

In addition to the therapeutic application of genetic material, genes can also be delivered alongside traditional chemotherapy drugs. Zhan et al. investigated the anti-glioblastoma effects of RGD-PEG-PEI/pORF-hTRAIL nanoparticle combined with CDX-PEG–PLA-PTX micelle (paclitaxel loaded CDX-poly(ethylene glycol)–block-poly(lactic acid) micelle). When administered the same dosages, the survival time of the intracranial glioblastoma-bearing model mice was significantly longer in the co-delivery (33.5 days) treated group than that of the groups solely treated with CDX-PEG–PLA-PTX (25.5 days), RGD-PEG-PEI/pORF-hTRAIL [24.5 days), or physiological saline (21.5 days)]. This research proved the high efficacy for co-delivery of tumor necrosis factor-related apoptosis-inducing ligand (TRAIL) and PTX in the intervention of intracranial glioblastoma by employing tumor-targeted gene carrier RGD-PEG-PEI and brain-targeted micelle CDX-PEG–PLA, respectively (Zhan et al., 2012).

OTHERS

Curcumin (Cur), a natural polyphenol of *Curcuma longa*, has been widely researched for its antitumor activities. However, the poor aqueous solubility and low biological availability have limited its further application. Zheng et al. fabricated Cur-loaded PEG–PLA micelles. The preparation of Cur-MPEG-PLA was very simple and fast. Besides, the micelle group showed a sustained release behavior of Cur and an enhanced toxicity on C6 and U251 glioma cells *in vitro*. Moreover, compared to free Cur, they induced more apoptosis on C6 glioma cells.

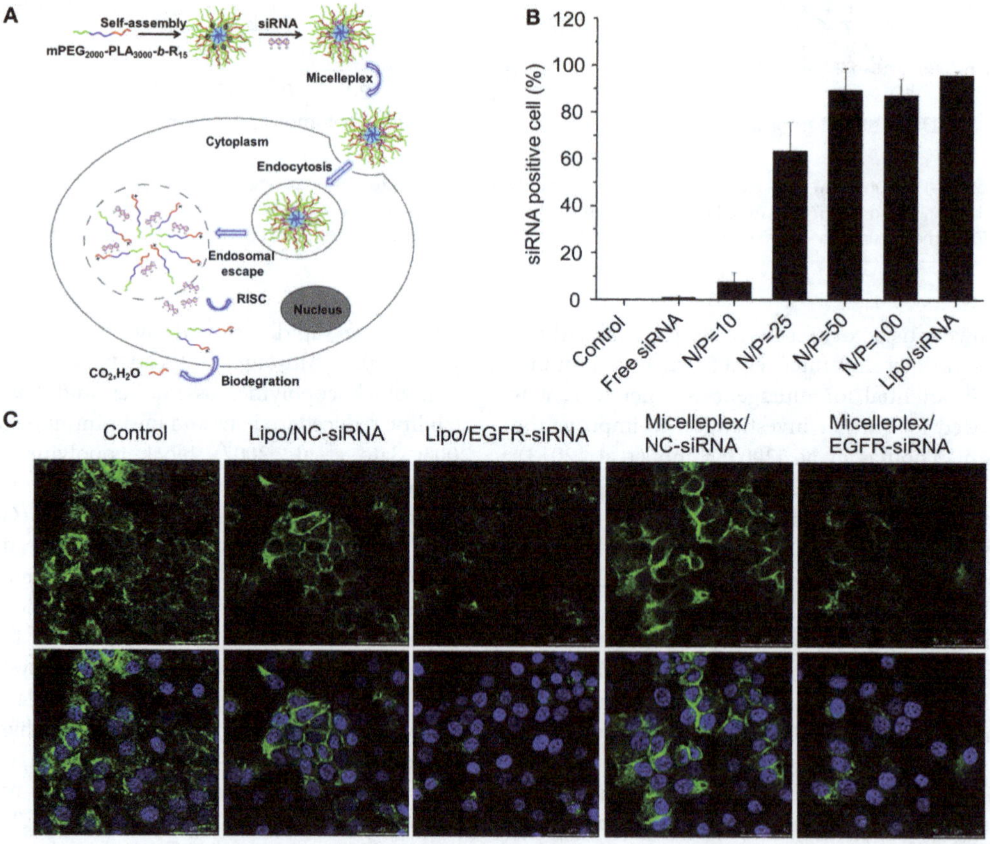

FIGURE 5 | (A) Schematic illustration of biodegradable cationic micelles for delivering siRNA into cancer cells. **(B)** siRNA-positive cells after treated with different FAM-siRNA formulations. **(C)** Confocal microscopic observation of EGFR silencing effect in MCF-7 cells. Reproduced with permission from Zhao et al. (2012).

The Cur-loaded micelles also effectively improved the anti-glioma activity of Cur *in vivo* (Zheng et al., 2016) (**Figure 6**). In another study, researchers constructed Cur-loaded pH-sensitive MPEG–PLAPAE micelles. These micelles could shrink from 171.0 nm to 22.6 nm and could increase their surface charge to 24.8 mV, which significantly improved the cell uptake of Cur by MCF-7 cells. Moreover, these micelles also exhibited excellent antitumor efficiency *in vivo* (Yu et al., 2014). The antitumor activity of Cur-loaded PEG–PLA micelles were also reported in other studies (Yang et al., 2012c; Kumari et al., 2016, 2017).

Antivascular therapy is a distinctive form of cancer treatment. It can cause a selective and rapid shutdown of the tumor vasculature, thus resulting in extensive cancer cell death. Wang et al. developed $\alpha_v\beta_3$ integrin-targeting peptide (RGD) functionalized polymeric micelles (RFPMs) based on the use of poly(ethylene glycol)-*block*-poly(D,L-lactide) (PEG–PLA). DOX was conjugated to the PEG–PLA micelle core and combretastatin A4 was physically encapsulated into the micelles (RFPMs-DOX-CA4). The micelles exhibited sequential release kinetics, resulting in sequential killing of endothelial cells and tumor cells *in vitro*. In B16-F10 tumor-bearing mice, RFPMs-DOX-CA4 showed stronger tumor growth inhibition and significantly higher survival rate compared to other treatment groups (Wang et al., 2011).

CONCLUSIONS

In the last few decades, polymeric micelles have become one of the most promising nano-delivery systems for the treatment of cancers have been used for the delivery of a variety of cargoes, from conventional chemotherapeutic drugs to specific therapeutic agents and biological macromolecules. Among various polymeric micelles, PEG–PLA based micelles have been intensively studied because of their excellent biodegradability and biocompatibility. Genexol-PM has already been approved for breast cancer treatment in South Korea. With the progressive development of cancer treatment methods, such as photodynamic therapy, photothermal therapy, immunotherapy, and gene therapy, PEG–PLA micelles are being increasingly applied in combination with these treatments. It is worth noting that besides primary passive targeting through the EPR, there is a clear shift toward the utilization of micelles which can be modified for active targeting, controlled delivery of therapeutic agents reliant on the unique tumor microenvironment or external environment, and combination of more than one type of therapeutic payload.

This review has discussed various examples of PEG–PLA micelles being applied in a variety of therapeutic applications for the treatment of cancers. These micelles contain a wide range of modifications including primary modification for passive

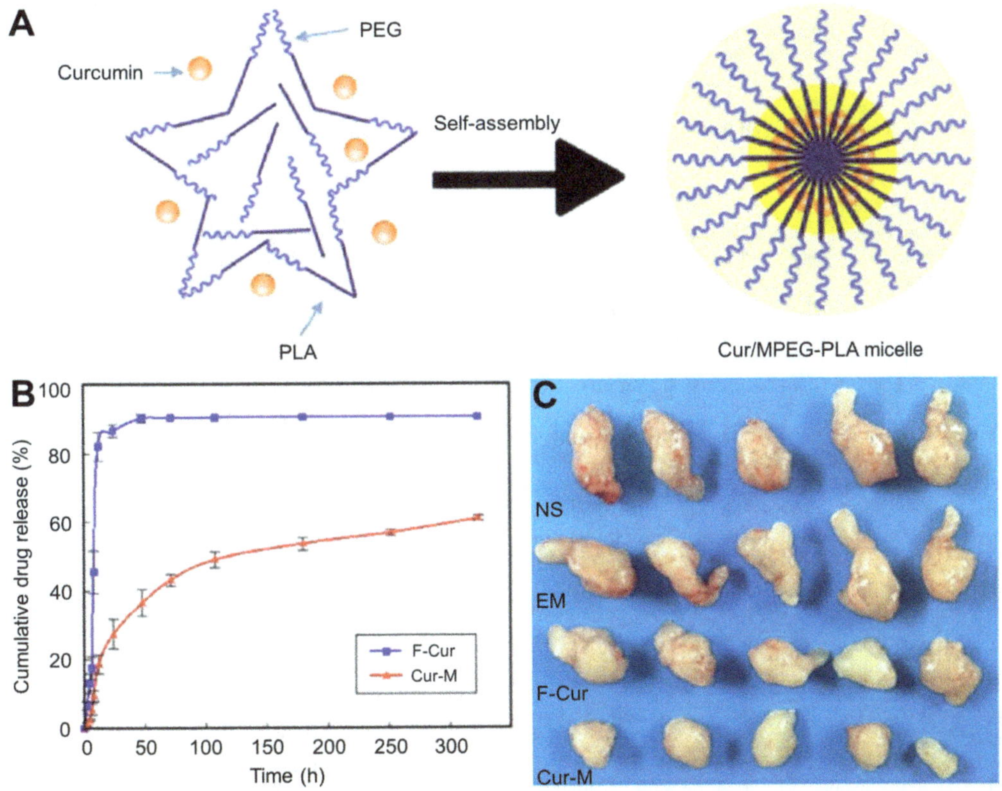

FIGURE 6 | (A) Preparation of Cur/MPEG–PLA micelles. **(B)** *In vitro* release study and **(C)** representative images of subcutaneous tumors in each treatment group. Reproduced with permission from Zheng et al. (2016).

targeting, incorporation of targeting ligands, responsiveness to the tumor microenvironment, and the mixing of micelles with drugs and other therapeutic agents. Among them, multifunctional PEG–PLA micelles have gained immense attention due to their versatility in simultaneously incorporating various agents (e.g., chemotherapeutic drugs and RNAi) and their ability to achieve multiple modifications (e.g., active targeting, passive targeting, and response to stimuli) to enhance cancer therapy.

It is promising to be hopeful about the future of PEG–PLA micelles given their inherent advantages. However, it should be noted that the safety of these novel concepts is a major concern. Rollerova et al. validated that PEG-*b*-PLA NPs might interfere with the activation and function of the hypothalamic-pituitary-gonadal (HPG) axis, which might relate to the nanoreprotoxicity of PEG-*b*-PLA NPs at both the central neuroendocrine and gonadal levels (Rollerova et al., 2015). In addition, PEG-*b*-PLA NPs also could cause neuroendocrine disrupting effect in the neonatal female rats (Scsukova et al., 2015). Dvoráková et al. indicated a possible age-related association between the oxidative stress and neonatal PEG-b-PLA administration (Dvoráková et al., 2017). Therefore, the PEG–PLA micelles still need to be carefully studied in several animal models and eventually in human patients.It is known that the simpler the structure of a system, the easier it is to translate. In the future, we should bear this in mind to design more "active" targeting and simple structures of PEG–PLA micellar drug delivery systems. It is promising that PEG–PLA micelles will play an increasingly important role in the wide range of treatment methods against cancer.

AUTHOR CONTRIBUTIONS

JW and SL produced the first draft. SC and DL revised the manuscript. DL, YH, and JG proposed the outline of the article and revised the draft before submission. CW revised the draft carefully. In additional all authors provided final approval of the manuscript.

ACKNOWLEDGMENTS

This work was financially supported by the National Natural Science Foundation of China (Grant Nos. 51673190, 51603204, 51303174, 51473165, 51390484, and 51520105004) and the Science and Technology Development Program of Jilin Province (Grant Nos. 20160204015SF and 20160204018SF).

REFERENCES

Allen, T. M. (2002). Ligand-targeted therapeutics in anticancer therapy. *Nat. Rev. Cancer* 2, 750–763. doi: 10.1038/nrc903

Allen, T. M., and Cullis, P. R. (2004). Drug delivery systems: entering the mainstream. *Science* 303, 1818–1822. doi: 10.1126/science.1095833

Alton, E. (2007). Progress and prospects: gene therapy clinical trials (part 1). *Gene Ther.* 14, 1439–1447. doi: 10.1038/sj.gt.3303001

Amjad, M. W., Kesharwani, P., Amin, M. C. I. M., and Iyer, A. K. (2017). Recent advances in the design, development, and targeting mechanisms of polymeric micelles for delivery of siRNA in cancer therapy. *Prog. Polym. Sci.* 64, 154–181. doi: 10.1016/j.progpolymsci.2016.09.008

Brannon-Peppas, L., and Blanchette, J. O. (2012). Nanoparticle and targeted systems for cancer therapy. *Adv. Drug Deliver. Rev.* 64, 206–212. doi: 10.1016/j.addr.2012.09.033

Brichard, V. G., and Lejeune, D. (2007). GSK's antigen-specific cancer immunotherapy programme: pilot results leading to Phase III clinical development. *Vaccine* 25, B61–B71. doi: 10.1016/j.vaccine.2007.06.038

Chabner, B. A., and Roberts, T. G. (2005). Chemotherapy and the war on cancer. *Nat. Rev. Cancer* 5, 65–72. doi: 10.1038/nrc1529

Cheever, M. A., and Higano, C. S. (2011). PROVENGE (Sipuleucel-T) in prostate cancer: the first FDA-approved therapeutic cancer vaccine. *Clin. Cancer Res.* 17, 3520–3526. doi: 10.1158/1078-0432.CCR-10-3126

Chen, J., Yang, M., Zhang, Q., Cho, E. C., Cobley, C. M., Kim, C., et al. (2010). Gold nanocages: a novel class of multifunctional nanomaterials for theranostic applications. *Adv. Funct. Mater.* 20, 3684–3694. doi: 10.1002/adfm.201001329

Cheng, R., Feng, F., Meng, F., Deng, C., Feijen, J., and Zhong, Z. (2011). Glutathione-responsive nano-vehicles as a promising platform for targeted intracellular drug and gene delivery. *J. Control. Release* 152, 2–12. doi: 10.1016/j.jconrel.2011.01.030

Cho, H., Gao, J., and Kwon, G. S. (2016). PEG-b-PLA micelles and PLGA-b-PEG-b-PLGA sol-gels for drug delivery. *J. Control. Release* 240, 191–201. doi: 10.1016/j.jconrel.2015.12.015

Chuan, X., Song, Q., Lin, J., Chen, X., Zhang, H., Dai, W., et al. (2014). Novel free-paclitaxel-loaded redox-responsive nanoparticles based on a disulfide-linked poly (ethylene glycol)–drug conjugate for intracellular drug delivery: synthesis, characterization, and antitumor activity *in vitro* and *in vivo*. *Mol. Pharm.* 11, 3656–3670. doi: 10.1021/mp500399j

Coumes, F., Huang, C. Y., Huang, C. H., Coudane, J., Domurado, D., Li, S., et al. (2015). Design and development of immunomodulatory antigen delivery systems based on peptide/PEG–PLA conjugate for tuning immunity. *Biomacromolecules* 16, 3666–3673. doi: 10.1021/acs.biomac.5b01150

Danafar, H., Rostamizadeh, K., Davaran, S., and Hamidi, M. (2017). Drug-conjugated PLA–PEG–PLA copolymers: a novel approach for controlled delivery of hydrophilic drugs by micelle formation. *Pharm. Dev. Technol.* 22, 947–957. doi: 10.3109/10837450.2015.1125920

Das, R. H., and Verma, N. (2016). Silencing the disease messengers: progress and prospects in developing nucleic acid based therapeutics. *RNAi Technol.* 5, 85–96.

Davis, M. E., and Shin, D. M. (2008). Nanoparticle therapeutics: an emerging treatment modality for cancer. *Nat. Rev. Drug Disco.* 7, 771–782. doi: 10.1038/nrd2614

De Gregorio, E., and Rappuoli, R. (2014). From empiricism to rational design: a personal perspective of the evolution of vaccine development. *Nat. Rev. Immunol.* 14, 505–514. doi: 10.1038/nri3694

Ding, H., Sumer, B. D., Kessinger, C. W., Dong, Y., Huang, G., Boothman, D. A., et al. (2011a). Nanoscopic micelle delivery improves the photophysical properties and efficacy of photodynamic therapy of protoporphyrin IX. *J. Control. Release* 151, 271–277. doi: 10.1016/j.jconrel.2011.01.004

Ding, H., Yu, H., Dong, Y., Tian, R., Huang, G., Boothman, D. A., et al. (2011b). Photoactivation switch from type II to type I reactions by electron-rich micelles for improved photodynamic therapy of cancer cells under hypoxia. *J. Control. Release* 156, 276–280. doi: 10.1016/j.jconrel.2011.08.019

Dou, S., Yang, X. Z., Xiong, M. H., Sun, C. Y., Yao, Y. D., Zhu, Y. H., et al. (2014). ScFv-decorated PEG-PLA-based nanoparticles for enhanced siRNA delivery to Her2+ breast cancer. *Adv. Healthc. Mater.* 3, 1792–1803. doi: 10.1002/adhm.201400037

Dranoff, G. (2004). Cytokines in cancer pathogenesis and cancer therapy. *Nat. Rev. Cancer* 4, 11–22. doi: 10.1038/nrc1252

Dvoráková, M., Rollerová, E., Scsuková, S., Bujnáková Mlynarčíková, A., Laubertová, L., and Žitnanová, I. (2017). Effect of neonatal exposure to poly (ethylene glycol)-block-poly (lactic acid) nanoparticles on oxidative state in infantile and adult female rats. *Oxid. Med. Cell Long.* 2017:7430435. doi: 10.1155/2017/7430435

Fang, J., Zhang, K., Jia, J., Wang, Z., and Hu, Q. (2015). Preparation and characterization of N-phthaloyl-chitosan-g-(PEO–PLA–PEO) as a potential drug carrier. *RSC Adv.* 5, 99418–99424. doi: 10.1039/C5RA12984B

Fang, S., Lin, J., Li, C., Huang, P., Hou, W., Zhang, C., et al. (2017). Dual-stimuli responsive nanotheranostics for multimodal imaging guided trimodal synergistic therapy. *Small* 13. doi: 10.1002/smll.201602580

Feng, X. R., Ding, J. X., Gref, R., and Chen, X. S. (2017). Poly (β-cyclodextrin)-mediated polylactide-cholesterol stereo complex micelles for controlled drug delivery. *Chinese J. Polym. Sci.* 35, 693–699. doi: 10.1007/s10118-017-1932-7

Geng, J., Sun, C., Liu, J., Liao, L. D., Yuan, Y., Thakor, N., et al. (2015). Biocompatible conjugated polymer nanoparticles for efficient photothermal tumor therapy. *Small* 11, 1603–1610. doi: 10.1002/smll.201402092

Gerweck, L. E., Vijayappa, S., and Kozin, S. (2006). Tumor pH controls the *in vivo* efficacy of weak acid and base chemotherapeutics. *Mol. Cancer Ther.* 5, 1275–1279. doi: 10.1158/1535-7163.MCT-06-0024

Ginn, S. L., Alexander, I. E., Edelstein, M. L., Abedi, M. R., and Wixon, J. (2013). Gene therapy clinical trials worldwide to 2012–an update. *J. Gene Med.* 15, 65–77. doi: 10.1002/jgm.2698

Grigsby, C. L., and Leong, K. W. (2010). Balancing protection and release of DNA: tools to address a bottleneck of non-viral gene delivery. *J. R Soc. Interface* 7, S67–S82. doi: 10.1098/rsif.2009.0260

He, C. F., Wang, S. H., Yu, Y. J., Shen, H. Y., Zhao, Y., Gao, H. L., et al. (2016). Advances in biodegradable nanomaterials for photothermal therapy of cancer. *Cancer Biol. Med.* 13, 299–312. doi: 10.20892/j.issn.2095-3941.2016.0052

Hobbs, S. K., Monsky, W. L., Yuan, F., Roberts, W. G., Griffith, L., Torchilin, V. P., et al. (1998). Regulation of transport pathways in tumor vessels: role of tumor type and microenvironment. *Proc. Natl. Acad. Sci. U.S.A.* 95, 4607–4612. doi: 10.1073/pnas.95.8.4607

Hoffman, H. A., Chakrabarti, L., Dumont, M. F., Sandler, A. D., and Fernandes, R. (2014). Prussian blue nanoparticles for laser-induced photothermal therapy of tumors. *RSC Adv.* 4, 29729–29734. doi: 10.1039/C4RA05209A

Hofmann, C. L., O'Sullivan, M. C., Detappe, A., Yu, Y., Yang, X., Qi, W., et al. (2017). NIR-emissive PEG-b-TCL micelles for breast tumor imaging and minimally invasive pharmacokinetic analysis. *Nanoscale* 9, 13465–13476. doi: 10.1039/C7NR02363D

Huang, M., Leng, C., Liu, S., Chen, H., Sia, C., and Chong, P. (2011). *Vaccine Delivery Systems Based on Amphiphilic Bioresorbable Polymers and Their Role in Vaccine Immunogenicity.* New York, NY: Nova Science Publishers. Available online at: https://www.novapublishers.com/catalog/product_info.php?products_id=25428

Hubbell, J. A. (2003). Enhancing drug function. *Science* 300, 595–596. doi: 10.1126/science.1083625

Hwa Kim, S., Hoon Jeong, J., Chul Cho, K., Wan Kim, S., and Gwan Park, T. (2005). Target-specific gene silencing by siRNA plasmid DNA complexed with folate-modified poly (ethylenimine). *J. Control. Release* 104, 223–232. doi: 10.1016/j.jconrel.2005.02.006

Ikada, Y., Jamshidi, K., Tsuji, H., and Hyon, S. H. (1987). Stereocomplex formation between enantiomeric poly (lactides). *Macromolecules* 20, 904–906. doi: 10.1021/ma00170a034

Jaque, D., Martínez Maestro, L., Del Rosal, B., Haro-Gonzalez, P., Benayas, A., Plaza, J. L., et al. (2014). Nanoparticles for photothermal therapies. *Nanoscale* 6, 9494–9530. doi: 10.1039/C4NR00708E

Jiang, L., Vader, P., and Schiffelers, R. (2017). Extracellular vesicles for nucleic acid delivery: progress and prospects for safe RNA-based gene therapy. *Gene Ther.* 24, 157–166. doi: 10.1038/gt.2017.8

Jin, Q., Cai, Y., Li, S., Liu, H., Zhou, X., Lu, C., et al. (2017). Edaravone-encapsulated agonistic micelles rescue ischemic brain tissue by tuning blood-brain barrier permeability. *Theranostics* 7, 884–898. doi: 10.7150/thno.18219

Juarranz, Á., Jaén, P., Sanz-Rodríguez, F., Cuevas, J., and González, S. (2008). Photodynamic therapy of cancer. Basic principles and applications. *Clin. Transl. Oncol.* 10, 148–154. doi: 10.1007/s12094-008-0172-2

Kumari, P., Muddineti, O. S., Rompicharla, S. V., Ghanta, P., Karthik, B. B. N. A., Ghosh, B., et al. (2017). Cholesterol-conjugated poly (D, L-lactide)-based micelles as a nanocarrier system for effective delivery of curcumin in cancer therapy. *Drug Deliv.* 24, 209–223. doi: 10.1080/10717544.2016.1245365

Kumari, P., Swami, M. O., Nadipalli, S. K., Myneni, S., Ghosh, B., and Biswas, S. (2016). Curcumin delivery by poly (Lactide)-based co-polymeric micelles: an *in vitro* anticancer study. *Pharm. Res. Dordr.* 33, 826–841. doi: 10.1007/s11095-015-1830-z

Leader, B., Baca, Q. J., and Golan, D. E. (2008). Protein therapeutics: a summary and pharmacological classification. *Nat. Rev. Drug Disco.* 7, 21–39. doi: 10.1038/nrd2399

Ledford, H. (2014). T-cell therapy extends cancer survival to years. *Nature* 516:156. doi: 10.1038/516156a.

Lee, K. S., Chung, H. C., Im, S. A., Park, Y. H., Kim, C. S., Kim, S. B., et al. (2008). Multicenter phase II trial of Genexol-PM, a Cremophor-free, polymeric micelle formulation of paclitaxel, in patients with metastatic breast cancer. *Breast Cancer Res. Tr.* 108, 241–250. doi: 10.1007/s10549-007-9591-y

Li, C., Wang, W., Xi, Y., Wang, J., Chen, J. F., Yun, J., et al. (2016a). Design, preparation and characterization of cyclic RGDfK peptide modified poly (ethylene glycol)-block-poly (lactic acid) micelle for targeted delivery. *Mat. Sci. Eng. C* 64, 303–309. doi: 10.1016/j.msec.2016.03.062

Li, S. Y., Liu, Y., Xu, C. F., Shen, S., Sun, R., Du, X. J., et al. (2016b). Restoring anti-tumor functions of T cells via nanoparticle-mediated immune checkpoint modulation. *J. Control. Release* 231, 17–28. doi: 10.1016/j.jconrel.2016.01.044

Li, X., Yang, X., Lin, Z., Wang, D., Mei, D., He, B., et al. (2015). A folate modified pH sensitive targeted polymeric micelle alleviated systemic toxicity of doxorubicin (DOX) in multi-drug resistant tumor bearing mice. *Eur. J. Pharm. Sci.* 76, 95–101. doi: 10.1016/j.ejps.2015.04.018

Liang, H., Ren, X., Qian, J., Zhang, X., Meng, L., Wang, X., et al. (2016). Size-shifting micelle nanoclusters based on a cross-linked and pH-sensitive framework for enhanced tumor targeting and deep penetration features. *ACS Appl. Mater. Inter.* 8, 10136–10146. doi: 10.1021/acsami.6b00668

Liu, X., Tao, H., Yang, K., Zhang, S., Lee, S. T., and Liu, Z. (2011). Optimization of surface chemistry on single-walled carbon nanotubes for *in vivo* photothermal ablation of tumors. *Biomaterials* 32, 144–151. doi: 10.1016/j.biomaterials.2010.08.096

Long, L. X., Zhao, J., Li, K., He, L. G., Qian, X. M., Liu, C. Y., et al. (2016). Synthesis of star-branched PLA-b-PMPC copolymer micelles as long blood circulation vectors to enhance tumor-targeted delivery of hydrophobic drugs *in vivo*. *Mater. Chem. Phys.* 180, 184–194. doi: 10.1016/j.matchemphys.2016.05.062

Luo, C., Wang, Y., Chen, Q., Han, X., Liu, X., Sun, J., et al. (2012). Advances of paclitaxel formulations based on nanosystem delivery technology. *Mini-Rev. Med. Chem.* 12, 434–444. doi: 10.2174/138955712800493924

Luo, J., Solimini, N. L., and Elledge, S. J. (2009). Principles of cancer therapy: oncogene and non-oncogene addiction. *Cell* 136, 823–837. doi: 10.1016/j.cell.2009.02.024

Ma, Y., Liang, X., Tong, S., Bao, G., Ren, Q., and Dai, Z. (2013). Gold nanoshell nanomicelles for potential magnetic resonance imaging, light-triggered drug release, and photothermal therapy. *Adv. Funct. Mater.* 23, 815–822. doi: 10.1002/adfm.201201663

Mebrouk, K., Chotard, F., Goff-Gaillard, C. L., Arlot-Bonnemains, Y., Fourmigué, M., and Camerel, F. (2015). Water-soluble nickel-bis (dithiolene) complexes as photothermal agents. *Chem. Commun.* 51, 5268–5270. doi: 10.1039/C4CC08231A

Meng, F., Hennink, W. E., and Zhong, Z. (2009). Reduction-sensitive polymers and bioconjugates for biomedical applications. *Biomaterials* 30, 2180–2198. doi: 10.1016/j.biomaterials.2009.01.026

Merdan, T., Kopecek, J., and Kissel, T. (2002). Prospects for cationic polymers in gene and oligonucleotide therapy against cancer. *Adv. Drug Deliver. Rev.* 54, 715–758. doi: 10.1016/S0169-409X(02)00046-7

Moghimi, S. M., Symonds, P., Murray, J. C., Hunter, A. C., Debska, G., and Szewczyk, A. (2005). A two-stage poly (ethylenimine)-mediated cytotoxicity: implications for gene transfer/therapy. *Mol. Ther.* 11, 990–995. doi: 10.1016/j.ymthe.2005.02.010

Mohme, M., Riethdorf, S., and Pantel, K. (2017). Circulating and disseminated tumour cells-mechanisms of immune surveillance and escape. *Nat. Rev. Clin. Oncol.* 14, 155–167. doi: 10.1038/nrclinonc.2016.144

Moret, I., Esteban Peris, J., Guillem, V. M., Benet, M., Revert, F., Dasí, F., et al. (2001). Stability of PEI–DNA and DOTAP–DNA complexes: effect of alkaline pH, heparin and serum. *J. Control. Release* 76, 169–181. doi: 10.1016/S0168-3659(01)00415-1

Moy, A. J., and Tunnell, J. W. (2017). Combinatorial immunotherapy and nanoparticle mediated hyperthermia. *Adv. Drug Deliver. Rev.* 114, 175–183. doi: 10.1016/j.addr.2017.06.008

Mykhaylyk, O., Antequera, Y. S., Vlaskou, D., and Plank, C. (2007). Generation of magnetic nonviral gene transfer agents and magnetofection *in vitro*. *Nat. Protoc.* 2, 2391–2411. doi: 10.1038/nprot.2007.352

Niu, Y. Q., He, T., Song, J., Chen, S. P., Liu, X. Y., Chen, Z. G., et al. (2017). A new AIE multi-block polyurethane copolymer material for subcellular microfilament imaging in living cells. *Chem. Commun.* 53, 7541–7544. doi: 10.1039/C7CC02555F

Ogawara, K., Shiraishi, T., Araki, T., Watanabe, T., Ono, T., and Higaki, K. (2016). Efficient anti-tumor effect of photodynamic treatment with polymeric nanoparticles composed of polyethylene glycol and polylactic acid block copolymer encapsulating hydrophobic porphyrin derivative. *Eur. J. Pharm. Sci.* 82, 154–160. doi: 10.1016/j.ejps.2015.11.016

Paszko, E., Ehrhardt, C., Senge, M. O., Kelleher, D. P., and Reynolds, J. V. (2011). Nanodrug applications in photodynamic therapy. *Photodiagn. Photodyn.* 8, 14–29. doi: 10.1016/j.pdpdt.2010.12.001

Peng, L. H., Huang, Y. F., Zhang, C. Z., Niu, J., Chen, Y., Chu, Y., et al. (2016). Integration of antimicrobial peptides with gold nanoparticles as unique non-viral vectors for gene delivery to mesenchymal stem cells with antibacterial activity. *Biomaterials* 103, 137–149. doi: 10.1016/j.biomaterials.2016.06.057

Puntawee, S., Theerasilp, M., Reabroi, S., Saeeng, R., Piyachaturawat, P., Chairoungdua, A., et al. (2016). Solubility enhancement and *in vitro* evaluation of PEG-b-PLA micelles as nanocarrier of semi-synthetic andrographolide analogue for cholangiocarcinoma chemotherapy. *Pharm. Dev. Technol.* 21, 437–444. doi: 10.3109/10837450.2015.1016619

Rollerova, E., Jurcovicova, J., Mlynarcikova, A., Sadlonova, I., Bilanicova, D., Wsolova, L., et al. (2015). Delayed adverse effects of neonatal exposure to polymeric nanoparticle poly (ethylene glycol)-block-polylactide methyl ether on hypothalamic–pituitary–ovarian axis development and function in Wistar rats. *Reprod. Toxicol.* 57, 165–175. doi: 10.1016/j.reprotox.2015.07.072

Salcher, E. E., and Wagner, E. (2010). Chemically programmed polymers for targeted DNA and siRNA transfection. *Top. Curr. Chem.* 296, 227–249. doi: 10.1007/128_2010_69

Sato, A., Choi, S. W., Hirai, M., Yamayoshi, A., Moriyama, R., Yamano, T., et al. (2007). Polymer brush-stabilized polyplex for a siRNA carrier with long circulatory half-life. *J. Control. Release* 122, 209–216. doi: 10.1016/j.jconrel.2007.04.018

Savić, R., Eisenberg, A., and Maysinger, D. (2006). Block copolymer micelles as delivery vehicles of hydrophobic drugs: micelle–cell interactions. *J. Drug Target.* 14, 343–355. doi: 10.1080/10611860600874538

Schmaljohann, D. (2006). Thermo-and pH-responsive polymers in drug delivery. *Adv. Drug Deliver. Rev.* 58, 1655–1670. doi: 10.1016/j.addr.2006.09.020

Scott, A. M., Wolchok, J. D., and Old, L. J. (2012). Antibody therapy of cancer. *Nat. Rev. Cancer* 12, 278–287. doi: 10.1038/nrc3236

Scsukova, S., Mlynarcikova, A., Kiss, A., and Rollerova, E. (2015). Effect of polymeric nanoparticle poly (ethylene glycol)-block-poly (lactic acid)(PEG-b-PLA) on *in vitro* luteinizing hormone release from anterior pituitary cells of infantile and adult female rats. *Neuro. Endocrinol. Lett.* 36, 88–94.

Sharifi, S., Behzadi, S., Laurent, S., Forrest, M. L., Stroeve, P., and Mahmoudi, M. (2012). Toxicity of nanomaterials. *Chem. Soc. Rev.* 41, 2323–2343. doi: 10.1039/C1CS15188F

Shi, L., Song, X. B., Wang, Y., Wang, K. T., Liu, P., Pang, B., et al. (2016). Docetaxel-conjugated monomethoxy-poly (ethylene glycol)-b-poly (lactide)(mPEG-PLA) polymeric micelles to enhance the therapeutic efficacy in oral squamous cell carcinoma. *RSC Adv.* 6, 42819–42826. doi: 10.1039/C6RA03332F

Shukla, V., Dalela, M., Vij, M., Weichselbaum, R., Kharbanda, S., Ganguli, M., et al. (2017). Systemic delivery of the tumor necrosis factor gene to tumors by a novel dual DNA-nanocomplex in a nanoparticle system. *Nanomed. Nanotechnol.* 13, 1833–1839. doi: 10.1016/j.nano.2017.03.004

Sun, C., Lee, J. S., and Zhang, M. (2008). Magnetic nanoparticles in MR imaging and drug delivery. *Adv. Drug Delive. Rev.* 60, 1252–1265. doi: 10.1016/j.addr.2008.03.018

Sun, T., Qi, J., Zheng, M., Xie, Z., Wang, Z., and Jing, X. (2015). Thiadiazole molecules and poly (ethylene glycol)-block-polylactide self-assembled nanoparticles as effective photothermal agents. *Colloid. Surface. B* 136, 201–206. doi: 10.1016/j.colsurfb.2015.09.020

Szakács, G., Paterson, J. K., Ludwig, J. A., Booth-Genthe, C., and Gottesman, M. M. (2006). Targeting multidrug resistance in cancer. *Nat. Rev. Drug Discov.* 5, 219–234. doi: 10.1038/nrd1984

Tannock, I. F., and Rotin, D. (1989). Acid pH in tumors and its potential for therapeutic exploitation. *Cancer Res.* 49, 4373–4384.

Tao, Z., Dang, X., Huang, X., Muzumdar, M. D., Xu, E. S., Bardhan, N. M., et al. (2017). Early tumor detection afforded by *in vivo* imaging of near-infrared II fluorescence. *Biomaterials* 134, 202–215. doi: 10.1016/j.biomaterials.2017.04.046

Tefit, J. N., and Serra, V. (2011). Outlining novel cellular adjuvant products for therapeutic vaccines against cancer. *Expert Rev. Vaccines* 10, 1207–1220. doi: 10.1586/erv.11.84

Thomas, C. E., Ehrhardt, A., and Kay, M. A. (2003). Progress and problems with the use of viral vectors for gene therapy. *Nat. Rev. Genet.* 4, 346–358. doi: 10.1038/nrg1066

Tian, J., Zhou, J., Shen, Z., Ding, L., Yu, J. S., and Ju, H. (2015). A pH-activatable and aniline-substituted photosensitizer for near-infrared cancer theranostics. *Chem. Sci.* 6, 5969–5977. doi: 10.1039/C5SC01721A

Tian, Q., Tang, M., Sun, Y., Zou, R., Chen, Z., Zhu, M., et al. (2011). Hydrophilic flower-like CuS superstructures as an efficient 980 nm laser-driven photothermal agent for ablation of cancer cells. *Adv. Mater.* 23, 3542–3547. doi: 10.1002/adma.201101295

Wang, J., Xu, W., Ding, J., Lu, S., Wang, X., Wang, C., et al. (2015). Cholesterol-enhanced polylactide-based stereocomplex micelle for effective delivery of doxorubicin. *Materials* 8, 216–230. doi: 10.3390/ma8010216

Wang, S., Huang, P., Nie, L., Xing, R., Liu, D., Wang, Z., et al. (2013). Single continuous wave laser induced photodynamic/plasmonic photothermal therapy using photosensitizer-functionalized gold nanostars. *Adv. Mater.* 25, 3055–3061. doi: 10.1002/adma.201204623

Wang, X., He, C., Yang, Q., Tan, L., Liu, B., Zhu, Z., et al. (2017). Dynamic covalent linked triblock copolymer micelles for glutathione-mediated intracellular drug delivery. *Mater. Sci. Engi. C* 77, 34–44. doi: 10.1016/j.msec.2017.03.240

Wang, X., Zhang, J., Wang, Y., Wang, C., Xiao, J., Zhang, Q., et al. (2016). Multi-responsive photothermal-chemotherapy with drug-loaded melanin-like nanoparticles for synergetic tumor ablation. *Biomaterials* 81, 114–124. doi: 10.1016/j.biomaterials.2015.11.037

Wang, Y., Yang, T., Wang, X., Dai, W., Wang, J., Zhang, X., et al. (2011). Materializing sequential killing of tumor vasculature and tumor cells via targeted polymeric micelle system. *J. Control. Release* 149, 299–306. doi: 10.1016/j.jconrel.2010.10.027

Wei, H., Cheng, S. X., Zhang, X. Z., and Zhuo, R. X. (2009). Thermo-sensitive polymeric micelles based on poly (N-isopropylacrylamide) as drug carriers. *Prog. Polym. Sci.* 34, 893–910. doi: 10.1016/j.progpolymsci.2009.05.002

Wiseman, J. W., Goddard, C. A., McLelland, D., and Colledge, W. H. (2003). A comparison of linear and branched polyethylenimine (PEI) with DCChol/DOPE liposomes for gene delivery to epithelial cells *in vitro* and *in vivo*. *Gene Ther.* 10:1654. doi: 10.1038/sj.gt.3302050

Wu, X. L., Kim, J. H., Koo, H., Bae, S. M., Shin, H., Kim, M. S., et al. (2010). Tumor-targeting peptide conjugated pH-responsive micelles as a potential drug carrier for cancer therapy. *Bioconjugate Chem.* 21, 208–213. doi: 10.1021/bc9005283

Xiong, J., Meng, F., Wang, C., Cheng, R., Liu, Z., and Zhong, Z. (2011). Folate-conjugated crosslinked biodegradable micelles for receptor-mediated delivery of paclitaxel. *J. Mater. Chem.* 21, 5786–5794. doi: 10.1039/c0jm04410e

Yang, K., Wan, J., Zhang, S., Tian, B., Zhang, Y., and Liu, Z. (2012a). The influence of surface chemistry and size of nanoscale graphene oxide on photothermal therapy of cancer using ultra-low laser power. *Biomaterials* 33, 2206–2214. doi: 10.1016/j.biomaterials.2011.11.064.

Yang, K., Xu, H., Cheng, L., Sun, C., Wang, J., and Liu, Z. (2012b). *In vitro* and *in vivo* near-infrared photothermal therapy of cancer using polypyrrole organic nanoparticles. *Adv. Mater.* 24, 5586–5592. doi: 10.1002/adma.201202625

Yang, Q., Tan, L., He, C., Liu, B., Xu, Y., Zhu, Z., et al. (2015). Redox-responsive micelles self-assembled from dynamic covalent block copolymers for intracellular drug delivery. *Acta Biomater.* 17, 193–200. doi: 10.1016/j.actbio.2015.01.044

Yang, R., Zhang, S., Kong, D., Gao, X., Zhao, Y., and Wang, Z. (2012c). Biodegradable polymer-curcumin conjugate micelles enhance the loading and delivery of low-potency curcumin. *Pharm. Res. Dordr.* 29, 3512–3525. doi: 10.1007/s11095-012-0848-8

Yin, L., Yuvienco, C., and Montclare, J. K. (2017). Protein based therapeutic delivery agents: contemporary developments and challenges. *Biomaterials* 134, 91–116. doi: 10.1016/j.biomaterials.2017.04.036

Yu, Y., and Qiu, L. (2016). Optimizing particle size of docetaxel-loaded micelles for enhanced treatment of oral epidermoid carcinoma. *Nanomed. Nanotechnol.* 12, 1941–1949. doi: 10.1016/j.nano.2016.04.012

Yu, Y., Wu, T., Johnson-Buck, A., Li, L., and Su, X. (2016a). A two-layer assay for single-nucleotide variants utilizing strand displacement and selective digestion. *Biosens. Bioelectron.* 82, 248–254. doi: 10.1016/j.bios.2016.03.070

Yu, Y., Zhang, Q., Buscaglia, J., Chang, C. C., Liu, Y., Yang, Z., et al. (2016b). Quantitative real-time detection of carcinoembryonic antigen (CEA) from pancreatic cyst fluid using 3-D surface molecular imprinting. *Analyst* 141, 4424–4431. doi: 10.1039/c6an00375c

Yu, Y., Zhang, Q., Chang, C. C., Liu, Y., Yang, Z., Guo, Y., et al. (2016c). Design of a molecular imprinting biosensor with multi-scale roughness for detection across a broad spectrum of biomolecules. *Analyst* 141, 5607–5617. doi: 10.1039/c6an01157h

Yu, Y., Zhang, X., and Qiu, L. (2014). The anti-tumor efficacy of curcumin when delivered by size/charge-changing multistage polymeric micelles based on amphiphilic poly (β-amino ester) derivates. *Biomaterials* 35, 3467–3479. doi: 10.1016/j.biomaterials.2013.12.096

Yue, J., Liu, S., Wang, R., Hu, X., Xie, Z., Huang, Y., et al. (2012). Fluorescence-labeled immunomicelles: preparation, *in vivo* biodistribution, and ability to cross the blood–brain barrier. *Macromol. Biosci.* 12, 1209–1219. doi: 10.1002/mabi.201200037

Zhai, S., Hu, X., Hu, Y., Wu, B., and Xing, D. (2017). Visible light-induced crosslinking and physiological stabilization of diselenide-rich nanoparticles for redox-responsive drug release and combination chemotherapy. *Biomaterials* 121, 41–54. doi: 10.1016/j.biomaterials.2017.01.002

Zhan, C., Wei, X., Qian, J., Feng, L., Zhu, J., and Lu, W. (2012). Co-delivery of TRAIL gene enhances the anti-glioblastoma effect of paclitaxel *in vitro* and *in vivo*. *J. Control. Release* 160, 630–636. doi: 10.1016/j.jconrel.2012.02.022

Zhang, Q., Kaisti, M., Prabhu, A., Yu, Y., Song, Y. A., Rafailovich, M. H., et al. (2017). Polyaniline-functionalized ion-sensitive floating-gate FETs for the on-chip monitoring of peroxidase-catalyzed redox reactions. *Electrochimi. Acta* 261, 256–264. doi: 10.1016/j.electacta.2017.12.130

Zhang, Y., Wang, X., Wang, J., Zhang, X., and Zhang, Q. (2011). Octreotide-modified polymeric micelles as potential carriers for targeted docetaxel delivery to somatostatin receptor overexpressing tumor cells. *Pharm. Res. Dordr.* 28, 1167–1178. doi: 10.1007/s11095-011-0381-1

Zhang, Y., Zhang, Y., Hong, G., He, W., Zhou, K., Yang, K., et al. (2013). Biodistribution, pharmacokinetics and toxicology of Ag 2 S near-infrared quantum dots in mice. *Biomaterials* 34, 3639–3646. doi: 10.1016/j.biomaterials.2013.01.089

Zhang, Z., Wang, L., Wang, J., Jiang, X., Li, X., Hu, Z., et al. (2012). Mesoporous silica-coated gold nanorods as a light-mediated multifunctional theranostic platform for cancer treatment. *Adv. Mater.* 24, 1418–1423. doi: 10.1002/adma.201104714

Zhao, Z. X., Gao, S. Y., Wang, J. C., Chen, C. J., Zhao, E. Y., Hou, W. J., et al. (2012). Self-assembly nanomicelles based on cationic mPEG-PLA-b-Polyarginine (R 15) triblock copolymer for siRNA delivery. *Biomaterials* 33, 6793–6807. doi: 10.1016/j.biomaterials.2012.05.067

Zheng, S., Gao, X., Liu, X., Yu, T., Zheng, T., Wang, Y., et al. (2016). Biodegradable micelles enhance the antiglioma activity of curcumin *in vitro* and *in vivo*. *Int. J. Nanomed.* 11, 2721–2136. doi: 10.2147/IJN.S102450

12

DACHPt-Loaded Nanoparticles Self-assembled from Biodegradable Dendritic Copolymer Polyglutamic Acid-*b*-D-α-Tocopheryl Polyethylene Glycol 1000 Succinate for Multidrug Resistant Lung Cancer Therapy

Hsiang-I Tsai [1†], ***Lijuan Jiang*** [1†], ***Xiaowei Zeng*** [2], ***Hongbo Chen*** [2], ***Zihuang Li*** [3*], ***Wei Cheng*** [4], ***Jinxie Zhang*** [1], ***Jie Pan*** [5], ***Dong Wan*** [5], ***Li Gao*** [6], ***Zhenhua Xie*** [4], ***Laiqiang Huang*** [1,4*], ***Lin Mei*** [2] ***and Gan Liu*** [2*]

[1] School of Life Sciences, Tsinghua University, Beijing, China, [2] School of Pharmaceutical Sciences (Shenzhen), Sun Yat-sen University, Guangzhou, China, [3] Department of Radiation Oncology, Second Clinical Medicine College of Jinan University, Shenzhen Municipal People's Hospital, Shenzhen, China, [4] Division of Life and Health Sciences, Graduate School at Shenzhen, Tsinghua University, Shenzhen, China, [5] School of Environmental and Chemical Engineering, Tianjin Polytechnic University, Tianjin, China, [6] Department of Urology, Affiliated Hospital of Guilin Medical University, Guilin, China

***Correspondence:**
Zihuang Li
lizihuang2006@126.com
Laiqiang Huang
huanglq@sz.tsinghua.edu.cn
Gan Liu
liugan5@mail.sysu.edu.cn

[†]Co-first authors.

The clinical applications of platinum-based antitumor agents are still largely limited by severe side effects as well as multidrug resistance (MDR). To solve these problems, we developed an 1,2-diaminocyclohexane-platinum(II) (DACHPt)-loaded nanoparticle (NP-TPGS-Pt) by self-assembly of poly(amidoamine)-polyglutamic acid-*b*-D-α-tocopheryl polyethylene glycol 1000 succinate (PAM-PGlu-*b*-TPGS) and DACHPt. NP-TPGS-Pt showed robust stability and pH-responsive DACHPt release profile *in vitro* similar to the PEG-containing nanoparticle (NP-PEG-Pt). Meanwhile, in contrast with NP-PEG-Pt, NP-TPGS-Pt exhibited efficient nanoparticle-based cellular uptake by the Pt-resistant A549/DDP human lung cancer cells and caused much more cytotoxicity than free Oxaliplatin and NP-PEG-Pt. Finally, this NP-TPGS-Pt was proved to perform outstanding inhibition of Pt-resistant tumor growth, much superior than free Oxaliplatin and NP-PEG-Pt. Thus, this NP-TPGS-Pt provides a novel powerful nanomedicine platform for combatting multidrug resistant cancer.

Keywords: multidrug resistance, TPGS, dendritic copolymers, nanoparticles, DACHPt

INTRODUCTION

Up to now, platinum-based antitumor agents have been widely used to treat lung cancer, bladder cancer, gastric cancer, and ovarian cancer, etc. (Graham et al., 2000; Klein and Hambley, 2009; Wheate et al., 2010; Han and Smith, 2013; Harrach and Ciarimboli, 2015; Torre et al., 2015; Ma et al., 2017). However, their clinical outcomes are still largely limited by severe side effects (Nishiyama et al., 2001; Xiao et al., 2017) and multidrug resistance (Wang and Lippard, 2005; Li et al., 2015; Yin et al., 2017). Drug nanocarriers, which can prolong the *in vivo* half-life of drugs and promote the enrichment in solid tumors through the enhanced permeation and retention (EPR) effect, have been verified potentially applicable to antitumor therapy (Peer et al., 2007; Oberoi et al., 2013; Salomone, 2013; Wang and Guo, 2013; Huang et al., 2015; Xu et al., 2015; Li et al., 2017; Liu et al., 2017b). We have previously reported an unimolecular micelle (UM/DACHPt) prepared by loading antitumor agent 1,2-diaminocyclohexane-platinum(II) (DACHPt) with dendritic block copolymer PAM-PGlu-*b*-PEG (Liu et al., 2017a).Compared to micelles self-assembled from block copolymer, this micelle showed superior stability, thereby extending the *in vivo* half-life, enhancing antitumor effects and reducing side effects. Nevertheless, besides relieving side effects, platinum drug-loaded nanocarriers always need to meet the requirement for overcoming tumor multidrug resistance. Since the antitumor effects of unimolecular micelles are inferior to those of free drugs *in vitro*, they would hardly fulfill the requirement. Therefore, it is of great significance to optimize the nanocarrier structure to be both stable *in vivo* and multidrug-resistant.

As a soluble derivative of vitamin E, D-α-tocopheryl polyethylene glycol 1000 succinate (TPGS) is esterified from the acid group of vitamin E succinate and polyethylene glycol (PEG) 1000. It has been approved by FDA as a safe pharmaceutical excipient (Mu and Feng, 2003; Zhang et al., 2012; Guo et al., 2013; Tan et al., 2017). It is well-documented that TPGS could enhance cellular uptake (Zhang and Feng, 2006; Zeng et al., 2013), and inhibit P-glycoprotein to circumvent drug resistance via interfering with the structure and function of mitochondria (Dintaman and Silverman, 1999; Zhu et al., 2014; Wang et al., 2015; Bao et al., 2017). In addition, our previous work has reported that surface modification of PLGA nanoparticles (NPs) with TPGS prolonged the half-life of drugs *in vivo* and facilitated their cellular uptake (Zeng et al., 2013). Thus we ensure that conjugating TPGS with PAM-PGlu rather than PEG would not only maintain the stability of nanocarrier, but also enhance the cellular uptake and overcome drug resistance. As far as we know, no such PAM-PGlu-*b*-TPGS was reported to prepare DACHPt-loaded nanoparticles.

Thus, we designed a novel TPGS-containing dendritic polymer PAM-PGlu-*b*-TPGS to prepare DACHPt-loaded NP-TPGS-Pt. PAM-PGlu-*b*-TPGS consisted of dendritic molecule PAMAM-G3, DACHPt-chelating agent PGlu and polymer TPGS (**Figure 1**). We then determined the size, zeta potential, drug loading content, encapsulation efficiency, *in vitro* stability and drug release behaviors of NP-TPGS-Pt. Meanwhile, the cellular uptake and *in vitro* cytotoxicity of NP-TPGS-Pt were evaluated by using non-small cell lung cancer cell line A549 and resistant A549/DDP cell line. Finally, the antitumor effects of NP-TPGS-Pt on the A549/DDP model were assessed.

EXPERIMENTAL SECTION

Materials

Carboxyl-terminated D-α-tocopheryl polyethylene glycol 1000 succinate (cTPGS) was synthesized in our previous work [21]. BLG-NCA was purchased from Kangmanlin chemicals (Nanjing, China). PAMAM-NH_2-G3 (PAM-NH_2, M_w = 6900 Da), CF_3COOH, HBr/HAc (w/V 33%), $DACHPtCl_2$ and Oxaliplatin were purchased from Aladdin Industrial (Shanghai, China). All the chemicals were commercially available and used as received. A549 and A549/DDP cells were obtained from American Type Culture Collection (ATCC). Fetal bovine serum (FBS), RPMI1640 media and penicillin/streptomycin were both purchased from Gibco. Female Balb/C nude mice (~18 g, 7 weeks old) were purchased from Guangdong Province Medical Animal Center and fed in a SPF (specific pathogen free) class experimental animal room. This study was carried out in accordance with the recommendations of the Care and Use of laboratory animals of Tsinghua University, the Administrative Committee on Animal Research in Tsinghua University. The protocol was approved by the Administrative Committee on Animal Research in Tsinghua University.

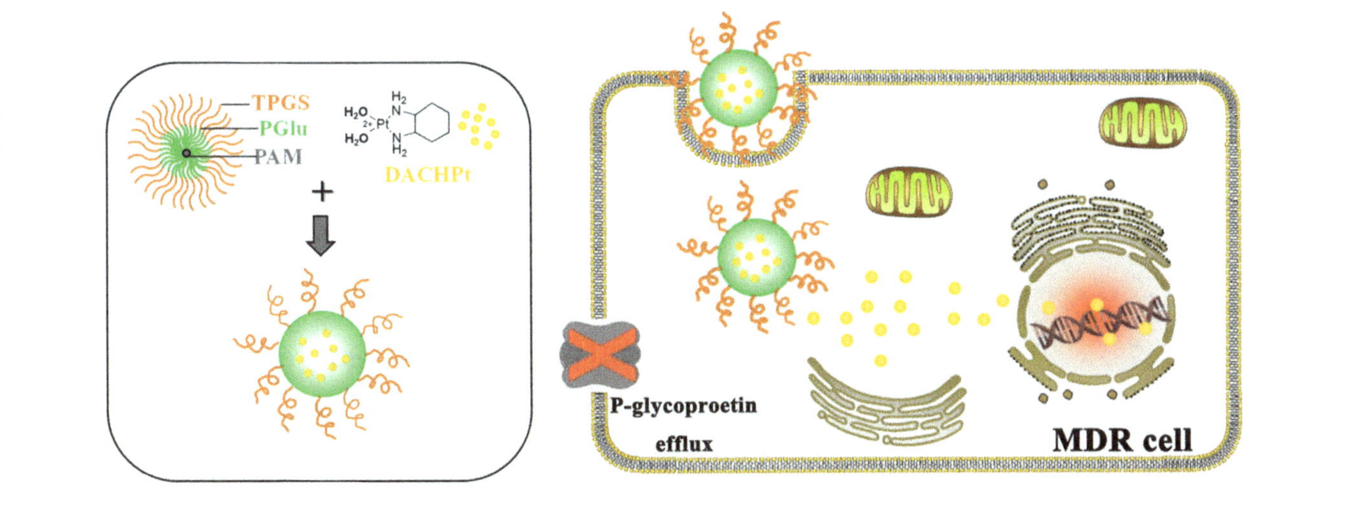

FIGURE 1 | Schematic illustration of overcoming the resistance of A549/DDP cells by NP-TPGS-Pt.

Synthesis of Dendritic Block Copolymer PAM-PGlu-*b*-TPGS

As shown in **Figure 2**, firstly, PAM-$PBLG_{384}$-NH_2 was synthesized according to our previous work (Liu et al., 2017a). Then PAM-PBLG-NH_2 (1 g) was reacted with excess TPGS-COOH and EDC at 4°C for 2 h to obtain the dendritic block copolymer PAM-PBLG-*b*-TPGS. The degree of polymerization of TPGS in PAM-PBLG-NH_2 was verified by ^{1}H-NMR spectroscopy (Varian UNITY-plus 400 M nuclear magnetic resonance spectrometer, solvent: $CDCl_3$). After that, 20 mL trifluoroacetic acid dissolving PAM-PBLG-*b*-TPGS was added in 2 mL hydrogen bromide (HBr) (33% in acetic acid) and stirred for 1 h at room temperature. Then the solution was neutralized by sodium hydroxide (NaOH) and dialyzed against distilled water (DI water) using a dialysis membrane with molecular weight cutoff (MWCO) of 5 kDa. The aqueous solution of purified product was lyophilized to obtain PAM-PGlu-*b*-TPGS.

Preparation of DACHPt-Loaded Nanoparticles

DACHPt-loaded nanoparticles were prepared similar to our previous work. Briefly, PAM-PGlu-*b*-TPGS solution was separately mixed with the DACHPt aqueous solution (Molar ratio Glu/ DACHPt = 3/1) and reacted for 72 h. The formed nanoparticles were purified by ultrafiltration using Centricon Plus-20 centrifugal filter units (MWCO 50 KDa, Millipore, MA, USA).

Characterization of DACHPt-Loaded Nanoparticles

The size distribution and zeta potential of DACHPt-loaded nanoparticles were measured using Zetasizer Nano ZS90 (Malvern Instruments Ltd., UK). Before measurement, the freshly prepared nanoparticles were diluted as needed. All measurements were carried out at 25°C. The data were obtained as the average of three measurements.

The morphology of nanoparticles were then observed by transmission electron microscopy (TEM, Tecnai G2 20, FEI Company, Oregon, USA). One microliter of the sample solution was placed on the resulting grids and dried in the air.

To measure the drug loading content (LC) and drug encapsulation efficiency (EE) of the DACHPt-loaded nanoparticles, a predefined amount of nanoparticles were dissolved in 1 mL water. The Pt concentration in the nanoparticles was quantified by Inductively coupled plasma mass spectrometry (ICP-MS, Xseries II, Thermoscientific, USA). The LC and EE of DACHPt-loaded nanoparticles were calculated according to

$$\mathrm{LC}\ (\%) = \frac{\text{amout of DACHPt in the nanoparticles}}{\text{amount of the nanoparticles}} \times 100\%$$

$$\mathrm{EE}\ (\%) = \frac{\text{amount of DACHPt in the nanoparticles}}{\text{amount of feeding DACHPt}} \times 100\%$$

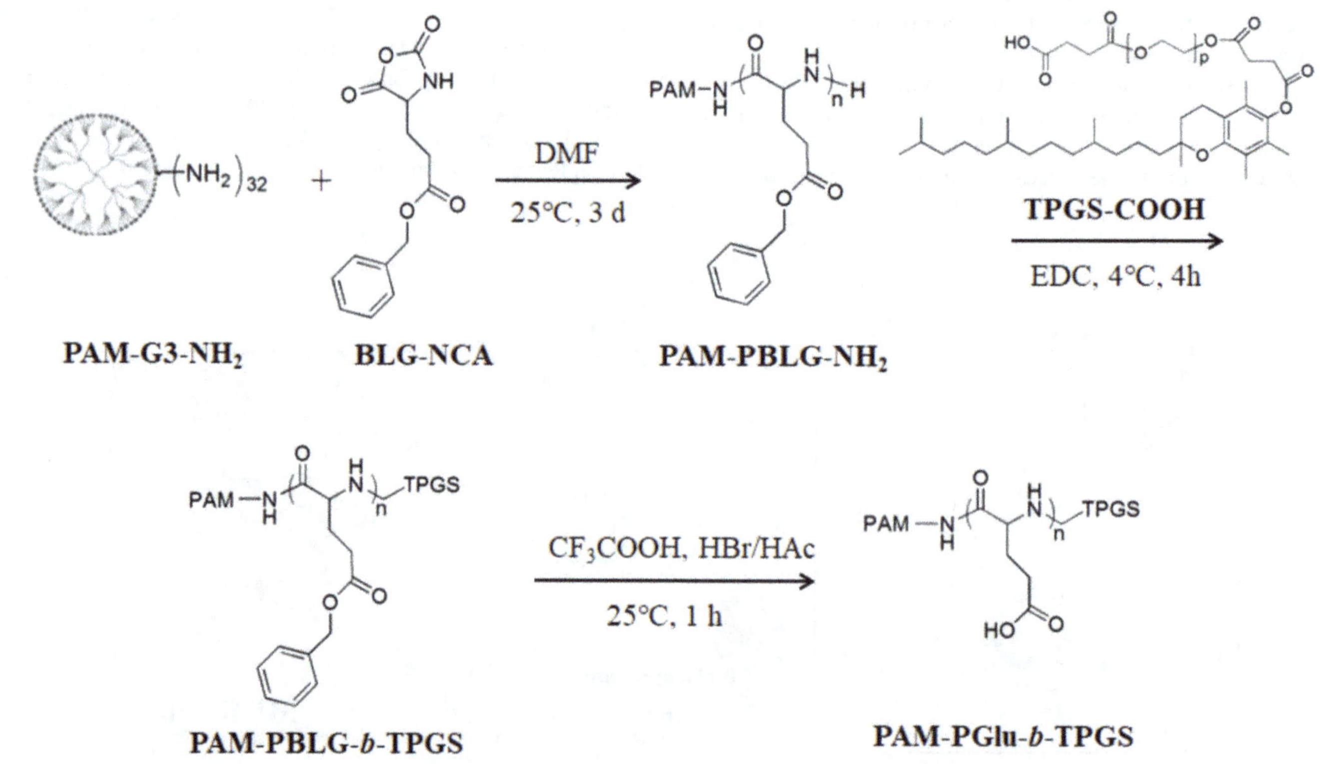

FIGURE 2 | Synthesis of the dendritic block copolymer PAM-PGlu-*b*-TPGS.

In Vitro Drug Release Study

The stability of NP-TPGS-Pt in cell culture media including 10% FBS at 25°C was evaluated by DLS. The DACHPt release profile of the nanoparticles was monitored by the dialysis method. Firstly, 1 ml of NP-TPGS-Pt was placed into the dialysis bag (MWCO 5 kDa) and immersed in 30 ml of cell culture media including 10% FBS (pH 7.4 and 5.5) at 37°C. The media outside was taken out at defined periods, and the concentrations of Pt were measured by ICP-MS.

Cellular Uptake Study

In this study, 5-Aminofluorescein-labeled NP-PEG-Pt, and NP-TPGS-Pt as the model fluorescent probe to investigate the uptake by A549 cells and A549/DDP cells. A549 cells and A549/DDP cells were cultured as described previously (Liu et al., 2017a). The cellular uptake experiments of 5-Aminofluorescein-NPs were performed using CLSM. A549 cells and A549/DDP cells ($1*10^5$ cells/well) were seeded in 12-well culture plates and cultured overnight in RPMI1640 with 10% FBS. On the following day, the cells were washed once with PBS and incubated with 5-AF-NP-PEG-Pt, and 5-AF-NP-TPGS-Pt in 10% serum containing the media for 3 h at 37°C. The cells were observed using a CLSM (Olympus Fluoview FV-1000, Tokyo, Japan) using an imaging software. The images of the cells were captured with differential interference contrast channel, and the images of 5-Aminofluorescein-NPs and the nuclei of DAPI-stained cells were recorded with following channels: blue channel (DAPI) excited at 340 nm and green channel (5-Aminofluorescein) excited at 488 nm.

MTT Assay

The 50% growth inhibitory concentrations (IC_{50}) of free Oxaliplatin, NP-PEG-Pt, and NP-TPGS-Pt in the A549 and A549/DDP cells were measured by the MTT assay. After incubated in a 96-well culture plate (10^4 cells/well) for 24 h, A549 cells were then exposed to 10, 20, 40, 100, and 200 μM oxaliplatin or DACHPt-loaded nanoparticles (on a platinum basis) for another 24, 48, and 72 h. At each point of time, The MTT solution was added, and cell viability was measured in a Bio-Rad 680 microplate reader by formazan absorbance at 490 nm.

In Vivo Antitumor Efficacy

After randomly divided into four groups ($n = 5$), the nude mice were built with human A549 xenograft tumor model by injection of 1.5×10^6 A549/DDP cells (100 μL) subcutaneous at the right axilla of each mouse. Before initiating treatment, tumors were observed frequently and allowed to grow to ~50 mm^3 in volume. Mice were injected intravenously five times via tail vein on days 0, 4, 8, 12, and 16 with saline, Oxaliplatin and DACHPt-loaded nanoparticles (6 mg/kg on a Pt basis). The antitumor efficacy was determined in accordance with the tumor volume (V), which was calculated similar to our previous work. The body weights of mice were simultaneously measured to evaluate the systemic toxicity. The results were considered statistically significant if two-tailed P-values were < 0.05.

Statistical Analysis

All of the experiments were carried out at least three times. The Data are expressed as mean ± *SD* unless noted otherwise and analyzed for significance using Student's t-test. Probability value (P) < 0.05 indicates statistically significant. $^*P < 0.05$; $^{**}P < 0.01$.

RESULTS AND DISCUSSION

Synthesis and Characterizations of Dendritic Copolymer PAM-PGlu-*b*-TPGs

The chemical structure of dendritic copolymer PAM-PGlu-*b*-TPGS was validated by ^1H NMR spectroscopy. **Figure 3A** shows the ^1H NMR spectrum of PAM-PBLG-*b*-TPGS, in which a, b, c, d, e, and g represent the characteristic peaks of methylene group (CH_2) in PAM, -C(O)C*H*(CH_2)NH-, -CHC$H_2$$CH_2$C(O)-, -CH$CH_2CH_2$C(O)- and C_6H_5CH_2- in PBLG, as well as CH_2 of PEG in TPGS, demonstrating the successful linking of TPGS. The number of TPGS in each dendritic molecule was 30 by calculating the areas of peaks e and g. As exhibited in **Figure 3B**, the characteristic peak of benzyl group in BLG disappears, suggesting that the deprotection was successful and PAM-PGlu-*b*-TPGS had been successfully prepared.

Afterwards, we obtained NP-TPGS-Pt by complexing PAM-PGlu-*b*-TPGS with DACHPt. The NPs had a narrow monodisperse distribution and the average hydrodynamic diameter of ~85.3 nm (**Figure 4A**). TEM presented that NF-TPGS-Pt were uniformly distributed spherical particles with the size of about 60 nm, being consistent with the DLS results (**Figure 4B**). In the meantime, we prepared NP-PEG-Pt with PAM-PGlu-*b*-PEG and DACHPt as control (**Table 1**).

Stability and Drug Release Study

Then we determined the *in vitro* stability of NP-TPGS-Pt. The size of NP-TPGS-Pt remained stable after 14 consecutive days of culture in cell medium (**Figure 5A**), indicating that it holds robust stability.

As evidenced by ICP-MS, the drug loading content of NP-TPGS-Pt was 26.3% (**Table 1**). Subsequently, we tested the *in vitro* release of DACHPt from NP-TPGS-Pt. In a previous study, we found that Pt release was accelerated in a chloride ion-containing environment under acidic conditions. Thus, we herein compared such release from NP-TPGS-Pt at pH 7.4 and 5.5. At pH 7.4, the drug release rate from NP-TPGS-Pt was only 20% after 96 h (**Figure 5B**), revealing that these NPs were fairly stable under physiological conditions and drug hardly leaked. On the other hand, NP-TPGS-Pt managed to rapidly release DACHPt at pH 5.5, predicting that they may work so inside tumor cells.

Cellular Uptake

It is well-established that drug delivery into cells through uptake of nanocarrier can well escape efflux protein-mediated transport, thereby overcoming multidrug resistance (Wei et al., 2015). Accordingly, we first studied the cellular uptake of NP-TPGS-Pt with confocal laser scanning microscopy (CLSM). We covalently linked NP-PEG-Pt and NP-TPGS-Pt with 5-aminofluorescein (AF), and observed their endocytosis by A549 and A549/DDP

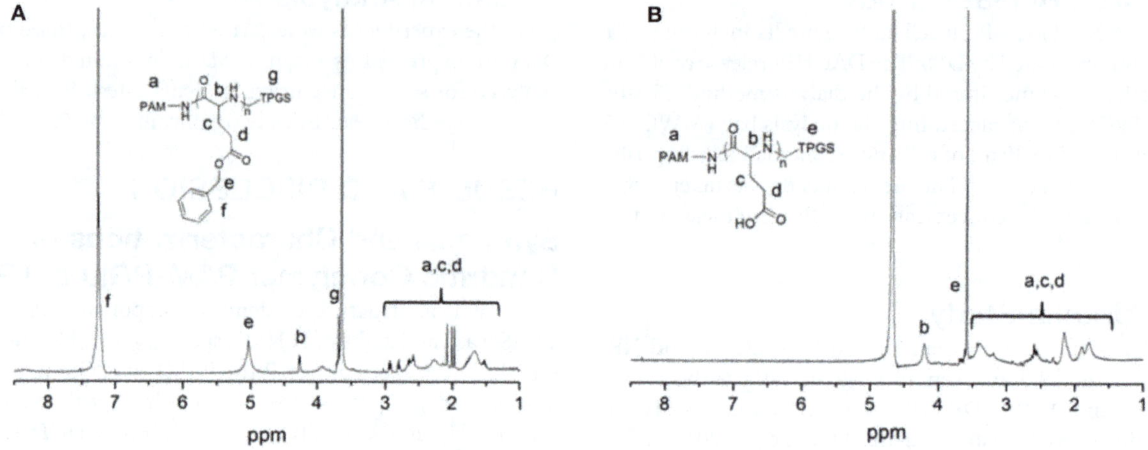

FIGURE 3 | (A) ^{1}H-NMR spectra of PAM-PBLG$_{384}$-NH$_2$ in $CDCl_3$, and (B) PAM-PGlu$_{384}$-*b*-(TPGS)$_{30}$ in D_2O.

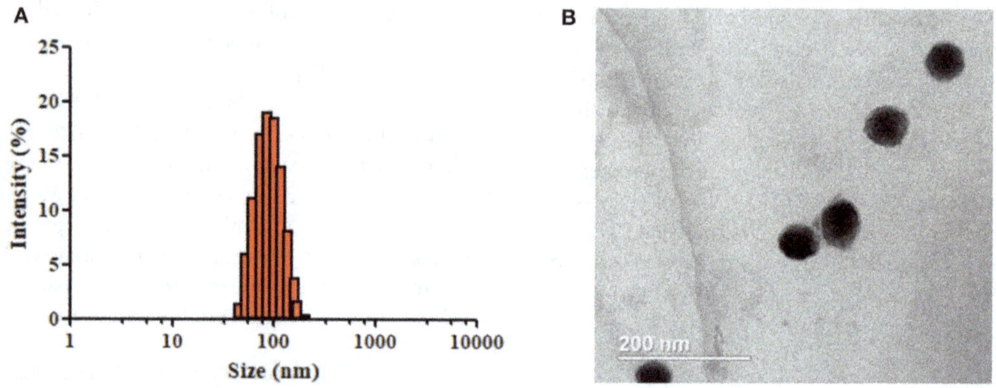

FIGURE 4 | (A) Size distribution and (B) TEM image of NP-TPGS-Pt.

cells. After 3 h, A549 cells emitted obvious fluorescence of NP-TPGS-Pt-AF (green), but the NP-PEG-Pt-AF group barely showed signal (**Figure 6A**), because intracellular fluorescence originated from NPs to which AF was covalently linked. Collectively, TPGS modification substantially promoted the cellular uptake of nanocarrier, whereas PEG hardly underwent uptake due to the apparent shielding effect. Given that the fluorescence signal of AF (green) in A549/DDP cells was almost equivalent to that of A549 cells, NP-TPGS-Pt was also subjected to uptake by A549/DDP cells (**Figure 6B**).

Then we further quantified the cellular uptake efficiency of NP-TPGS-Pt at 3 h. As presented in **Figure 6C**, the NP-PEG-Pt uptake efficiencies of A549 and A549/DDP cells are lower than 20%, while those for NP-TPGS-Pt reach as high as 60%. In short, drug-resistant cells were still capable of efficient uptake of NP-TPGS-Pt (**Figure 6D**).

In Vitro Cytotoxicity

To demonstrate the ability of NP-TPGS-Pt to kill tumor cells, especially the drug-resistant ones, we performed MTT assay using A549 and A549/DDP cells. Meanwhile, free Oxaliplatin, NP-PEG-Pt and drug-free NP-TPGS were employed as controls. A549 and A549/DDP cells were treated by different concentrations of drugs for 24 and 48 h. After 24 h of culture, Oxaliplatin significantly killed A549 cells, whereas NP-PEG-Pt also exerted much weaker effects (**Figure 7A**), being in agreement with the above cellular uptake efficiencies. However, NP-TPGS-Pt worked more effectively than Oxaliplatin did. Moreover, the IC_{50} values of Oxaliplatin and NP-PEG-Pt were 98.8 and 214.0 μM, respectively, but that of NP-TPGS-Pt was merely 45.4 μM (**Table 2**). With increasing culture time, although the antitumor effects of the

TABLE 1 | Characterization of DACHPt-loaded nanoparticles.

NPs	Dh (nm)	PDI	ZP (mV)	LC (%)	EE (%)
NP-TPGS-Pt	85.3 ± 3.6	0.16	−16.3 ± 1.7	26.3 ± 1.5	75 ± 3.7
NP-PEG-Pt	55.3 ± 2.4	0.13	−20.3 ± 2.0	24.3 ± 1.1	71 ± 3.4

PDI, polydispersity index; ZP, zeta potential; LC, loading content; EE, encapsulation efficiency.

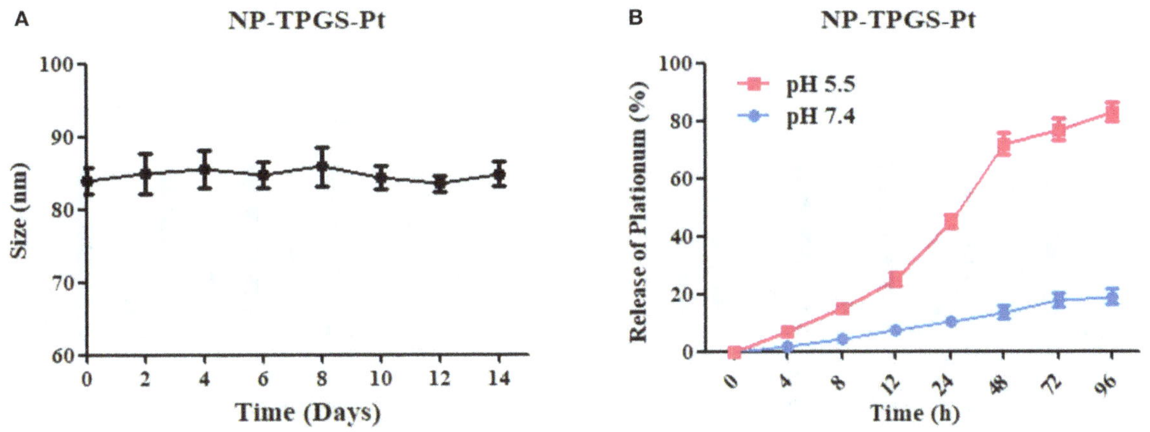

FIGURE 5 | (A) DACHPt-loaded NPs incubated in medium containing 10% FBS maintained their sizes for 14 days. **(B)** Accumulative release of DACHPt-loaded NPs in media containing 10% FBS with different pH-values. The result was reported as the average of three measurements.

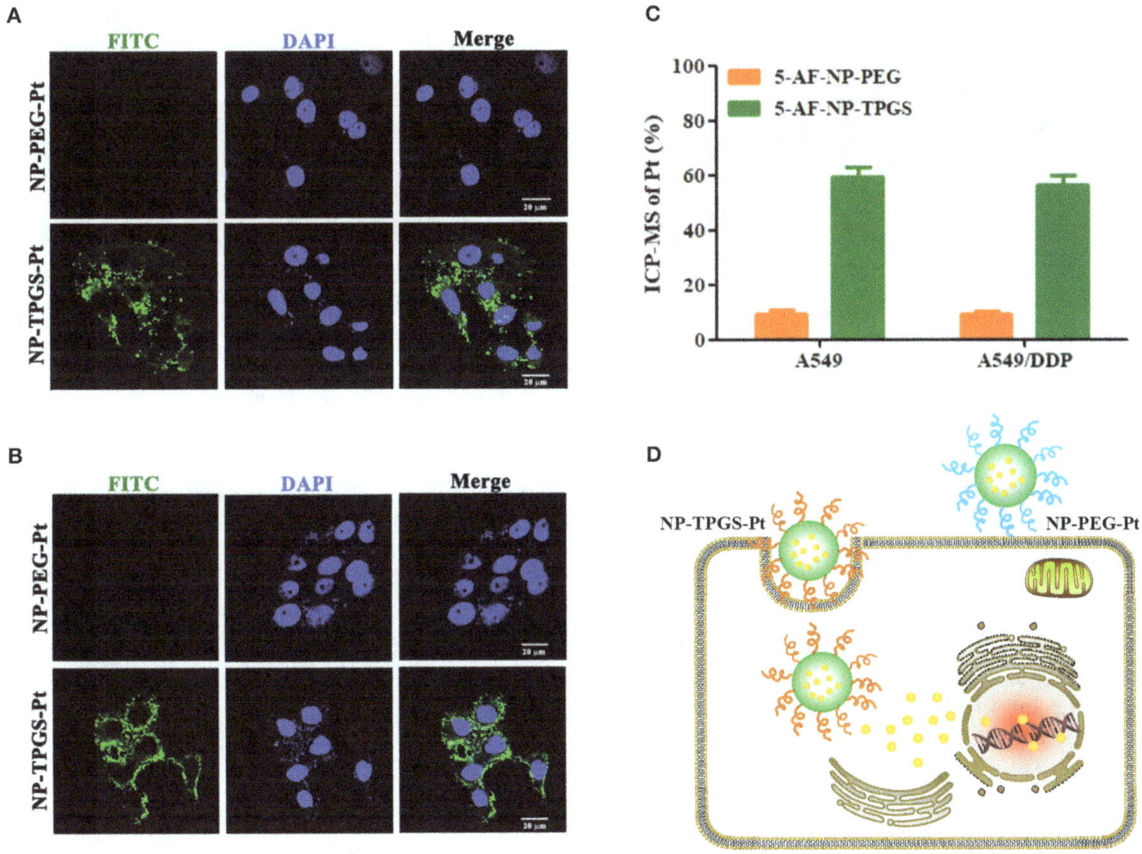

FIGURE 6 | Cellular uptake of NP-TPGS-Pt by A549 andA549/DDP cells. **(A,B)** CLSM images in A549 and A549/DDP cells, **(C)** Cellular uptake efficiency of A549 and A549/DDP cells after incubation with NP-PEG-Pt and NP-TPGS-Pt for 3 h. **(D)** An illustration for cell uptake in A549/DDP cells. (Scale bar: 20 µm).

three Oxaliplatin formulations were significantly boosted, the outcomes of NP-TPGS-Pt were significantly superior to those of Oxaliplatin and NP-PEG-Pt (**Figure 7B**). Taken together, modifying NP surface with TPGS increased the cytotoxicity through efficient uptake and persistent drug release.

On the other hand, Oxaliplatin killed A549/DDP cells far less effectively than A549 cells. Since the IC_{50} values of

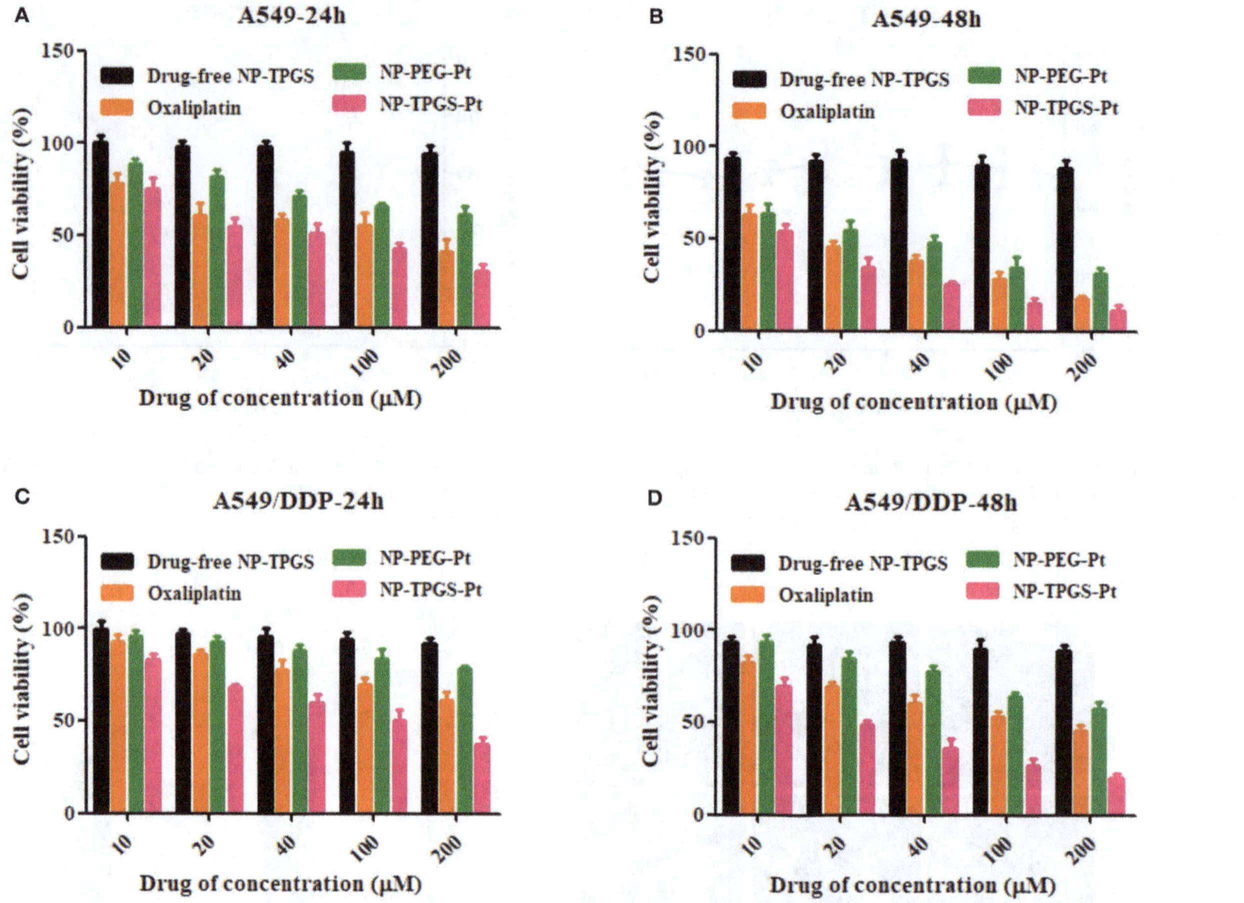

FIGURE 7 | Cell viability of A549 and A549/DDP cells incubated with the TPGS/DACHPt compared with that of oxaliplatin, NP-PEG-Pt and NP-TPGS-Pt at the same Oxaliplatin dose and that of the drug-free TPGS with the same polymer concentrations: **(A,B)** A549 cells for 24 and 48 h. **(C,D)** A549/DDP cells for 24 and 48 h.

Oxaliplatin at 24 and 48 h were 347.4 and 118.6 μM, respectively, A549/DDP cells were indeed strongly drug-resistant. Likewise, the antitumor effects of NP-PEG-Pt were inferior to those of Oxaliplatin. In contrast, the IC_{50} values of NP-TPGS-Pt at 24 and 48 h were 85.4 and 23.1 μM, respectively which were much lower than those of Oxaliplatin (**Figures 7C,D**), and slightly lower than those against A549 cells. Hence, NP-TPGS-Pt could overcome the drug resistance of cells. Additionally, MTT assay disclosed no influence of DACHPt-free NP-TPGS on cell growth, so they were highly biosafe and thus applicable to practice.

TABLE 2 | IC_{50} values of Oxaliplatin, NP-PEG-Pt and NP-TPGS-Pt against A549 and A549/DDP cells following 24 and 48 h of incubation.

	Time (h)	IC_{50} (μM)		
		Oxaliplatin	**NP-PEG-Pt**	**NP-TPGS-Pt**
A549	24	98.8 ± 8.4	214.0 ± 2.0	45.4 ± 2.7
	48	16.1 ± 1.1	31.1 ± 2.6	9.8 ± 0.8
A549/DDP	24	347.4 ± 10.2	–	85.4 ± 8.7
	48	118.6 ± 9.8	235.2 ± 10.8	23.1 ± 3.5

In Vivo Antitumor Effects

Given the positive results above, we ultimately evaluated the *in vivo* antitumor effects of NP-TPGS-Pt. The mice xenografted with A549/DDP cells were injected with normal saline, Oxaliplatin, NP-PEG-Pt and NP-TPGS-Pt respectively every 4 days, five times in total. After 20 days of treatment, the average tumor volumes of saline, Oxaliplatin and NP-PEG-Pt groups grew to 408.8, 337.3, and 278.8 mm^3, respectively, but that of the NP-TPGS-Pt group only increased to 188.7 mm^3 (**Figure 8A**). Clearly, NP-TPGS-Pt markedly inhibited tumor growth, with better outcomes than those of Oxaliplatin and NP-PEG-Pt. Besides, the body weights of NP-TPGS-Pt-treated mice and the other three groups were similar, without obvious changes (**Figure 8B**). After 20 days of treatment, all mice were sacrificed, from which tumors were collected. **Figures 8C,D** show the morphologies and average body weights of all tumors, both confirming the outstanding antitumor effects of NP-TPGS-Pt. Overall, NP-TPGS-Pt were able to solve tumor multidrug resistance.

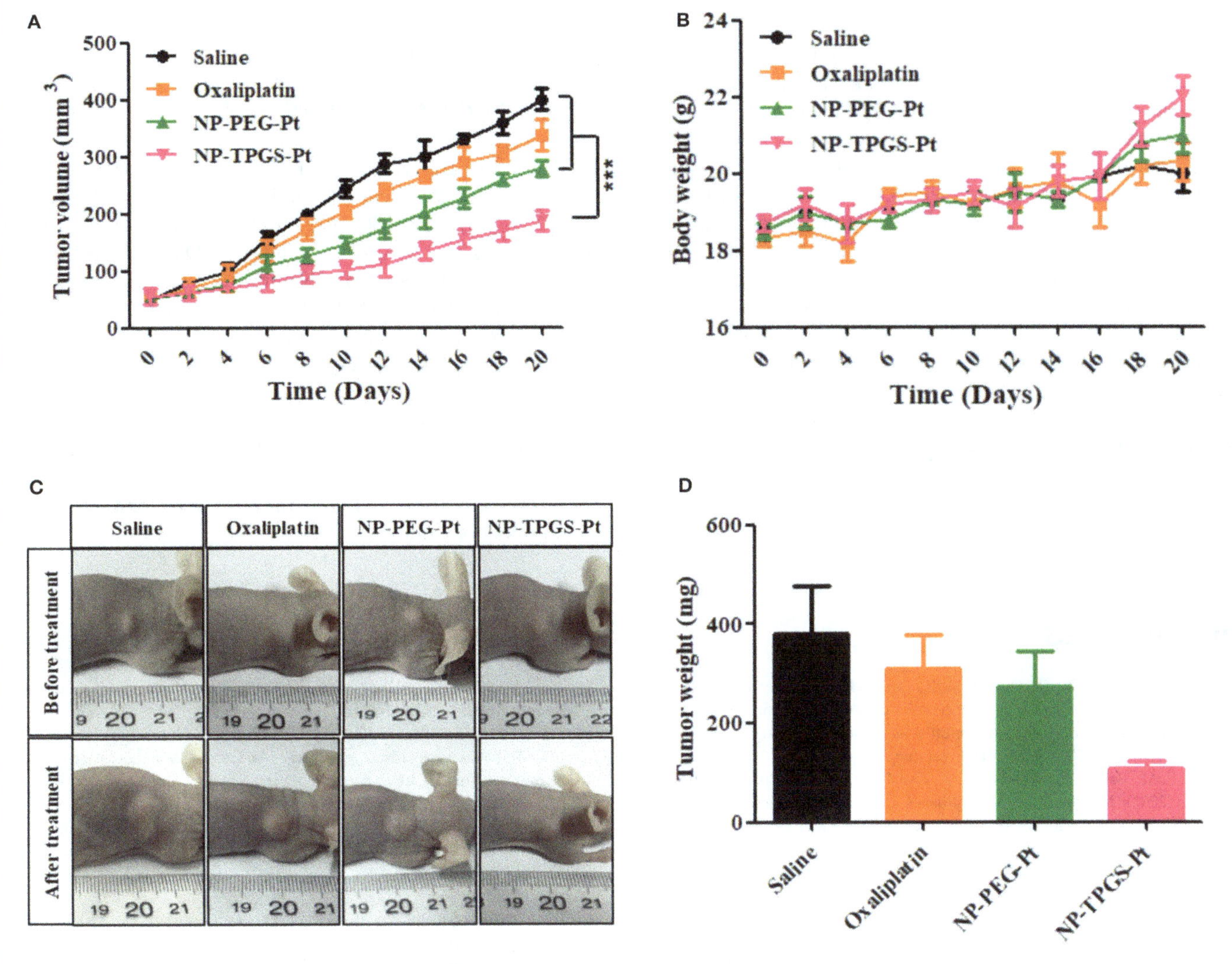

FIGURE 8 | Influence of DACHPt formulations on antitumor effects **(A)**, and changes of body weight **(B)** of A549/DDP xenograft-bearing nude mice. Images **(C)** and weights **(D)** of tumors resected from each group of sacrificed mice on the last day.

DISCUSSION AND CONCLUSIONS

In our previous research (Liu et al., 2017a), we developed the DACHPt-loaded UM (UM/DACHPt) dendritic block copolymer for micelles formulation of small molecular anti-tumor drugs and characterized the properties of the nanoparticle *in vitro*. Since the antitumor effects of unimolecular micelles are inferior to those of free drugs *in vitro*, they would hardly fulfill the requirement. Therefore, to optimize the nanocarrier structure to be both stable *in vivo* and multidrug-resistant. Indeed, TPGS has been reported to inhibit P-glycoprotein mediated multi-drug resistance (MDR) in tumor cells, which may reduce the excretion of drugs (Collnot et al., 2007; Zeng et al., 2013).

From the DLS results (**Figure 4A** and **Table 1**), we obtained NP-TPGS-Pt by complexing PAM-PGlu-b-TPGS with DACHPt. The NPs had a narrow monodisperse distribution and the average hydrodynamic diameter of ~85.3 nm. The size of NP-TPGS-Pt was much larger than which of NP-PEG-Pt. Because of PEG is completely hydrophilic polymers, PEG-b-PGlu could interact with DACHPt to be unimolecular micelles, therefore the size and the dendritic block copolymers itself size didn't big changed. But TPGS has certain hydrophobic, after PEG-b-PGlu interact with DACHPt, TPGS would induce the accumulation of the dendritic block copolymers, so the final particle size of NP-TPGS-Pt was bigger than NP-PEG-Pt. In other reports also showed TPGS dendritic block copolymers gathered into 100 nanometers in micelle (Zeng et al., 2013). And in TEM presented that NF-TPGS-Pt were uniformly distributed spherical particles with the size of about 60 nm, being consistent with the DLS results (**Figure 4B**). The particle size measured by TEM was smaller than that by DLS, because DLS detected the hydrodynamic diameter in aqueous solution in which the hydrophilic TPGS layer expanded while TEM was performed by using dry NPs.

Previous reports found that Pt release was accelerated in a chloride ion-containing environment under acidic conditions (Song et al., 2012). In **Figure 5**, the drug release rate from

NP-TPGS-Pt was only 20% after 96 h, revealing that these NPs were fairly stable under physiological conditions and drug hardly leaked. We observed the acid environment could accelerate the Pt release, because the accelerated release at acidic pH may be due to the protonation of carboxylic groups of PGlu, which weakens the drug and micelles coupling.

In conclusion, we successfully synthesized the dendritic block copolymer PAM-PGlu-*b*-TPGS which was thereafter self-assembled into nanoparticles by chelating the potent antitumor agent DACHPt. This TPGS-coated nanocarrier had robust stability and underwent nanoparticle-based cellular uptake by drug-resistant cancer cells, eventually remarkably suppressing the growth of these cells and drug-resistant tumors *in vivo*. Hence, the nanocarrier provides a novel strategy for treating multidrug-resistant tumors.

AUTHOR CONTRIBUTIONS

GL, LH, and ZL designed the research project; H-IT and LJ had full controlled the experiments, data analysis, and preparation of article; XZ, HC, WC, JZ, JP, DW, LG, ZX, and LM were involved in planning the analysis and drafting the article. The final draft article was approved by all the authors.

ACKNOWLEDGMENTS

The authors are grateful for the financial support from National Natural Science Foundation of China (81771966, 51703258, 31270019,21506161, 21646010, 81660425, 81670141), Guangdong Natural Science Funds for Distinguished Young Scholar (2014A030306036), Natural Science Foundation of Guangdong Province (2015A030313848, 2015A030313846), Guangdong Special Support Program, Science and Technology Planning Project of Guangdong Province (2016A020217001), Science, Technology & Innovation Commission of Shenzhen Municipality (JCYJ20160301152300347, JCYJ20160428182427603, JCYJ20150518162154828), the Fundamental Research Funds for the Central Universities (No. 17ykjc05), and Project of scientific research and technology development of Guilin City (20170226).

REFERENCES

Bao, Y. L., Kong, M., Gao, X. Q., Yin, M. X., Deng, H., Tan, Q., et al. (2017). pH-, redox dual-sensitive poly(beta-amino ester)-g-TPGS copolymer nanoparticles for drug delivery and inhibition of multidrug resistance in cancer. *React. Funct. Polym.* 120, 131–138. doi: 10.1016/j.reactfunctpolym.2017.09.013

Collnot, E. M., Baldes, C., Wempe, M. F., Kappl, R., Hüttermann, J., Hyatt, J. A., et al. (2007). Mechanism of inhibition of P-glycoprotein mediated efflux by vitamin E TPGS: influence on ATPase activity and membrane fluidity. *Mol. Pharm.* 4, 465–474. doi: 10.1021/mp060121r

Dintaman, J. M., and Silverman, J. A. (1999). Inhibition of P-glycoprotein by D-alpha-tocopheryl polyethylene glycol 1000 succinate (TPGS). *Pharm. Res.* 16, 1550–1556. doi: 10.1023/A:1015000503629

Graham, M. A., Lockwood, G. F., Greenslade, D., Brienza, S., Bayssas, M., and Gamelin, E. (2000). Clinical pharmacokinetics of oxaliplatin: a critical review. *Clin. Cancer Res.* 6, 1205–1218.

Guo, Y., Luo, J., Tan, S. W., Otieno, B. O., and Zhang, Z. P. (2013). The applications of vitamin E TPGS in drug delivery. *Eur. J. Pharm. Sci.* 49, 175–186. doi: 10.1016/j.ejps.2013.02.006

Han, Y., and Smith, M. T. (2013). Pathobiology of cancer chemotherapy-induced peripheral neuropathy (CIPN). *Front. Pharmacol.* 4:156. doi: 10.3389/fphar.2013.00156

Harrach, S., and Ciarimboli, G. (2015). Role of transporters in the distribution of platinum-based drugs. *Front. Pharmacol.* 6:85. doi: 10.3389/fphar.2015.00085

Huang, K., Shi, B., Xu, W., Ding, J., Yang, Y., Liu, H., et al. (2015). Reduction-responsive polypeptide nanogel delivers antitumor drug for improved efficacy and safety. *Acta Biomater.* 27, 179–193. doi: 10.1016/j.actbio.2015.08.049

Klein, A. V., and Hambley, T. W. (2009). Platinum drug distribution in cancer cells and tumors. *Chem. Rev.* 109, 4911–4920. doi: 10.1021/cr9001066

Li, B., Li, Q., Mo, J., and Dai, H. (2017). Drug-loaded polymeric nanoparticles for cancer stem cell targeting. *Front. Pharmacol.* 8:51. doi: 10.3389/fphar.2017.00051

Li, Y., Deng, Y., Tian, X., Ke, H., Guo, M., Zhu, A., et al. (2015). Multipronged design of light-triggered nanoparticles to overcome cisplatin resistance for efficient ablation of resistant tumor. *ACS Nano* 9, 9626–9637. doi: 10.1021/acsnano.5b05097

Liu, G., Gao, H., Zuo, Y., Zeng, X., Tao, W., Tsai, H. I., et al. (2017a). DACHPt-loaded unimolecular micelles based on hydrophilic dendritic block copolymers for enhanced therapy of lung cancer. *ACS Appl. Mater. Interfaces* 9, 112–119. doi: 10.1021/acsami.6b11917

Liu, G., Tsai, H. I., Zeng, X., Zuo, Y. X., Tao, W., Han, J., et al. (2017b). Phosphorylcholine-based stealthy nanocapsules enabling tumor microenvironment-responsive doxorubicin release for tumor suppression. *Theranostics* 7, 1192–1203. doi: 10.7150/thno.17881

Ma, P., Xiao, H. H., Yu, C., Liu, J. H., Cheng, Z. Y., Song, H. Q., et al. (2017). Enhanced cisplatin chemotherapy by iron oxide nanocarrier-mediated generation of highly toxic reactive oxygen species. *Nano Lett.* 17, 928–937. doi: 10.1021/acs.nanolett.6b04269

Mu, L., and Feng, S. S. (2003). A novel controlled release formulation for the anticancer drug paclitaxel (Taxol (R)): PLGA nanoparticles containing vitamin E TPGS. *J. Control. Release* 86, 33–48. doi: 10.1016/S0168-3659(02)00320-6

Nishiyama, N., Kato, Y., Sugiyama, Y., and Kataoka, K. (2001). Cisplatin-loaded polymer-metal complex micelle with time-modulated decaying property as a novel drug delivery system. *Pharm. Res.* 18, 1035–1041. doi: 10.1023/A:1010908916184

Oberoi, H. S., Nukolova, N. V., Kabanov, A. V., and Bronich, T. K. (2013). Nanocarriers for delivery of platinum anticancer drugs. *Adv. Drug Deliv. Rev.* 65, 1667–1685. doi: 10.1016/j.addr.2013.09.014

Peer, D., Karp, J. M., Hong, S., FaroKHzad, O. C., Margalit, R., and Langer, R. (2007). Nanocarriers as an emerging platform for cancer therapy. *Nat. Nanotechnol.* 2, 751–760. doi: 10.1038/nnano.2007.387

Salomone, S. (2013). PLGA: the smart therapeutics goods carrier. *Front. Pharmacol.* 4:20. doi: 10.3389/fphar.2013.00020

Song, W., Li, M., Tang, Z., Li, Q., Yang, Y., Liu, H., et al. (2012). Methoxypoly(ethylene glycol)-block-Poly(L-glutamic acid)-loaded cisplatin and a combination with iRGD for the treatment of non-small-cell lung cancers. *Macromol. Biosci.* 12, 1514–1523. doi: 10.1002/mabi.201200145

Tan, S., Zou, C., Zhang, W., Yin, M., Gao, X., and Tang, Q. (2017). Recent developments in d-alpha-tocopheryl polyethylene glycol-succinate-based nanomedicine for cancer therapy. *Drug Deliv.* 24, 1831–1842. doi: 10.1080/10717544.2017.1406561

Torre, L. A., Bray, F., Siegel, R. L., Ferlay, J., Lortet-Tieulent, J., and Jemal, A. (2015). Global cancer statistics, 2012. *CA Cancer J. Clin.* 65, 87–108. doi: 10.3322/caac.21262

Wang, D. F., Rong, W. T., Lu, Y., Hou, J., Qi, S. S., Xiao, Q., et al. (2015). TPGS(2k)/PLGA nanoparticles for overcoming multidrug resistance by interfering mitochondria of human alveolar adenocarcinoma cells. *ACS Appl. Mater. Interfaces* 7, 3888–3901. doi: 10.1021/am508340m

Wang, D., and Lippard, S. J. (2005). Cellular processing of platinum anticancer drugs. *Nat. Rev. Drug Discov.* 4, 307–320. doi: 10.1038/nrd1691

Wang, X., and Guo, Z. (2013). Targeting and delivery of platinum-based anticancer drugs. *Chem. Soc. Rev.* 42, 202–224. doi: 10.1039/C2CS35259A

Wei, T., Chen, C., Liu, J., Liu, C., Posocco, P., Liu, X., et al. (2015). Anticancer drug nanomicelles formed by self-assembling amphiphilic dendrimer to combat cancer drug resistance. *Proc. Natl. Acad. Sci. U.S.A.* 112, 2978–2983. doi: 10.1073/pnas.1418494112

Wheate, N. J., Walker, S., Craig, G. E., and Oun, R. (2010). The status of platinum anticancer drugs in the clinic and in clinical trials. *Dalton Trans.* 39, 8113–8127. doi: 10.1039/c0dt00292e

Xiao, H., Qi, R., Li, T., Awuah, S. G., Zheng, Y., Wei, W., et al. (2017). Maximizing synergistic activity when combining RNAi and platinum-based anticancer agents. *J. Am. Chem. Soc.* 139, 3033–3044. doi: 10.1021/jacs.6b12108

Xu, W., Ding, J., Xiao, C., Li, L., Zhuang, X., and Chen, X. (2015). Versatile preparation of intracellular-acidity-sensitive oxime-linked polysaccharide-doxorubicin conjugate for malignancy therapeutic. *Biomaterials* 54, 72–86. doi: 10.1016/j.biomaterials.2015.03.021

Yin, M. X., Bao, Y. L., Gao, X. Q., Wu, Y. P., Sun, Y., Zhao, X. Y., et al. (2017). Redox/pH dual-sensitive hybrid micelles for targeting delivery and overcoming multidrug resistance of cancer. *J. Mater. Chem. B* 5, 2964–2978. doi: 10.1039/C6TB03282F

Zeng, X., Tao, W., Mei, L., Huang, L., Tan, C., and Feng, S. S. (2013). Cholic acid-functionalized nanoparticles of star-shaped PLGA-vitamin E TPGS copolymer for docetaxel delivery to cervical cancer. *Biomaterials* 34, 6058–6067. doi: 10.1016/j.biomaterials.2013.04.052

Zhang, Z. P., and Feng, S. S. (2006). The drug encapsulation efficiency, *in vitro* drug release, cellular uptake and cytotoxicity of paclitaxel-loaded poly(lactide)-tocopheryl polyethylene glycol succinate nanoparticles. *Biomaterials* 27, 4025–4033. doi: 10.1016/j.biomaterials.2006.03.006

Zhang, Z. P., Tan, S. W., and Feng, S. S. (2012). Vitamin E TPGS as a molecular biomaterial for drug delivery. *Biomaterials* 33, 4889–4906. doi: 10.1016/j.biomaterials.2012.03.046

Zhu, H. J., Chen, H. B., Zeng, X. W., Wang, Z. Y., Zhang, X. D., Wu, Y. P., et al. (2014). Co-delivery of chemotherapeutic drugs with vitamin E TPGS by porous PLGA nanoparticles for enhanced chemotherapy against multi-drug resistance. *Biomaterials* 35, 2391–2400. doi: 10.1016/j.biomaterials.2013.11.086

13

Ceramide-Graphene Oxide Nanoparticles Enhance Cytotoxicity and Decrease HCC Xenograft Development: A Novel Approach for Targeted Cancer Therapy

***Shi-Bing Wang*[1,2†], *Ying-Yu Ma*[2†], *Xiao-Yi Chen*[1], *Yuan-Yuan Zhao*[1] and *Xiao-Zhou Mou*[1,2*]**

[1] Key Laboratory of Tumor Molecular Diagnosis and Individualized Medicine of Zhejiang Province, Zhejiang Provincial People's Hospital, People's Hospital of Hangzhou Medical College, Hangzhou, China, [2] Clinical Research Institute, Zhejiang Provincial People's Hospital, People's Hospital of Hangzhou Medical College, Hangzhou, China

***Correspondence:**
Xiao-Zhou Mou
mouxz@zju.edu.cn

† These authors have contributed equally to this work

Despite substantial efforts to develop novel therapeutic strategies for treating hepatocellular carcinoma (HCC), the effectiveness and specificity of available drugs still require further improvement. Previous work has shown that exogenous ceramide can play a key role in inducing the apoptotic death of cancer cells, however, the poor water-solubility of this compound has hampered its use for cancer treatment. In the present study, we used polyethylene glycol (PEG) and polyethylenimine (PEI) co-conjugated ultra-small nano-GO (NGO-PEG-PEI) loaded with C6-ceramide (NGO-PEG-PEI/Cer) as a strategy for HCC treatment. We assessed the biological role of NGO-PEG-PEI/Cer, and we assessed its antitumor efficacy against HCC both *in vitro* and *in vivo* in combination with the chemotherapeutic drug sorafenib. We found that NGO-PEG-PEI significantly enhanced the cellular uptake of C6-ceramide. By investigating the mechanism of cellular delivery, we determined that the internalization of NGO-PEG-PEI/Cer progressed primarily via a clathrin-mediated mechanism. The combination of NGO-PEG-PEI/Cer and sorafenib exhibited synergy between these two drugs. Further work revealed that NGO-PEG-PEI/Cer may play a role in subverting multidrug resistance (MDR) in HCC cells by inactivating MDR and Akt signaling. NGO-PEG-PEI/Cer also significantly inhibited tumor growth and improved survival times *in vivo*, and the synergetic effect of NGO-PEG-PEI/Cer combined with sorafenib was also observed in drug-resistant HCC xenografts. In conclusion, our NGO-PEG-PEI nanocomposite is an effective nano-platform for loading C6-ceramide for therapeutic use in treating HCC, exhibiting high cancer cell killing potency in this tumor model. The NGO-PEG-PEI/Cer/sorafenib combination additionally represents a promising potential therapeutic strategy for the treatment of drug-resistant HCC.

Keywords: hepatocellular carcinoma, graphene oxide, ceramide, apoptosis, drug-resistant

INTRODUCTION

Hepatocellular carcinoma (HCC) is the third most common cause of cancer-related death globally, accounting for approximately 80% of all types of primary liver cancer (Torre et al., 2015). Currently, HCC treatment is largely focused on a combination of surgery, chemotherapy, drug-targeted therapy and radiofrequency ablation as appropriate. These comprehensive treatments can significantly improve prognosis and prolong the life span of patients (Forner et al., 2012). Unfortunately, the majority of patients diagnosed with HCC are not eligible for surgery, leaving systemic therapy as the primary treatment option in those patients with advanced disease (Lencioni et al., 2016; Yu, 2016). Although conventional anticancer drugs have been used for the treatment of HCC, their high toxicity and relative non-specificity impede long-term application (Keating and Santoro, 2009). In addition, several clinical studies have demonstrated that conventional cytotoxic chemotherapy has low response rates and severe side effects (Thomas et al., 2008). Therefore, targeted drug delivery strategies and targeted therapeutics are the current key topics of research interest among those seeking to treat this deadly disease.

Ceramide, the simplest of the sphingolipids, is composed of a sphingosine base and amide-linked acyl chains varying in length from C14 to C26 (Ponnusamy et al., 2010). Ceramides have been reported to act as bioeffectors capable of mediating various cellular processes, including proliferation and apoptosis of cancer cells (Alphonse et al., 2013; Camacho et al., 2013). Work has revealed that ceramide has numerous effects on cell function, with the potential to induce cell growth arrest, senescence, apoptosis, and autophagy (Hannun and Obeid, 2008). Interestingly, ceramide can also mediate alternative pre-mRNA splicing, thereby enabling cells to express pro-apoptotic isoforms of bcl-x and caspase-9 (Chalfant et al., 2002; Massiello and Chalfant, 2006). Given these findings, ceramide has attracted tremendous attention in the field of cancer therapy as a potentially powerful tumor suppressor (Henry et al., 2013). C6-ceramide in particular has been widely used for the treatment of malignant tumors (Tagaram et al., 2011; Overbye et al., 2017). For example, Adiseshaiah et al. found that the synergistic combination therapy of nanoliposomal C6-ceramide and vinblastine is associated with a disruption of autophagy in HCC and colorectal cancer (Adiseshaiah et al., 2013). Tagaram et al. also demonstrated that ceramide induces p-AKT-dependent apoptosis in human HCC cells *in vitro* and suppresses xenograft tumor growth *in vivo* (Tagaram et al., 2011), exerting an inherent tumor-killing effect. However, ceramide is highly hydrophobic, which largely limits its application *in vivo*, necessitating the search for a suitable carrier for ceramide delivery that does not restrict its pharmacological effects.

Recently, nanoparticle therapy has been identified as a potential multi-modal approach to enhance therapeutic efficacy and reduce side effects associated with cancer treatment (Davis et al., 2008; Goncalves et al., 2013; Tao et al., 2017a, 2018). Nanoparticles are associated with a more targeted localization to tumors and an active mode cellular uptake, making it possible to achieve controlled-release drug delivery and specific gene transfection (Davis et al., 2008; Tao et al., 2013; Zhu et al., 2018). Graphene, a class of two-dimensional carbon nanomaterials with desirable physical and chemical properties, has attracted great interest in many different fields including biomedicine (Feng and Liu, 2011; Chen et al., 2012). Nano-graphene oxide (NGO) is reported to act as potential nano-platform for the delivery of anticancer chemotherapy drugs and genes (Zhang et al., 2010; Zhang L. et al., 2011). NGO was reported to be suitable for loading doxorubicin (DOX) at rates as high as 235% (the weight ratio of loaded drug to carriers) (de Melo-Diogo et al., 2018). However, the toxicology of NGO has been focused recently, which showed that its cellular toxicity *in vitro* is closely related to its surface functionalization (Hu et al., 2011). Zhang et al. developed DOX-loaded NGO-PEG (Polyethylene Glycol) as a strategy for chemo-photothermal synergistic therapy in one system, which significantly enhanced the therapeutic efficacy of cancer treatment *in vivo* and *in vitro* (Zhang W. et al., 2011).

NGO has great potential for use as delivery vehicles designed to enhance cancer treatment, So our collaborator developed PEG and PEI (Polyethylenimine) co-conjugated ultra-small nano-GO (NGO-PEG-PEI) as a novel gene delivery carrier, and found that it showed excellent stability against salts and serum (Feng et al., 2013). In the present study, we used these nanoparticles for loading C6-ceramide, and we found that this formulation allows C6-ceramide to travel through the bloodstream and target tumor cells via enhanced cellular permeability and retention, facilitating its potential clinical use as a novel therapeutic strategy. Additionally, through *in vitro* and *in vivo* studies we also investigated the antitumor efficacy and molecular mechanisms of NGO-PEG-PEI/Cer combined with other chemotherapy drugs in HCC.

MATERIALS AND METHODS

Synthesis and Characterization of NGO-PEG-PEI/Cer

NGO-PEG-PEI was kindly provided by Dr. Kai Yang at the School of Radiation Medicine and Protection (SRMP) of Soochow University (Suzhou, China). Briefly, GO was obtained by oxidation of graphite following the modified Hummers method. Preparation of NGO-PEG-PEI was performed according to previous description (Feng et al., 2013). A mixture of GO solution (0.5 mg/ml) with 6-armed amine-terminated PEG (0.5 mg/ml) was under sonication for 5 min. Then EDC (0.5 mg/ml) was added, after another 5 min sonication, the mixture was stirred gently for 10 min at room temperature. The mixture was stirred for 6 h at room temperature following the second time addition of EDC (1 mg/ml) after being sonicated with PEI (2.5 mg/ml) for 5 min. After that, the mixture was washed with deionized water by 100 nm Milli-Q membrane filter (Millipore, Bedford, MA, United States) 3 times, and we obtained NGO-PEG-PEI re-suspended in water.

NBD C6-ceramide (6-((N-(7-Nitrobenz-2-Oxa-1,3-Diazol-4-yl)amino)hexanoyl)Sphingosine) (N1154, Thermo Fisher Scientific, MA, United States) solution with gradient concentration was prepared and its absorbance at 536 nm was measured. The standard curve was drawn according to different concentrations. Then C6-ceramide was mixed with a certain concentration of NGO-PEG-PEI solution in equal volume and oscillated overnight. After centrifuging for 30 min at 8000 rpm, the absorbance of supernatant was determined, and the concentration of free drug in supernatant was obtained according to the standard curve. Then NGO-PEG-PEI/Cer was prepared according to the maximum loading of C6-ceramide carried by NGO-PEG-PEI.

After loadinging the C6-Ceramide with NGO-PEG-PEI, PBS was added to make the final volume of 1.0 ml. The average size and zeta potential of the NGO-PEG-PEI/Cer complex were then measured with dynamic laser scattering (DLS) and a Zetasizer 3000HS particle analyzer (Malvern Instrument Inc., Worcestershire, United Kingdom), respectively. The sizes and zeta potential values were presented as the average values of three measurements.

Cell Culture and Maintenance

The human HCC cell lines HepG2, HuH7, and PLC/PRF/5 were purchased from the Cell Bank of Type Culture Collection of Chinese Academy of Sciences (Shanghai, China). HuH7-SR is sorafenib-resistant HuH7 cell line, which was retained in our lab. All the cell lines were authenticated by short-tandem repeat profiling and cultured in Dulbecco's Modified Eagle's Medium (GIBCO, Carlsbad, CA, United States) supplemented with 10% heat inactivated fetal bovine serum (GIBCO). Cells were incubated in a 5% CO_2 humidified incubator at 37°C.

Cell Uptake of NGO-PEG-PEI/Cer

HCC cells were plated into 6-well plates at a density of 1×10^5 cells/well and incubated with NGO-C6 in dulbecco's modified eagle's medium (DMEM) containing 10% fetal bovine serum. The cells were rinsed by PBS and then collected. The uptake ratio of NGO-PEG-PEI/Cer by HCC cells was measured by flow cytometry (Beckman, NJ, United States)) using NBD labeled on NGO-PEG-PEI/Cer. The whole procedures were operated in dark place.

Cell Viability Assay

For cell proliferation analysis, cells were dispensed in 96-well culture plates at a density of 5 × 103 cells/well. After attachment, cells were treated with Ceramide-C6, NGO-PEG-PEI/Cer, Sorafenib or combination therapy with NGO-PEG-PEI/Cer and Sorafenib at given concentration and time. The medium added with PBS was a blank control. Cell survival rate was evaluated by a standard 3-(4,5-dimethylthiazol-2-yl)-2,5-diphenyltetrazolium bromide (MTT) assay (Sigma, St. Louis, MO, United States), Medium was removed and fresh medium containing MTT (5 mg/ml) was added to each well. The cells were incubated at 37°C for 4 h, after draw off the supernatant of each well carefully and then an equal volume 150 μl of dimethyl sulfoxide (DMSO) was added to each well and mixed thoroughly on concentrating table for 10 min. The absorbance from the plates was read at 595 nm with Cytation 3 Multi-Mode Reader (BioTek, Vermont, United States).

Cell Apoptosis Assay

Apoptosis staining Kit containing Annexin V- fluoresceine isothiocyanate (FITC)/Propidium iodide (PI) (KeyGene Biotech, Nanjing, China) was used to detect cell apoptosis according to the manufacture's protocol. Cells were stained with 5 μl Annexin V-FITC and 5 μl PI after 48 h of treatment of NGO-PEG-PEI, C6 or NGO-PEG-PEI/Cer and then keep in dark at room temperature for 15 min. After that, these cells were analyzed by flow cytometer (Novo cyte 3130, ACEA Biosciences, Santiago, CA, United States).

Western Blotting Analysis

Cells were harvested in lysis buffer (Beyotime, China) involving 1% Complete Mini-Protease Inhibitor Cocktail (Roche Diagnosis, Switzerland). Protein extractions were quantified using the bicinchoninic acid (BCA) kit (Thermo scientific, MA) and heated for 10 min at 100°C. Thirty microgram of protein was resolved in 12% SDS-PAGE and transferred to nitrocellulose membrane (Millipore, Germany). After blocked for 1 h at 37°C, the membranes were immunobloted with different antibodies overnight at 4°C. Antibodies against Caspase-8, Caspase-9, Caspase-3, recombinant poly ADP ribose polymerase (PARP), P-glycoprotein (P-gp), multidrug resistance 1 (MDR1), AKT serine/threonine kinase 1 (Akt), jun proto-oncogene (c-Jun), glyceraldehyde-3-phosphate dehydrogenase (GAPDH) were purchased from Abcam (Shanghai, China). Antibodies against Caspase-8 (1:1000), Caspase-9 (1:1000), Caspase-3 (1:1000), PARP (1:500), XIAP (1:1000), cIAP-1 (1:1000), cIAP-2 (1:1000), Survivin (1:1000), livin(1:1000), P-gp(1:500), and MDR1 (1:1000) were purchased from EMD Millipore Corporation (Billerica, MA, United States). Membranes were then washed with TBST and incubated with Horseradish Peroxidase (HRP)-conjugated goat anti-rabbit or anti-mouse antibody (1:5000) for 1 h at room temperature. Finally, blots were detected using ChemiDoc^{TM} MP Imaging System (Bio-Rad) with a SuperEnhancedchemiluminescence detection kit (Applygen, Beijing, China).

Clonogenic Assay

The ability of the HCC cells to generate *in vitro* colonies was determined using clonogenic assay. Briefly, cells were incubated six-well plates at a concentration of 500 cells/well after treatment with NGO-PEG-PEI, C6 and NGO-PEG-PEI/Cer. The medium was regularly changed for 2 weeks until colony formation. Then the colonies were gently washed with phosphate buffer saline (PBS) after the supernatants removed, fixed with cold methanol for 20 min, and stained with crystal violet 0.1% in PBS at room temperature for 10 min followed by air-drying.

Images were captured and the total number of colonies/well was counted.

In vivo Antitumor Effect and Systemic Toxicity

Male Balb/c mice (6 weeks old) were obtained from Laboratory Animal Center of Zhejiang Chinese Medical University (Hangzhou, China). Tumor bearing mice were established by subcutaneous injection of 5 × 10^6 HCC cells (HuH7 or HuH7-SR) in 200 μl PBS into the flank region of Balb/c mice. The dimension of tumors was monitored by digital calipers. Average tumor volume is about 90 mm^3. Then the mice were randomized into 4 different treatment groups (7 mice per group): control group (PBS), NGO-PEG-PEI group, C6-ceramide group, NGO-PEG-PEI/Cer group. Then the mice bearing tumors in different groups were intravenous injected with PBS, NGO-PEG-PEI, C6-ceramide, NGO-PEG-PEI/Cer, respectively. After treatment, tumor volumes were tracked every 3 days by digital caliper measurements.

Control and nanocomposites-treated mice were sacrificed at 18 days after treatment. Major organs of those mice were collected, fixed in 4% formalin, conducted with paraffin embedded sections, stained with hematoxylin and eosin (H&E) and immuhistochemistry, and examined under a digital microscope.

This study was carried out in accordance with the recommendations of Laboratory Animal Center of Zhejiang Chinese Medical University, and the project was approved by the ethics committee of Zhejiang Provincial People's Hospital.

Statistical Analysis

The Statistical Package for the Social Sciences (version 13.0; SPSS Inc., Chicago, IL, United States) was used to perform all statistical analyses. Continuous data were analyzed using paired *t*-test or Wilcoxon rank test. Categorical data were analyzed using χ^2 or Fisher's exact test. Survival analysis was estimated by Kaplan–Meier method accompanying the log-rank test to calculate differences between the curves.

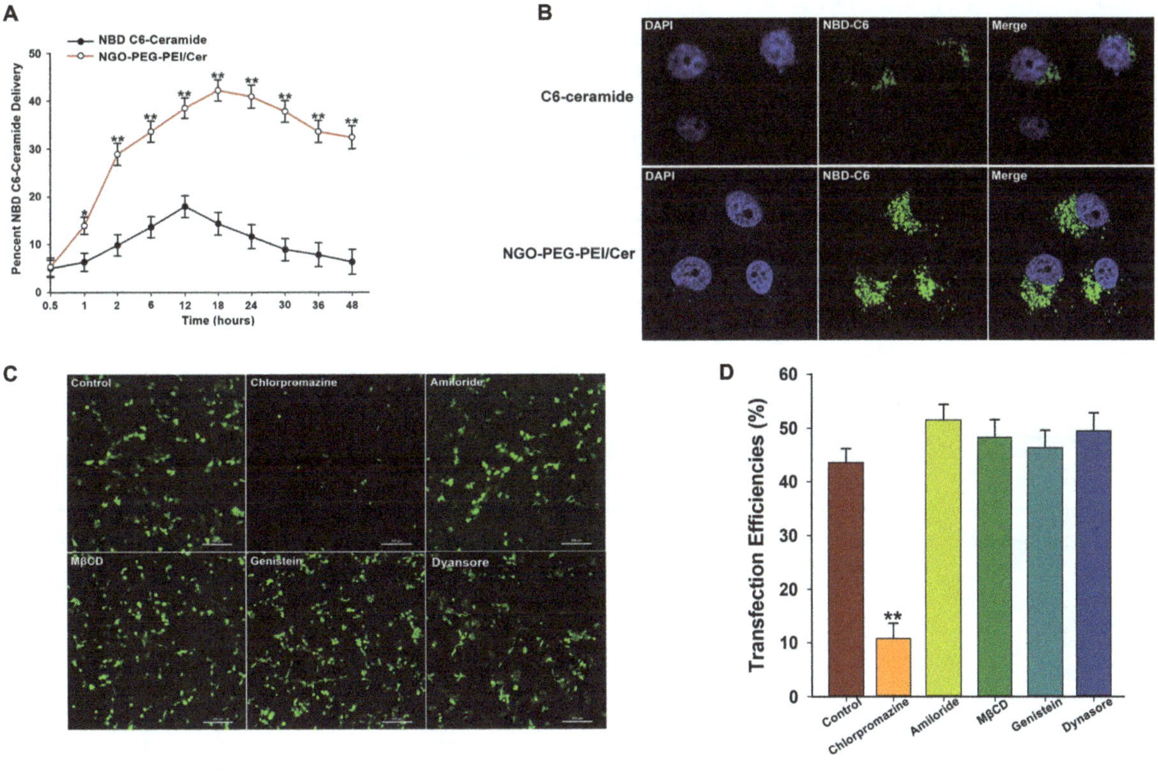

FIGURE 1 | Characterization of NGO-PEG-PEI/Cer complex *in vitro*. **(A)** *In vitro* pharmacokinetics of C6-ceramide delivery by fluorescence spectrophotometry. NGO-PEG-PEI delivery of C6-ceramide resulted in a greater cellular accumulation of C6-ceramide as a function of time relative to naked C6-ceramide administration in the presence of 10% FBS. NGO-PEG-PEI were formulated with trace C6-ceramide to determine the kinetics of ceramide delivery to HCC cells. The total counts of NGO-PEG-PEI and naked C6-ceramide added to the cells were set at 100%. Error bars were based on triplicate samples, *$p < 0.05$, **$p < 0.01$ when comparing NGO-PEG-PEI/Cer accumulation with naked C6-ceramide accumulation. **(B)** Cell confocal microscopic images of NBD C6-ceramide (green) and cell nuclei (blue) were collected from HepG2 cells treated with NGO-PEG-PEI/Cer or C6-Ceramide. **(C)** To confirm the mechanisms of cellular uptake of the NGO-PEG-PEI/Cer complexes, cells were pre-treated for 30 min with inhibitors diluted in FBS-free media at the indicated concentrations. NGO-PEG-PEI/Cer complexes were then added in the absence or presence of inhibitors for an additional 2 h. Complexes were then removed and replaced with fresh 5% FBS-containing media and incubated for 24 h. Green fluorescence was observed by **(C)** fluorescence microscopy and **(D)** flow cytometry. Error bars were based on triplicate samples. **$P < 0.01$ versus control.

For all tests, P-values were obtained from two-tailed statistical tests and p-values less than 0.05 were considered statistically significant.

RESULTS

Synthesis and Characterization of NGO-PEG-PEI/Cer Nanoparticles

Graphene oxide (GO) has been extensively explored in nanomedicine for its excellent physiochemical, electrical, and optical properties. In this study, polyethylene glycol (PEG) and polyethylenimine (PEI) were covalently conjugated to GO via amide bonds, yielding a physiologically stable dual-polymer-functionalized nano-GO conjugate (NGO-PEG-PEI) of ultra-small size. The synthesis and characterization of the NGO-PEG-PEI has been reported elsewhere (Feng et al., 2013). The NGO-PEG-PEI/Cer nanoparticles were generated via electrostatic interaction between the positively charged cationic NGO-PEG-PEI and the negatively charged C6-ceramide surface (**Supplementary Figure 1**). To determine optimal conditions for generating the NGO-PEG-PEI/Cer complex, the absorbance of the NGO-PEG-PEI/Cer were measured with various concentrations of the C6-Ceramide by UV Spectrophotometer. The size distribution and zeta potentials of the NGO-PEG-PEI/Cer complex were measured with various concentrations of the DA3 polymer by DLS and a zeta potential analyzer, respectively (**Supplementary Figure 1**).

We incorporated trace amounts of C6-ceramide into NGO-PEG-PEI formulations to quantify the amount of NGO-PEG-PEI/Cer delivery compared with naked C6-ceramide administration. Pharmacokinetic studies revealed that NGO-PEG-PEI formulations delivered C6-ceramide more effectively and efficiently than did mock administration of C6-ceramide in the presence of 10% FBS (**Figure 1A**). NGO-PEG-PEI delivery resulted in a threefold increase in ceramide accumulation in HepG2 cells, with a maximal accumulation observed at approximately 18 h. Additionally, confocal microscopy demonstrated that NGO-PEG-PEI/Cer nanoparticles were present in the cytoplasm and enhanced transduction efficiency of C6-Ceramide in cancer cells (**Figure 1B**).

We next investigated the mechanism by which C6-ceramide is released or transferred from NGO-PEG-PEI vehicles into cellular membranes. To elucidate the mechanism of cellular delivery of NGO-PEG-PEI/Cer, we studied the effects of inhibitors of various endocytotic mechanisms, including chlorpromazine (clathrin inhibitor), amiloride (actin inhibitor), methyl-β-cyclodextrin (MβCD, caveolae inhibitor), genistein (PTK inhibitor), and dynasore (dynamin inhibitor). Cells without inhibitor pretreatment were studied as controls under the same experimental conditions. Relative green fluorescence levels were measured after transduction with NGO-PEG-PEI/Cer complexes, and the experimental results suggested that the cell entry process for NGO-PEG-PEI is via clathrin-mediated endocytosis, as chlorpromazine led to a 32.36% inhibition of internalization (**Figures 1C,D**).

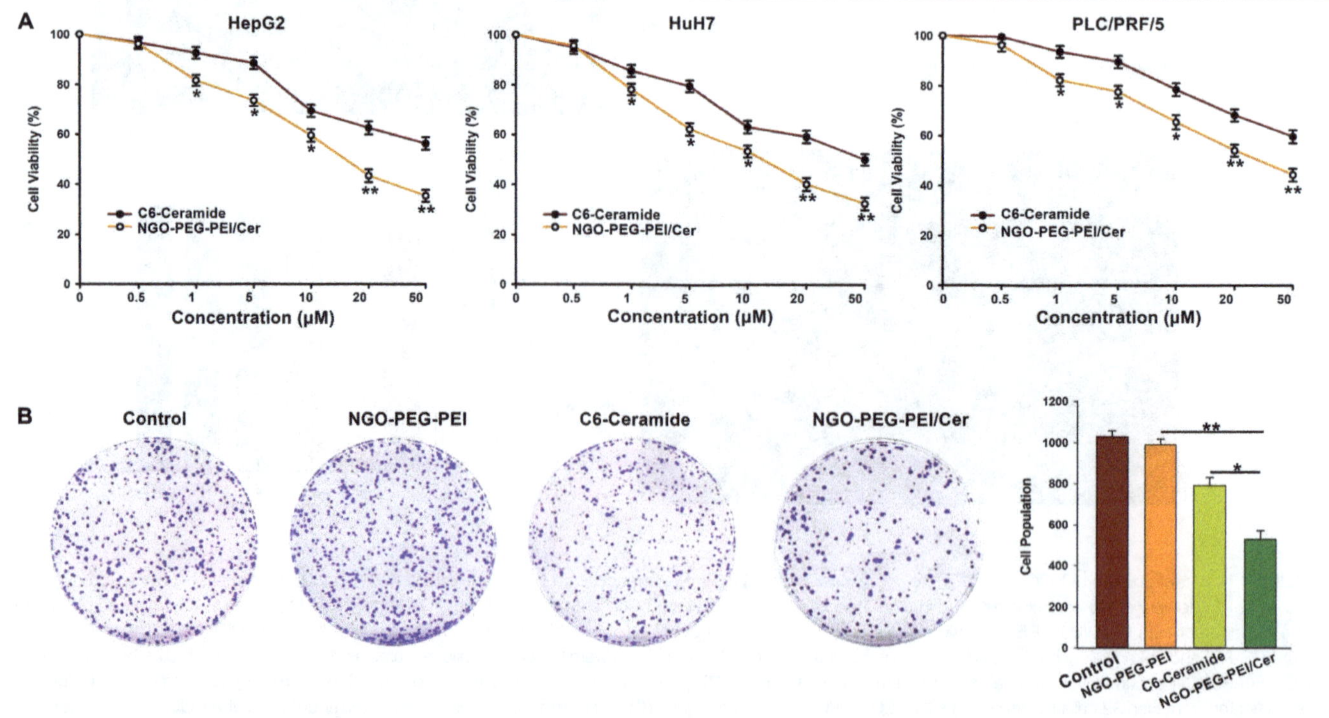

FIGURE 2 | *In vitro* anti-tumor activity of NGO-PEG-PEI/Cer. **(A)** Cells were seeded in 96-well plates and infected with NGO-PEG-PEI/CER or C6-ceramide at a series of concentrations. Cell viability was determined by MTT cell proliferation assays at 48 h post-infection. The results were presented as mean ± SD of three separate experiments. **(B)** Clonogenic formation of HepG2 cells treated by NGO-PEG-PEI/Cer. $^{*}P < 0.05$, $^{**}P < 0.01$.

In vitro Antitumor Activity of NGO-PEG-PEI/Cer

A 3-(4,5-dimethylthiazol-2-yl)-2,5-diphenyltetrazolium bromide (MTT) assay was performed 48 h post-infection with NGO-PEG-PEI/Cer to evaluate the cytotoxicity of the nanocomposites in the HepG2, HuH7 or PLC/PRF/5 cell lines in the presence of 10% FBS. The results indicated a significantly higher inhibition of cell growth in cells treated with NGO-PEG-PEI/Cer relative to those treated with C6-ceramide in a dose-dependent fashion (**Figure 2A**).

To further confirm the inhibitory effect of NGO-PEG-PEI/Cer on the proliferation of HCC cells, we conducted a clone formation assay and found that NGO-PEG-PEI/Cer could effectively inhibit the proliferation of HCC cells (**Figure 2B**).

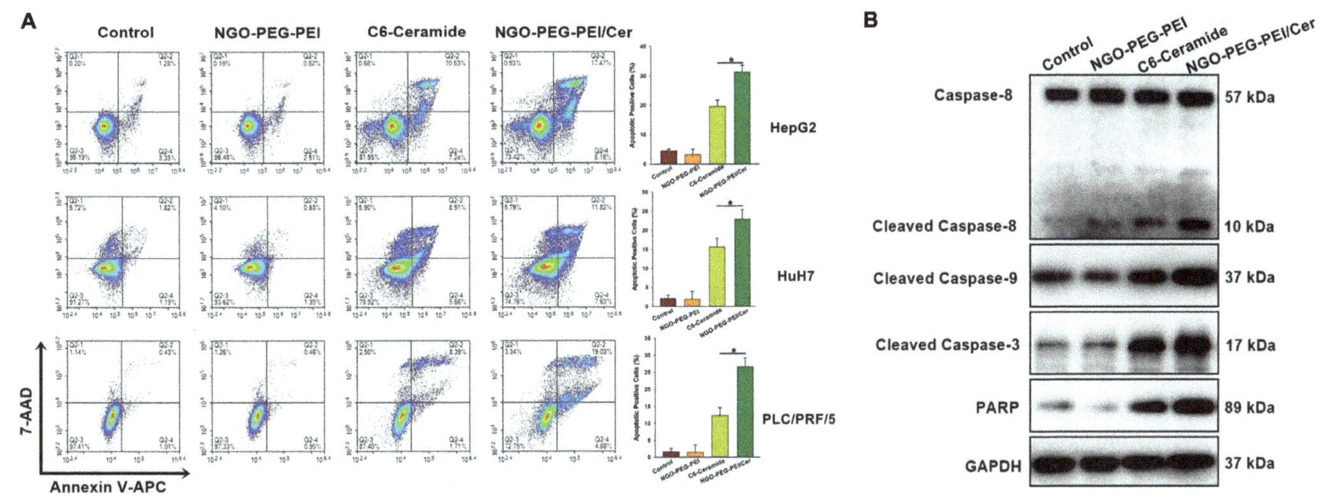

FIGURE 3 | NGO-PEG-PEI/CER induced apoptosis in HCC cells *in vitro*. **(A)** Apoptosis was analyzed via Annexin V-FITC/PI double staining. HepG2, HuH7, or PLC/PRF/5 cells were infected with NGO-PEG-PEI/Cer (10 μM), C6-ceramide (10 μM), or NGO-PEG-PEI (100 μg/ml) for 24 h. Florescence was then analyzed by flow cytometry. Data are presented as mean ± SD of three separate experiments. **(B)** HepG2 cells were infected with NGO-PEG-PEI/Cer (10 μM), C6-ceramide (10 μM), or NGO-PEG-PEI (100 μg/ml) for 24 h. Whole cell extracts were prepared and immunoblotted to detect caspase pathway activation. GAPDH was used as a loading control. *$P < 0.05$.

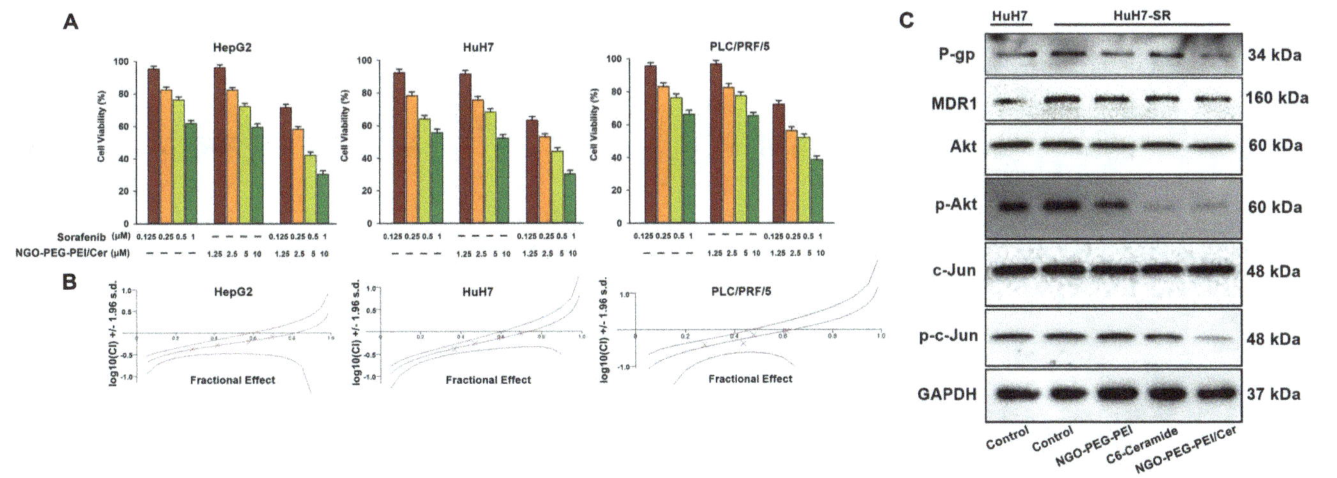

FIGURE 4 | NGO-PEG-PEI/Cer enhances sorafenib-mediated growth inhibition in HCC cells. **(A)** Cells were treated with NGO-PEG-PEI/Cer and/or sorafenib for 48 h, and cell viability was then determined by MTT assay. Data are presented as mean ± SD of three separate experiments. **(B)** The potential synergistic effect of sorafenib combined with NGO-PEG-PEI/Cer on HCC cells was assessed by Chou–Talalay Combination Index (CI) analysis using the CalcuSyn software. The middle curve line indicates the simulated combination index values, which are expressed as the log10 (CI) ± 1.96 SD, encircled by two lines of algebraic evaluation of the 95% confidence intervals. The log10 (CI) values attained at given fractional affects represent an antagonism between the treatments when >0, an additive efficiency when equal to 0 and a synergism when <0. This was quantified by CIN analysis and expressed as CIN versus fraction affected. Where calculable, 95% confidence intervals are shown. **(C)** The sorafenib-resistant HuH7 cell line (HuH7-SR) was used to illuminate the mechanism by which NGO-PEG-PEI/Cer may influence sorafenib-resistant HCC. NGO-C6(10 μM), C6-ceramide (10 μM), or NGO (100 μg/ml) was used to treat HuH7-SR cells. Uninfected cells served as control. Forty eight hours later, whole cell extracts were prepared and immunoblotted. GAPDH was used as a loading control.

NGO-PEG-PEI/Cer Treatment Induces Apoptosis *in vitro*

To address the underlying mechanism by which NGO-PEG-PEI/Cer induces cytotoxicity, we evaluated NGO-PEG-PEI/Cer associated apoptosis *in vitro* by flow cytometry. We observed significant increases in apoptosis in the HepG2, HuH7 or PLC/PRF/5 cell lines treated with NGO-PEG-PEI/Cer relative to those threated with C6-ceramide, NGO-PEG-PEI or PBS (**Figure 3A**).

We further evaluated apoptosis by assessing the expression of apoptosis-related proteins in HepG2 cells at 48 h post-infection using Western blotting analysis. The results indicated a significant increase in the activation of caspases 3, 8, and 9, and increased PARP cleavage in NGO-PEG-PEI/Cer-treated cells (**Figure 3B**). Taken together, these findings indicated that NGO-PEG-PEI/Cer effectively induced apoptosis via caspase activation.

Combined Treatment With Sorafenib and NGO-PEG-PEI/Cer Results in Synergistic Efficacy

To determine whether NGO-PEG-PEI/Cer enhances the cytotoxic effect of sorafenib, we analyzed the viability of HCC cells after co-treatment with NGO-PEG-PEI/Cer and sorafenib. The HepG2, HuH7, and PLC/PRF/5 cells were treated with

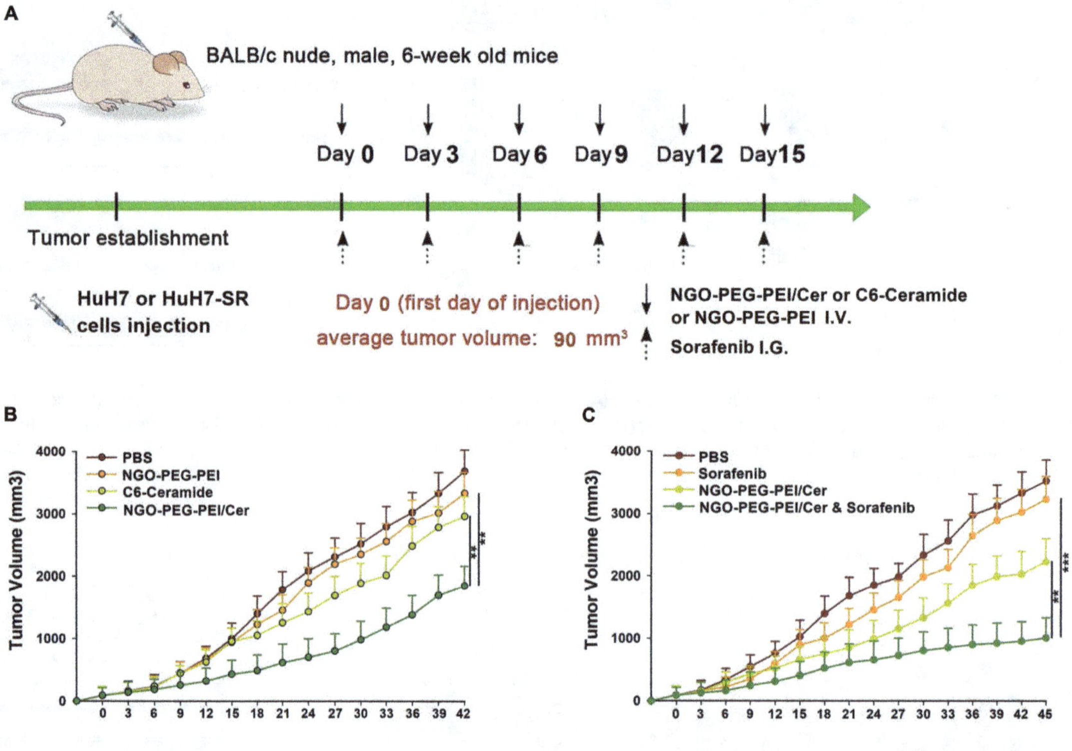

FIGURE 5 | Antitumor efficacy of NGO-PEG-PEI/Cer and synergistic effects of sorafenib and NGO-PEG-PEI/Cer *in vivo*. **(A)** Schematic of experimental timeline. BALB/c athymic nude mice implanted with HuH7 or HuH7-SR tumor xenografts were intravenously injected with PBS (100 μl), C6-ceramide 5 mg/kg), or NGO-PEG-PEI/Cer (5 mg/kg) every 3 days for a total of 6 times, or intragastric administration with a single dose of sorafenib (10 mg/kg) every 3 days for 6 times, or with a combination of sorafenib and NGO-PEG-PEI/Cer at the same conditions as above. **(B,C)** Tumor volumes were measured at different times after treatment. Data are presented as mean ± standard error ($n = 6$). *$P < 0.05$; **$P < 0.01$; and ***$P < 0.001$, one-way analysis of variance (ANOVA) and multiple comparisons. **(D,E)** Images show the inhibitory effects of each treatment on tumor growth based on survival.

sorafenib (0.125, 0.25, 0.5, or 1 μM) with or without NGO-PEG-PEI/Cer (1.25, 2.5, 5, or 10 μM). The combination of NGO-PEG-PEI/Cer with sorafenib significantly inhibited cell growth as compared with treatment with sorafenib or NGO-PEG-PEI/Cer alone (**Figure 4A**). Next, the synergistic effects of sorafenib combined with NGO-PEG-PEI/Cer on HCC cells were quantified by combination index (CIN) analysis and expressed as CIN versus fraction affected in **Figure 4B**. These results revealed that the combination of sorafenib and NGO-PEG-PEI/Cer has a synergistic tumor killing effect.

These results raised the question of the mechanism by which NGO-PEG-PEI/Cer influences sorafenib-resistant HCC cell lines. Therefore, we generated a sorafenib-resistant HuH7 cell line (HuH7-SR) and assessed the expression of multidrug resistance-related proteins or Akt, phospho-Akt, c-Jun, phospho-c-Jun of these HuH7-SR cells treated with NGO-PEG-PEI/Cer, C6-ceramide, or NGO-PEG-PEI by Western blot analysis in the presence of 10% FBS. Compared with the sensitive HuH7 cells, HuH7-SR cells exhibited markedly elevated levels of multidrug resistance-related proteins (P-gp and MDR1) and Akt, phospho-Akt, c-Jun, phospho-c-Jun. Our results further demonstrate that NGO-PEG-PEI/Cer has the capacity to reduce levels of multidrug resistance-related proteins and Akt, phospho-Akt, c-Jun, phospho-c-Jun (**Figure 4C**). Taken together, these findings indicated a synergistic repressive effect of the combination of sorafenib and NGO-PEG-PEI/Cer treatment on HCC cell proliferation.

Enhanced Cytotoxic Effect of Co-treatment With Sorafenib and NGO-PEG-PEI/Cer *in vivo*

We developed two hepatoma carcinoma tumor xenograft mouse models using the HuH7 cells and HuH7-SR cells in BALB/c athymic nude mice to evaluate the effects of NGO-PEG-PEI/Cer treatment or co-treatment with sorafenib and NGO-PEG-PEI/Cer *in vivo* (**Figure 5A**). Anti-tumor efficacy was evaluated by plotting tumor growth curves over a 42 or 45 days observation period. The mean tumor volume was significantly decreased in mice injected with sorafenib, NGO-PEG-PEI/Cer, and the combination therapy relative with those injected with PBS (**Figures 5B,C**). Furthermore, co-treatment of sensitive HuH7 and HuH7-SR cells with sorafenib and NGO-PEG-PEI/Cer was more effective than sorafenib ($P = 0.001$ and 0.002, respectively) and NGO-PEG-PEI/Cer alone ($P = 0.001$ and 0.003, respectively). Co-treatment with sorafenib and NGO-PEG-PEI/Cer was also associated with a higher survival rate than treatment with PBS, sorafenib, or NGO-PEG-PEI/Cer (**Figures 5D,E**).

The tumor histopathological changes were further evaluated by hematoxylin and eosin (H&E) staining and immunohistochemistry (IHC). The combined treatment with sorafenib and NGO-PEG-PEI/Cer resulted in greater cytotoxicity than either single treatment as evidenced by H&E staining. Moreover, very high Caspase-3 expression was evident in the tumor tissues from mice which received the combined treatment based on IHC staining with an anti-Caspase-3 antibody (**Figure 6**). Results from this experiment showed significantly higher rates of apoptosis in the combination treatment group when compared with either individual treatment (**Figure 6**).

DISCUSSION

Ceramide is reported to modulate cell death, cycle arrest, metastasis, stress responses, and pro-inflammatory responses in cancer cells (Saddoughi and Ogretmen, 2013; Kitatani et al., 2016), especially in HCC (Morales et al., 2007). Despite its key role in regulating tumor cell growth and death, its cell impermeability and its tendency to undergo precipitation in aqueous solutions have limited the use of ceramide as a therapeutic agent.

With the development of nanotechnology, application of nanomedicine in drug delivery becomes an area of rapid growth and advancement given its significant ability to enhance therapeutic efficacy, minimize side effects of drugs, and enhance drug bioavailability *in vivo* (Chen et al., 2016; Taghdisi et al., 2016; Tao et al., 2016, 2017b). Therefore, many nanomaterials – namely liposomes, micelles, dendrimers, carbon nanotubes, polymers, inorganic metallic nanolayers, and graphene oxides – have been explored in efforts to design nanocarriers for different drugs (Elgadir et al., 2015; Pattni et al., 2015). Recently, NGO has been explored in the field of biomedicine, which was found to be promising for drug delivery (Huang et al., 2012; Jayakumar et al., 2012). It is attractive in part due to its ease of synthesis, controlled particle size, and high surface area for drug loading. Although NGO without additional surface coatings appears

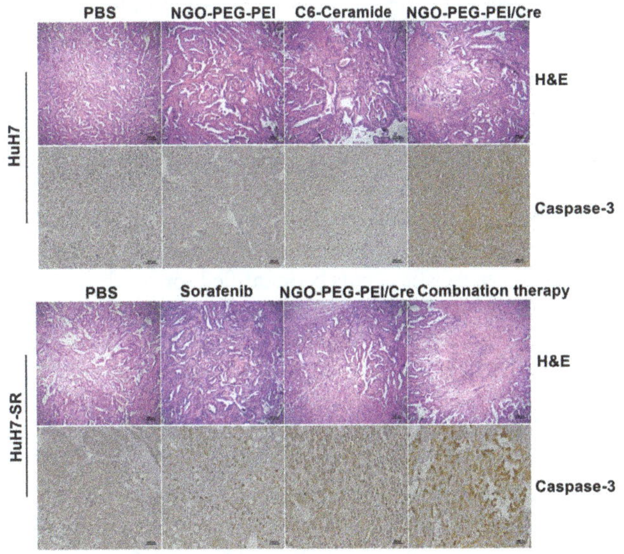

FIGURE 6 | Histopathological analysis. Subcutaneous HuH7 or HuH7-SR tumors were collected 18 days after injection, and sections were analyzed by the indicated methods. H&E staining showed that tumor tissues treated with the NGO-PEG-PEI/Cer or combination of sorafenib and NGO-PEG-PEI/Cer exhibited the greatest amount of cell death. An immunohistochemical analysis demonstrated there was strong expression of caspase-3 in xenografts treated with NGO-PEG-PEI/Cer as well as in those from the combined therapy group.

to exhibit dose-dependent toxicity, well functionalized NGO with biocompatible coatings such as PEG has been found to reduce obvious toxicity (Yang et al., 2013a,b). Other studies have explored the use of NGO for DNA plasmid and siRNA delivery after being functionalized by PEI (Feng et al., 2011; Zhang L. et al., 2011). Our collaborator also found that PEG and PEI functionalized NGO may enhance gene delivery (Feng et al., 2013). In the present study, we used NGO-PEG-PEI to carry C6, and we determined that the maximum drug loading capacity of 100 μg/ml NGO-PEG-PEI was 56 μM C6-ceramide. Next, in order to verify the enhanced intracellular trafficking of NGO-PEG-PEI/Cer, we assessed the cell uptake of NBD labeled NGO-PEG-PEI/Cer. Our results revealed that NGO-PEG-PEI significantly enhanced the cellular uptake of C6 and resulted in a threefold increase in ceramide accumulation with a maximal accumulation observed after approximately 18 h, which revealed that NGO-PEG-PEI formulations delivered C6-ceramide more effectively and efficiently. The mechanism of cellular delivery was also explored, established that this intracellular internalization of NGO-PEG-PEI/Cer progressed mainly via a clathrin-mediated mechanism.

C6-ceramide was cytotoxic and anti-proliferative when employed against a panel of human melanoma cells (Jiang et al., 2016), as well as against cervical cancer and colon cancer cells (Overbye et al., 2017). Nanoliposomal C6-ceramide has also been reported to induce cell apoptosis of HCC cells *in vitro*, concomitant with an accumulation of cells in the G2 phase of the cell cycle (Tagaram et al., 2011). In the present study, cell viability and toxicity were also detected after treatment with NGO-PEG-PEI/Cer, and our results showed that NGO-PEG-PEI/Cer exhibited high tumor cell killing potency as it was capable of both reducing HCC cell proliferation and increasing apoptosis. These findings thus suggest that NGO-PEG-PEI/Cer may induce potent, specific antitumor cytotoxicity.

Sorafenib, which is the first multi-target, multi-kinase inhibitor to be developed, is systematically used in the treatment of advanced liver cancer and has been proven to be effective (Wilhelm et al., 2006; Cheng et al., 2009). However, many patients do not respond to sorafenib, or they develop drug resistance after several months of sorafenib treatment. Therefore, it is urgent that enhancers or synergistic agents be identified for combination use with sorafenib to improve the clinical treatment of HCC. In our study, NGO-PEG-PEI/Cer combined with sorafenib was utilized for treating HCC, and the CI50 was determined to establish a synergistic effect. Our results showed that combination treatment with both drugs showed clear synergism effects superior to single drug treatment. NGO-PEG-PEI/Cer combined with sorafenib displayed an overall CI50 value <1, confirming the synergy between these two drugs. Further work revealed that the NGO-PEG-PEI/Cer/sorafenib combination may exert anti-multidrug resistance (anti-MDR) activities in HCC cells by significant inactivation of MDR and Akt signaling. These results illustrated that NGO-PEG-PEI/Cer combined with sorafenib can mediate an efficient synergistic therapeutic effect for antitumor therapy in drug-resistant HCC.

To evaluate the effects of NGO-PEG-PEI-C6 on HCC tumor-bearing mouse xenografts, survival time and tumor volume were evaluated, revealing that NGO-PEG-PEI/Cer significantly delayed tumor growth and improved survival times. Li et al. previously found that injection of nanoliposome-loaded C6-ceramide slowed tumor growth by reducing proliferation and increasing apoptosis in HCC (Li et al., 2018), suggesting that delivery system of ceramide via nanoparticle may be an effective strategy for the treatment of human HCC *in vitro* and *in vivo*. The synergetic effects of NGO-PEG-PEI/Cer combined with sorafenib were also evident in our mouse model, with evidence of tumor growth inhibition and improved overall survival improvement in mice receiving the combination regimen. These findings suggest that the NGO-PEG-PEI/Cer/sorafenib combination represents a potential therapeutic strategy for the treatment of drug-resistant HCC *in vivo*.

In summary, using nanotechnology-based advances in drug delivery, we utilized NGO-PEG-PEI nanocomposites as an effective nano-platform for loading C6-ceramide for therapeutic treatment of HCC. This formulated composite exhibited excellent anti-cancer efficacy *in vitro* and in *vivo*, facilitating its potential clinical use. Furthermore, combined treatment with NGO-PEG-PEI/Cer and sorafenib achieved a superior therapeutic effect in drug-resistant HCC, suggesting that NGO-PEG-PEI/Cer has great potential to treat drug-resistant HCC when used as a synergistic agent in combination with sorafenib.

AUTHOR CONTRIBUTIONS

X-ZM conceived and designed the experiments. S-BW and Y-YM carried out the majority of experiments and drafted the manuscript. X-YC analyzed the results and revised the manuscript. Y-YZ collected and analyzed the data. All authors read and approved the final manuscript.

FUNDING

This work was supported by the Zhejiang Provincial Natural Science Foundation of China (No. LQ16H160017 to Y-YM, No. LY17H180010 to X-YC), the National Natural Science Foundation of China (No. 81672430 to X-ZM, No. 81602706 to S-BW), Funds of Science Technology Department of Zhejiang Province (No. LGF18H160026 to Y-YZ).

SUPPLEMENTARY MATERIAL

FIGURE S1 | Synthesis and characterization of NGO-PEG-PEI/Cer. **(A)** The zeta potential value of the NGO-PEG-PEI were measured. **(B)** A schematic illustration showing the synthesis of NGO-PEG-PEI conjugate and the preparation of NGO-PEG-PEI/Cer complex. **(C)** The absorbance of the NGO-PEG-PEI/Cer were measured with various concentrations of the C6-Ceramide by UV Spectrophotometer. **(D)** The average size (nm) of the NGO-PEG-PEI/Cer complex was measured.

REFERENCES

Adiseshaiah, P. P., Clogston, J. D., McLeland, C. B., Rodriguez, J., Potter, T. M., Neun, B. W., et al. (2013). Synergistic combination therapy with nanoliposomal C6-ceramide and vinblastine is associated with autophagy dysfunction in hepatocarcinoma and colorectal cancer models. *Cancer Lett.* 337, 254–265. doi: 10.1016/j.canlet.2013.04.034

Alphonse, G., Maalouf, M., Battiston-Montagne, P., Ardail, D., Beuve, M., Rousson, R., et al. (2013). p53-independent early and late apoptosis is mediated by ceramide after exposure of tumor cells to photon or carbon ion irradiation. *BMC Cancer* 13:151. doi: 10.1186/1471-2407-13-151

Camacho, L., Meca-Cortes, O., Abad, J. L., Garcia, S., Rubio, N., Diaz, A., et al. (2013). Acid ceramidase as a therapeutic target in metastatic prostate cancer. *J. Lipid Res.* 54, 1207–1220. doi: 10.1194/jlr.M032375

Chalfant, C. E., Rathman, K., Pinkerman, R. L., Wood, R. E., Obeid, L. M., Ogretmen, B., et al. (2002). De novo ceramide regulates the alternative splicing of caspase 9 and Bcl-x in A549 lung adenocarcinoma cells. Dependence on protein phosphatase-1. *J. Biol. Chem.* 277, 12587–12595. doi: 10.1074/jbc.M112010200

Chen, G., Roy, I., Yang, C., and Prasad, P. N. (2016). Nanochemistry and nanomedicine for nanoparticle-based diagnostics and therapy. *Chem. Rev.* 116, 2826–2885. doi: 10.1021/acs.chemrev.5b00148

Chen, G. Y., Pang, D. W., Hwang, S. M., Tuan, H. Y., and Hu, Y. C. (2012). A graphene-based platform for induced pluripotent stem cells culture and differentiation. *Biomaterials* 33, 418–427. doi: 10.1016/j.biomaterials.2011.09.071

Cheng, A. L., Kang, Y. K., Chen, Z., Tsao, C. J., Qin, S., Kim, J. S., et al. (2009). Efficacy and safety of sorafenib in patients in the asia-pacific region with advanced hepatocellular carcinoma: a phase III randomised, double-blind, placebo-controlled trial. *Lancet Oncol.* 10, 25–34. doi: 10.1016/S1470-2045(08)70285-7

Davis, M. E., Chen, Z. G., and Shin, D. M. (2008). Nanoparticle therapeutics: an emerging treatment modality for cancer. *Nat. Rev. Drug Discov.* 7, 771–782. doi: 10.1038/nrd2614

de Melo-Diogo, D., Costa, E. C., Alves, C. G., Lima-Sousa, R., Ferreira, P., Louro, R. O., et al. (2018). POxylated graphene oxide nanomaterials for combination chemo-phototherapy of breast cancer cells. *Eur. J. Pharm. Biopharm.* 131, 162–169. doi: 10.1016/j.ejpb.2018.08.008

Elgadir, M. A., Uddin, M. S., Ferdosh, S., Adam, A., Chowdhury, A. J. K., and Sarker, M. Z. I. (2015). Impact of chitosan composites and chitosan nanoparticle composites on various drug delivery systems: A review. *J. Food Drug Anal.* 23, 619–629. doi: 10.1016/j.jfda.2014.10.008

Feng, L., and Liu, Z. (2011). Graphene in biomedicine: opportunities and challenges. *Nanomedicine* 6, 317–324. doi: 10.2217/nnm.10.158

Feng, L., Yang, X., Shi, X., Tan, X., Peng, R., Wang, J., et al. (2013). Polyethylene glycol and polyethylenimine dual-functionalized nano-graphene oxide for photothermally enhanced gene delivery. *Small* 9, 1989–1997. doi: 10.1002/smll.201202538

Feng, L., Zhang, S., and Liu, Z. (2011). Graphene based gene transfection. *Nanoscale* 3, 1252–1257. doi: 10.1039/c0nr00680g

Forner, A., Llovet, J. M., and Bruix, J. (2012). Hepatocellular carcinoma. *Lancet* 379, 1245–1255. doi: 10.1016/S0140-6736(11)61347-0

Goncalves, G., Vila, M., Portoles, M. T., Vallet-Regi, M., Gracio, J., and Marques, P. A. (2013). Nano-graphene oxide: a potential multifunctional platform for cancer therapy. *Adv. Healthc. Mater.* 2, 1072–1090. doi: 10.1002/adhm.201300023

Hannun, Y. A., and Obeid, L. M. (2008). Principles of bioactive lipid signalling: lessons from sphingolipids. *Nat. Rev. Mol. Cell. Biol.* 9, 139–150. doi: 10.1038/nrm2329

Henry, B., Moller, C., Dimanche-Boitrel, M. T., Gulbins, E., and Becker, K. A. (2013). Targeting the ceramide system in cancer. *Cancer Lett.* 332, 286–294. doi: 10.1016/j.canlet.2011.07.010

Hu, W., Peng, C., Lv, M., Li, X., Zhang, Y., Chen, N., et al. (2011). Protein corona-mediated mitigation of cytotoxicity of graphene oxide. *ACS Nano* 5, 3693–3700. doi: 10.1021/nn200021j

Huang, X., Qi, X., Boey, F., and Zhang, H. (2012). Graphene-based composites. *Chem. Soc. Rev.* 41, 666–686. doi: 10.1039/c1cs15078b

Jayakumar, M. K., Idris, N. M., and Zhang, Y. (2012). Remote activation of biomolecules in deep tissues using near-infrared-to-UV upconversion nanotransducers. *Proc. Natl. Acad. Sci. U.S.A.* 109, 8483–8488. doi: 10.1073/pnas.1114551109

Jiang, F., Jin, K., Huang, S., Bao, Q., Shao, Z., Hu, X., et al. (2016). Liposomal C6 ceramide activates protein phosphatase 1 to inhibit melanoma cells. *PLoS One* 11:e0159849. doi: 10.1371/journal.pone.0159849

Keating, G. M., and Santoro, A. (2009). Sorafenib: a review of its use in advanced hepatocellular carcinoma. *Drugs* 69, 223–240. doi: 10.2165/00003495-200969020-00006

Kitatani, K., Usui, T., Sriraman, S. K., Toyoshima, M., Ishibashi, M., Shigeta, S., et al. (2016). Ceramide limits phosphatidylinositol-3-kinase C2beta-controlled cell motility in ovarian cancer: potential of ceramide as a metastasis-suppressor lipid. *Oncogene* 35, 2801–2812. doi: 10.1038/onc.2015.330

Lencioni, R., Llovet, J. M., Han, G., Tak, W. Y., Yang, J., Guglielmi, A., et al. (2016). Sorafenib or placebo plus TACE with doxorubicin-eluting beads for intermediate stage HCC: the space trial. *J. Hepatol.* 64, 1090–1098. doi: 10.1016/j.jhep.2016.01.012

Li, G., Liu, D., Kimchi, E. T., Kaifi, J. T., Qi, X., Manjunath, Y., et al. (2018). Nanoliposome C6-ceramide increases the anti-tumor immune response and slows growth of liver tumors in mice. *Gastroenterology* 154, 1024.e9–1036.e9. doi: 10.1053/j.gastro.2017.10.050

Massiello, A., and Chalfant, C. E. (2006). SRp30a (ASF/SF2) regulates the alternative splicing of caspase-9 pre-mRNA and is required for ceramide-responsiveness. *J. Lipid Res.* 47, 892–897. doi: 10.1194/jlr.C600003-JLR200

Morales, A., Lee, H., Goni, F. M., Kolesnick, R., and Fernandez-Checa, J. C. (2007). Sphingolipids and cell death. *Apoptosis* 12, 923–939. doi: 10.1007/s10495-007-0721-0

Overbye, A., Holsaeter, A. M., Markus, F., Skalko-Basnet, N., Iversen, T. G., Torgersen, M. L., et al. (2017). Ceramide-containing liposomes with doxorubicin: time and cell-dependent effect of C6 and C12 ceramide. *Oncotarget* 8, 76921–76934. doi: 10.18632/oncotarget.20217

Pattni, B. S., Chupin, V. V., and Torchilin, V. P. (2015). New developments in liposomal drug delivery. *Chem. Rev.* 115, 10938–10966. doi: 10.1021/acs.chemrev.5b00046

Ponnusamy, S., Meyers-Needham, M., Senkal, C. E., Saddoughi, S. A., Sentelle, D., Selvam, S. P., et al. (2010). Sphingolipids and cancer: ceramide and sphingosine-1-phosphate in the regulation of cell death and drug resistance. *Future Oncol.* 6, 1603–1624. doi: 10.2217/fon.10.116

Saddoughi, S. A., and Ogretmen, B. (2013). Diverse functions of ceramide in cancer cell death and proliferation. *Adv. Cancer Res.* 117, 37–58. doi: 10.1016/B978-0-12-394274-6.00002-9

Tagaram, H. R., Divittore, N. A., Barth, B. M., Kaiser, J. M., Avella, D., Kimchi, E. T., et al. (2011). Nanoliposomal ceramide prevents in vivo growth of hepatocellular carcinoma. *Gut* 60, 695–701. doi: 10.1136/gut.2010.216671

Taghdisi, S. M., Danesh, N. M., Lavaee, P., Emrani, A. S., Hassanabad, K. Y., Ramezani, M., et al. (2016). Double targeting, controlled release and reversible delivery of daunorubicin to cancer cells by polyvalent aptamers-modified gold nanoparticles. *Mater. Sci. Eng. C Mater. Biol. Appl.* 61, 753–761. doi: 10.1016/j.msec.2016.01.009

Tao, W., Ji, X., Xu, X., Islam, M. A., Li, Z., Chen, S., et al. (2017a). Antimonene quantum dots: synthesis and application as near-infrared photothermal agents for effective cancer therapy. *Angew. Chem. Int. Ed. Engl.* 56, 11896–11900. doi: 10.1002/anie.201703657

Tao, W., Zhu, X., Yu, X., Zeng, X., Xiao, Q., Zhang, X., et al. (2017b). Black phosphorus nanosheets as a robust delivery platform for cancer theranostics. *Adv. Mater.* 29:1603276. doi: 10.1002/adma.201603276

Tao, W., Ji, X., Zhu, X., Li, L., Wang, J., Zhang, Y., et al. (2018). Two-dimensional antimonene-based photonic nanomedicine for cancer theranostics. *Adv. Mater.* 30:e1802061. doi: 10.1002/adma.201802061

Tao, W., Zeng, X., Liu, T., Wang, Z., Xiong, Q., Ouyang, C., et al. (2013). Docetaxel-loaded nanoparticles based on star-shaped mannitol-core PLGA-TPGS diblock copolymer for breast cancer therapy. *Acta Biomater.* 9, 8910–8920. doi: 10.1016/j.actbio.2013.06.034

Tao, W., Zeng, X., Wu, J., Zhu, X., Yu, X., Zhang, X., et al. (2016). Polydopamine-based surface modification of novel nanoparticle-aptamer bioconjugates for in vivo breast cancer targeting and enhanced therapeutic effects. *Theranostics* 6, 470–484. doi: 10.7150/thno.14184

Thomas, M. B., O'Beirne, J. P., Furuse, J., Chan, A. T., Abou-Alfa, G., and Johnson, P. (2008). Systemic therapy for hepatocellular carcinoma: cytotoxic chemotherapy, targeted therapy and immunotherapy. *Ann. Surg. Oncol.* 15, 1008–1014. doi: 10.1245/s10434-007-9705-0

Torre, L. A., Bray, F., Siegel, R. L., Ferlay, J., Lortet-Tieulent, J., and Jemal, A. (2015). Global cancer statistics, 2012. *CA Cancer J. Clin.* 65, 87–108. doi: 10.3322/caac.21262

Wilhelm, S., Carter, C., Lynch, M., Lowinger, T., Dumas, J., Smith, R. A., et al. (2006). Discovery and development of sorafenib: a multikinase inhibitor for treating cancer. *Nat. Rev. Drug Discov.* 5, 835–844. doi: 10.1038/nrd2130

Yang, K., Feng, L., Shi, X., and Liu, Z. (2013a). Nano-graphene in biomedicine: theranostic applications. *Chem. Soc. Rev.* 42, 530–547. doi: 10.1039/c2cs35342c

Yang, K., Li, Y., Tan, X., Peng, R., and Liu, Z. (2013b). Behavior and toxicity of graphene and its functionalized derivatives in biological systems. *Small* 9, 1492–1503. doi: 10.1002/smll.201201417

Yu, S. J. (2016). A concise review of updated guidelines regarding the management of hepatocellular carcinoma around the world: 2010-2016. *Clin. Mol. Hepatol.* 22, 7–17. doi: 10.3350/cmh.2016.22.1.7

Zhang, L., Lu, Z., Zhao, Q., Huang, J., Shen, H., and Zhang, Z. (2011). Enhanced chemotherapy efficacy by sequential delivery of siRNA and anticancer drugs using PEI-grafted graphene oxide. *Small* 7, 460–464. doi: 10.1002/smll.201001522

Zhang, W., Guo, Z., Huang, D., Liu, Z., Guo, X., and Zhong, H. (2011). Synergistic effect of chemo-photothermal therapy using PEGylated graphene oxide. *Biomaterials* 32, 8555–8561. doi: 10.1016/j.biomaterials.2011.07.071

Zhang, L., Xia, J., Zhao, Q., Liu, L., and Zhang, Z. (2010). Functional graphene oxide as a nanocarrier for controlled loading and targeted delivery of mixed anticancer drugs. *Small* 6, 537–544. doi: 10.1002/smll.200901680

Zhu, X., Ji, X., Kong, N., Chen, Y., Mahmoudi, M., Xu, X., et al. (2018). Intracellular mechanistic understanding of 2d mos2 nanosheets for anti-exocytosis-enhanced synergistic cancer therapy. *ACS Nano* 12, 2922–2938. doi: 10.1021/acsnano.8b00516

14

Dual-Responsive Core Cross-Linking Glycopolymer-Drug Conjugates Nanoparticles for Precise Hepatocarcinoma Therapy

Jing Wu, Jiayi Yuan, Baotong Ye, Yaling Wu, Zheng Xu, Jinghua Chen and Jingxiao Chen**

Key Laboratory of Carbohydrate Chemistry and Biotechnology, Ministry of Education, School of Pharmaceutical Sciences, Jiangnan University, Wuxi, China

***Correspondence:**
Jinghua Chen
chenjinghua@jiangnan.edu.cn
Jingxiao Chen
tomchenjx@jiangnan.edu.cn

Nanoparticles (NPs) have demonstrated a potential for hepatocarcinoma therapy. However, the effective and safe NP-mediated drug transportation is still challenging due to premature leakage and inaccurate release of the drug. Herein, we designed a series of core cross-linking galactose-based glycopolymer-drug conjugates (GPDs) NPs with both redox-responsive and pH-sensitive characteristics to target and program drug release. Glycopolymer is comprised of galactose-containing units, which gather on the surface of GPD NPs and exhibit specific recognition to hepatocarcinoma cells, which over-express the asialoglycoprotein receptor. GPD NPs are stable in a normal physiological environment and can rapidly release the drug in hepatocarcinoma cells, which are reductive and acidic, by combining disulfide bond cross-linked core, as well as boronate ester-linked hydrophilic glycopolymer chain and the hydrophobic drug.

Keywords: glycopolymer, redox-responsive, pH-sensitive, hepatocarcinoma therapy, ASGPR

INTRODUCTION

Human hepatocellular carcinoma (HCC) is a common type of primary liver cancer and is diagnosed in more than half a million people worldwide (de Souza et al., 2015). At present, HCC has received increasing attention because of its important effect on the physiological functions of the liver, high lethality, and the growing incidences in many regions (Torre et al., 2015). Chemotherapy is a common HCC treatment strategy that is limited because it is always accompanied by dose-limiting toxicity, high rate of tumor recurrence, and drug resistance (Dutta and Mahato, 2017; Kuruvilla et al., 2017). Moreover, the phagocytosis of Kupffer cells hinders the accuracy and efficacy of chemotherapeutics (Lahmar et al., 2016). To date, nanotechnology is applied to address these problems and has obtained effective molecular-level diagnosis (Mura et al., 2013; Lim et al., 2015). It also serves as vectors, sensors, and targeting agents to achieve optimal efficacy in precise drug transportation because of its potential to alter the biodistribution and pharmacokinetics of drugs (Tao et al., 2013, 2015, 2016; Li et al., 2016; Zhang et al., 2017; Dai et al., 2018). In addition, some nanomaterials, which are known as theranostic nanosystem, provide a novel approach to obtain ideal efficacy by combining diagnosis and treatment together (Tao et al., 2017a,b; Zhu et al., 2018). However, the clinical application of the nanoparticle (NP)-mediated treatment is still challenging due to the premature drug leakage and inaccurate drug release in dilute bloodstream, thereby resulting in serious systemic side-effects to normal tissues and cells (Tao et al., 2014; Tibbitt et al., 2016; Chen et al., 2017; Rosenblum et al., 2018).

Over the past decades, neoplasm pathophysiology gradually reveals distinctive hallmarks of the tumor from normal tissues (Hanahan and Weinberg, 2000; Hanahan and Weinberg, 2011; Flavahan et al., 2017). To the best of our knowledge, hepatic galactose/*N*-acetylglucosamine receptor, also known as asialoglycoprotein receptor (ASGPR), is specifically exposed on the surface of hepatoma cells with a considerably high amount (Rigopoulou et al., 2012; Lepenies et al., 2013). Thus, ASGPR is used as an autoantigen to achieve targeted hepatopathy therapy through specific recognition of galactose (Fu et al., 2015). Moreover, tumor microenvironment, such as acidity (Dong et al., 2013; Du et al., 2015), hypoxia (Wilson and Hay, 2011; Semenza, 2017), high level of glutathione (GSH) (Dutta et al., 2017), and overexpressed enzymes (Zhu et al., 2012; Chen et al., 2015), inspires rational design of smart NPs to respond to various biochemical and physicochemical stimuli (Fleige et al., 2012). To achieve this goal, researchers introduced cleavable linkages (Ma and Tian, 2014), such as pH-sensitive bonds [e.g., boronate ester (Liu et al., 2013; Chen et al., 2016) and "Schiff" base (Chen et al., 2014)] and redox-responsive linkages [e.g., disulfide (Yu et al., 2014; Xu et al., 2017) and Se–Se bonds (Xu et al., 2013)] to construct NPs, which not only distinguishes carcinoma cells from normal cells but also regulates the drug release procedure and precisely meets the mechanisms of various agents, such as extracellular and intracellular release (Ding et al., 2017; Shi et al., 2017). Therefore, to realize a reliable and efficient NP-mediated HCC treatment, stable loading of hydrophobic agents in the blood circulation without leakage, selective transport, and release of the drug into hepatoma cells are necessary.

Herein, we developed a core cross-linking glycopolymer-drug conjugates (GPDs) NPs with unique dual-responsive characteristics to achieve selective transportation and program release of anticancer drug for HCC treatment (**Figure 1**). Inspired by the specific recognition between ASGPR and galactose (D'Souza and Devarajan, 2015), and the cluster glycoside effect (Dimick et al., 1999; Lundquist and Toone, 2002), which can effectively improve the affinity of carbohydrate ligands for their protein receptors, we employed galactose to build glycopolymer to obtain enhanced ASGPR-mediated hepatoma cellular binding and internalization. A disulfide bond was introduced to the side-chain of glycopolymer via a dynamically covalent boronate ester between galactose moieties and phenylboronic acid, which exhibits pH-regulated characteristics. Subsequently, hydrophobic model anticancer drug doxorubicin (DOX) was conjugated with the glycopolymer to form a series of amphiphilic conjugates through a self-eliminating disulfide bond (Satyam, 2008; Roy et al., 2015). This process ensures the traceless release of DOX, thereby keeping the original chemical structure and pharmacological action of DOX. Moreover, the hydrophobic core of the self-assembly GPD NPs was interiorly cross-linked through disulfide bond to stabilize the architecture and avoid drug leakage in the physiological environment. The GSH level in the cytosol of cancer cells is much higher than that in normal cells or extracellular fluid (Wang et al., 2013). Thus, by incorporating both redox-responsive and pH-sensitive characteristics into the GPD NPs, DOX can be accurately and programmatically released from the NPs in the cytoplasm of hepatoma cells, which are reductive and acidic.

MATERIALS AND METHODS

Materials

β-*D*-Galactose pentaacetate (98%) was purchased from Alfa Aesar (China) Chemical Co. Ltd. 2-Hydroxyethyl methacrylate (HEMA, 97%) was obtained from J&K Scientific Ltd. (China). Boron trifluoride diethyletherate ($BF_3{\cdot}Et_2O$, 98%) was purchased from Aladdin Reagent (Shanghai) Co., Ltd. 4-Cyano-4-(phenylcarbonothioylthio)pentanoic acid (CPA, >97%), GSH, and 2,2′-Azobis(2-methylpropionitrile) (AIBN) were purchased from Sigma-Aldrich (China) Inc. 4-Mercaptophenylboronic acid (MPBA, >95%) was obtained from Energy Chemical Co. (China). DOX hydrochloride (DOX·HCl, 99%) was provided by Beijing HvsF United Chemical Materials Co., Ltd. (China) and used as received. AIBN was recrystallized from ethanol before use. All other chemical regents and solvents were purchased from Shanghai Chemical Reagent Co. (China) and of analytical reagent grade, used directly. Dulbecco's modified Eagle's medium (DMEM), Roswell Park Memorial Institute (RPMI) 1640 medium, fetal bovine serum (FBS), penicillin-streptomycin, and Lysotracker green DND-26 were purchased from Thermo Fisher Scientific (United States). 3-(4,5-dimethylthiazol-2-yl)-2,5-diphenyltetrazolium bromide (MTT), trypsin, and 4,6-diamidino-2-phenylindole (DAPI) staining solution were obtained from Beyotime Biotechnology Co., Ltd. (China).

Synthesis of 2-[(2,3,4,6-tetra-*O*-acetyl-β-*D*-galactopyranosyl)oxy]ethyl Methacrylate (GalAc-EMA)

β-*D*-galactose pentaacetate (5.0 g, 13 mmol) and HEMA (1.3 ml, 10 mmol) were dissolved in 50 ml dichloromethane (DCM) in an ice bath under N_2 atmosphere, and $BF_3{\cdot}Et_2O$ (4.4 ml, 34 mmol) was added dropwise into the solution. After stirring at 0°C for 2 h, the mixture was moved to room temperature continued to be stirred overnight. Afterwards, the suspension was filtrated and the filtrate was washed with DI water and saturated NaCl solution for three times, then, dried over anhydrous magnesium sulfate. The product was obtained and purified by column chromatography (silica gel, DCM/ethyl acetate, 4/1). Yield: 73% (light yellow viscous liquid). The chemical structure of GalAc-EMA was identified with ^1H NMR spectrum on an AVANCE III (Bruker, Germany) equipment (Supplementary Figures 1, 2).

Synthesis of polyGal-EMA (PGal)

GalAc-EMA (1.00 g, 2.17 mmol), CPA (24.3 mg, 0.09 mmol), and AIBN (2.8 mg, 0.02 mmol) were dissolved in 2 ml anhydrous dimethyl sulfoxide (DMSO). The mixture was degassed with a freeze-vacuum-thaw cycle for three times under N_2 atmosphere. Then, the reaction was stirred at 75°C for 24 h. Afterwards,

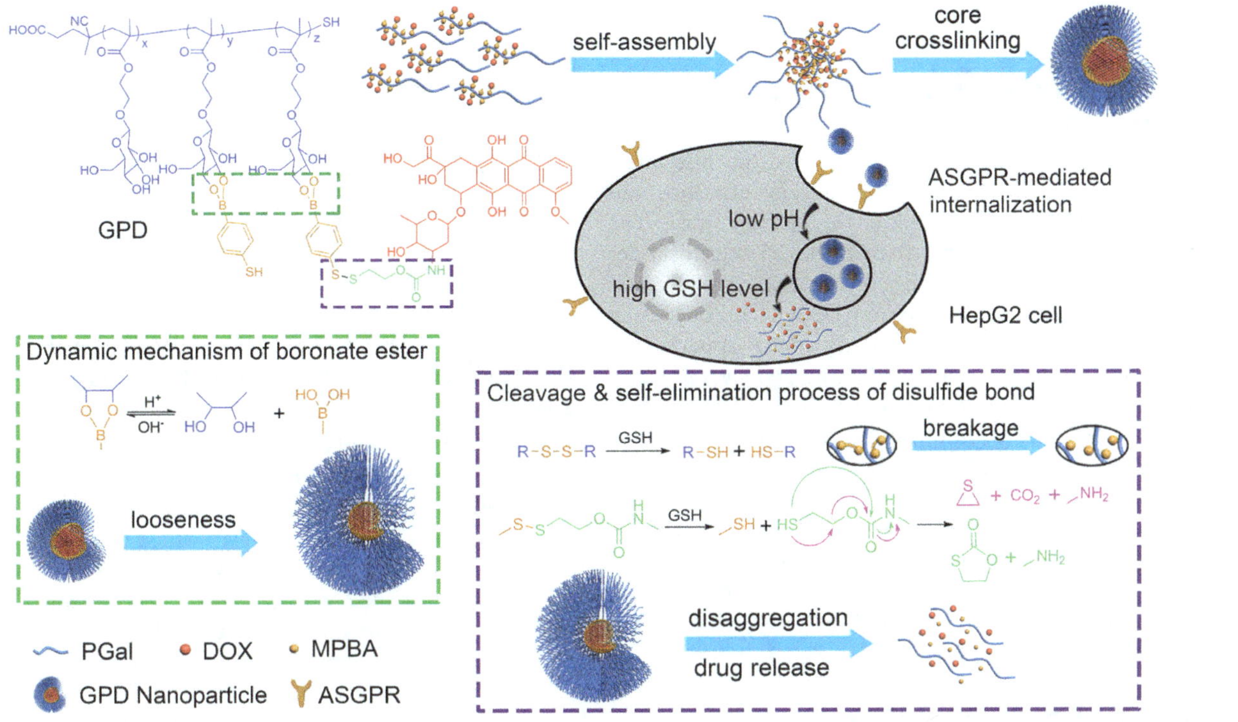

FIGURE 1 | Construction of galactose-based glycopolymer-DOX conjugates (GPDs) NPs for selective HCC therapy. The redox- and pH responsive mechanisms were designed to achieve program drug release in cancer cells.

TABLE 1 | Characterizations of GPDs and GPD NPs.

GPD	Molar ratio of units Gal-EMA/MPBA/DOX		GPC measurements			DL (wt%)	TEM estimated size (nm)	DLS measurements		
	Feeding ratio	Calculated ratio[a]	M_w (Da)	M_n (Da)	PDI			Size (nm)	PDI	ζ-potential (mV)
GPD1	10:3:1	10.4:3.2:1	10,115	7964	1.27	8.9	176.3 ± 10.5	279.7	0.41	0.01
GPD2	7:2:1	7.4:2.3:1	10,879	9142	1.19	10.2	107.3 ± 6.6	134.1	0.21	−0.03
GPD3	7:3:1	7.2:3.3:1	11,559	9796	1.18	12.4	98.6 ± 7.9	113.8	0.14	0.02
GPD4	8:3:2	4.2:1.2:1	12,643	10,279	1.23	16.5	21.4 ± 3.9	59.2	0.16	0.00

[a] *The ratio was calculated form the characteristic peak area integration of ^1H NMR spectra.*

the mixture was cooled down and the product (PGalAc) was precipitated in cold diethyl ether. The product was collected by centrifugation and dried under vacuum. Yield: 92% (pink solid, Supplementary Figure 3).

PolyGal (PGal) was obtained by deprotecting the acetyl group of PGalAc. Briefly, 0.5 g of PGalAc was dissolved in 50 ml DCM, and 1 ml CH_3OH solution of CH_3ONa (30%) was added dropwise. After stirring at room temperature for 20 min, the solution was adjusted to neutral pH using dilute HCl (1 M). The solution was then dialyzed with DI water for 48 h, and the PGal was collected by freeze-drying. Yield: 63% (white solid, Supplementary Figure 4).

Synthesis of Glycopolymer-DOX Conjugates (GPDs)

PolyGal (45 mg, 0.1 mmol) was dissolved in 5 ml anhydrous DMSO and the solution was degassed with N_2 for 30 min. Then, 5 ml degassed DMSO solution of MPBA and disulfide-activated DOX (DOX-ss-Py), the synthesis route and ^1H NMR spectrum (shown in Supplementary Figures 5, 6) was added dropwise. The molar ratio of PGal, MPBA, and DOX-ss-Py was adjusted to obtain a series of GPDs with different hydrophilic/hydrophobic balances (**Table 1**). The mixture was stirred at room temperature for 12 h and poured into an ammonium bicarbonate solution (pH 8.5). After dialyzing in the dialysis tube (molecular weight cut-off, MWCO: 3.5 kDa) with ammonium bicarbonate solution for 24 h, the product was collected by freeze-drying, and the degrees of substitution (DS) of the pendant group were evaluated from ^1H NMR spectra (Supplementary Figures 7, 8). In addition, DOX was directly connected with PGal through succinic anhydride to form a covalent linked PGal-DOX conjugate (GDC) as the control. The drug loading (DL) amount of GPDs was determined using UV–vis spectrophotometer on a UV-2550 (Shimadzu, Japan) equipment at 480 nm in DMF, and the DL values were calculated as follows: DL (%) = (mass of DOX) × 100/(mass of GPDs).

Preparation and Characterizations of GPD NPs

Glycopolymer-drug conjugates were dissolved in phosphate buffer solution (PBS, pH 7.4) at different concentrations and incubated at 37°C for 1 h to allow the self-assembly. The concentration of GPDs was optimized to be 0.5 mg/ml under the evaluation of average size and size distribution of the formed GPD NPs by dynamic light scattering (DLS) technique using a Zetasizer Nano ZS (Malvern, United Kingdom) apparatus at 37°C. The stability of GPD NPs was estimated by recording the variation of size distribution at different times in the PBS (pH 7.4 or 5.5) with or without GSH (10 mM) at 37°C. The morphology of the GPD NPs was observed by transmission electron microscopy (TEM) on a JEM-2100 (JEOL, Japan) instrument with an acceleration voltage of 200 kV. The samples were prepared by dripping a drop of solution onto a copper grid, dried naturally and then followed by negatively staining with phosphotungstic acid solution (0.2%, w/v), and dried in the air.

In Vitro Drug Release Assay

The solution of GPD3 NPs (1 mg/ml, 2 ml) was put into dialysis tubes (MWCO: 3.5 kDa) and immersed into 10 ml of PBS (pH 7.4 or 5.5, with or without 10 mM of GSH) at 37°C, respectively, to simulate the drug release behavior in different physiological conditions. After each sampling at the assigned time intervals, the buffer was replaced with the corresponding fresh medium. The amount of released drug in the medium was determined by UV–vis spectrophotometer at 480 nm. The cumulative release ratio of drug (%) = (mass of released drug) × 100/(mass of total drug). Each value was averaged from three independent trials. The GDC NPs and DOX non-covalently loaded GDC (DOX@GDC) NPs were used as the control.

Cell Culture

Human hepatocyte carcinoma cell line (HepG2 cells) and transformed African green monkey SV40-transformed kidney fibroblast cell line (COS7 cells) were incubated in DMEM complete medium, and human gastric adenocarcinoma cell line (MGC-803 cells) was incubated in RPMI 1640 complete medium at 37°C in a humidified atmosphere containing 5% CO_2. The medium contains 10% FBS and 1% (penicillin–streptomycin, 100 U/ml).

Cytotoxicity Assay *in Vitro*

The cytotoxicity of GPD3 NPs was performed against HepG2, MGC-803, and COS7 cells by MTT assay. Briefly, cells were seeded in 96-well plates at a density of 5000 cells per well with 100 μl of complete culture medium. After cells were cultured to the logarithmic phase, the solutions of GPD3 NPs with various concentrations were added into the well. The cells were cultivated for 48 h, and then, the culture medium was replaced with 100 μl of MTT solution (0.5 mg/ml in PBS) and incubated at 37°C for 4 h. The medium was removed and 150 μl of DMSO was added to each well for dissolving the formazan. The optical density (OD) was measured at 570 nm using Multiskan MK3 microplate reader (Thermo, United States). The relative cell viability was calculated as follows: Cell viability (%) = OD_{sample} × 100/$OD_{control}$, each date was obtained from the average value of three independent trials. The cytotoxicity induced by DOX·HCl was measured as the positive control, using 5% DMSO as the co-solvent.

Confocal Laser Scanning Microscope (CLSM) Observation and Flow Cytometry Analysis

HepG2, MGC-803, and COS7 cells were seeded in confocal dishes at 1×10^5 cells per well, respectively. Then, each type of cells was incubated with GPD3 NPs (equivalent to 10 mg/l free DOX) for 2 and 4 h. The cells were carefully washed with PBS three times and fixed with 4% paraformaldehyde for 15 min. Subsequently, the cells were stained with DAPI (0.2 μg/ml) for 30 min and washed with PBS three times. Afterwards, the cells were viewed under a TCS SP8 confocal laser scanning microscope (CLSM, Leica, Germany).

For the quantitative analysis, three types of cells were seeded in six-well plates and incubated for 24 h, and the medium was replaced with the medium solution of GPD3 NPs (equivalent to 5 mg/l free DOX). After incubating for 1, 2, and 4 h, the cells were washed with PBS (pH 7.4) carefully for three times and collected by trypsinization. Then, the cells were resuspended in 0.5 ml of PBS (pH 7.4) and quantitatively analyzed by flow cytometry, using FACSCalibur flow cytometer (BD Biosciences, United States). The number of cells collected was 20,000, and each experiment was performed with three independent trials. To identify the ASGPR-mediated internalization of GPD3 NPs, HepG2 cells were pre-incubated with 0.5 ml of galactose solution (2 mg/ml) or PGal (the monomer units amount was equivalent to 2 mg/ml of galactose). After 2 h incubation, the GPD3 NPs solution (equivalent to 5 mg/l free DOX) was directly added into the plate. The cells were continuously incubated for 2 or 4 h. Then, the plate was carefully washed with PBS (pH 7.4) and the mean fluorescent intensity (MFI) was measured by flow cytometer.

Intracellular Distribution Assay

HepG2 cells (4×10^4 cell/well) were seeded in dishes and incubated in RPMI 1640 (1 ml) containing 10% FBS for 24 h. Then, GPD3 NPs (equivalent to 5 mg/l DOX) dispersed in the culture medium were added and the cells were incubated at 37°C for 2, 4, and 8 h. After removing the medium and washing with PBS (pH 7.4) three times, the cells were fixed with 4% paraformaldehyde. Afterwards, the cells were successively stained with 0.5 ml of LysoTracker-Green DND-26 (50 nM) for 30 min and 0.5 ml of DAPI Solution (0.2 μg/ml) for 15 min. Then, the cells were carefully washed with PBS and observed by CLSM. Free DOX was employed as the positive control and incubated for 4 h.

RESULTS AND DISCUSSION

Preparation and Characterizations of GPDs

First, GalAc-EMA and DOX-ss-Py were successfully synthesized (Kularatne et al., 2010; Kumar et al., 2015), and their chemical structures were identified with ^{1}H NMR spectra (see details in the Supporting Information). Then, we employed a classical reversible addition-fragmentation chain transfer (RAFT) polymerization method and used GalAc-EMA as the monomer to synthesize a galactose-based glycopolymer, PGal. Subsequently, thiol group was introduced into the side-chain of PGal through a dynamically covalent interaction between a diol group of galactose units and a phenylboronic acid group of MPBA in a mildly alkaline condition (Deshayes et al., 2013). Afterward, DOX was connected with PGal through a designed disulfide bond, which is a redox-responsive linkage with self-eliminating characteristic (Santra et al., 2011; Li et al., 2015). A series of GPDs were received by adjusting the molar ratio of three units, that is, Gal-EMA, MPBA, and DOX. Moreover, the amount of MPBA was higher than that of DOX moiety in our design to set aside a portion of thiol group for disulfide cross-linking. As shown in **Table 1**, the molar ratios of three units of GPDs calculated from their characteristic peak area integrations of ^{1}H NMR spectra (Supplementary Figure 8) exhibited close values in comparison with their feeding ratios. These results indicated that the components of GPDs were easy to be tuned by varying the feeding ratio of the three units. In addition, GPC measurements indicated that the molecular weight of four GPDs were close to 10 kDa with narrow distributions, where their polydispersity values were lower than 1.3. These results showed a controllable nature of RAFT polymerization. The DL values of four GPDs measured using the UV–vis spectroscopy were 8.9, 10.2, 12.4, and 16.5%. These values were consistent with the results calculated from the ^{1}H NMR. Among the four GPD samples, GPD3 and GPD4 possessed higher content of DOX than the other two samples. Thus, their molecular weights were relatively higher than that of GPD1 and GPD2. Theoretically, these GPDs exhibited amphiphilic characteristic because galactose is hydrophilic, while DOX moieties show hydrophobic nature. These results demonstrated the hydrophilic/hydrophobic balance of the designed GPDs can be adjusted by varying the molar ratio of three units, which regulated the self-assembly behavior of GPDs to some extent.

Morphology of GPD NPs

After synthesis, we separately dissolved four GPDs in PBS (pH 7.4) to allow the self-assembly of GPDs to form various NPs. As shown in **Figure 2**, all four GPDs formed homogeneous spherical NPs in an aqueous solution. The mean diameter of four GPDs estimated from the TEM images were 176.3 ± 10.5, 107.3 ± 6.6, 98.6 ± 7.9, and 21.4 ± 3.9 nm (**Table 1**). As discussed above, the self-assembly of GPDs was regulated by varying their hydrophilic/hydrophobic balance depending on the proportions of MPBA and DOX moieties in the GPDs. The average size of GPD NPs showed decreasing trend with increasing amount of MPBA and DOX. Among the four samples, GPD3 and GPD4 have higher DOX contents and stronger hydrophobicity, thereby leading these two GPDs to form more uniform NPs than the other samples. This phenomenon is attributed to the fact that hydrophobic moieties, that is, MPBA and DOX, gathered at the core region and drive self-assembly to form NPs. Thus, the increasing hydrophobicity of GPDs increased the kernel density, reduced the critical aggregation concentration, and stabilized the architecture of NPs, thereby resulting in the decrease in particle size. Additionally, the average sizes of four GPD NPs measured from DLS were 279.7, 134.1, 113.8, and 59.2 nm (Supplementary Figure 9), thereby showing comparable results with those of TEM observation. DLS measured average size was a litter higher than the estimated average size from the TEM images. However, the difference was reduced with the increasing amount of MPBA. These results were attributed to the thiol group on MPBA charge of the core cross-linking. Thus, the increasing amount of MPBA improved the stability of core region of GPD NPs, thereby resulting in the decreasing difference of the size between hydration state for DLS and dry state in TEM observation. In addition, the ζ-potential value of four GPD NPs exhibited that their surface charges were nearly neutral, thereby indicating that hydrophilic galactose moieties coated on the surface of these NPs. Considering the DOX loading amount and the average size in aqueous medium, we chose GPD3 as the sample for the next study.

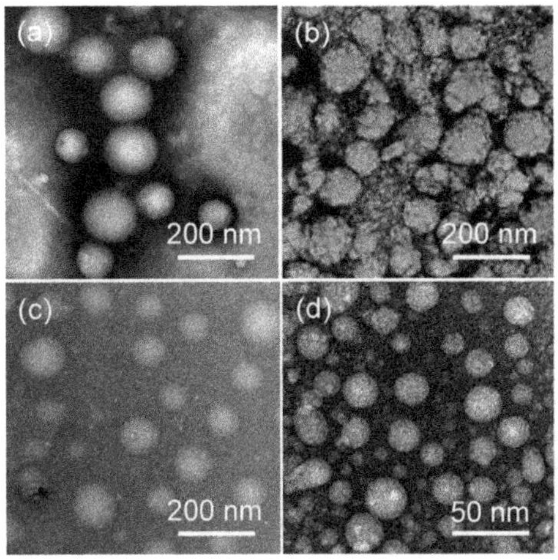

FIGURE 2 | Transmission electron microscopy (TEM) images of self-assembly **(a)** GPD1, **(b)** GPD2, **(c)** GPD3, and **(d)** GPD4 NPs in PBS (pH 7.4).

Stability and Environmental Sensitivity of GPD NPs

The stability and sensitivity of the self-assembly GPD NPs, which are relative to the long-term circulation and programmed drug transportation, are important for the clinical trial of polymer-drug conjugates. Thus, we evaluated the stability of GPD3 NPs in different milieus to simulate the process in various physiological environments. As shown in **Figure 3**, the TEM images illustrated that GPD3 NPs kept their morphologies

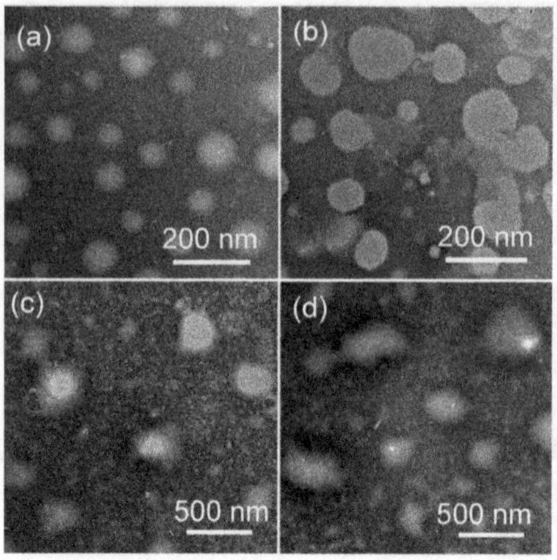

FIGURE 3 | Transmission electron microscopy (TEM) images of the morphologic variation of GPD3 NPs after immersing in **(a)** PBS (pH 7.4), **(b)** PBS (pH 7.4) containing GSH (10 mM), PBS (pH 5.5) **(c)** without, or **(d)** with GSH (10 mM) for 6 h.

in PBS (pH 7.4, **Figure 3a**) but gradually disaggregated in reductive environment (**Figure 3b**), acidic milieu (**Figure 3c**), or the condition with both reductive and acidic characteristics (**Figure 3d**). NPs were increased in size from approximately 100 nm in PBS (pH 7.4) to approximately 200 nm in a reductive solution and continuously increased to 500 nm or more in acidic mediums and acidic buffers containing 10 mM GSH. These results demonstrated that GPD3 NPs exhibited different disaggregation rates and responsiveness levels with a variation of environments. We further employed DLS to detect the disaggregation process of GPD3 NPs in these aforementioned environments, as shown in **Figure 4**. GPD3 NPs exhibited a stable narrow size distribution in PBS (pH 7.4) after 24 h (**Figure 4A**), and this situation lasted for 2 weeks during the measurement (Supplementary Figure 10), thereby showing an outstanding stability of GPD3 NPs. However, the size of GPD3 NPs varied with the alternative environments, showing comparable regular feature with the results illustrated in TEM images. In the reductive and alkalescent solutions, GPD3 NPs loosened, and their average size increased with increasing time (**Figure 4B**) because of the breakage of disulfide bond, which is responsible for core cross-linking of GPD NPs. This process was similar to that in the acidic medium (**Figure 4C**), which leads to the fracture of boronate ester. Moreover, the size was increased intensively in the environment possessing both reducibility and acidity (**Figure 4D**) than in the above-mentioned two conditions. This variation was derived from our designed dual responsive strategy, which obtained precise drug release. In the inner hydrophobic core of GPD NPs, DOX was connected to PGal through disulfide bond and boronate ester. Between the hydrophobic core and hydrophilic shell, excess disulfide bond was employed to cross-link the core region. Thus, GPD NPs showed favorable stability in PBS (pH 7.4), which simulates normal physiological environment. Given that disulfide bond shows responsivity to reductive condition (Yu et al., 2014; Xu et al., 2017), and boronate ester is sensitive to low pH (Chen et al., 2016), GPD NPs became far more unstable in the environment with both reductive and acidic conditions, corresponding to the cytoplasmic and endosomal environment of cancer cells. Therefore, the designed GPD NPs may exhibit a rapid disaggregation in the simulated environment in the cancer cells, which are reductive and acidic, thereby showing programmed drug release feature.

In Vitro Drug Release Assay

To evaluate the stimuli-responsive drug release of GPD3 NPs, we investigated the DOX release in four different conditions to simulate physiologically biochemical milieus. As shown in **Figure 5A**, GPD3 NPs exhibited different release characteristics in four different conditions. In normal physiological and low-pH conditions, the DOX release rate was lower than 20% for over 200 h. However, the DOX release rate was rapidly increased to more than 70% in the medium containing GSH to induce reductive environment. In particular, the release rate exhibited nearly an idea zero-order release pattern for the first 100 h. Meanwhile, the total release rate was further increased beyond 80% in the acidic solution containing GSH. However, the GDC NP control group showed insignificant difference among the four different conditions (**Figure 5B**). The total release amount of DOX was lower than 20% because the DOX was connected with PGal through covalent bonds that is, ester and amide bonds, and it showed insensitivity to GSH and low pH. Nevertheless, the DOX in the GDC NP group showed not only insensitive release feature but also fast release in all four conditions (**Figure 5C**). Considering that the DOX was non-covalently loaded at the hydrophobic core region of GDC NPs, the release of DOX was dependent on the free diffusion of DOX molecules from the inner core to the outer region, thereby leading to undesired release at pH 7.4. Moreover, the release rate of DOX was higher in acidic conditions than that at pH 7.4. This result is due to the fact that the hydrophobic DOX loaded at the core region becomes hydrophilic in low pH, thereby improving the release rate. These results demonstrated that GPD3 NPs possessed favorable responsive drug release characteristics, which was highly relative to the presence of GSH because the core region is cross-linked by disulfide bond. Even in an acidic medium, the release of DOX was limited by the shield of disulfide bond cross-linked network. Given that the endosomal environment is acidic, and the cytoplasm of cancer cells has a higher level of GSH (approximately 20-fold than that in normal cells), thereby exhibiting a reductive environment. These results indicated that GPD3 NPs may exhibit a specifically programmed release during the transportation in cancer cells.

In Vitro Cytotoxicity Assay

To evaluate the cytotoxicity of GPD3 NPs, we employed COS7, HepG2, and MGC-803 cells in the investigation, as shown in **Figure 6**. The IC50 values of free DOX against three types of cells were all lower than 0.25 mg/l (**Figure 6A**). We found that free DOX exhibited insignificant difference against three types of cells. In addition, the viability of HepG2 cells was higher than that of COS7 and MGC-803 cells. The chemotherapeutic

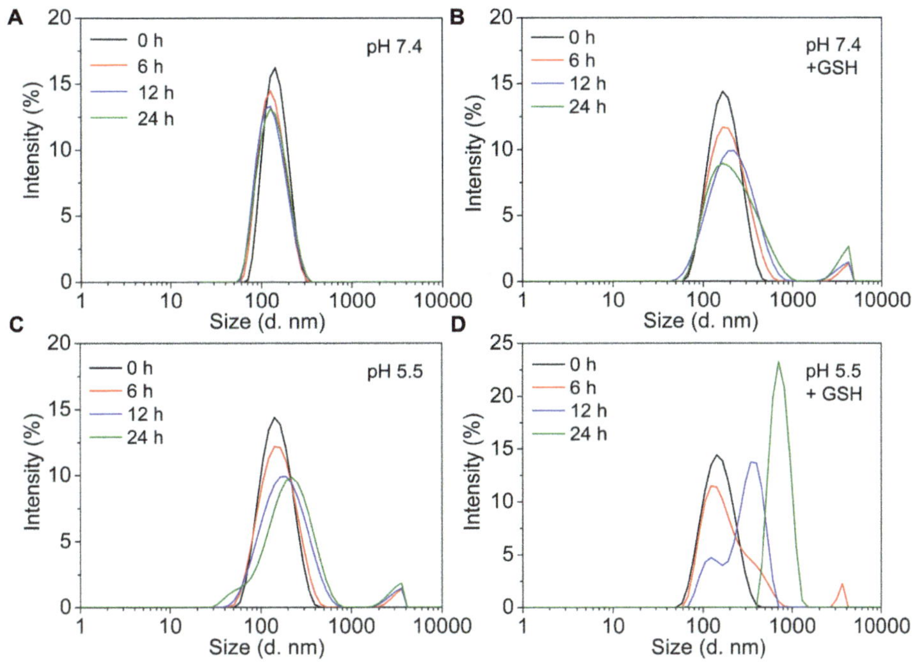

FIGURE 4 | The variation of size distributions of GPD3 NPs after immersing in **(A)** PBS (pH 7.4), **(B)** PBS (pH 7.4) containing GSH (10 mM), PBS (pH 5.5) **(C)** without, or **(D)** with GSH (10 mM) for different periods.

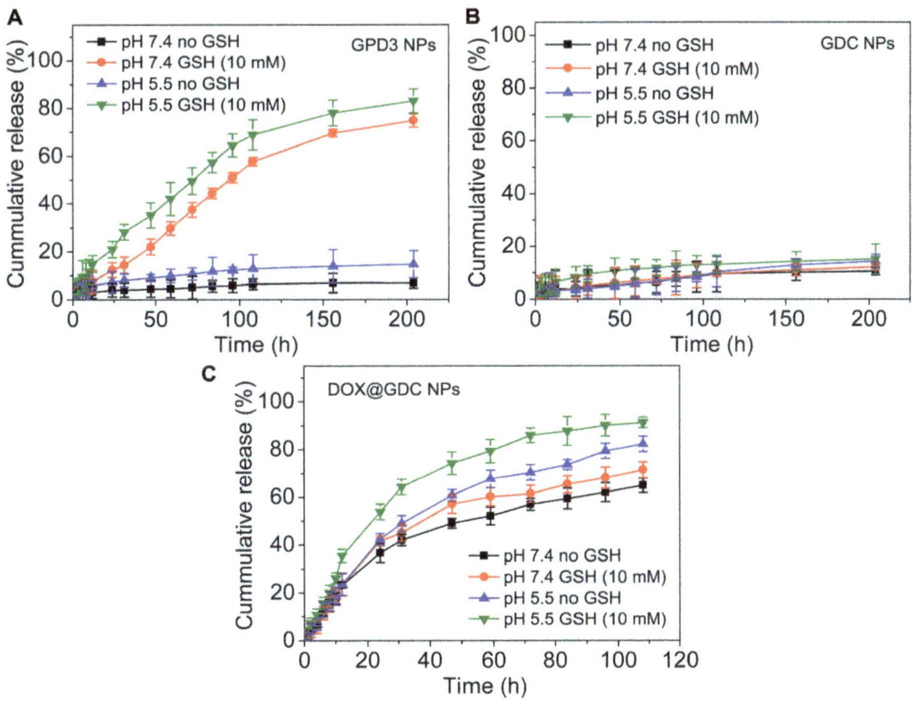

FIGURE 5 | *In vitro* DOX release profiles of **(A)** GPD3 NPs, **(B)** GDC NPs, and **(C)** DOX@GDC NPs in different conditions simulated various physiological environments.

agent can barely distinguish between the target and non-target cells. This result is the main reason why chemotherapy is always accompanied with serious systemic toxicity. However, our designed GPD3 NPs showed selective toxicity against the three aforementioned cells (**Figure 6B**). The IC50 value was higher than 2 mg/l against COS7 cells, but only 0.32 mg/l against HepG2

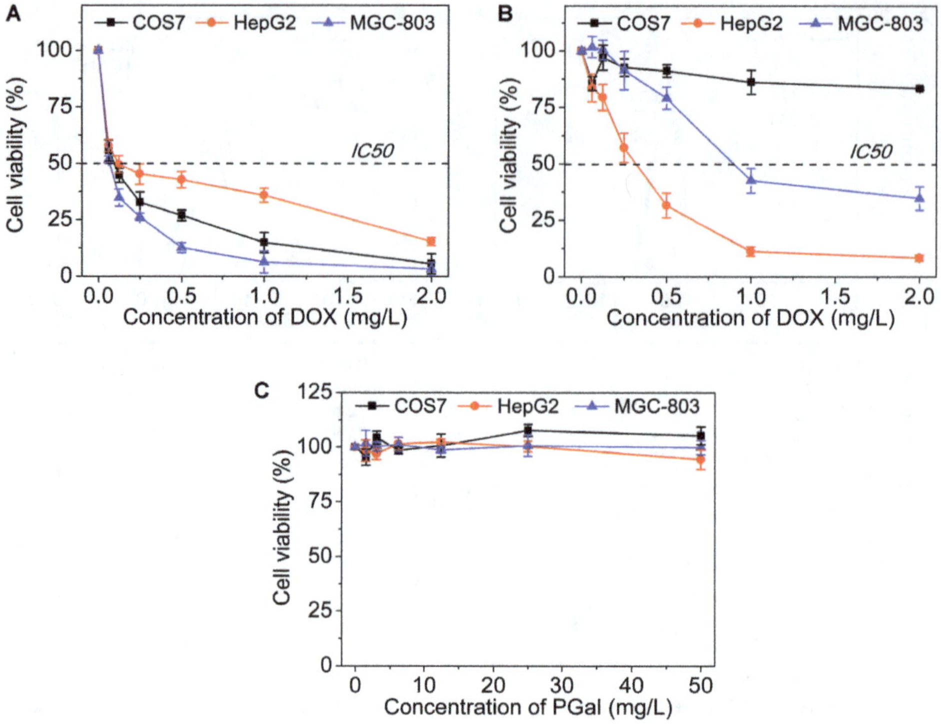

FIGURE 6 | Cell viability of **(A)** free DOX, **(B)** GPD3 NPs, and **(C)** PGal against COS7, HepG2, and MGC-803 cells.

cells, and 0.89 mg/l against MGC-803 cells. The cell viability of COS7 cells were higher than those of HepG2 and MGC-803 cancer cells. In addition, HepG2 cells exhibited the highest sensitivity to GPD3 NPs among the cells employed. Considering that PGal was non-toxic (**Figure 6C**), the cell inhibition was highly derived from the conjugated DOX. These phenomena occurred because HepG2 cell is a typical type of HCC, on which a higher amount of ASPGR is exposed. However, MGC-803 cell is a kind of gastric carcinoma cell and COS7 cell is a fibroblast-like cell. These mean ASPGR is non-expressed on both MGC-803 and COS7 cells, thereby resulting in non-recognition of the designed GPD NPs. Therefore, GPD3 NPs can efficiently and selectively deliver anticancer drug DOX to HCC cells and protect normal and non-target cells, showing potential in HCC therapy.

Cellular Uptake

To investigate the reason for the selective inhibition of GPD3 NPs against different cells, we used CLSM to observe the internalization of GPD3 NPs to different cells, as shown in **Figure 7**. Among these cells, we found brighter red fluorescence localized in HepG2 cells than those of COS7 and MGC-803 cells. Since red fluorescent DOX moieties were connected with PGal, these results showed that a higher amount of GPD3 NPs was internalized into HepG2 cells. Additionally, the red fluorescence in COS7 and MGC-803 cells showed insignificant variation with increasing incubation time. However, the fluorescent intensity was continuously increased in HepG2 cells. This phenomenon was due to the increasing amount of internalized GPD3 NPs and aggregation-caused quenching (ACQ) of DOX, which gathered at the hydrophobic core region of GPD3 NPs. As the DOX was gradually released into the cytoplasm of cells over the incubation time, the fluorescent intensity was increased with decreasing ACQ effect. These results were also consistent with the results in the drug release assay. We further used flow cytometry to quantitatively estimate the fluorescent intensity in different cells, as shown in **Figure 8A**. For the first 1 h, the MFI in three cells showed insignificant differences. However, the MFI value in HepG2 cells was increased with time and became nearly twofold when compared with that in COS7 and MGC-803 cells after 4 h. These results indicated that GPD3 NPs can selectively transport DOX to HepG2 cells and cause efficient cell inhibition. We hypothesized that this difference was due to the specific recognition between galactose, which coated on the surface of GPD NPs, and ASGPR exposed on HepG2 cells, thereby resulting in ASGPR-mediated internalization. Generally, ASGPR facilitates binding and uptake of circulating asialoglycoproteins through the recognition of the exposed terminal galactose (Lepenies et al., 2013). Nevertheless, autoimmune hepatitis, including HCC-induced inflammation, may lead to the suppression of ASGPR binding to asialoglycoproteins by the stimulatory effects of cytokines, such as interferon-γ, interleukin-2, and tumor necrosis factor, resulting in the exposure and increasing amount of ASGPR on the cell surface (Geijtenbeek and Gringhuis, 2009; Rigopoulou et al., 2012; Kuruvilla et al., 2017). Therefore, the designed GPD3 NPs, which were coated with galactose moieties on their surface, can be specifically internalized by HepG2 cells. However, the internalization of GPD3 NPs by COS7 cells and MGC-803 cancer cells was limited because ASGPR

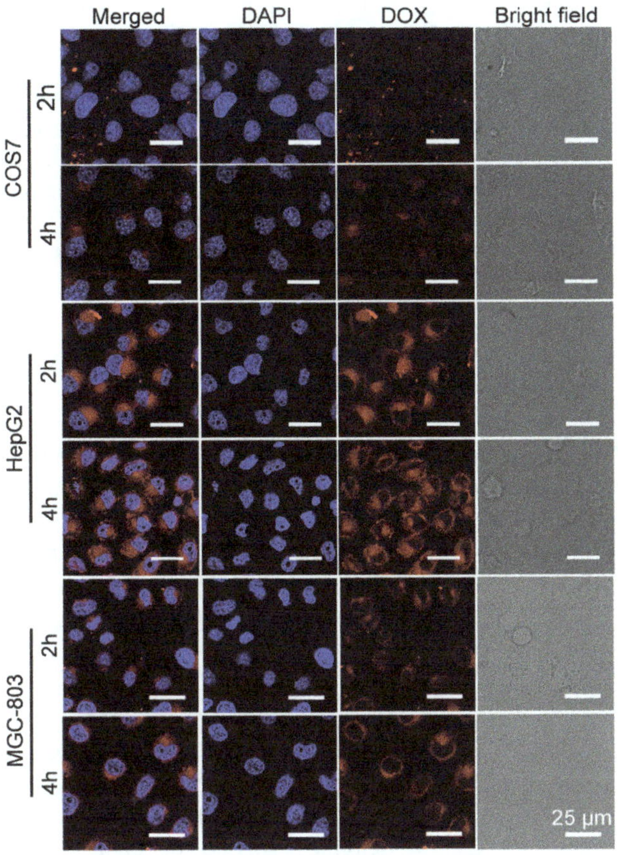

FIGURE 7 | Cellular uptake of GPD3 NPs in COS7, HepG2, and MGC-803 cells after incubation of 2 and 4 h observed by CLSM. The cell nuclei were stained with blue probe DAPI.

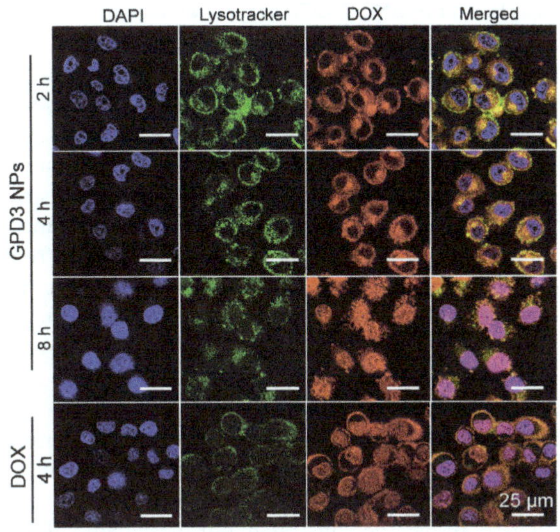

FIGURE 9 | Cell distributions of GPD3 NPs (equivalent to 5 mg/l DOX) in HepG2 cells after incubation for different periods. Cell nuclei were stained with DAPI (blue), lysosomes, and endosomes were labeled with Lysotracker Green DND-26 (green). HepG2 cells incubated with free DOX (5 mg/l) was used as the control.

is not expressed on normal and gastric cancer cells, thereby showing a selective characteristic. To verify this hypothesis, we employed galactose and PGal as inhibition agents to decrease the internalization of GPD3 NPs in HepG2 cells (**Figure 8B**). We found that GPD3 NPs uptake was inhibited by both galactose and PGal. However, the internalization of free DOX was not influenced by these two inhibitors because they can bind with ASGPR and block the ASGPR-mediated pathway of GPD3 NPs. However, the inhibitor was unable to inhibit the free diffusion of the small molecular agent DOX. Given that the conjugated DOX was connected with GPD and encapsulated in the core of NPs, the above-mentioned results indicated that the drug was transported into the cells by the ASGPR-mediated pathway. We also found that PGal exhibited higher inhibition efficiency than that of galactose. This result was attributed to the documented cluster glycoside effect, which improved the binding ability of PGal to ASGPR (Dimick et al., 1999; Lundquist and Toone, 2002). These results not only indicated that our designed GPD NPs can be specifically internalized by HCC cells, but also revealed that glycopolymer-based GPD NPs can exhibit selective and enhanced internalization to HepG2 cells.

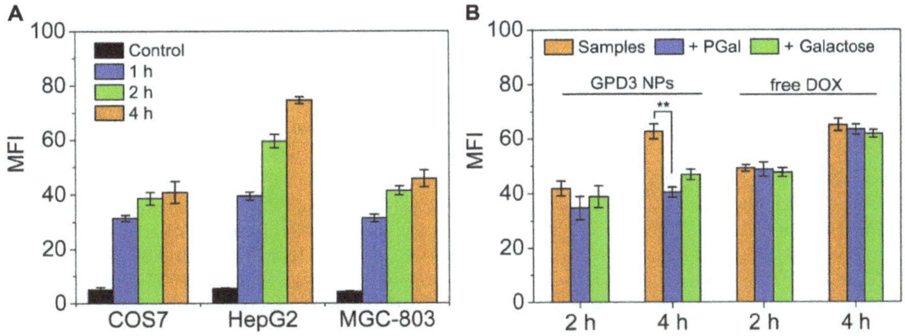

FIGURE 8 | Mean fluorescent intensity (MFI) of **(A)** COS7, HepG2, and MGC-803 cells incubated with GPD3 NPs (equivalent to 10 mg/l of DOX) for different periods. **(B)** HepG2 cells incubated with GPD3 NPs (equivalent to 5 mg/l of DOX) and free DOX (5 mg/l) under the inhibition of galactose (2 mg/ml) and PGal (equibalent to 2 mg/ml of galactose). $^{**}p < 0.05$.

Distribution Assay of GPD NPs

To observe the distribution of GPD3 NPs in HepG2 cells, we employed lysotracker as the fluorescent probe to label endosomes and lysosomes in the cells. As shown in **Figure 9**, we found that the intensity of red fluorescence was increased in cells for the first 2 and 4 h. However, the colocalization of red and green fluorescence indicated that GPD3 NPs were mainly distributed in endosomes and lysosomes for the first 2 h. These subcellular units are acidic; thus, NPs will enlarge and escape from the endosomes and lysosomes. Afterward, we found that the red fluorescence was distributed in cytoplasm after 4 h, which verified our hypothesis mentioned above. To the best of our knowledge, GSH is overexpressed in cytoplasm of cancer cells with both reducibility and acidity. Therefore, DOX would be rapidly released out from GPD3 NPs. Subsequently, red fluorescence was colocalized with blue fluorescence after 8 h, indicating that the drug was internalized into the cell nuclei stained with DAPI. These results demonstrated our designed GPD3 NPs exhibited a programmed drug transportation characteristic. For free DOX, the red fluorescence directly distributed in the cells and concentrated upon cell nuclei after coincubation for 4 h. This result was attributed to the fact that internalization of small molecular drug primarily depends on free diffusion, thereby showing rapid but non-selective characteristic.

CONCLUSION

In summary, we have designed and prepared a series of dual-responsive GPD NPs for precise HCC therapy. GPD NPs possessed an adjustable size corresponding to the DL amount, thereby varying the hydrophilic/hydrophobic balance of amphiphiles. The model drug DOX was conjugated on the galactose-functionalized glycopolymer through the use of self-eliminating disulfide bond and boronate ester as linkages, thereby showing both redox-responsive and pH-sensitive characteristics. Moreover, the core cross-linking strategy stabilized GPD NPs in a normal physiological environment. However, performing rapid drug release feature in the milieu resulted in both reductivity and acidity. In addition, the transportation of the drug showed a programmed drug characteristic. Simultaneously, GPD NPs can be specifically internalized into HepG2 cells through an ASPGR-mediated pathway by the recognition of galactose, which coated on the surface of GPD NPs. Thus, these GPD NPs have potential uses in precise HCC therapy.

AUTHOR CONTRIBUTIONS

JW developed the main study. JY and BY helped in completing the synthesis. YW and ZX took part in the cell experiments and analysis. JhC and JxC drafted the manuscript and developed the study design. All authors have given final approval for this paper to be published.

FUNDING

This work was supported by National Natural Science Foundation of China (21574059 and 51303068), Fundamental Research Funds for the Central Universities (JUSRP51709A), National First-Class Discipline Program of Light Industry Technology and Engineering (LITE2018-20), and Top-notch Academic Programs Project of Jiangsu Higher Education Institutions (PPZY2015B146).

REFERENCES

Chen, H., Zhang, W., Zhu, G., Xie, J., and Chen, X. (2017). Rethinking cancer nanotheranostics. *Nat. Rev. Mater.* 2:17024. doi: 10.1038/natrevmats.2017.24

Chen, J. X., Liu, W., Zhang, M., and Chen, J. H. (2014). Heparosan based negatively charged nanocarrier for rapid intracellular drug delivery. *Int. J. Pharm.* 473, 493–500. doi: 10.1016/j.ijpharm.2014.07.045

Chen, J. X., Shi, Y., Zhang, Y. R., Teng, L. P., and Chen, J. H. (2016). One-pot construction of boronate ester based pH-responsive micelle for combined cancer therapy. *Colloids Surf. B Biointerfaces* 143, 285–292. doi: 10.1016/j.colsurfb.2016.03.053

Chen, W. H., Luo, G. F., Lei, Q., Jia, H. Z., Hong, S., Wang, Q. R., et al. (2015). MMP-2 responsive polymeric micelles for cancer-targeted intracellular drug delivery. *Chem. Commun.* 51, 465–468. doi: 10.1039/c4cc07563c

Dai, Q., Bertleff-Zieschang, N., Braunger, J. A., Björnmalm, M., Cortez-Jugo, C., and Caruso, F. (2018). Particle targeting in complex biological media. *Adv. Healthc. Mater.* 7:1700575. doi: 10.1002/adhm.201700575

de Souza, P. C., Ranjan, A., and Towner, R. A. (2015). Nanoformulations for therapy of pancreatic and liver cancers. *Nanomedicine* 10, 1515–1534. doi: 10.2217/nnm.14.231

Deshayes, S., Cabral, H., Ishii, T., Miura, Y., Kobayashi, S., Yamashita, T., et al. (2013). Phenylboronic acid-installed polymeric micelles for targeting sialylated epitopes in solid tumors. *J. Am. Chem. Soc.* 135, 15501–15507. doi: 10.1021/ja406406h

Dimick, S. M., Powell, S. C., McMahon, S. A., Moothoo, D. N., Naismith, J. H., and Toone, E. J. (1999). On the meaning of affinity: cluster glycoside effects and concanavalin A. *J. Am. Chem. Soc.* 121, 10286–10296. doi: 10.1021/ja991729e

Ding, L., Zhu, X., Wang, Y., Shi, B., Ling, X., Chen, H., et al. (2017). Intracellular fate of nanoparticles with polydopamine surface engineering and a novel strategy for exocytosis-inhibiting, lysosome impairment-based cancer therapy. *Nano Lett.* 17, 6790–6801. doi: 10.1021/acs.nanolett.7b03021

Dong, D. W., Xiang, B., Gao, W., Yang, Z. Z., Li, J. Q., and Qi, X. R. (2013). pH-responsive complexes using prefunctionalized polymers for synchronous delivery of doxorubicin and siRNA to cancer cells. *Biomaterials* 34, 4849–4859. doi: 10.1016/j.biomaterials.2013.03.018

D'Souza, A. A., and Devarajan, P. V. (2015). Asialoglycoprotein receptor mediated hepatocyte targeting-strategies and applications. *J. Control. Release* 203, 126–139. doi: 10.1016/j.jconrel.2015.02.022

Du, J., Lane, L. A., and Nie, S. (2015). Stimuli-responsive nanoparticles for targeting the tumor microenvironment. *J. Control. Release* 219, 205–214. doi: 10.1016/j.jconrel.2015.08.050

Dutta, K., Hu, D., Zhao, B., Ribbe, A. E., Zhuang, J., and Thayumanavan, S. (2017). Templated self-assembly of a covalent polymer network for intracellular protein delivery and traceless release. *J. Am. Chem. Soc.* 139, 5676–5679. doi: 10.1021/jacs.7b01214

Dutta, R., and Mahato, R. I. (2017). Recent advances in hepatocellular carcinoma therapy. *Pharmacol. Ther.* 173, 106–117. doi: 10.1016/j.pharmthera.2017.02.010

Flavahan, W. A., Gaskell, E., and Bernstein, B. E. (2017). Epigenetic plasticity and the hallmarks of cancer. *Science* 357:eaal2380. doi: 10.1126/science.aal2380

Fleige, E., Quadir, M. A., and Haag, R. (2012). Stimuli-responsive polymeric nanocarriers for the controlled transport of active compounds: concepts and applications. *Adv. Drug Deliv. Rev.* 64, 866–884. doi: 10.1016/j.addr.2012.01.020

Fu, L., Sun, C., and Yan, L. (2015). Galactose targeted pH-responsive copolymer conjugated with near infrared fluorescence probe for imaging of intelligent drug delivery. *ACS Appl. Mater. Interfaces* 7, 2104–2115. doi: 10.1021/am508291k

Geijtenbeek, T. B., and Gringhuis, S. I. (2009). Signalling through C-type lectin receptors: shaping immune responses. *Nat. Rev. Immunol.* 9, 465–479. doi: 10.1038/nri2569

Hanahan, D., and Weinberg, R. A. (2000). The hallmarks of cancer. *Cell* 100, 57–70.

Hanahan, D., and Weinberg, R. A. (2011). Hallmarks of cancer: the next generation. *Cell* 144, 646–674. doi: 10.1016/j.cell.2011.02.013

Kularatne, S. A., Venkatesh, C., Santhapuram, H. K. R., Wang, K., Vaitilingam, B., Henne, W. A., et al. (2010). Synthesis and biological analysis of prostate-specific membrane antigen-targeted anticancer prodrugs. *J. Med. Chem.* 53, 7767–7777. doi: 10.1021/jm100729b

Kumar, S., Maiti, B., and De, P. (2015). Carbohydrate-conjugated amino acid-based fluorescent block copolymers: their self-assembly, pH responsiveness, and/or lectin recognition. *Langmuir* 31, 9422–9431. doi: 10.1021/acs.langmuir.5b02245

Kuruvilla, S. P., Tiruchinapally, G., Elazzouny, M., and Elsayed, M. E. H. (2017). N-Acetylgalactosamine-targeted delivery of dendrimer-doxorubicin conjugates influences doxorubicin cytotoxicity and metabolic profile in hepatic cancer cells. *Adv. Healthc. Mater.* 6:1601046. doi: 10.1002/adhm.201601046

Lahmar, Q., Keirsse, J., Laoui, D., Movahedi, K., van Overmeire, E., and van Ginderachter, J. A. (2016). Tissue-resident versus monocyte-derived macrophages in the tumor microenvironment. *Biochim. Biophys. Acta* 1865, 23–34. doi: 10.1016/j.bbcan.2015.06.009

Lepenies, B., Lee, J., and Sonkaria, S. (2013). Targeting C-type lectin receptors with multivalent carbohydrate ligands. *Adv. Drug Deliv. Rev.* 65, 1271–1281. doi: 10.1016/j.addr.2013.05.007

Li, D., Kordalivand, N., Fransen, M. F., Ossendorp, F., Raemdonck, K., Vermonden, T., et al. (2015). Reduction-sensitive dextran nanogels aimed for intracellular delivery of antigens. *Adv. Funct. Mater.* 25, 2993–3003. doi: 10.1002/adfm.201500894

Li, S., Liu, L., Rong, L., Qiu, W., Jia, H., Li, B., et al. (2016). A dual-FRET-based versatile prodrug for real-time drug release monitoring and in situ therapeutic efficacy evaluation. *Adv. Funct. Mater.* 25, 7317–7326. doi: 10.1002/adfm.201503262

Lim, E. K., Kim, T., Paik, S., Haam, S., Huh, Y. M., and Lee, K. (2015). Nanomaterials for theranostics: recent advances and future challenges. *Chem. Rev.* 115, 327–394. doi: 10.1021/cr300213b

Liu, H., Li, Y., Sun, K., Fan, J., Zhang, P., Meng, J., et al. (2013). Dual-responsive surfaces modified with phenylboronic acid-containing polymer brush to reversibly capture and release cancer cells. *J. Am. Chem. Soc.* 135, 7603–7609. doi: 10.1021/ja401000m

Lundquist, J. J., and Toone, E. J. (2002). The cluster glycoside effect. *Chem. Rev.* 102, 555–578.

Ma, X., and Tian, H. (2014). Stimuli-responsive supramolecular polymers in aqueous solution. *Acc. Chem. Res.* 47, 1971–1981. doi: 10.1021/ar500033n

Mura, S., Nicolas, J., and Couvreur, P. (2013). Stimuli-responsive nanocarriers for drug delivery. *Nat. Mater.* 12, 991–1003. doi: 10.1038/nmat3776

Rigopoulou, E. I., Roggenbuck, D., Smyk, D. S., Liaskos, C., Mytilinaiou, M. G., Feist, E., et al. (2012). Asialoglycoprotein receptor (ASGPR) as target autoantigen in liver autoimmunity: lost and found. *Autoimmun. Rev.* 12, 260–269. doi: 10.1016/j.autrev.2012.04.005

Rosenblum, D., Joshi, N., Tao, W., Karp, J. M., and Peer, D. (2018). Progress and challenges towards targeted delivery of cancer therapeutics. *Nat. Commun.* 9:1410. doi: 10.1038/s41467-018-03705-y

Roy, J., Nguyen, T. X., Kanduluru, A. K., Venkatesh, C., Lv, W., Reddy, P. V., et al. (2015). DUPA conjugation of a cytotoxic indenoisoquinoline topoisomerase I inhibitor for selective prostate cancer cell targeting. *J. Med. Chem.* 58, 3094–3103. doi: 10.1021/jm5018384

Santra, S., Kaittanis, C., Santiesteban, O. J., and Perez, J. M. (2011). Cell-specific, activatable, and theranostic prodrug for dual-targeted cancer imaging and therapy. *J. Am. Chem. Soc.* 133, 16680–16688. doi: 10.1021/ja207463b

Satyam, A. (2008). Design and synthesis of releasable folate-drug conjugates using a novel heterobifunctional disulfide-containing linker. *Bioorg. Med. Chem. Lett.* 18, 3196–3199. doi: 10.1016/j.bmcl.2008.04.063

Semenza, G. L. (2017). Hypoxia-inducible factors: coupling glucose metabolism and redox regulation with induction of the breast cancer stem cell phenotype. *EMBO J.* 36, 252–259. doi: 10.15252/embj.201695204

Shi, J., Kantoff, P. W., Wooster, R., and Farokhzad, O. C. (2017). Cancer nanomedicine: progress, challenges and opportunities. *Nat. Rev. Cancer* 17, 20–37. doi: 10.1038/nrc.2016.108

Tao, W., Ji, X., Xu, X., Islam, M. A., Li, Z., Chen, S., et al. (2017a). Antimonene quantum dots: synthesis and application as near-infrared photothermal agents for effective cancer therapy. *Angew. Chem. Int. Ed. Engl.* 56, 11896–11900. doi: 10.1002/anie.201703657

Tao, W., Zeng, X., Liu, T., Wang, Z., Xiong, Q., Ouyang, C., et al. (2013). Docetaxel-loaded nanoparticles based on star-shaped mannitol-core PLGA-TPGS diblock copolymer for breast cancer therapy. *Acta Biomater.* 9, 8910–8920. doi: 10.1016/j.actbio.2013.06.034

Tao, W., Zeng, X., Wu, J., Zhu, X., Yu, X., Zhang, X., et al. (2016). Polydopamine-based surface modification of novel nanoparticle-aptamer bioconjugates for in vivo breast cancer targeting and enhanced therapeutic effects. *Theranostics* 6, 470–484. doi: 10.7150/thno.14184

Tao, W., Zeng, X., Zhang, J., Zhu, H., Chang, D., Zhang, X., et al. (2014). Synthesis of cholic acid-core poly(ε-caprolactone-ran-lactide)-b-poly(ethylene glycol) 1000 random copolymer as a chemotherapeutic nanocarrier for liver cancer treatment. *Biomater. Sci.* 2, 1262–1274. doi: 10.1039/C4BM00134F

Tao, W., Zhang, J., Zeng, X., Liu, D., Liu, G., Zhu, X., et al. (2015). Blended nanoparticle system based on miscible structurally similar polymers: a safe, simple, targeted, and surprisingly high efficiency vehicle for cancer therapy. *Adv. Healthc. Mater.* 4, 1203–1214. doi: 10.1002/adhm.201400751

Tao, W., Zhu, X., Yu, X., Zeng, X., Xiao, Q., Zhang, X., et al. (2017b). Black phosphorus nanosheets as a robust delivery platform for cancer theranostics. *Adv. Mater.* 29:1603276. doi: 10.1002/adma.201603276

Tibbitt, M. W., Dahlman, J. E., and Langer, R. (2016). Emerging frontiers in drug delivery. *J. Am. Chem. Soc.* 138, 704–717. doi: 10.1021/jacs.5b09974

Torre, L. A., Bray, F., Siegel, R. L., Ferlay, J., Lortet-Tieulent, J., and Jemal, A. (2015). Global cancer statistics, 2012. *CA Cancer J. Clin.* 65, 87–108. doi: 10.3322/caac.21262

Wang, J., Sun, X., Mao, W., Sun, W., Tang, J., Sui, M., et al. (2013). Tumor redox heterogeneity-responsive prodrug nanocapsules for cancer chemotherapy. *Adv. Mater.* 25, 3670–3676. doi: 10.1002/adma.201300929

Wilson, W. R., and Hay, M. P. (2011). Targeting hypoxia in cancer therapy. *Nat. Rev. Cancer* 11, 393–410. doi: 10.1038/nrc3064

Xu, H., Cao, W., and Zhang, X. (2013). Selenium-containing polymers: promising biomaterials for controlled release and enzyme mimics. *Acc. Chem. Res.* 46, 1647–1658. doi: 10.1021/ar4000339

Xu, W., Ding, J., and Chen, X. (2017). Reduction-responsive polypeptide micelles for intracellular delivery of antineoplastic agent. *Biomacromolecules* 18, 3291–3301. doi: 10.1021/acs.biomac.7b00950

Yu, S., Ding, J., He, C., Cao, Y., Xu, W., and Chen, X. (2014). Disulfide cross-linked polyurethane micelles as a reduction-triggered drug delivery system for cancer therapy. *Adv. Healthc. Mater.* 3, 752–760. doi: 10.1002/adhm.201300308

Zhang, P., Wang, Y., Lian, J., Shen, Q., Wang, C., Ma, B., et al. (2017). Engineering the surface of smart nanocarriers using a pH-/thermal-/GSH-responsive polymer zipper for precise tumor targeting therapy in vivo. *Adv. Mater.* 29:1702311. doi: 10.1002/adma.201702311

Zhu, L., Kate, P., and Torchilin, V. P. (2012). Matrix metalloprotease 2-responsive multifunctional liposomal nanocarrier for enhanced tumor targeting. *ACS Nano* 6, 3491–3498. doi: 10.1021/nn300524f

Zhu, X., Ji, X., Kong, N., Chen, Y., Mahmoudi, M., Xu, X., et al. (2018). Intracellular mechanistic understanding of 2D MoS2 nanosheets for anti-exocytosis enhanced synergistic cancer therapy. *ACS Nano* 12, 2922–2938. doi: 10.1021/acsnano.8b00516

15

Significant Suppression of Non-Small-Cell Lung Cancer by Hydrophobic Poly(ester amide) Nanoparticles with High Docetaxel Loading

Xing Chen[1†], Lili Zhao[2†], Yang Kang[3†], Zhiyu He[1], Fei Xiong[1], Xiang Ling[1] and Jun Wu[1*]*

[1] *Key Laboratory of Sensing Technology and Biomedical Instrument of Guangdong Province, School of Engineering, Sun Yat-sen University, Guangzhou, China,* [2] *Digestive Endoscopy Center, Jiangsu Province Hospital, Nanjing, China,* [3] *Key Laboratory of Mountain Ecological Restoration and Bioresource Utilization, Chengdu Institute of Biology, Chinese Academy of Sciences, Chengdu, China*

***Correspondence:**
Jun Wu
wujun29@mail.sysu.edu.cn
Xiang Ling
lingx23@mail.sysu.edu.cn*

† These authors have contributed equally to this work.

Non-small-cell lung cancer (NSCLC) accounts for over 85% of clinical lung cancer cases, which is the leading cause of cancer-related death. To develop new therapeutic strategy for NSCLC, a library of L-phenylalanine-based poly(ester amide) (Phe-PEA) polymers was synthesized and assembled with docetaxel (Dtxl) to form Dtxl-loaded Phe-PEA nanoparticles (NPs). The hydrophobic Phe-PEA polymers were able to form NPs by nanoprecipitation method and the characterization results showed that the screened Dtxl-8P4 NPs have small particle size (~100 nm) and high Dtxl loading (~20 wt%). *In vitro* experiments showed that Dtxl-8P4 NPs were rapidly trafficked into cancer cells, then effectively escaped from lysosomal degradation and achieved significant tumor cell inhibition. *In vivo* results demonstrated that Dtxl-8P4 NPs with prolonged blood circulation could efficiently deliver Dtxl to A549 tumor sites, leading to reduced cell proliferation, block metastasis, and increase apoptosis, then persistent inhibition of tumor growth. Therefore, Phe-PEA NPs are able to load high amount of hydrophobic drugs and could be a promising therapeutic approach for NSCLC and other cancer treatments.

Keywords: cancer, docetaxel, hydrophobicity, nanoparticle, poly(ester amide)

INTRODUCTION

Being ranked the majority of lung cancer, non-small-cell lung cancer (NSCLC) causes human death due to its relative insensitiveness to chemotherapy (Jemal et al., 2008; Umar et al., 2012). More than 60% of NSCLC patients are diagnosed to have advanced or metastatic tumors, which are unsuitable for surgical resection with curative intent (Tong, 2006; Pao and Chmielecki, 2010). Thus, alternative therapeutic platforms to control or inhibit tumor development are highly desired. Docetaxel (Dtxl) is of the chemotherapy drug class taxane, structurally similar to paclitaxel, but more effective as the inhibitor of microtubule depolymerization (Bissery, 1995). In the past decades, Taxotere has emerged as one of the most important cytotoxic agents, with proven clinical efficacy against many cancers including NSCLC (Kintzel et al., 2006; Baker et al., 2009). However, the use of

Dtxl in this formulation with non-ionic surfactant Tween 80 and 13% ethanol leads to several well-known adverse reactions due to either the agents itself (e.g., neutropenia, anemia, nephrotoxicity, neurotoxicity, and musculoskeletal toxicity) or the solvent system (e.g., hypersensitivity and fluid retention) (Persohn et al., 2005). Side effects of commercial Taxotere have considerably overshadowed its clinical application.

Nanoparticles (NPs) have been extensively reported for their prominent superiorities that can be delivered to specific sites by size-dependent passive targeting (Matsumura and Maeda, 1986; Pan et al., 2011a,b, 2012; Bertrand et al., 2014; Deng et al., 2016; Lu et al., 2016; Zhao et al., 2016; Li et al., 2017; Lin et al., 2017; Liu et al., 2017; Shi et al., 2017). Among them, numerous nanoplatforms have been utilized to deliver Dtxl for improved cancer treatment (Tao et al., 2014; Bowerman et al., 2017; Laura et al., 2017). However, the clinical application of most reported platforms is hindered by the low loading capacity of Dtxl (Guo and Huang, 2014). Thus, the carrier material with reasonable hydrophobicity is urgently needed (Chu et al., 2013). Amino acid-based poly(ester amide) polymers with both ester and amide blocks on their backbones have been widely studied over many years (Wu et al., 2012a,b; Wu and Chu, 2013), as they possess not only good biodegradability and biocompatibility but also tunable physicochemical properties, especially hydrophobicity (Wu et al., 2011, 2015; Yu et al., 2014), which may be promising for developing NPs with high Dxtl loading.

Hence, we postulated that the novel design of hydrophobic L-phenylalanine-poly(ester amide) (Phe-PEA) polymer NPs with higher Dtxl loading could bring about more effective antitumor efficiency with better *in vivo* tolerance. In this paper, Phe-PEA polymers comprised of phenylalanine, diacid, and diol were synthesized and used because of their excellent NP formation and drug loading capability. Dtxl-loaded Phe-PEA polymer NPs were prepared by nanoprecipitation and the physicochemical characteristics were determined. After optimization, Dtxl-8P4 NPs with attractive uptake kinetics and strong cytotoxicity were found to greatly improve circulation retention, then enhance therapeutic effects for A549 tumors with less systemic toxicity (**Figure 1**).

MATERIALS AND METHODS

Materials and Reagents

L-Phenylalanine, 1,4-butanediol, 1,6-hexanediol, adipoyl dichloride, sebacoyl dichloride, toluene-4-sulfonic acid monohydrate, and *p*-nitrophenol were purchased from Sigma–Aldrich and used without further purification. DMSO, acetone, toluene, triethylamine, ethyl acetate, and methanol were purchased from Aladdin. Dtxl was purchased from LC Laboratories. Taxotere® was purchased from Sanofi Aventis. Dil was purchased from Thermo Fisher Scientific, United States. 1,2-distearoyl-*sn*-glycero-3-phosphoethanolamine-*N*-[methoxy-(polyethylene glycol)-3000] (ammonium salt) (DSPE-PEG 3000) was purchased from Avanti Polar Lipids. F-12K, EMEM, trypsin-EDTA, fetal bovine serum (FBS), penicillin–streptomycin solution, phosphate-buffered saline (PBS), and water were provided by Gibco®.

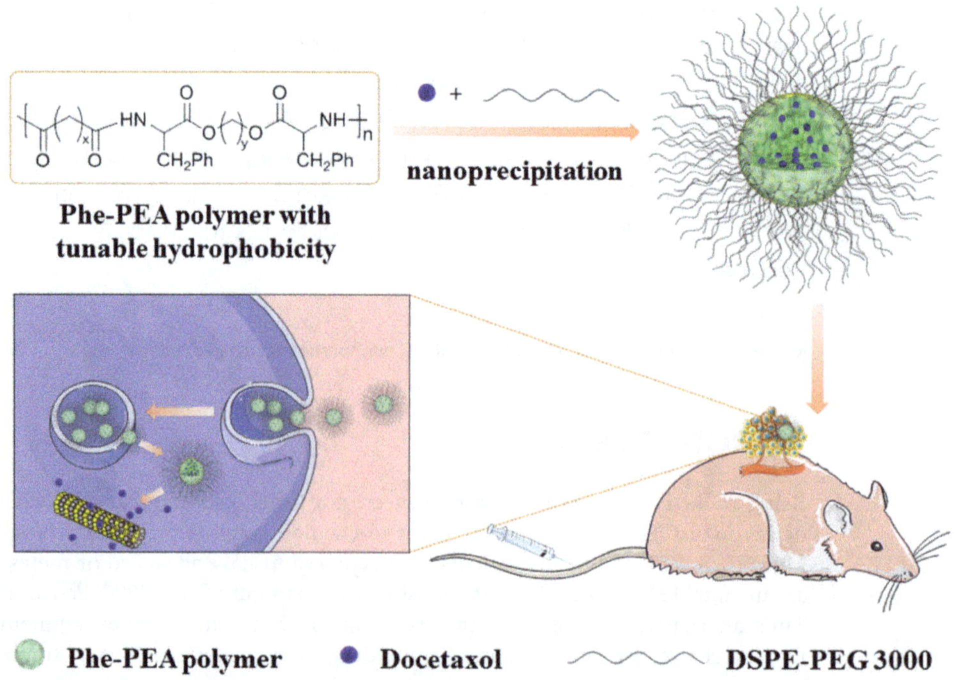

FIGURE 1 | Representative scheme for preparation of Dtxl-8P4 NPs and introduction of *in vivo* and intracellular delivery.

Synthesis of Monomers and Polymers

The synthesis of Phe-PEA polymers was divided into following steps (Katsarava et al., 1999): (i) preparation of di-*p*-nitrophenyl esters of dicarboxylic acid (monomer I) by condensation reaction; (ii) preparation of toluene-4-sulfonic acid salts of bis(Phe) alkylene diesters (monomer II) via solid–liquid reaction; (iii) preparation of Phe-PEA polymers through solution polycondensation (**Figure 2**). Synthetic details of monomers I and II could be found in previous reports (Wu and Chu, 2012), while Phe-PEA polymers (yield > 80%) were obtained by optimized protocols (Fonseca et al., 2014): monomers I (5 mmol) and II (5 mmol) in dry DMSO (8 ml) were mixed well by vortex and kept at 120°C under vigorous stirring, then triethylamine (15 mmol) was drop-wisely added to get a uniform yellow solution. The mixture was kept at 80°C overnight without stirring and resulting polymers were precipitated by adding cold ethyl acetate, washed with methanol, and dried under vacuum.

Here, two kinds of monomers I were prepared: di-*p*-nitrophenyl adipate (N4, $x = 4$) and di-*p*-nitrophenyl sebacate (N8, $x = 8$). Two kinds of monomers II were prepared: toluene-4-sulfonic acid salts of bis(Phe) butane diesters (Phe-4, $y = 4$) and toluene-4-sulfonic acid salts of bis(Phe) hexane diesters (Phe-6, $y = 6$). Phe-PEA polymers (x-Phe-y) were prepared by solution polycondensation of monomers I and II at various combinations and summarized in **Table 1**, where x was the numbers of methylene in diacid and y was the numbers of methylene in diol. Chemical structures of above monomers and polymers were confirmed by ^{1}H-NMR (Avance III, Bruker, Switzerland). All the spectra were the same as previously reported (**Supplementary Figure S1**) (Katsarava et al., 1999).

For measuring of molecular weight (MW) of Phe-PEAs, gel permeation chromatography (GPC) method was used and the PEA solutions were prepared at a concentration of 1 mg/ml in a tetrahydrofuran (THF) solution. The MWs of Phe-PEAs were determined from a standard curve generated from polystyrene standards with MWs ranging from 841.7 to 2.93 kDa that were chromatographed under the same conditions as the samples. The standard curve was generated from a third-order polynomial fit of the polystyrene standard MWs (**Table 2**).

Preparation and Characterization of Nanoparticles (NPs)

Dtxl-8P4 NPs were prepared by nanoprecipitation method: 6 mg of 8-Phe-4 polymer and a certain amount of Dtxl (10, 20, or 30 wt% of NPs) was dissolved in 0.2 ml of DMSO. Next, the mixture was dropwise added to 10 ml of aqueous solution containing DSPE-PEG 3000 (20 wt% of

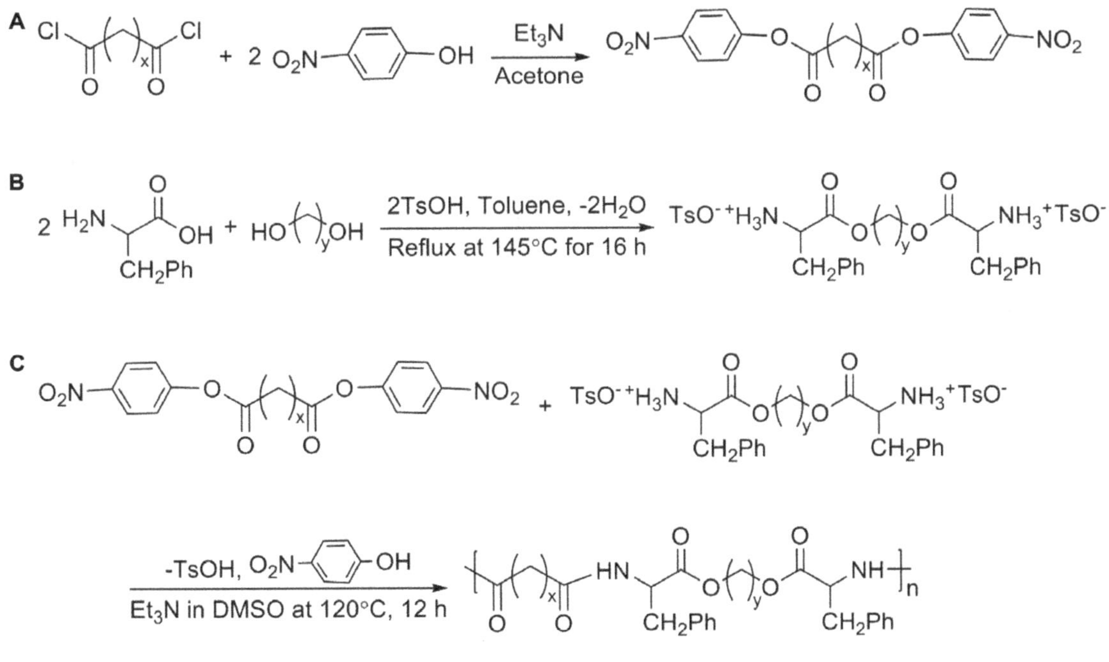

FIGURE 2 | Synthetic routes of Phe-PEA polymers.

TABLE 1 | Phe-PEA polymers and their corresponding NPs.

Monomer I	Monomer II	Phe-PEA polymers	Formed NPs	Particle size (nm)	Polydispersity index	Zeta potential (mV)	Dtxl loading (%)
N4	Phe-4	4-Phe-4	Dtxl-4P4 NPs	154.4 ± 2.7	0.253 ± 0.013	−23.56 ± 2.05	6.7 ± 0.7
N4	Phe-6	4-Phe-6	Dtxl-4P6 NPs	128.6 ± 5.6	0.133 ± 0.005	−26.10 ± 1.13	7.5 ± 0.6
N8	Phe-4	8-Phe-4	Dtxl-8P4 NPs	86.2 ± 0.5	0.125 ± 0.029	−26.39 ± 1.54	8.9 ± 0.9
N8	Phe-6	8-Phe-6	Dtxl-8P6 NPs	67.1 ± 1.2	0.220 ± 0.016	−28.92 ± 0.77	8.5 ± 1.0

TABLE 2 | Molecular mass characteristics of Phe-PEA polymers.

PEA	Mn (10^3 Da)	Mw (10^3 Da)	PDI
4-Phe-4	19.2	23.3	1.21
4-Phe-6	18.7	24.9	1.33
8-Phe-4	22.4	26.8	1.20
8-Phe-6	21.7	27.0	1.24

NPs) under vigorously stirring. The remaining free molecules and organic solvent were removed by washing with PBS twice using Amicon Ultra-15 centrifugal filters (MWCO 100 KDa, Millipore, United States). Finally, Dtxl-8P4 NPs were dispersed in 1.0 ml of PBS for further use. 8P4 NPs were prepared without Dtxl and used as blank control. Dtxl-4P4, Dtxl-4P6, or Dtxl-8P6 NPs were prepared by the similar procedure using 6 mg of 4-Phe-4, 4-Phe-6, or 8-Phe-6 polymer and fixed feeding of Dtxl (10 wt% of NPs). Dil-8P4 NPs were prepared by mixing pre-determined amounts of 8-Phe-4 polymer, Dtxl, and Dil (3 wt% of NPs) in DMSO, then following above nanoprecipitation procedure. Particle size and zeta potential of NPs were measured by dynamic light scattering (DLS, Zetasizer Nano-ZS90, Malvern, United Kingdom). Morphology of NPs was visualized by transmission electron microscopy (TEM, Tecnai G2 Spirit, FEI, United States).

Docetaxel loading capacity of NPs was determined by Agilent 1260 HPLC with a ZORBAX Extend-C18 column at the temperature of 30°C and a flow rate of 1.0 ml/min (mobile phase, water:acetonitrile = 50:50). The injection volume was 20 μl for each sample. The UV detection wavelength was 232 nm and Dtxl loading was calculated using following equation:

$$\text{Loading capacity \%} = \frac{\text{Weight of loaded drugs}}{\text{Weight of polymers} + \text{Weight of loaded drugs}} \times 100.$$

In Vitro Release Profiles

Dtxl-8P4 NPs were transferred to dialysis bags (MWCO 3500 Da, Spectrum, United States) and immersed in PBS (pH 5.0 or 7.4). Dtxl release was conducted at 37°C with constant stirring at 100 rpm. At specific time intervals, 1 ml of the sample solution was collected and replaced with equal volume of fresh PBS.

The amounts of Dtxl were analyzed by UPLC-MS/MS (TSQ Quantum Access Max, Thermo Fisher Scientific, United States) with following MS ionization parameters: positive ESI mode; spray voltage, 3500 V; ion source temperature, 300°C; collision energy, 0 eV. The analytes were quantified by using Multiple Reaction Monitoring (MRM) to monitor ion transitions *m/z* of 830.2–303.7. Chromatography was performed via Agilent 1100 HPLC with an Ultimate XB-C18 column at the temperature of 40°C and a flow rate of 0.2 ml/min (mobile phase, 0.1% formic acid:methanol = 40:60). The gradient elution was 60% methanol at 0–0.30 min, 60–100% methanol at 0.30–0.50 min, 100% methanol at 0.50–2.00 min, 100–60% methanol at 2.00–2.50 min, and 60% methanol at 2.50–5.00 min.

Cell Culture

A549, PC3, and DU145 cells were purchased from American Type Culture Collection (ATCC) and cultured by recommended protocols from the manufacturer. Cells were grown in the corresponding medium, supplemented with 10% FBS and 1% penicillin–streptomycin solution, maintained at 37°C and 5% CO_2.

Cellular Uptake

A549 cells were seeded in six-well plates (20,000 cells per well) and incubated with 1 ml of complete medium for 24 h. Dil-8P4 NPs at different concentrations were added. At selected time points, cells were washed with cold PBS twice, harvested by trypsinization, centrifuged, and resuspended in 4% formaldehyde, then analyzed by flow cytometer (FACSCalibur, BD, United States).

Cellular Internalization

A549 cells were seeded in 35-mm dishes (20,000 cells per well) and incubated with 1 ml of complete medium for 24 h. Dil-8P4 NPs were added. At selected time points, cells were washed with cold PBS twice and fixed with 4% formaldehyde at 37°C for 15 min. Subsequently, cells were washed with PBS twice again and stained with LysoTracker green and Hoechst 33342, then observed under an FV3000 confocal laser scanning microscope (CLSM, Olympus, Japan).

Cytotoxicity

Cytotoxicity was evaluated with AlamarBlue Cell Viability Assay (Thermo Fisher Scientific, United States) against A549, PC3, and DU145 cells. Cells were seeded in 96-well plates (5000 cells per well) and incubated with 0.1 ml of complete medium for 24 h. Cells were incubated with different concentrations of 8P4 NPs, Taxotere, or Dtxl-8P4 NPs. At selected time points, cells were treated according to manufacturer's protocol using a microplate reader (Synergy4, Bio Tek Instruments, United States).

Animals

BALB/c mice (male, 4–5 weeks old), nude mice (female, 4 weeks old), and SD rats (male, 200–220 g) were provided by the Laboratory Animal Center of Sun Yat-sen University. This animal study was carried out in accordance with the recommendations of "the guidelines of the Experimental Laboratory Animal Committee of Sun Yat-sen University and the National Institutes of Health's Guide for the Care and Use of Laboratory Animals."

TABLE 3 | Dtxl-8P4 NPs at different Dtxl feeding.

Dtxl feeding (%)	Particle size (nm)	Polydispersity index	Zeta potential (mV)	Dtxl loading (%)
10	86.2 ± 0.5	0.125 ± 0.029	−26.39 ± 1.54	8.9 ± 0.9
20	99.7 ± 4.7	0.078 ± 0.011	−28.65 ± 2.98	15.7 ± 1.3
30	172.4 ± 2.0	0.189 ± 0.004	−29.44 ± 2.57	19.6 ± 1.1

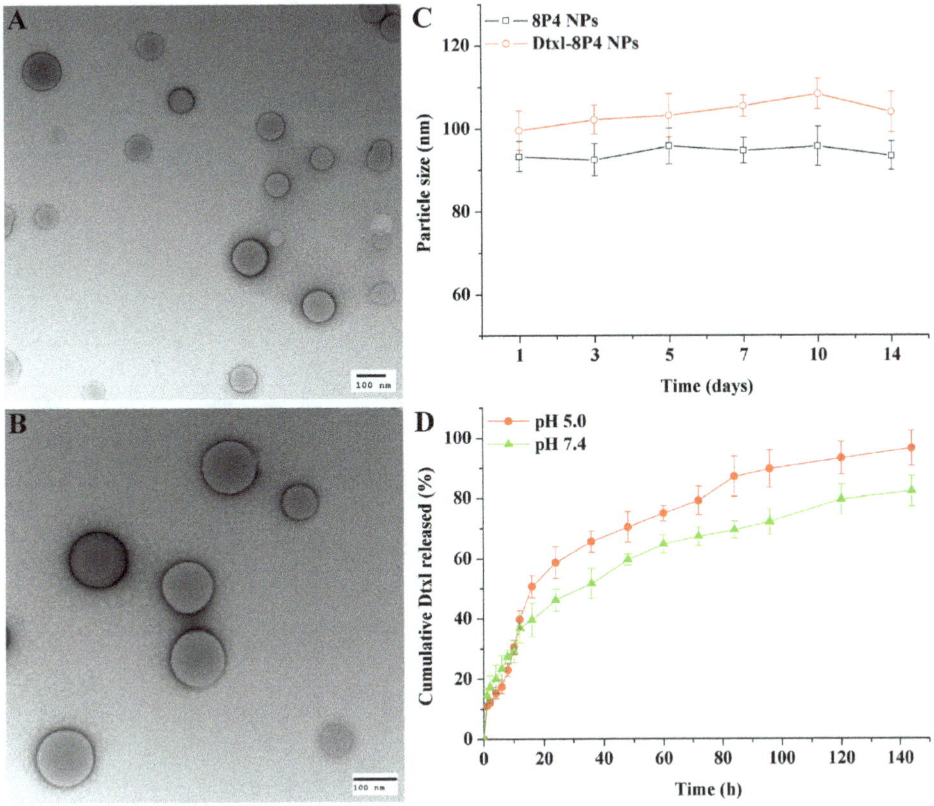

FIGURE 3 | TEM images of **(A)** 8P4 NPs and **(B)** Dtxl-8P4 NPs. **(C)** Particle size of 8P4 NPs and Dtxl-8P4 NPs. **(D)** The cumulative release profiles of Dtxl-8P4 NPs.

The animal protocol was approved by the "Experimental Laboratory Animal Committee of Sun Yat-sen University."

The human pulmonary carcinoma xenograft model was established by subcutaneously injecting A549 cell suspension (2,000,000 cells in medium and Matrigel) into the back region of nude mice. As the volume of xenograft tumor reached ~100 mm^3, mice were used for following experiments.

Pharmacokinetics

SD rats ($n = 3$ per group) were intravenously injected with either (i) PBS, (ii) Taxotere, or (iii) Dtxl-8P4 NPs at a dose of 5 mg Dtxl/kg, respectively. At pre-determined time points, blood was withdrawn from retro-orbital plexus and plasma was collected. Dtxl concentrations were analyzed by UPLC-MS/MS with the same chromatographic condition as described above. Hundred microliters of plasma was mixed with 10 μl of Dtxl, followed by adding 500 μl of methyl tert-butyl ether, vortexed, and centrifuged at 12,000 rpm for 10 min. The supernatant was evaporated and re-constituted with mobile phase. Pharmacokinetic parameters were calculated with Phoenix WinNonlin 6.3 program (Pharsight Corporation, St. Louis, MO, United States).

Histology Analysis

BALB/c mice ($n = 5$ per group) was intravenously injected with either (i) PBS, (ii) 8P4 NPs, (iii) Taxotere, or (iv) Dtxl-8P4 NPs at a dose of 5 mg Dtxl/kg every 7 days. After 39 days, all the mice were sacrificed and major organs (heart, liver, spleen, lung, kidneys) were excised for hematoxylin and eosin (HE) staining. Slides were observed under a fully automated upright microscope (DM6000 B, Leica, Germany).

In Vivo Antitumor Efficacy

A549 tumor-bearing nude mice ($n = 5$ per group) was intravenously injected with either (i) PBS, (ii) 8P4 NPs, (iii) Taxotere at a maximum tolerated dosage (MTD) of 5 mg Dtxl/kg, (iv) Dtxl-8P4 NPs at a dose of 5 mg Dtxl/kg, or (v) Dtxl-8P4 NPs at a dose of 10 mg Dtxl/kg every 7 days. Body weights and tumor volumes were recorded every 2 days. Tumor volume was calculated as follows:

$$\text{Volume} = \text{length} \times \text{width}^2/2.$$

HE, IHC, and TUNEL

A549 tumor-bearing nude mice ($n = 5$ per group) was intravenously injected with either (i) PBS, (ii) 8P4 NPs, (iii) Taxotere, or (iv) Dtxl-8P4 NPs at a dose of 5 mg Dtxl/kg every 7 days. After 39 days, tumors were quickly excised for HE and IHC. Slices were incubated with primary antibodies of CD31 and MMP2 (Cell Signaling) and HRP/DAB Detection IHC Kit (Abcam) according to the manufacturers' instructions.

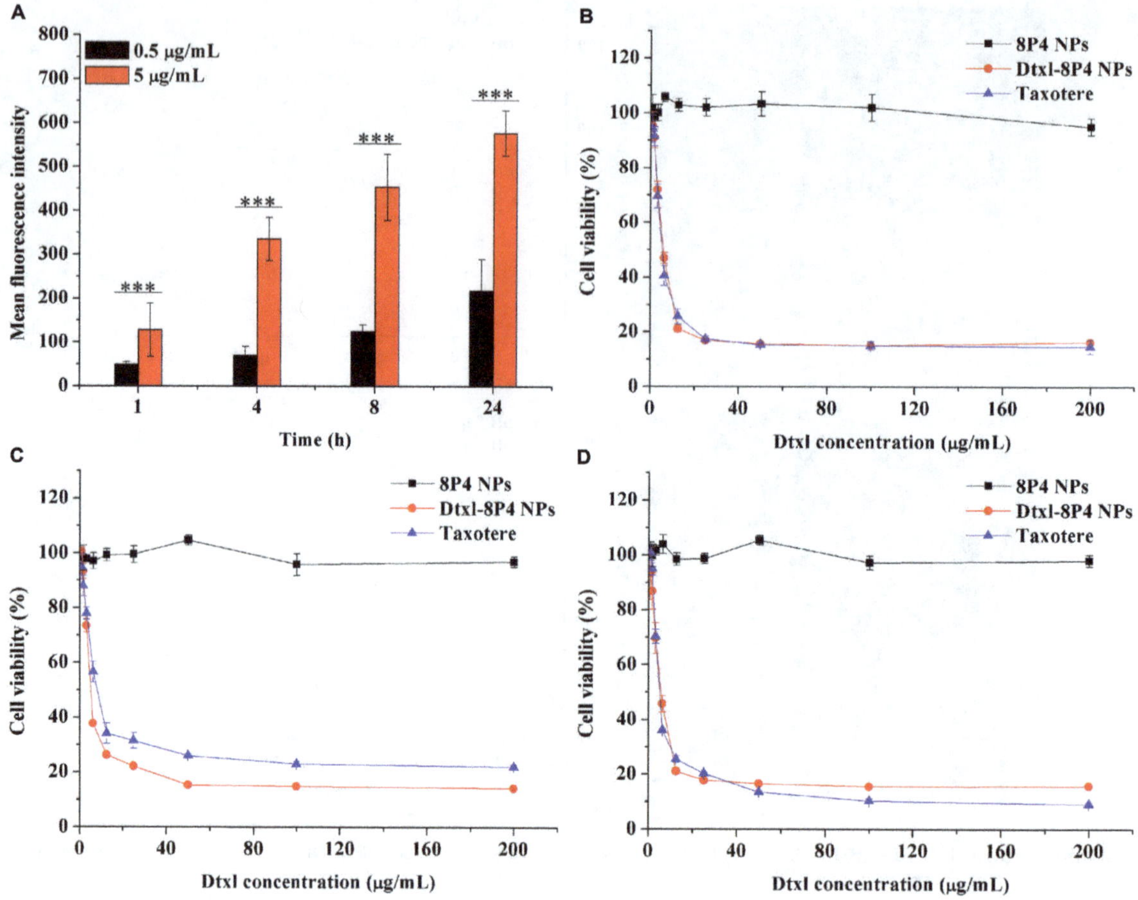

FIGURE 4 | (A) Fluorescence intensity of A549 cells incubated with Dil-8P4 NPs. **(B–D)** Cytotoxicity of Dtxl-8P4 NPs and Taxotere against **(B)** A549, **(C)** DU145, and **(D)** PC3 cells after exposure for 48 h.

Terminal deoxynucleotidyl transferase-mediated deoxyuridine triphosphate nick end labeling (TUNEL) was performed according to the instruction of In Situ Cell Death Detection Kit (Roche).

Statistical Analysis

Results were expressed as mean ± SD and repeated at least three times. Two-tailed Student's *t*-test was applied to analyze the statistical significance of difference between two groups, one-way analysis of variance (ANOVA) was used for multiple groups. Statistical significance was set at $^{*}p < 0.05$, $^{**}p < 0.01$, and $^{***}p < 0.001$.

RESULTS

The Hydrophobic Nature of Phe-PEA Polymers Induced Formation of Dtxl-8P4 NPs with Small Particle Size and High Dtxl Loading

L-Phenylalanine-based poly(ester amide) polymers were prepared by solution polycondensation of monomers I and II at various combinations. By introducing diacid or diol segments with different alkyl chains, the hydrophobic nature of Phe-PEA polymers changed accordingly. As the length of alkyl chain increased, the hydrophobicity as well as loading capacity of polymers enhanced, while the formed NPs tended to possess smaller size, which might be caused by the formation of more dehydrated and compacted cores via hydrophobic force. Due to high drug loading, satisfying entrapment efficiency and reliable stability, Dtxl-8P4 NPs were selected for the following experiments (**Table 3**).

Transmission electron microscopy images showed that the loading of a relatively higher amount of Dtxl (~16 wt%) into 8P4 NPs did not significantly alter the spherical morphology of NPs, but slightly increased their particle size (**Figures 3A–C**).

Dtxl-8P4 NPs Exhibited Attractive Uptake Kinetics and Strong Cytotoxicity *in Vitro*

In vitro release profiles were obtained by representing the percentage of Dtxl released with respect to the amount of drug loaded into NPs. **Figure 3D** demonstrated a sustained-release phase, in which ca. 82.3 and 96.5% of Dtxl were released from Dtxl-8P4 NPs in 144 h at pH 7.4 and 5.0, respectively. This

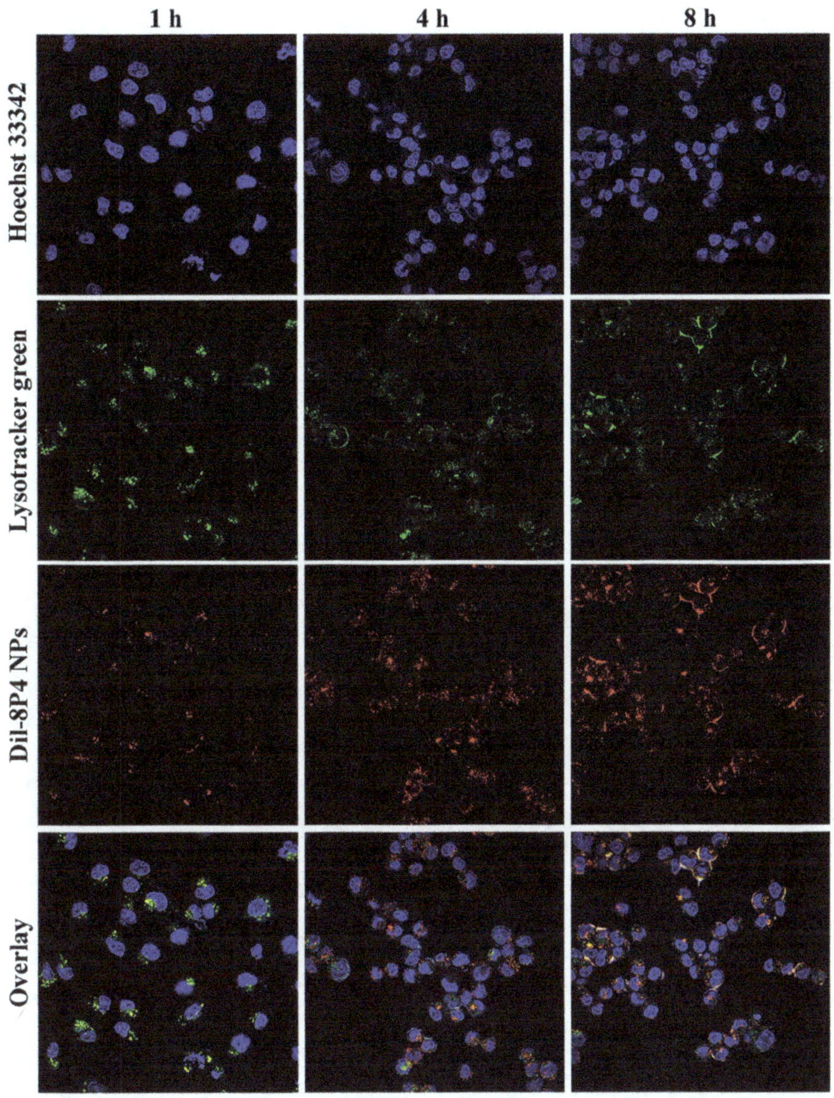

FIGURE 5 | Confocal laser scanning microscope images of A549 cells incubated with 5 mg/ml Dil-8P4 NPs. The nuclei and endosome were stained with Hoechst 33342 (blue) and LysoTracker green (green), respectively (60× objectives).

sustained release could mainly result from the erosion and degradation of the components of NPs. Importantly, no burst effect was observed, further confirming that Dtxl incorporated into 8P4 NPs was likely to remain association with NPs and be taken up into cells as the form of particles rather than free drugs.

Cellular internalization of NPs was performed by labeling A549 cells with a specific fluorescent probe, Dil, which was entrapped into 8P4 NPs at a minor amount to minimize the effect on intracellular trafficking. As displayed in **Figure 4A**, prolonging incubation time or increasing incubation concentration of Dil-8P4 NPs resulted in higher internalization, suggesting time- and concentration-dependent manners. After *trans*-membrane transport, Dil-8P4 NPs were found to co-localize with endosomes within 1 h, confirming a relatively fast cellular uptake (**Figure 5**). After that, the red fluorescence was mainly observed in cytoplasm, effectively avoiding the fate of lysosomal degradation.

As a next step, *in vitro* cytotoxicity of Dtxl-8P4 NPs was tested against A549, PC3, and DU145 cells by AlamarBlue (**Figures 4B–D**). The viability of cells treated with Dtxl-8P4 NPs did not demonstrate a significant difference compared with Taxotere at low drug levels, but the inhibiting activity of NPs increased at high drug levels. In addition, blank 8P4 NPs without Dtxl had a negligible toxic effect at all test concentrations.

Dtxl-8P4 NPs Enhanced Therapeutic Effects for A549 Tumors with Less Systemic Toxicity

In order to verify whether Dtxl-8P4 NPs impaired major organs, pathological examination was evaluated in healthy BALB/c mice (**Figure 6**). Taxotere caused severe hepatotoxicity with several structural and metabolic changes, i.e., vacuolar degeneration

TABLE 4 | Pharmacokinetic parameters of Dtxl after intravenous injection of Dtxl-8P4 NPs or Taxotere.

Model type	Parameter	Unit	Dtxl-8P4 NPs	Taxotere
Non-compartment model	$AUC_{0\rightarrow inf}$	h*mg/l	30.069 ± 2.722	6.438 ± 0.549
	$AUMC_{0\rightarrow inf}$	h*h*mg/l	2034.456 ± 193.682	266.471 ± 0.443
	CL	μl/h/kg	0.166 ± 0.017	0.777 ± 0.039
	V_{ss}	μl/kg	12.965 ± 2.578	40.705 ± 6.394
	$MRT_{0\rightarrow inf}$	h	67.660 ± 8.233	41.390 ± 5.081
Two-compartment model	A	mg/l	1.287 ± 0.120	2.300 ± 0.287
	α	1/h	1.424 ± 0.331	7.492 ± 2.101
	B	mg/l	0.691 ± 0.092	0.800 ± 0.185
	β	1/h	0.039 ± 0.012	0.583 ± 0.186
	$t_{1/2\alpha}$	h	0.487 ± 0.113	0.093 ± 0.026
	$t_{1/2\beta}$	h	17.779 ± 5.324	1.190 ± 0.380
	k_{10}	1/h	0.106 ± 0.023	1.845 ± 0.373
	k_{12}	1/h	0.834 ± 0.191	3.863 ± 1.214
	k_{21}	1/h	0.523 ± 0.158	2.366 ± 0.875

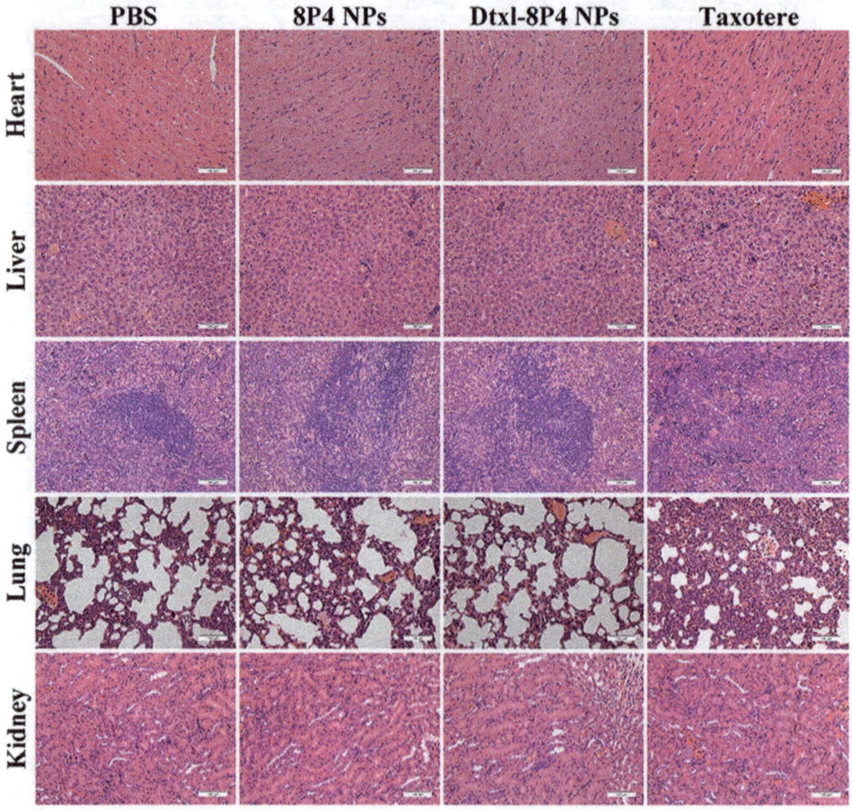

FIGURE 6 | Histopathological analysis of major organs from BALB/c mice (n = 5 per group) treated with PBS, 8P4 NPs, Dtxl-8P4 NPs, and Taxotere (20× objectives).

and inflammatory cell infiltration; splenic nodule atrophy; pulmonary hemorrhage; and tubular dilation with flattening of renal epithelium cells. However, no any noticeable histological alternations were captured in Dtxl-8P4 NPs as well as PBS and 8P4 NPs groups, confirming good biocompatibility.

The plasma Dtxl concentrations vs. time profiles were shown in **Figure 7A**. Pharmacokinetics presented the remarkably enhanced retention of Dtxl-8P4 NPs in blood circulation, whereas Taxotere exhibited the rapid elimination from circulation system. Non-compartmental and two-compartmental analysis showed significant changes in pharmacokinetic parameters of Dtxl (**Table 4**). Area under the curve ($AUC_{0\rightarrow inf}$), area under the first moment curve ($AUMC_{0\rightarrow inf}$), and mean residence time (MRT_{0-inf}) of NPs

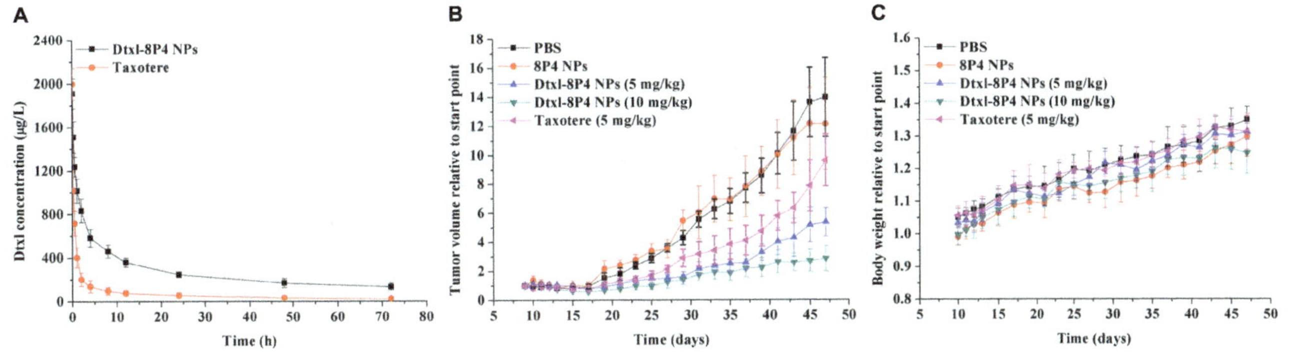

FIGURE 7 | (A) Pharmacokinetics after intravenous injection of Dtxl-8P4 NPs and Taxotere at a dose of 5 mg Dtxl/kg (n = 3 per group). **(B)** Tumor growth and **(C)** body weight curves of A549 tumor-bearing nude mice (n = 5 per group) treated with PBS, 8P4 NPs, Dtxl-8P4 NPs, and Taxotere.

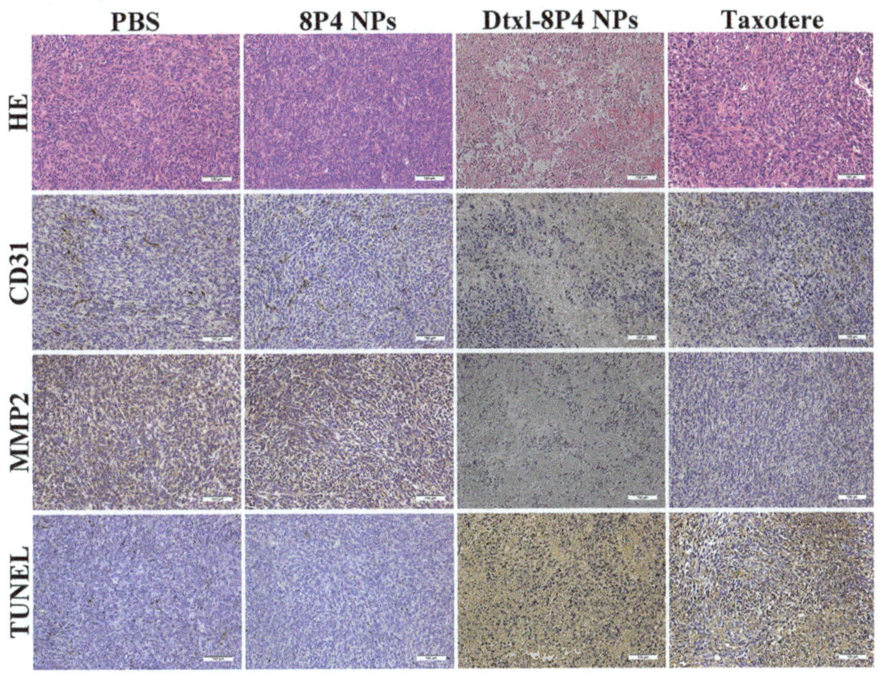

FIGURE 8 | HE staining analysis, CD31 and MMP2 expression and TUNEL examination of tumors from A549 tumor-bearing nude mice (n = 5 per group) treated with PBS, 8P4 NPs, Dtxl-8P4 NPs, and Taxotere after a schedule of multiple doses (20× objectives).

were 4.7-, 7.6-, and 1.6-fold higher than Taxotere, while clearance (CL) and volume of distribution (V_{ss}) were reduced by 78.6 and 68.1%, respectively. $t_{1/2}$ of distribution and elimination phase was all dramatically extended compared with Taxotere.

To prove the potential of Dtxl-8P4 NPs for tumor growth suppression, a schedule of multiple dosing was applied since day 9 after A549 tumor implantation (**Figures 7B,C**). PBS and 8P4 NPs groups exhibited rapid tumor growth, whereas MTD for weekly dosing of Taxotere significantly delayed tumor growth. In comparison, a better tumor inhibition with sustaining weight gain was observed in mice receiving equal dosing of Dtxl-8P4 NPs. What's more, the most aggressive treatment with double dosing of chemotherapy suppressed tumor growth for longer but barely induced weight loss, probably due to biocompatible Dtxl-8P4 NPs prevented the random drug release in the body and enhanced therapeutic efficacy of Dtxl.

Dtxl-8P4 NPs Effectively Suppressed Proliferation, Metastasis, and Apoptosis of Tumors

The pathology of tumor tissues revealed coincident results (**Figure 8**). For the vigorous growth of tumors in PBS and 8P4 NPs groups, nuclei and cytoplasm presented a blue-pink interlaced image on the whole section. Once tumors underwent apoptosis, nuclei disappeared and cytoplasm became an amorphous mass of necrotic material. The destructed tumor area of Dtxl-8P4 NPs accounted for the highest percentage among all the groups, further revealing the enhanced chemotherapeutic efficiency of NPs. Besides, the histological analysis of proliferation, metastasis, and apoptosis for tumors treated with rounds of chemotherapy was carried out through IHC and TUNEL. Dtxl-8P4 NPs greatly suppressed the expression of CD31 and MMP2, compared with other groups, verifying that tumor proliferation and metastasis were effectively restricted (Giatromanolaki et al., 1997; Bjorklund and Koivunen, 2005; Kim et al., 2009; Jacob and Prekeris, 2015). The administration of PBS or 8P4 NPs caused negligible TUNEL-positive staining, while Dtxl-8P4 NPs resulted in the most remarkable apoptosis of tumors, emphasizing the great efficacy of NPs.

DISCUSSION

In summary, amino acid-based Phe-PEA polymers were synthesized and formulated with Dtxl to construct Dtxl-loaded Phe-PEA polymer NPs. The hydrophobic nature of polymers contributed to the installation of high hydrophobic payloads. Dtxl-8P4 NPs showed the small particle size ~100 nm with high loading capacity ~20 wt%, a low burst effect, and a sustained drug release *in vitro*. Cytotoxicity of Dtxl-8P4 NPs against tumor cells was superior to Taxotere would be attributed to the rapid cellular uptake and effective lysosomal escape. The better antitumor efficacy and less systemic toxicity of Dtxl-8P4 NPs might be attributed to extended blood circulation and high Dtxl loading. Thus, Dtxl-8P4 NPs could be promising as a novel formulation of Dtxl in cancer chemotherapy to fight against NSCLC.

AUTHOR CONTRIBUTIONS

XC and LZ conceived and directed the study. YK, ZH, and FX performed syntheses and spectroscopic studies. XC and YK co-wrote the paper. XL and JW oversaw the project and contributed to the execution of the experiments and interpretation of the results. All authors contributed to the characterizations and discussion and reviewed and approved the final paper.

FUNDING

This work was supported by the Thousand Talents Plan for Young Professionals, the National Natural Science Foundation of China (21704104), West Light Foundation of the Chinese Academy of Sciences (Y7C1021100), the Science and Technology Planning Project of Guangdong Province (2016A010103015), and the Science and Technology Program of Guangzhou (201707010094).

ACKNOWLEDGMENTS

We appreciate the valuable and insightful thoughts from all the members of the Wu Laboratory.

REFERENCES

Baker, J., Ajani, J., Scotte, F., Winther, D., Martin, M., Aapro, M. S., et al. (2009). Docetaxel-related side effects and their management. *Eur. J. Oncol. Nurs.* 13, 49–59. doi: 10.1016/j.ejon.2008.10.003

Bertrand, N., Wu, J., Xu, X., Kamaly, N., and Farokhzad, O. C. (2014). Cancer nanotechnology: the impact of passive and active targeting in the era of modern cancer biology. *Adv. Drug Deliv. Rev.* 66, 2–25. doi: 10.1016/j.addr.2013.11.009

Bissery, M. C. (1995). Preclinical pharmacology of docetaxel. *Eur. J. Cancer* 31(Suppl. 4), S1–S6. doi: 10.1016/0959-8049(95)00357-O

Bjorklund, M., and Koivunen, E. (2005). Gelatinase-mediated migration and invasion of cancer cells. *Biochim. Biophys. Acta* 1755, 37–69. doi: 10.1016/j.bbcan.2005.03.001

Bowerman, C. J., Byrne, J. D., Chu, K. S., Schorzman, A. N., Keeler, A. W., Sherwood, C. A., et al. (2017). Docetaxel-Loaded PLGA nanoparticles improve efficacy in taxane-resistant triple-negative breast cancer. *Nano Lett.* 17, 242–248. doi: 10.1021/acs.nanolett.6b03971

Chu, K. S., Schorzman, A. N., Finniss, M. C., Bowerman, C. J., Peng, L., Luft, J. C., et al. (2013). Nanoparticle drug loading as a design parameter to improve docetaxel pharmacokinetics and efficacy. *Biomaterials* 34, 8424–8429. doi: 10.1016/j.biomaterials.2013.07.038

Deng, Y., Li, E., Cheng, X., Zhu, J., Lu, S., Ge, C., et al. (2016). Facile preparation of hybrid core–shell nanorods for photothermal and radiation combined therapy. *Nanoscale* 8, 3895–3899. doi: 10.1039/c5nr09102k

Fonseca, A. C., Gil, M. H., and Simoes, P. N. (2014). Biodegradable poly(ester amide)s – A remarkable opportunity for the biomedical area: review on the synthesis, characterization and applications. *Prog. Polym. Sci.* 39, 1291–1311. doi: 10.1016/j.progpolymsci.2013.11.007

Giatromanolaki, A., Koukourakis, M. I., Theodossiou, D., Barbatis, K., O'byrne, K., Harris, A. L., et al. (1997). Comparative evaluation of angiogenesis assessment with anti-factor-VIII and anti-CD31 immunostaining in non-small cell lung cancer. *Clin. Cancer Res.* 3, 2485–2492.

Guo, S., and Huang, L. (2014). Nanoparticles containing insoluble drug for cancer therapy. *Biotechnol. Adv.* 32, 778–788. doi: 10.1016/j.biotechadv.2013.10.002

Jacob, A., and Prekeris, R. (2015). The regulation of MMP targeting to invadopodia during cancer metastasis. *Front. cell Dev. Biol.* 3:4. doi: 10.3389/fcell.2015.00004

Jemal, A., Thun, M. J., Ries, L. A., Howe, H. L., Weir, H. K., Center, M. M., et al. (2008). Annual report to the nation on the status of cancer, 1975–2005, featuring trends in lung cancer, tobacco use, and tobacco control. *J. Natl. Cancer Inst.* 100, 1672–1694. doi: 10.1093/jnci/djn389

Katsarava, R., Beridze, V., Arabuli, N., Kharadze, D., Chu, C. C., and Won, C. Y. (1999). Amino acid-based bioanalogous polymers. Synthesis, and study of regular poly(ester amide)s based on bis(α-amino acid) α,ω-alkylene diesters, and aliphatic dicarboxylic acids. *J. Polym. Sci. A Polym. Chem.* 37, 391–407. doi: 10.1002/(SICI)1099-0518(19990215)37:4<391::AID-POLA3>3.0.CO;2-E

Kim, S. J., Kim, J. S., Papadopoulos, J., Wook Kim, S., Maya, M., Zhang, F., et al. (2009). Circulating monocytes expressing CD31: implications for acute and chronic angiogenesis. *Am. J. Pathol.* 174, 1972–1980. doi: 10.2353/ajpath.2009.080819

Kintzel, P. E., Michaud, L. B., and Lange, M. K. (2006). Docetaxel-associated epiphora. *Pharmacotherapy* 26, 853–867. doi: 10.1592/phco.26.6.853

Laura, G., Inmaculada, P., Cristina, T., Jesús, R., Francesco, S., Carmen, O., et al. (2017). Docetaxel-loaded nanoparticles assembled from β-cyclodextrin/calixarene giant surfactants: physicochemical properties and cytotoxic effect in prostate cancer and glioblastoma cells. *Front. Pharmacol.* 8:249. doi: 10.3389/fphar.2017.00249

Li, B., Li, Q., Mo, J., and Dai, H. (2017). Drug-loaded polymeric nanoparticles for cancer stem cell targeting. *Front. Pharmacol.* 8:51. doi: 10.3389/fphar.2017.00051

Lin, X., Yan, S., Qi, S., Xu, Q., Han, S., Guo, L., et al. (2017). Transferrin-modified nanoparticles for photodynamic therapy enhance the antitumor efficacy of hypocrellin A. *Front. Pharmacol.* 8:815. doi: 10.3389/fphar.2017.00815

Liu, X., Zhang, X., Zhu, M., Lin, G., Liu, J., Zhou, Z., et al. (2017). PEGylated Au@Pt nanodendrites as novel theranostic agents for computed tomography imaging and photothermal/radiation synergistic therapy. *ACS Appl. Mater. Interfaces* 9, 279–285. doi: 10.1021/acsami.6b15183

Lu, B., Huang, X., Mo, J., and Zhao, W. (2016). Drug delivery using nanoparticles for cancer stem-like cell targeting. *Front. Pharmacol.* 7:84. doi: 10.3389/fphar.2016.00084

Matsumura, Y., and Maeda, H. (1986). A new concept for macromolecular therapeutics in cancer chemotherapy: mechanism of tumoritropic accumulation of proteins and the antitumor agent smancs. *Cancer Res.* 46, 6387–6392.

Pan, Y., Du, X., Zhao, F., and Xu, B. (2012). Magnetic nanoparticles for the manipulation of proteins and cells. *Chem. Soc. Rev.* 41, 2912–2942. doi: 10.1039/c2cs15315g

Pan, Y., Gao, Y., Shi, J., Wang, L., and Xu, B. (2011a). A versatile supramolecular hydrogel of nitrilotriacetic acid (NTA) for binding metal ions and magnetorheological response. *Chem. Sci.* 21, 6804–6806. doi: 10.1039/c1jm10822k

Pan, Y., Long, M., Li, X., Shi, J., Hedstrom, L., and Xu, B. (2011b). Glutathione (GSH)-decorated magnetic nanoparticles for binding glutathione-S-transferase (GST) fusion protein and manipulating live cells. *Chem. Sci.* 2, 945–948. doi: 10.1039/c1sc00030f

Pao, W., and Chmielecki, J. (2010). Rational, biologically based treatment of EGFR-mutant non-small-cell lung cancer. *Nat. Rev. Cancer* 10, 760–774. doi: 10.1038/nrc2947

Persohn, E., Canta, A., Schoepfer, S., Traebert, M., Mueller, L., Gilardini, A., et al. (2005). Morphological and morphometric analysis of paclitaxel and docetaxel-induced peripheral neuropathy in rats. *Eur. J. Cancer* 41, 1460–1466. doi: 10.1016/j.ejca.2005.04.006

Shi, J., Kantoff, P. W., Wooster, R., and Farokhzad, O. C. (2017). Cancer nanomedicine: progress, challenges and opportunities. *Nat. Rev. Cancer* 17, 20–37. doi: 10.1038/nrc.2016.108

Tao, W., Zeng, X. W., Zhang, J. X., Zhu, H. J., Chang, D. F., Zhang, X. D., et al. (2014). Synthesis of cholic acid-core poly(ϵ-caprolactone-*ran*-lactide)-b-poly(ethylene glycol) 1000 random copolymer as a chemotherapeutic nanocarrier for liver cancer treatment. *Biomater. Sci.* 2, 1262–1274. doi: 10.1039/C4BM00134F

Tong, A. W. (2006). Small RNAs and non-small cell lung cancer. *Curr. Mol. Med.* 6, 339–349. doi: 10.2174/156652406776894554

Umar, A., Dunn, B. K., and Greenwald, P. (2012). Future directions in cancer prevention. *Nat. Rev. Cancer* 12, 835–848. doi: 10.1038/nrc3397

Wu, J., and Chu, C. C. (2012). Block copolymer of poly(ester amide) and polyesters: synthesis, characterization, and in vitro cellular response. *Acta Biomater.* 8, 4314–4323. doi: 10.1016/j.actbio.2012.07.027

Wu, J., and Chu, C. C. (2013). Water insoluble cationic poly(ester amide)s: synthesis, characterization and applications. *J. Mater. Chem. B* 1, 353–360. doi: 10.1039/C2TB00070A

Wu, J., Mutschler, M. A., and Chu, C. C. (2011). Synthesis and characterization of ionic charged water soluble arginine-based poly(ester amide). *J. Mater. Sci. Mater. Med.* 22, 469–479. doi: 10.1007/s10856-011-4243-5

Wu, J., Wu, D. Q., Mutschler, M. A., and Chu, C. C. (2012a). Cationic hybrid hydrogels from amino-acid-based poly(ester amide): fabrication, characterization, and biological properties. *Adv. Funct. Mater.* 22, 3815–3823. doi: 10.1002/adfm.201103147

Wu, J., Yamanouchi, D., Liu, B., and Chu, C. C. (2012b). Biodegradable arginine-based poly(ether ester amide)s as a non-viral DNA delivery vector and their structure-function study. *J. Mater. Chem.* 22, 18983–18991. doi: 10.1039/c2jm33753c

Wu, J., Zhao, L., Xu, X., Bertrand, N., Choi, W. I., Yameen, B., et al. (2015). Hydrophobic cysteine poly(disulfide)-based redox-hypersensitive nanoparticle platform for cancer theranostics. *Angew. Chem. Int. Ed. Engl.* 54, 9218–9223. doi: 10.1002/anie.201503863

Yu, J. Y., Lin, F., Lin, P. P., Gao, Y. H., and Becker, M. L. (2014). Phenylalanine-based poly(ester urea): synthesis, characterization, and *in vitro* degradation. *Macromolecules* 47, 121–129. doi: 10.1021/ma401752b

Zhao, H., Lin, Z. Y., Yildirimer, L., Dhinakar, A., Zhao, X., and Wu, J. (2016). Polymer-based nanoparticles for protein delivery: design, strategies and applications. *J. Mater. Chem. B* 4, 4060–4071. doi: 10.1039/C6TB00308G

16

Icariin Activates Autophagy via Down-Regulation of the NF-κB Signaling-Mediated Apoptosis in Chondrocytes

Bobin Mi[1], Junqing Wang[2], Yi Liu[1], Jing Liu[1], Liangcong Hu[1], Adriana C. Panayi[3], Guohui Liu[1]* and Wu Zhou[1]*

[1] Department of Orthopaedics, Union Hospital, Tongji Medical College, Huazhong University of Science and Technology, Wuhan, China, [2] State Key Laboratory of Molecular Vaccinology and Molecular Diagnostics & Center for Molecular Imaging and Translational Medicine, School of Public Health, Xiamen University, Xiamen, China, [3] Addenbrooke's Hospital, University of Cambridge School of Clinical Medicine, Cambridge, United Kingdom

***Correspondence:**
Guohui Liu
liuguohui@hust.edu.cn
Wu Zhou
wuzhoutjmu1986@163.com

Osteoarthritis (OA) is a common chronic and degenerative joint condition that is mainly characterized by cartilage degradation, osteophyte formation, and joint stiffness. The NF-κB signaling pathway in inflammation, autophagy, and apoptosis plays a prominent role in the progression of OA. Icariin, a prenylated flavonol glycoside extracted from Epimedium, have been proven to exert anti-osteoporotic and anti-inflammatory effects in OA. However, the action mechanisms of its effect on chondrocytes have yet to be elucidated. In the present study, we demonstrated that the *in vitro* therapeutic effects of icariin on rat chondrocytes in a dose-dependent manner. We found that TNF-α induced the production of IL-1, IL-6, IL-12, reactive oxygen species (ROS), nitric oxide (NO), Caspase-3, and Caspase-9 in chondrocytes. We also provided evidence that TNF-α inhibited autophagy markers (Atg 5, Atg 7) and prevented LC3 I translate to LC3 II. Furthermore, TNF-α induced matrix metalloproteinase (MMP)3 and MMP9 expression. The negative effects of TNF-α on chondrocytes can be partially blocked by treating with icariin or ammonium pyrrolidinedithiocarbamate (PDTC, an NF-κB inhibitor). The present study data also suggested that icariin suppressed both TNF-α-stimulated p65 nuclear translocation and IκBα protein degradation. These results indicated that icariin protected against OA by suppressing inflammatory cytokines and apoptosis, through activation of autophagy via NF-κB inhibition. In conclusion, icariin appears to favorably modulate autophagy and apoptosis in chondrocytes making it a promising compound for cartilage tissue engineering in the treatment of OA.

Keywords: icariin, tissue engineering, autophagy, apoptosis, chondrocytes

INTRODUCTION

Osteoarthritis (OA) is a chronic degenerative joint disease that occurs mostly in the elderly (Glyn-Jones et al., 2015). As the population ages, the occurrence of OA increases and, consequently, finding an effective treatment is imperative. The capacity of chondrocytes to regenerate normal cartilage matrix architecture declines with aging, resulting in cartilage degradation and erosion

(Blanco et al., 2011). In the cases of OA, various changes occur in the cartilage including inflammation, oxidative stress, loss of cartilage matrix, autophagy, and apoptosis.

During the progression of OA, the increased expression of inflammatory cytokines (such as TNF-α and IL-1β) in articular cartilage and synovium contribute to the degradation and erosion of cartilage (Raman et al., 2018). At the same time, autophagy and apoptosis occur in the progression of OA. Autophagy is necessary for maintaining the cell's metabolism and homeostasis, and for cellular quality control by clearing waste or damaged proteins and organelles (Galluzzi et al., 2014). The dysregulation of autophagy that happens with OA contributes to the degeneration of the articular cartilage (Vasheghani et al., 2015). The importance of autophagy in preventing age-related OA has been demonstrated by the increasing number of studies on the topic (Duarte, 2015; Loeser et al., 2016). In addition, more and more evidences suggest that increased chondrocyte apoptosis induces cartilage degeneration in OA (Kobayashi et al., 2016). Thus, activation of autophagy and inhibition of apoptosis in chondrocytes may limit OA progress.

Recently, various biomaterials, such as hydrogels, have been used as drug delivery systems to regulate chondrocyte autophagy (Chen et al., 2016). Driven by the rapid progression of nanomedicine and nanotechnology (Tao et al., 2015, 2017a; Ding et al., 2017; Rosenblum et al., 2018), compounds have been increasingly studied in the context of regeneration medicine and tissue engineering. However, few compounds are reported to be useful for tissue engineering in cartilage repair. Icariin is a well-known compound extracted from Herba Epimedil, with a wide range of pharmacological effects, including anti-inflammatory, anti-atherosclerotic, and anti-oxidative properties (Fang and Zhang, 2017; Wang G.Q. et al., 2017; Xiong et al., 2017). Recently, icariin-mediated chondroprotective effects have attracted growing attention. Icariin protects against OA by inhibiting overexpression of metalloproteinase 13 (MMP-13) and proinflammatory cytokines in chondrocytes (Zeng et al., 2014). In addition to inhibiting H_2O_2-induced human umbilical vein endothelial cell apoptosis, icariin suppresses NF-κB signaling in macrophages (Wang and Huang, 2005; Chen et al., 2010). The effect of icariin on chondrocyte autophagy and apoptosis, however, remains unclear.

In this study, we investigate whether icariin has chondroprotective effects against TNF-α-induced cell death. These effects might be closely related with autophagy activation and apoptosis inhibition. In addition, we explore the underlying mechanisms of icariin-mediated cell autophagy and apoptosis.

MATERIALS AND METHODS

Reagent, Antibodies, and Ethics Statement

Icariin was purchased from Sigma-Aldrich (MO, United States). Cell Counting Kit-8 (CCK8) was purchased from MedChemExpress (NJ, United States). Antibodies against ATG5, ATG7, LC3, p65, phosphorylated p65 (p-p65), IκBα, MMP3, MMP9 were purchased from Abcam (Cambridge, United Kingdom). Antibody against GAPDH was purchased from Cell Signaling Technology, Inc. (MA, United States). The NF-κB inhibitor pyrrolidinedithiocarbamate (PDTC) was purchased from Abcam (Cambridge, United Kingdom). Enzyme-linked immunosorbent assay (ELISA) kits were purchased from Bio-Swamp Life Science (Shanghai, China). The Sprague-Dawley (SD) rat was purchased from The Center of Experimental Animal, Tongji Medical College, Huazhong University of Science and Technology. All experimental procedures were approved by the Institutional Animal Care and Use Committee at Tongji Medical College, Huazhong University of Science and Technology.

Cell Isolation and Culture

Chondrocytes were isolated from the articular cartilage of 7–10-day-old male SD rats. Briefly, pieces of articular cartilage were digested with 0.25 mg/mL trypsin for 30 min and 2 mg/mL collagenase type II for 8 h at 37°C. After digestion, isolated chondrocytes were passed through a 180-μm filter and the cells were centrifuged and washed with PBS several times. The cells were then isolated and stained with trypan blue to evaluate cell viability. Chondrocytes with viability greater than 85% were cultured in Dulbecco's modified Eagle's medium (DMEM) containing 10% fetal bovine serum (FBS) and 100 IU/ml penicillin, 100 μg/ml streptomycin at 37°C, 5% CO_2. When the cells were treated with 50 ng/ml TNF-α, 10 μM icariin, 10 μM PDTC, icariin or PDTC were added to the medium 2 h prior to TNF-α addition. In the autophagic flux assay, 0.1 μm bafilomycin A1 was added to the medium 1 h prior to icariin or PDTC addition. In the experiments, chondrocytes were treated with PBS (control), TNF-α, icariin with TNF-α, or PDTC with TNF-α for 24 h. All experiments were conducted in triplicate.

Cytotoxicity Assay

Rat chondrocytes were seeded in 96-well plates (5×10^3 cells/well) overnight, followed by treatment with various concentrations of icariin for 24 h, 48 h, and 72 h at 37°C in an atmosphere containing 5% CO_2. Following this, 10 μl CCK8 solution was added to each well and the cells were cultured at 37°C for 2 h. The OD value was then measured with a microplate reader (Thermo Fisher Scientific, United States) at 450 nm.

ELISA

Chondrocytes were seeded onto a 24-well plate at 2×10^4 cells per well. Following 24 h incubation, cells were treated with PBS, TNF-α, icariin with TNF-α, or PDTC with TNF-α. The supernatants were collected after 24 h incubation and the levels of IL-1, IL-6, and IL-12 were quantified using the ELISA kits.

Western Blot

Total proteins were extracted using cold RIPA buffer containing protease inhibitor (Boster Biological Technology, Ltd., Wuhan, China). Proteins were quantified using the bicinchoninic acid protein assay kit (BCA kit) according to the manufacturer's instructions. Equal amount of proteins (10 μg) were separated by 10% SDS-PAGE and transferred to polyvinylidene fluoride (PVDF) membranes (Millipore, United States). Membranes were blocked in 5% bull serum albumin (BSA, Sigma, United States) in TBST for 2 h, then incubated with primary antibody at 4°C overnight. The primary antibodies were as follows: p65 (1:2000), p-p65 (1:2000), IκBα (1:5000), ATG5 (1:5000), ATG7 (1:10000), LC3 (1:3000), MMP3 (1:10000), MMP9 (1:10000), and GAPDH (1:1000). After washing with TBST (50 mM Tris PH 8.0, 150 mM NaCl, 0.01% Tween-20) three times, the membrane was incubated with HRP-conjugated corresponding secondary antibodies (Goat Anti-Rabbit IgG, 1:10000) for 1 h at room temperature. Following washing, the immunoreactive proteins were visualized with the ECL western detection kit (Thermo Fisher Scientific, United States). The band density was quantified using TANON GIS software (Tanon, Shanghai, China).

Reverse Transcription-Quantitative (RT-q) PCR

Total RNA from chondrocytes was extracted using Trizol reagent (Thermo Fisher Scientific, United States). Total RNA was reverse-transcribed to cDNA with RT Master Mix (Takara Japan). The RT-PCR was performed with SYBR Master Mix using StepOne-Plus system (ABI, United States) under the following conditions: denature at 95°C for 30 s, anneal at 60°C for 1 min and extend at 95°C for 5 s. The gene expression was analyzed by $2^{-\Delta\Delta Ct}$ method using GAPDH as the internal control. The primer sequences were as follows: ATG5, forward (5′-AA CGAGAAGCAGAGCCA-3′) and reverse (5′-ATGCCAT TTCAGGGGTG-3′); ATG7, forward (5′-GAAGAACCAGAAA GGAGG-3′) and reverse (5′-CAGGCACTTGACAGACAC-3′); Bax, forward (5′-TGGTTGCCCTCTTCTA-3′) and reverse (5′CACCCTGGTCTTGGAT-3′); Bcl-2 forward (5′-CACAG AGGGGCTACGAGT-3′) and reverse (5′-CAGGCTGGAAGG AGAAGA-3′); GAPDH, forward (5′-CAAGTTCAACGGCA CAG-3′) and reverse (5′-CCAGTAGACTC CACGAC AT-3′).

Transmission Electron Microscopy (TEM)

Collected cells were fixed with 2.5% glutaraldehyde for 24 h, which followed by fixed with 1% osmium tetroxide for 1 h at 4°C. After dehydrated with a series of ethanol concentrations (50, 70, 80, 90, and 100%) for 10-min intervals, the samples were incubated in a mixture of acetone and epoxy resin (v:v = 1:1) for 6 h, followed by incubation with pure epoxy resin for 4 h. After semi-thin sectioning, cells were stained with 0.5% toluidine blue and observed under the microscope. Finally, the ultra-section sections were observed using a TEM (Hitachi, Japan).

Cell Cycle Assay

Collected cells were washed and suspended in 0.3 mL PBS containing 10% FBS and 0.7 mL ethyl alcohol for 24 h at −20°C. The cells were then suspended with 0.1 mL RNase A (1 mg/mL) and 0.4 mL propidium iodide (PI) (50 μg/mL) for 10 min. The percentage of cells in the different stages was measured using Flow Cytometry.

Cell Apoptosis Assay

Collected cells were stained with a mixture of calcein-AM and PI solution for 20 min. Fluorescence images of cells were then recorded using an inverted fluorescent microscope. The percentages of cell death were evaluated by calculating the number of PI-stained (dead, red) and calcein-AM-stained (live, green) cells. The number of cells were counted in five random fields by three independent authors. The mean value of each measurement was used for analysis.

Measurement of ROS Production

The ROS level was measured using Reactive oxygen species assay kit (Nanjing Jiancheng Bioengineering Institute, Nanjing, China) according to the manufactures' instructions. Briefly, treated cells were incubated with 10 μM dichlorodihydrofluorescein diacetate (DCFH-DA) in the dark for 30 min. Then, the cells were rinsed with DMEM and analyzed on a flow cytometer with excitation wavelength of 500 nm and emission wavelength of 525 nm. ROS level in the experimental group was normalized to the control group.

Measurement of NO Production

NO production was detected with nitrate/nitrite colorimetric assay kit of Griess reaction (Nanjing Jiancheng Bioengineering Institute, Nanjing, China) according to the manufacturer's protocol. In brief, cultured medium was collected from treated cells and mixed with equal volume of Griess reagent. Following a 10-min incubation, absorbance was measured at 550 nm on a microplate reader (Thermo Fisher Scientific, United States).

Caspase-3 and Caspase-9 Activity Assay

Caspase-3 and caspase-9 was detected with Caspase colorimetric assay kit (Nanjing Jiancheng Bioengineering Institute, Nanjing, China). Briefly, collected cells were lysed in the provided lysis buffer. The absorbance was measured at 405 nm on a microplate reader (Thermo Fisher Scientific, United States).

Immunocytochemical Staining of p65

Cells were collected and washed with PBS, and then fixed with 4% paraformaldehyde for 15 min. After washing with PBS, the cells were blocked with 5% BSA for 2 h at 37°C. Then, p-p65 antibody (1:150) was added and incubated overnight at 4°C, followed by adding Max Vision TMHRP-polymer for 1 h, and followed by incubation with DAB for 5 min. The number of p65 in the nucleus was counted in five random fields by three independent authors. The mean value of each measurement was taken for analysis.

Statistical Analysis

Data were presented as means ± standard deviation (*SD*). Statistical analysis was performed in GraphPad Prism 6.0 (GraphPad Software, United States) using Student's *t*-test and one-way analysis variance (ANOVA). Statistical significance was considered when $P < 0.05$.

RESULTS

Cytotoxicity of Icariin on Chondrocytes

To determine whether icariin was toxic to chondrocytes, CCK8 assay was used after the cells had been treated with increasing concentration of icariin (0, 3, 5, 7, 10, 20 μM) for 24, 48, and 72 h. As shown in **Figure 1**, icariin promoted cell viability in a dose-dependent manner. The dose of 10 μM and 20 μM icariin had a similar beneficial effect on chondrocytes. (**Figure 1**) The dose of 10 μM was selected for the subsequent experiments.

Effects of Icariin on TNF-α-Induced Inflammatory Cytokines

There are various inflammatory cytokines involved in the pathologic process of OA. These cytokines, such as IL-1β, induce the production of the other inflammatory cytokines (Hong et al., 2014), leading to inflammatory milieu in chondrocytes. In the present study, we found that TNF-α induced the production of IL-1, IL-6, and IL-12 in chondrocytes. Such effects were partially blocked with the addition of icariin to TNF-α-treated cells (**Figure 2**), suggesting that icariin had an anti-inflammatory effect on chondrocytes.

Icariin Activates Autophagy in TNF-α-Treated Chondrocytes

To investigate the effect of icariin on the autophagy of chondrocytes, the autophagy markers Atg 5 and Atg 7 were detected. The western blot and PCR results showed that autophagy markers were significantly reduced in TNF-α-treated cells when compared with those cells co-treated with icariin and TNF-α, indicating that icariin protected against TNF-α-induced inhibition of autophagy (**Figures 3A–C**). In addition to Atg 5 and Atg 7, western blotting result of LC3 (a classic marker of autophagy) was also used to establish the effect of icariin on autophagy. Icariin significantly enhanced LC3-II level when adding to the TNF-α-treated cells (**Figure 3D**). During the late phase of autophagy, the fusion of lysosomes with autophagosomes may lead to a lower accumulation of LC3-II in the cytoplasm. To demonstrate this effect, bafilomycin A1 was added 24 h prior to cells co-treated with TNF-α and icariin to inhibit the fusion of lysosomes with autophagosomes. The level of LC3-II increased when bafilomycin A1 was added to the TNF-α-icariin-treated cells (**Figure 3D**), suggesting that autophagy may fail to detect when autophagosomes fusion with lysosomes. Furthermore, TEM images illustrated that the number

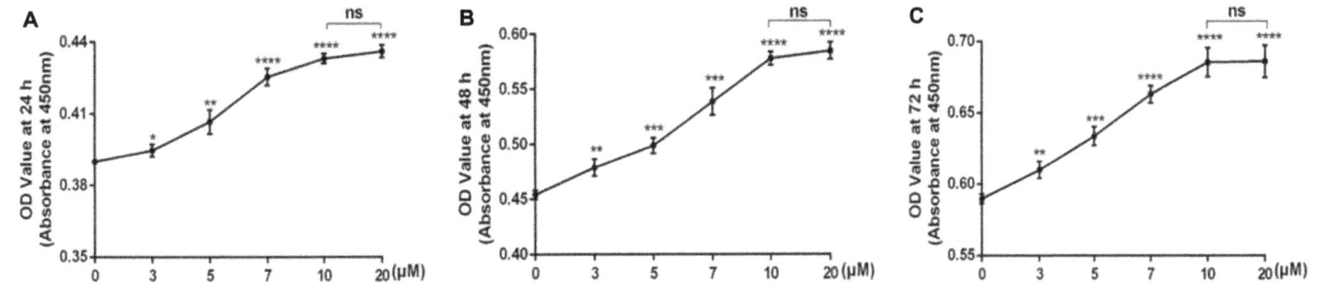

FIGURE 1 | (A–C) The cytotoxicity of icariin on chondrocytes was examined using the concentration of 0, 3, 5, 7, 10, and 20 μM after 24, 48, and 72 h of culture. Values were expressed as means ± SD. *$P < 0.05$, **$p < 0.01$, ***$p < 0.001$, ****$p < 0.0001$.

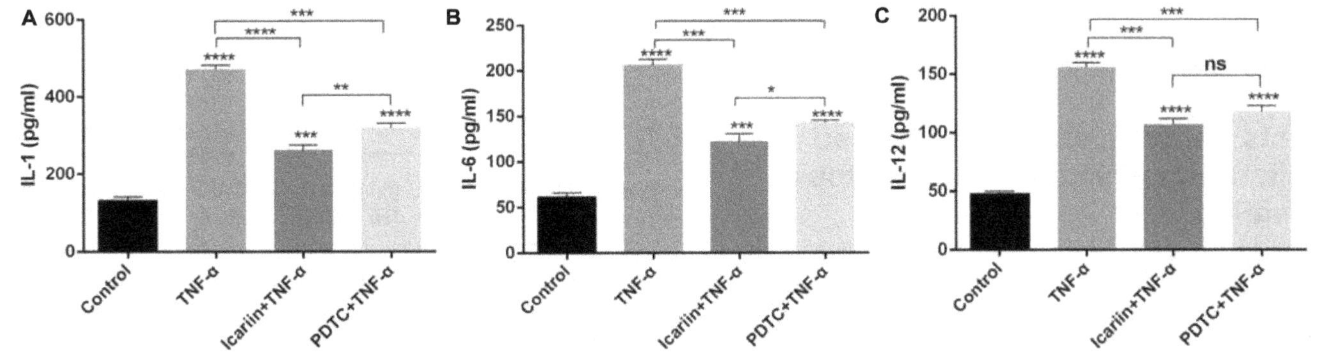

FIGURE 2 | Effect of PBS, TNF-α, icariin with TNF-α, and PDTC with TNF-α on the production of inflammatory cytokines. **(A–C)** TNF-α induced the production of IL-1, IL-6, and IL-12 in chondrocytes. Icariin or PDTC partially attenuated the TNF-α-induced inflammatory cytokines production. Values were expressed as means ± SD. *$P < 0.05$, **$p < 0.01$, ***$p < 0.001$, ****$p < 0.0001$.

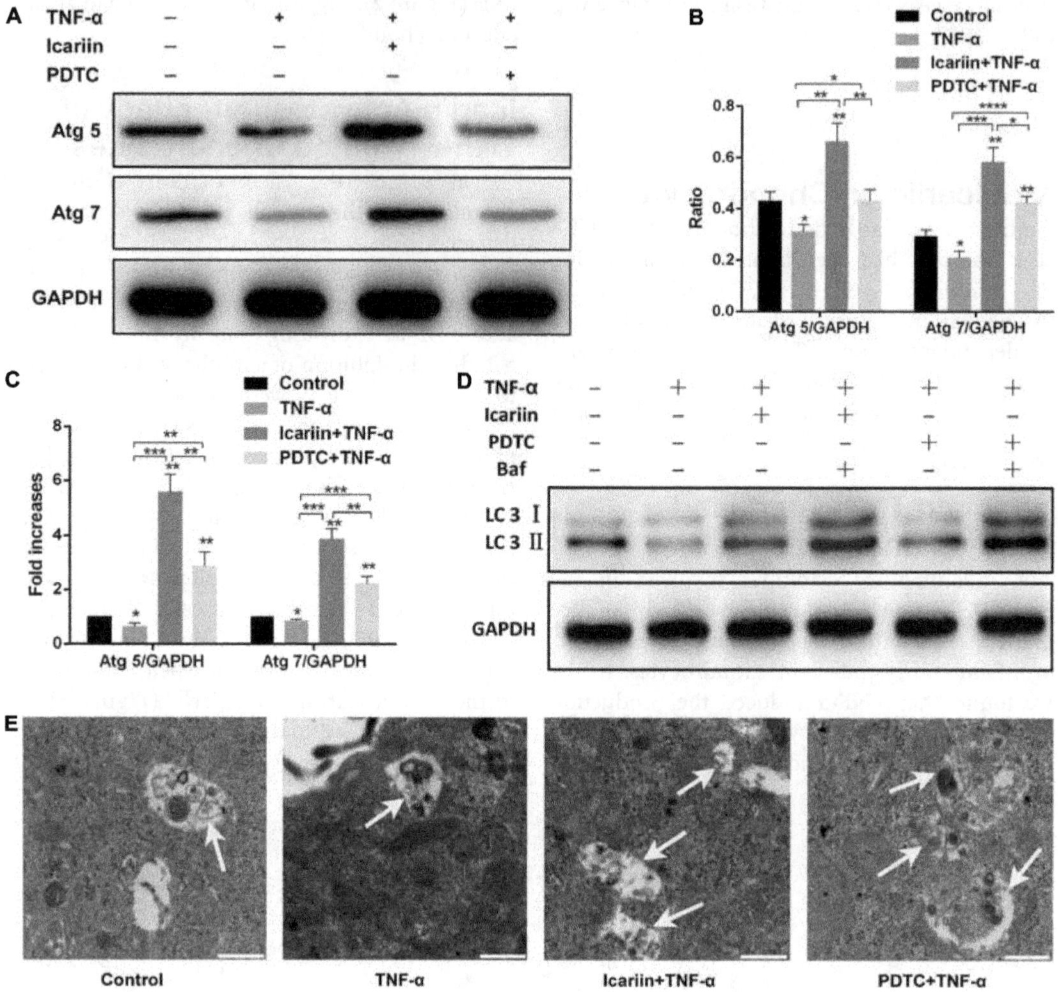

FIGURE 3 | Effect of PBS, TNF-α, icariin with TNF-α, and PDTC with TNF-α on the autophagy of chondrocytes. **(A–D)** Western blot and PCR analysis indicated that icariin and PDTC could partially reverse the TNF-α-induced inhibition of autophagy. Bafilomycin A1 significantly increased the LC3- II level in icariin-TNF-α-treated cells and in PDTC-TNF-α-treated cells. **(E)** Transmission electron microscopy from four groups. Autophagosomes in images are marked with black arrows. White arrow represents autophagosome in the cytoplasm. Scale bar = 500 nm. Values are expressed as means ± SD. **P* < 0.05, ***p* < 0.01, ****p* < 0.001, *****p* < 0.0001. Baf: Bafilomycin A1.

of autophagosomes in cells co-treated with icariin and TNF-α was higher than that cells treated solely with TNF-α (**Figure 3E**). These results indicated that icariin activated autophagy in TNF-α-treated chondrocytes.

Effects of Icariin on TNF-α-Induced Proliferation Inhibition and Apoptosis Activation

It is well known that inhibition of the proliferation rate correlates with decreased cell cycle progression in chondrocytes. We analyzed the cell cycle division of chondrocytes treated with PBS, TNF-α and icariin with TNF-α. According to the PI staining of flow cytometry analysis, TNF-α arrested chondrocytes in the G1 phase. However, the percentage of the cell population in the S phase increased from 22.27% to 26.11% when addition of icariin to the TNF-α-treated chondrocytes (**Figures 4A,B**). These results suggested that cell cycle progression might be delayed by TNF-α, a delay that is partially reversed by icariin treatment.

We also analyzed the effect of TNF-α on chondrocyte apoptosis by calcein-AM/PI double-staining and found that TNF-α significantly induced chondrocyte apoptosis. However, when icariin was added to TNF-α-treated cells, the percentage of cell death decreased from 46.33% to 24.33% (**Figures 4C,D**), suggesting that icariin protected against TNF-α-induced cell apoptosis. To further determine whether icariin affects the mitochondrial apoptosis pathway of chondrocytes, the anti-apoptotic protein Bcl-2 level and the pro-apoptotic Bax level were detected using western blot and PCR. TNF-α significantly inhibited Bcl-2 expression but induced Bax expression. These effects were partially blocked by icariin treatment (**Figures 5A–E**). Furthermore, the effect of that TNF-α-induced Caspase-3/9 activation in chondrocytes was blocked by addition of icariin. (**Figures 5F,G**).

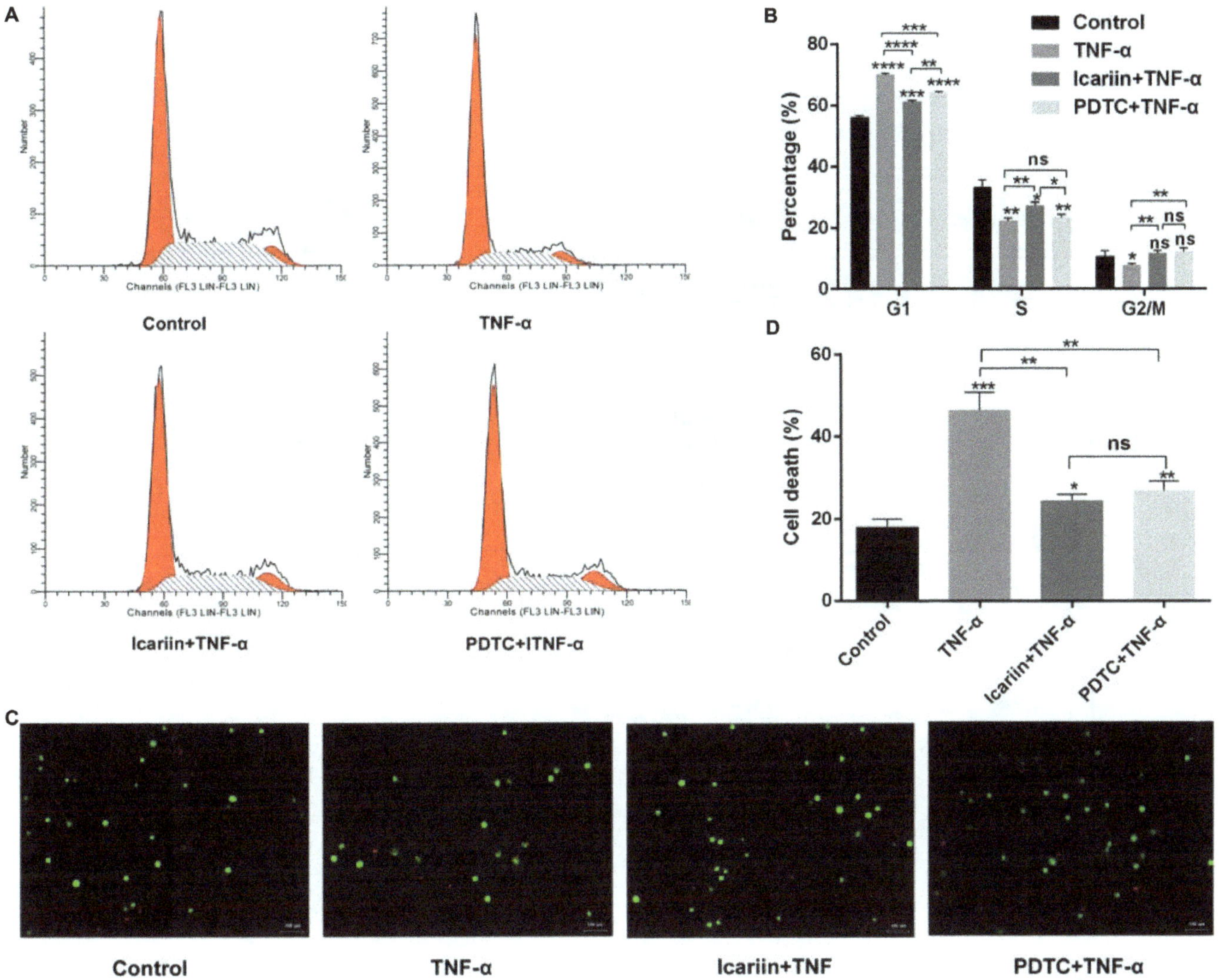

FIGURE 4 | Effect of PBS, TNF-α, icariin with TNF-α, and PDTC with TNF-α on cell cycle progression and apoptosis of chondrocytes. **(A)** The distribution of cell cycles after 24 h treatment. **(B)** TNF-α induced cell cycle arrest at the G1 phase. Icariin or PDTC induced TNF-α-treated cell cycle arrest at the S-G2/M phase. **(C)** Calcein-AM/PI double-staining of apoptotic cell death. **(D)** Analysis of apoptosis revealed that TNF-α induced chondrocyte apoptosis. Icariin or PDTC partially blocked the TNF-α-induced chondrocyte apoptosis. Magnification: 200×. Values are expressed as means ± *SD*. **P* < 0.05, ***p* < 0.01, ****p* < 0.001, *****p* < 0.0001.

Effect of Icariin on TNF-α-Induced NO and ROS Production and Catabolism in Chondrocytes

The level of NO and ROS is known to increase when chondrocytes are exposed to inflammatory cytokines. In the present study, we found that TNF-α significantly induced NO and ROS production, an effect which could be blocked by addition of icariin (**Figure 6**).

Disruption of homeostasis in cartilage metabolism impairs the extracellular matrix and chondrocytes, resulting in cartilage degradation. The excessive matrix catabolism was usually caused by excessive mechanical joint loading or inflammatory cytokines, which was reflected by the increased levels of matrix-degrading enzymes matrix metalloproteinase (MMP) family. In the present study, TNF-α induced the production of MMP 3 and MMP 9, an effect which could be blocked by addition of icariin (**Figure 7**). These results indicated that icariin inhibited NO and ROS production and reconstituted homeostasis of metabolism in chondrocytes.

Icariin Inhibits NF-κB Pathway Activated by TNF-α in Chondrocytes

In the present study, western blot results showed that TNF-α significantly increased the level of p-p65 and decreased the level of IκBα in chondrocytes when compared with the control group, suggesting that TNF-α stimulation of the NF-κB pathway (**Figures 8A,B**). This finding also proven by the result of immunocytochemical staining that the number of p65 translocate

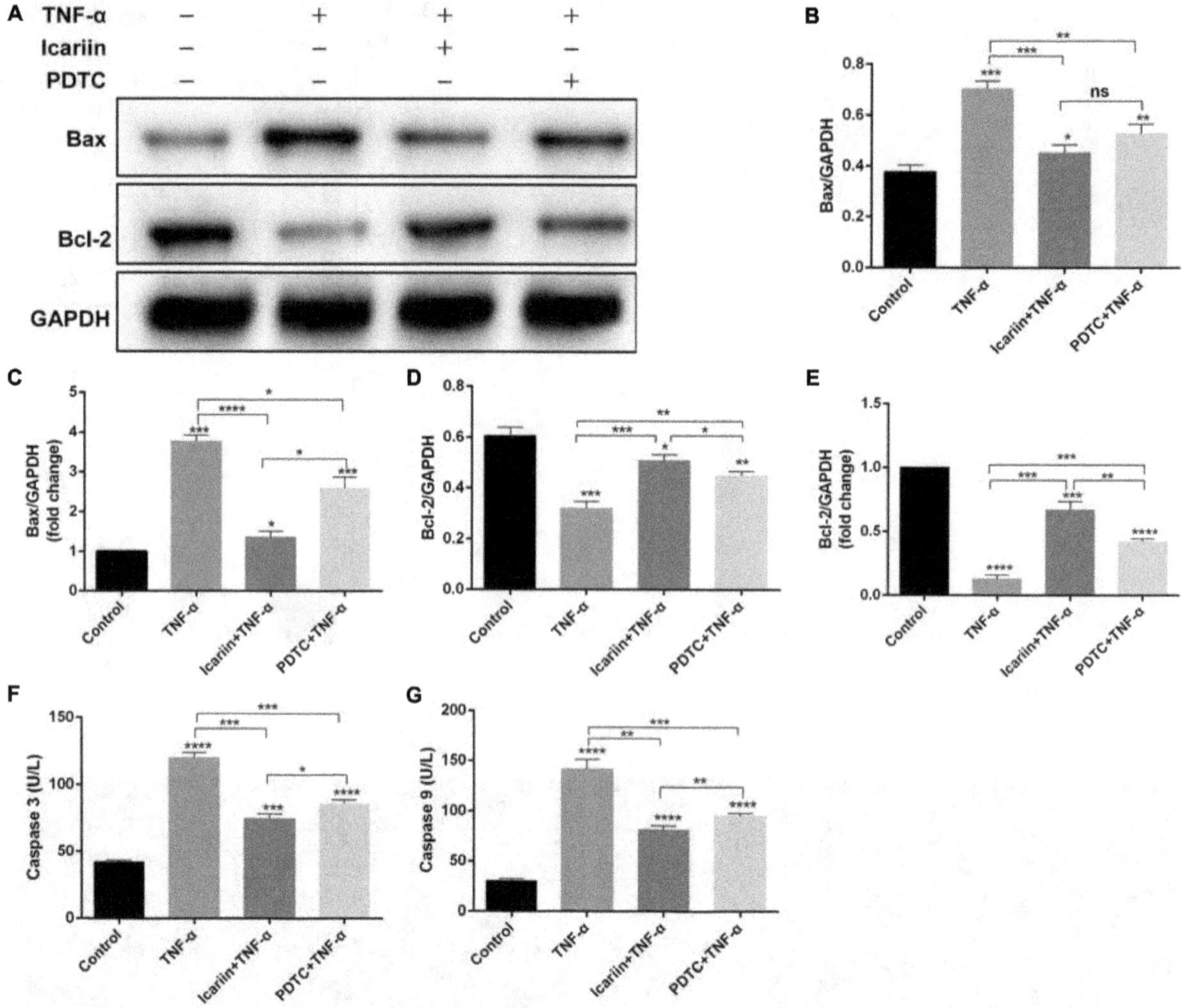

FIGURE 5 | Effect of PBS, TNF-α, icariin with TNF-α and PDTC with TNF-α on the apoptosis of chondrocytes. **(A–E)** Western blot and PCR analysis showed that the TNF-α group had a higher level of pro-apoptotic protein Bax and a lower level of anti-apoptotic protein Bcl-2 compared with the other three groups. **(F,G)** ELISA results showed that the level of Caspase-3/9 was higher in the TNF-α group than the other three groups. Values were expressed as means ± *SD*. $^{*}P < 0.05$, $^{**}p < 0.01$, $^{***}p < 0.001$, $^{****}p < 0.0001$.

to nucleus in TNF-α-treated cells is higher than the control group (**Figures 8C,D**). In contrast, icariin caused the TNF-α-induced p-p65 increase and IκBα degradation reversal. Furthermore, the number of p65 translated to the nucleus also decreased by addition of icariin to TNF-α-treated cells. (**Figure 8**).

Involvement of NF-κB Pathway in the Autophagy Activation and Apoptosis Inhibition Induced by DHA

The NF-κB pathway plays a crucial role in various pathogenesis process of OA. To investigate whether this pathway was involved in the TNF-α-induced negative effect on chondrocytes, we used an NF-κB inhibitor, PDTC. In the present study, we found that PDTC partially blocked the TNF-α-induced inflammatory cytokines production, proliferation and autophagy inhibition, apoptosis activation, and hypercatabolism. (**Figures 2–8**).

DISCUSSION

Inflammatory cytokines including TNF-α and IL-6 contribute to cartilage catabolism and degeneration in OA (Lai et al., 2014; Nasi et al., 2016). Excessive inflammatory cytokines inhibit autophagy activation, further increasing production of ROS and leading to cell death (Liu-Bryan and Terkeltaub, 2015). In the current study, we demonstrated that TNF-α suppressed autophagy in chondrocytes, which was reflected by the lower level of autophagy marker. Previous studies found that TNF-α inhibited the expression of Atg 5 and suppressed the conversion of LC3 I to II (Jiang et al., 2016). With Atg 5 knockdown, mice were more likely to develop OA with aging (Bouderlique et al., 2016), suggesting that activation of autophagy has a beneficial effect in preventing OA. When inflammatory cytokines release, the level of ROS and NO production increases, ultimately leading to chondrocyte apoptosis (Akuri et al., 2017). The present study

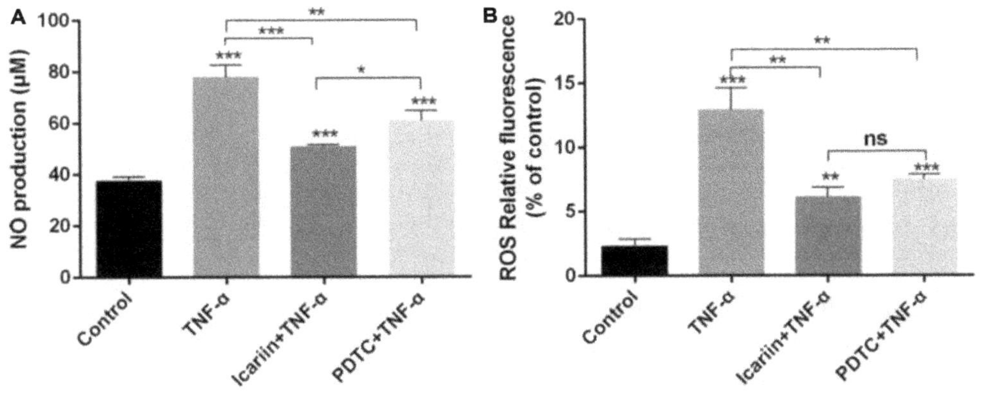

FIGURE 6 | Effect of PBS, TNF-α, icariin with TNF-α, and PDTC with TNF-α on the production levels of NO and ROS. **(A,B)** TNF-α induced the production of NO, ROS, an effect which could be reversed by adding icariin or PDTC treatment. Values were expressed as means ± SD. $^*P < 0.05$, $^{**}p < 0.01$, $^{***}p < 0.001$.

results consistent with previous studies which showed that TNF-α induced chondrocyte apoptosis via upregulated expression level of ROS and NO. In addition, previous studies, as well as the current study, have demonstrated that TNF-α induced the pro-apoptotic protein Bax production and reduced the anti-apoptotic protein Bcl-2 production, leading to hypercatabolism in chondrocytes (Ye et al., 2015). It should be noted that there are other proinflammatory cytokines contribute to the autophagy suppression and apoptosis induction in OA (Goldring and Otero, 2011). These cytokines may result in a synergistic effect in inhibiting autophagy and activating apoptosis during the pathological process of OA. Unfortunately, the present study reported that TNF-α further induced the production of other inflammatory cytokines. Therefore, it is necessary to regulate the inflammatory processes of OA. Indeed, treatments of OA with non-steroidal anti-inflammatory drugs that inhibit the release of proinflammatory cytokines is common practice (Urech et al., 2010).

The cytotoxic effects of icariin on other cell types have been investigated (Zhang et al., 2015). In the present study, icariin exhibited a positive effect on cell viability, in a dose-dependent manner. Both doses of 10 μM and 20 μM icariin showed similar effect on cell viability. Previous studies reported that icariin alleviated the inflammatory response in most cell types (Pan et al., 2017; Sun et al., 2018). In the present study, we demonstrated that icariin attenuated the production of inflammatory cytokines in chondrocytes. As overproduction of inflammatory cytokines inhibit autophagy activation (Qi et al., 2014), it is logical to suppose that icariin reverses the inflammatory cytokines-induced autophagy inhibition. Some studies reported that icariin plays a beneficial role on cell survival by inhibiting autophagy (Tang et al., 2015; Li et al., 2017). In the present study, however, we found that icariin blocked the TNF-α-induced autophagy inhibition in chondrocytes. This result may be attributed to its anti-inflammatory effect on chondrocytes. When autophagy activation, it could further suppress inflammatory response in chondrocytes (Ansari et al., 2017). Given that icariin and autophagy have both been shown to attenuate inflammatory response, this may act as a positive feedback loop to suppress TNF-α-induced inflammation. Along with the production of inflammatory cytokines was suppressed by icariin, so was apoptosis. In addition, the decreased level of NO and ROS induced by icariin also contribute to the inhibition of apoptosis and catabolism (Shen et al., 2015; Qiao et al., 2018). The apoptosis results were consistent with previous studies that support that icariin had protective effect against apoptosis (Deng et al., 2017). Consequently, icariin plays a dual role of autophagy activation and apoptosis inhibition in chondrocytes.

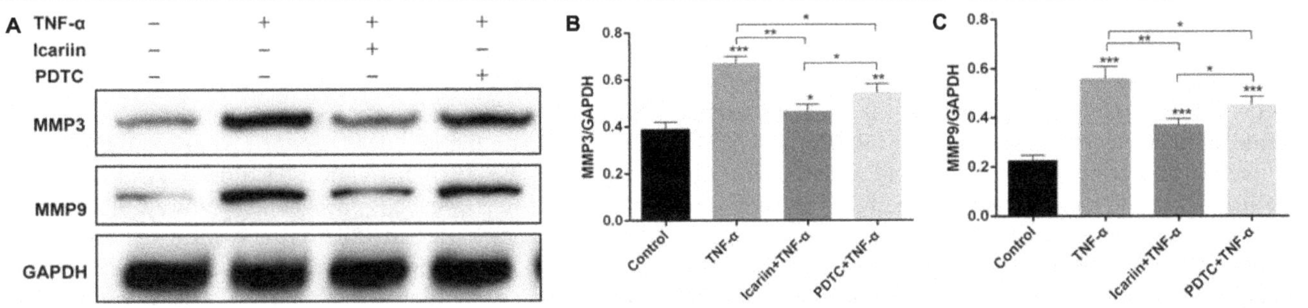

FIGURE 7 | Effect of PBS, TNF-α, icariin with TNF-α and PDTC with TNF-α on the catabolism of chondrocytes. **(A–C)** Western blot analysis showed that the levels of MMP3 and MMP9 were higher in the TNF-α group than the other three groups. Values were expressed as means ± SD. $^*P < 0.05$, $^{**}p < 0.01$, $^{***}p < 0.001$.

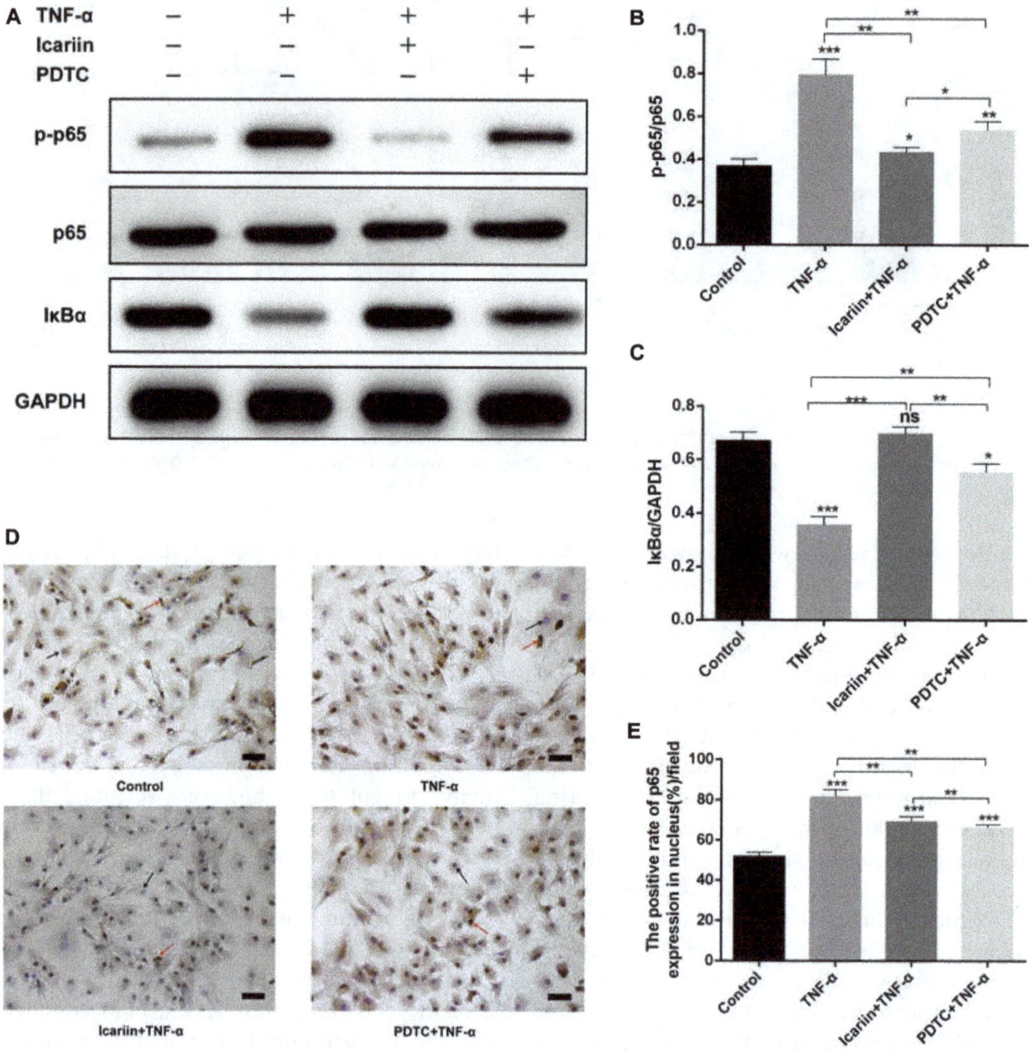

FIGURE 8 | Effect of PBS, TNF-α, icariin with TNF-α and PDTC with TNF-α on the NF-κB signaling pathway. **(A–C)** TNF-α significantly increased the level of *p*-p65 and decreased the level of IκBα, an effect which could be partially reversed by adding icariin or PDTC treatment. **(D,E)** More p65 translocated to the nucleus in TNF-α-stimulated cells, a process which was blocked with the addition of icariin or PDTC treatment. The black arrow indicated nucleus and red arrow indicated p65 translocated to the nucleus. Values were expressed as means ± SD. $^{*}P < 0.05$, $^{**}p < 0.01$, $^{***}p < 0.001$. Magnification: 200×. Scale Bar = 50 μm.

Previous studies reported that activation of the NF-κB signaling pathway induced pro-inflammatory cytokines release (Dubey et al., 2018). Exposure of chondrocytes to a variety of inflammatory cytokines lead to the degradation of IκB, allowing p65 translocate to the nucleus (Guo et al., 2015). The present study showed that TNF-α induced NF-κB pathway activation. Icariin is known to inhibit NF-κB signaling, leading to anti-inflammatory effect (Hua et al., 2018). Thus, the TNF-α-induced NF-κB activation was reversed with addition of icariin, suggesting that icariin had a negative effect on NF-κB activation. NF-κB plays a key role in both chondrocyte autophagy and apoptosis. When the NF-κB signaling pathway was activated by inflammatory cytokines, autophagy inhibition along with apoptosis activation appear, which play a synergetic effect on accelerating chondrocyte death (Jiang et al., 2016; Zhang et al., 2016). The results that autophagy markers significantly increased and apoptotic markers significantly decreased when addition of icariin or PDTC to the TNF-α-treated chondrocytes, suggested that icariin protected against OA by inhibiting the TNF-α-induced NF-κB signaling pathway activation. Interestingly, we noticed that icariin treatment had a better anti-inflammatory effect than PDTC treatment on TNF-α-treated cells in terms of IL-1 and IL-6. In addition, it also had a better reversal effect than PDTC, i.e., on the negative effect of TNF-α-induced autophagy inhibition and apoptosis activation. Previous studies reported that in addition to the NF-κB signaling pathway, other signaling pathways such as the MAPK/JNK and ERK pathways are also involved in the pathogenesis process of OA (Wang et al., 2018). In the future experiments, we would like to verify whether icariin protects against OA via these or other signaling pathways.

Tissue engineering is an evolving interdisciplinary field integrating medicine, material science, biochemistry, and biomedical engineering, which centered on development of biological alternates to restore and/or to improve tissue and organ function (Tao et al., 2013; Tao et al., 2016; Zhu et al., 2018). Along with the development of biomaterial, the drug delivery system has attracted more attention in the treatment of cancer, diabetes and OA (Tao et al., 2017b; Wang J. et al., 2017; Zhao et al., 2017; Maudens et al., 2018). Jiang et al. (2018) developed a poly (lactic-co-glycolic acid)-based nanoscale drug delivery system for the treatment of OA. Li et al. (2012) reported that icariin up-regulated the expressions of aggrecan, sox9, and collagen I of chondrocytes, features which make it a potential promoting compound for cartilage tissue engineering. Previous studies found that targeted microspheres loaded with icariin could exert colon-protective effects through reduction of the inflammatory response (Wang et al., 2016). Pan et al. (2016) also reported that icariin loaded biphasic-induced magnetic CS/nHA/MNP microcapsules is a useful drug delivery system for bone repair . Considering the various beneficial effects of icariin, it could be considered an excellent compound to be used in drug-delivery system. In the future studies, we plan to look for a good biocompatibility drug delivery system which is suitable to load icariin for the treatment of OA.

In conclusion, we demonstrated that icariin had no cytotoxic effects on chondrocytes up to the dose of 20 μM. TNF-α induced inhibition of autophagy and activation of apoptosis, and increased inflammatory cytokines, NO and ROS, as well as stimulating catabolism. These negative effects could be partially reversed by adding icariin to TNF-α-treated chondrocytes via inhibition of NF-κB signaling. Thus, the present study highlights that icariin induces autophagy activation and apoptosis inhibition of chondrocytes via suppression of the NF-κB signaling pathway. Future *in vivo* evaluation using macro-hydrogels to explore icariin's therapeutic potential in OA treatment is currently under way in our laboratory.

AUTHOR CONTRIBUTIONS

BM, WZ, and GL conceived and designed the experiments. JL, YL, and LH performed the experiments. BM and JW wrote the manuscript and made the same contribution to the manuscript. AP revised the language of the manuscript.

FUNDING

The study was supported by the Natural Science Foundation of Hubei Province (Grant No. WJ2017Q025), the Science and Technology Department of Hubei Province (Grant No. 2016CFB303), and the Free Innovation Research Fund of Wuhan Union Hospital.

REFERENCES

Akuri, M. C., Barbalho, S. M., Val, R. M., and Guiguer, E. L. (2017). Reflections about Osteoarthritis and *Curcuma longa*. *Pharmacogn. Rev.* 11, 8–12. doi: 10.4103/phrev.phrev_54_16

Ansari, M. Y., Khan, N. M., and Haqqi, T. M. (2017). A standardized extract of *Butea monosperma* (Lam.) flowers suppresses the IL-1beta-induced expression of IL-6 and matrix-metalloproteases by activating autophagy in human osteoarthritis chondrocytes. *Biomed. Pharmacother.* 96, 198–207. doi: 10.1016/j.biopha.2017.09.140

Blanco, F. J., Rego, I., and Ruiz-Romero, C. (2011). The role of mitochondria in osteoarthritis. *Nat. Rev. Rheumatol.* 7, 161–169. doi: 10.1038/nrrheum.2010.213

Bouderlique, T., Vuppalapati, K. K., Newton, P. T., Li, L., Barenius, B., and Chagin, A. S. (2016). Targeted deletion of Atg5 in chondrocytes promotes age-related osteoarthritis. *Ann. Rheum. Dis.* 75, 627–631. doi: 10.1136/annrheumdis-2015-207742

Chen, P., Xia, C., Mei, S., Wang, J., Shan, Z., Lin, X., et al. (2016). Intra-articular delivery of sinomenium encapsulated by chitosan microspheres and photo-crosslinked GelMA hydrogel ameliorates osteoarthritis by effectively regulating autophagy. *Biomaterials* 81, 1–13. doi: 10.1016/j.biomaterials.2015.12.006

Chen, S. R., Xu, X. Z., Wang, Y. H., Chen, J. W., Xu, S. W., Gu, L. Q., et al. (2010). Icariin derivative inhibits inflammation through suppression of p38 mitogen-activated protein kinase and nuclear factor-kappaB pathways. *Biol. Pharm. Bull.* 33, 1307–1313. doi: 10.1248/bpb.33.1307

Deng, X., Wu, W., Liang, H., Huang, D., Jing, D., Zheng, D., et al. (2017). Icariin prevents IL-1beta-induced apoptosis in human nucleus pulposus via the PI3K/AKT pathway. *Evid. Based Complement. Alternat. Med.* 2017:2198323. doi: 10.1155/2017/2198323

Ding, L., Zhu, X., Wang, Y., Shi, B., Ling, X., Chen, H., et al. (2017). Intracellular fate of nanoparticles with polydopamine surface engineering and a novel strategy for exocytosis-inhibiting, lysosome impairment-based cancer therapy. *Nano Lett.* 17, 6790–6801. doi: 10.1021/acs.nanolett.7b03021

Duarte, J. H. (2015). Osteoarthritis: autophagy prevents age-related OA. *Nat. Rev. Rheumatol.* 11:683. doi: 10.1038/nrrheum.2015.145

Dubey, S., Yoon, H., Cohen, M. S., Nagarkatti, P., Nagarkatti, M., and Karan, D. (2018). Withaferin A associated differential regulation of inflammatory cytokines. *Front. Immunol.* 9:195. doi: 10.3389/fimmu.2018.00195

Fang, J., and Zhang, Y. (2017). Icariin, an anti-atherosclerotic drug from chinese medicinal herb horny goat weed. *Front. Pharmacol.* 8:734. doi: 10.3389/fphar.2017.00734

Galluzzi, L., Pietrocola, F., Levine, B., and Kroemer, G. (2014). Metabolic control of autophagy. *Cell* 159, 1263–1276. doi: 10.1016/j.cell.2014.11.006

Glyn-Jones, S., Palmer, A. J., Agricola, R., Price, A. J., Vincent, T. L., Weinans, H., et al. (2015). Osteoarthritis. *Lancet* 386, 376–387. doi: 10.1016/S0140-6736(14)60802-3

Goldring, M. B., and Otero, M. (2011). Inflammation in osteoarthritis. *Curr. Opin. Rheumatol.* 23, 471–478. doi: 10.1097/BOR.0b013e328349c2b1

Guo, B., Yang, N., Borysiewicz, E., Dudek, M., Williams, J. L., Li, J., et al. (2015). Catabolic cytokines disrupt the circadian clock and the expression of clock-controlled genes in cartilage via an NFsmall ka, CyrillicB-dependent pathway. *Osteoarthr. Cartil.* 23, 1981–1988. doi: 10.1016/j.joca.2015.02.020

Hong, E. H., Song, J. Y., Lee, S. J., Park, I. C., Um, H. D., Park, J. K., et al. (2014). Low-dose gamma-radiation inhibits IL-1beta-induced dedifferentiation and inflammation of articular chondrocytes via blockage of catenin signaling. *IUBMB Life* 66, 128–137. doi: 10.1002/iub.1248

Hua, W., Zhang, Y., Wu, X., Kang, L., Tu, J., Zhao, K., et al. (2018). Icariin attenuates interleukin-1beta-induced inflammatory response in human nucleus pulposus cells. *Curr. Pharm. Des.* 23, 6071–6078. doi: 10.2174/1381612823666170615112158

Jiang, L. B., Meng, D. H., Lee, S. M., Liu, S. H., Xu, Q. T., Wang, Y., et al. (2016). Dihydroartemisinin inhibits catabolism in rat chondrocytes by activating autophagy via inhibition of the NF-kappaB pathway. *Sci. Rep.* 6:38979. doi: 10.1038/srep38979

Jiang, T., Kan, H. M., Rajpura, K., Carbone, E. J., Li, Y., and Lo, K. W. (2018). Development of targeted nanoscale drug delivery system for Osteoarthritic cartilage tissue. *J. Nanosci. Nanotechnol.* 18, 2310–2317. doi: 10.1166/jnn.2018.14311

Kobayashi, H., Chang, S. H., Mori, D., Itoh, S., Hirata, M., Hosaka, Y., et al. (2016). Biphasic regulation of chondrocytes by Rela through induction of anti-apoptotic and catabolic target genes. *Nat. Commun.* 7:13336. doi: 10.1038/ncomms13336

Lai, Y., Bai, X., Zhao, Y., Tian, Q., Liu, B., Lin, E. A., et al. (2014). ADAMTS-7 forms a positive feedback loop with TNF-alpha in the pathogenesis of osteoarthritis. *Ann. Rheum. Dis.* 73, 1575–1584. doi: 10.1136/annrheumdis-2013-203561

Li, D., Yuan, T., Zhang, X., Xiao, Y., Wang, R., Fan, Y., et al. (2012). Icariin: a potential promoting compound for cartilage tissue engineering. *Osteoarthr. Cartil.* 20, 1647–1656. doi: 10.1016/j.joca.2012.08.009

Li, H., Yuan, Y., Zhang, Y., Zhang, X., Gao, L., and Xu, R. (2017). Icariin inhibits AMPK-dependent autophagy and adipogenesis in adipocytes *In vitro* and in a model of graves' Orbitopathy *In vivo*. *Front. Physiol.* 8:45. doi: 10.3389/fphys.2017.00045

Liu-Bryan, R., and Terkeltaub, R. (2015). Emerging regulators of the inflammatory process in osteoarthritis. *Nat. Rev. Rheumatol.* 11, 35–44. doi: 10.1038/nrrheum.2014.162

Loeser, R. F., Collins, J. A., and Diekman, B. O. (2016). Ageing and the pathogenesis of osteoarthritis. *Nat. Rev. Rheumatol.* 12, 412–420. doi: 10.1038/nrrheum.2016.65

Maudens, P., Seemayer, C. A., Pfefferle, F., Jordan, O., and Allemann, E. (2018). Nanocrystals of a potent p38 MAPK inhibitor embedded in microparticles: therapeutic effects in inflammatory and mechanistic murine models of osteoarthritis. *J. Control. Release* 276, 102–112. doi: 10.1016/j.jconrel.2018.03.007

Nasi, S., So, A., Combes, C., Daudon, M., and Busso, N. (2016). Interleukin-6 and chondrocyte mineralisation act in tandem to promote experimental osteoarthritis. *Ann. Rheum. Dis.* 75, 1372–1379. doi: 10.1136/annrheumdis-2015-207487

Pan, L., Zhang, Y., Chen, N., and Yang, L. (2017). Icariin regulates cellular functions and gene expression of osteoarthritis patient-derived human fibroblast-like synoviocytes. *Int. J. Mol. Sci.* 18:2656. doi: 10.3390/ijms18122656

Pan, P., Chen, J., Fan, T., Hu, Y., Wu, T., and Zhang, Q. (2016). Facile preparation of biphasic-induced magnetic icariin-loaded composite microcapsules by automated in situ click technology. *Colloids Surf. B Biointerfaces* 140, 50–59. doi: 10.1016/j.colsurfb.2015.12.027

Qi, Y., Zhang, M., Li, H., Frank, J. A., Dai, L., Liu, H., et al. (2014). Autophagy inhibition by sustained overproduction of IL6 contributes to arsenic carcinogenesis. *Cancer Res.* 74, 3740–3752. doi: 10.1158/0008-5472.CAN-13-3182

Qiao, C., Ye, W., Li, S., Wang, H., and Ding, X. (2018). Icariin modulates mitochondrial function and apoptosis in high glucose-induced glomerular podocytes through G protein-coupled estrogen receptors. *Mol. Cell. Endocrinol.* doi: 10.1016/j.mce.2018.01.014 [Epub ahead of print].

Raman, S., FitzGerald, U., and Murphy, J. M. (2018). Interplay of inflammatory mediators with epigenetics and cartilage modifications in osteoarthritis. *Front. Bioeng. Biotechnol.* 6:22. doi: 10.3389/fbioe.2018.00022

Rosenblum, D., Joshi, N., Tao, W., Karp, J. M., and Dan, P. (2018). Progress and challenges towards targeted delivery of cancer therapeutics. *Nat. Commun.* 9:1410. doi: 10.1038/s41467-018-03705-y

Shen, C., Cai, G. Q., Peng, J. P., and Chen, X. D. (2015). Autophagy protects chondrocytes from glucocorticoids-induced apoptosis via ROS/Akt/FOXO3 signaling. *Osteoarthr. Cartil.* 23, 2279–2287. doi: 10.1016/j.joca.2015.06.020

Sun, X., Deng, X., Cai, W., Li, W., Shen, Z., Jiang, T., et al. (2018). Icariin inhibits LPS-induced cell inflammatory response by promoting GRalpha nuclear translocation and upregulating GRalpha expression. *Life Sci.* 195, 33–43. doi: 10.1016/j.lfs.2018.01.006

Tang, Y., Jacobi, A., Vater, C., Zou, L., Zou, X., and Stiehler, M. (2015). Icariin promotes angiogenic differentiation and prevents oxidative stress-induced autophagy in endothelial progenitor cells. *Stem Cells* 33, 1863–1877. doi: 10.1002/stem.2005

Tao, W., Ji, X., Xu, X., Islam, M. A., Li, Z., Chen, S., et al. (2017a). Antimonene quantum dots: synthesis and application as near-infrared photothermal agents for effective cancer therapy. *Angew. Chem.* 56, 11896–11900. doi: 10.1002/anie.201703657

Tao, W., Zhu, X., Yu, X., Zeng, X., Xiao, Q., Zhang, X., et al. (2017b). Black phosphorus nanosheets as a robust delivery platform for cancer theranostics. *Adv. Mater.* 29:1603276. doi: 10.1002/adma.201603276

Tao, W., Zeng, X., Liu, T., Wang, Z., Xiong, Q., Ouyang, C., et al. (2013). Docetaxel-loaded nanoparticles based on star-shaped mannitol-core PLGA-TPGS diblock copolymer for breast cancer therapy. *Acta Biomater.* 9, 8910–8920. doi: 10.1016/j.actbio.2013.06.034

Tao, W., Zeng, X., Wu, J., Zhu, X., Yu, X., Zhang, X., et al. (2016). Polydopamine-based surface modification of novel nanoparticle-aptamer bioconjugates for in vivo breast cancer targeting and enhanced therapeutic effects. *Theranostics* 6, 470–484. doi: 10.7150/thno.14184

Tao, W., Zhang, J., Zeng, X., Liu, D., Liu, G., Zhu, X., et al. (2015). Blended nanoparticle system based on miscible structurally similar polymers: a safe, simple, targeted, and surprisingly high efficiency vehicle for cancer therapy. *Adv. Healthc. Mater.* 4, 1203–1214. doi: 10.1002/adhm.201400751

Urech, D. M., Feige, U., Ewert, S., Schlosser, V., Ottiger, M., Polzer, K., et al. (2010). Anti-inflammatory and cartilage-protecting effects of an intra-articularly injected anti-TNF{alpha} single-chain Fv antibody (ESBA105) designed for local therapeutic use. *Ann. Rheum. Dis.* 69, 443–449. doi: 10.1136/ard.2008.105775

Vasheghani, F., Zhang, Y., Li, Y. H., Blati, M., Fahmi, H., Lussier, B., et al. (2015). PPARgamma deficiency results in severe, accelerated osteoarthritis associated with aberrant mTOR signalling in the articular cartilage. *Ann. Rheum. Dis.* 74, 569–578. doi: 10.1136/annrheumdis-2014-205743

Wang, G. Q., Li, D. D., Huang, C., Lu, D. S., Zhang, C., Zhou, S. Y., et al. (2017). Icariin reduces dopaminergic neuronal loss and microglia-mediated inflammation in vivo and in vitro. *Front. Mol. Neurosci.* 10:441. doi: 10.3389/fnmol.2017.00441

Wang, J., Tao, W., Chen, X., Farokhzad, O. C., and Liu, G. (2017). Emerging advances in nanotheranostics with intelligent bioresponsive systems. *Theranostics* 7, 3915–3919. doi: 10.7150/thno.21317

Wang, P., Mao, Z., Pan, Q., Lu, R., Huang, X., Shang, X., et al. (2018). Histone deacetylase-4 and histone deacetylase-8 regulate interleukin-1beta-induced cartilage catabolic degradation through MAPK/JNK and ERK pathways. *Int. J. Mol. Med.* 41, 2117–2127. doi: 10.3892/ijmm.2018.3410

Wang, Q. S., Wang, G. F., Zhou, J., Gao, L. N., and Cui, Y. L. (2016). Colon targeted oral drug delivery system based on alginate-chitosan microspheres loaded with icariin in the treatment of ulcerative colitis. *Int. J. Pharm.* 515, 176–185. doi: 10.1016/j.ijpharm.2016.10.002

Wang, Y. K., and Huang, Z. Q. (2005). Protective effects of icariin on human umbilical vein endothelial cell injury induced by H2O2 in vitro. *Pharmacol. Res.* 52, 174–182. doi: 10.1016/j.phrs.2005.02.023

Xiong, W., Zhang, W., Yuan, W., Du, H., Ming, K., Yao, F., et al. (2017). Phosphorylation of icariin can alleviate the oxidative stress caused by the duck hepatitis virus a through mitogen-activated protein kinases signaling pathways. *Front. Microbiol.* 8:1850. doi: 10.3389/fmicb.2017.01850

Ye, J., Wu, G., Li, X., Li, Z., Zheng, C., Liu, X., et al. (2015). Millimeter wave treatment inhibits apoptosis of chondrocytes via regulation dynamic equilibrium of intracellular free Ca (2+). *Evid. Based Complement. Alternat. Med.* 2015:464161. doi: 10.1155/2015/464161

Zeng, L., Wang, W., Rong, X. F., Zhong, Y., Jia, P., Zhou, G. Q., et al. (2014). Chondroprotective effects and multi-target mechanisms of Icariin in IL-1 beta-induced human SW 1353 chondrosarcoma cells and a rat osteoarthritis model. *Int. Immunopharmacol.* 18, 175–181. doi: 10.1016/j.intimp.2013.11.021

Zhang, D., Wang, Z., Sheng, C., Peng, W., Hui, S., Gong, W., et al. (2015). Icariin prevents amyloid beta-induced apoptosis via the PI3K/Akt pathway in PC-12 cells. *Evid. Based Complement. Alternat. Med.* 2015:235265. doi: 10.1155/2015/235265

Zhang, H. B., Zhang, Y., Chen, C., Li, Y. Q., Ma, C., and Wang, Z. J. (2016). Pioglitazone inhibits advanced glycation end product-induced matrix metalloproteinases and apoptosis by suppressing the activation of MAPK and NF-kappaB. *Apoptosis* 21, 1082–1093. doi: 10.1007/s10495-016-1280-z

Zhao, L., Huang, Q., Liu, Y., Wang, Q., Wang, L., Xiao, S., et al. (2017). Boronic acid as glucose-sensitive agent regulates drug delivery for diabetes treatment. *Materials* 10:E170. doi: 10.3390/ma1002 0170

Zhu, X., Ji, X., Kong, N., Chen, Y., Mahmoudi, M., Xu, X., et al. (2018). Intracellular mechanistic understanding of 2D MoS2 nanosheets for anti-exocytosis-enhanced synergistic cancer therapy. *ACS Nano* 12, 2922–2938. doi: 10.1021/acsnano.8b00516

17

Lipid Nanoparticles-Encapsulated YF4: A Potential Therapeutic Oral Peptide Delivery System for Hypertension Treatment

Shengnan Zhao[1†], Jinhua Li[1,2†], Yang Zhou[1,2†], Lingjing Huang[3], Yanfei Li[3], Juanjuan Xu[3], Chunmei Fu[3], Xia Guo[2*] and Jian Yang[1*]*

[1] School of Applied Chemistry and Biological Technology, Shenzhen Polytechnic, Shenzhen, China, [2] Key Laboratory of Birth Defect and Related Disorders of Women and Children, Department of Pediatric Hematology/Oncology, West China Second University Hospital, Sichuan University, Chengdu, China, [3] Key Laboratory of Drug Targeting and Drug Delivery System (Ministry of Education), West China School of Pharmacy, Sichuan University, Chengdu, China

***Correspondence:**
Chunmei Fu
fuchunmei@scu.edu.cn
Xia Guo
guoxkl@163.com
Jian Yang
jiany@szpt.edu.cn

† These authors have contributed equally to this work

Drugs are administered orally in the clinical treatment of hypertension. Antihypertensive peptides have excellent angiotensin converting enzyme inhibitors activity *in vitro*. However, the poor oral bioavailability and therapeutic effect of antihypertensive peptides were mainly caused by rapid degradation in gastrointestinal and the short circulation time in blood, which remain to be further optimized. Therefore, the novel oral peptide delivery system is urged to improve the oral absorption and efficacy of peptide drugs. In this work, Tyr-Gly-Leu-Phe (YF4)-loaded lipid nanoparticles (YF4-LNPs) combined the advantages of polymer nanoparticles and liposomes were developed, which could greatly enhance the oral bioavailability and ameliorate the sustained release of peptide drug. YF4 loaded nanoparticles (YF4-NPs) were firstly prepared by a double-emulsion internal phase/organic phase/external phase (W1/O/W2) solvent evaporation method. YF4-NPs were further coated by membrane hydration-ultrasonic dispersion method to obtain the YF4-LNPs. The optimal YF4-LNPs showed a small particle size of 227.3 ± 3.8 nm, zeta potential of -7.27 ± 0.85 mV and high entrapment efficiency of $90.28 \pm 1.23\%$. Transmission electronic microscopy analysis showed that the core-shell lipid nanoparticles were spherical shapes with an apparent lipid bilayer on the surface. Differential scanning calorimetry further proved that YF4 was successfully entrapped into YF4-LNPs. The optimal preparation of YF4-LNPs exhibited sustained release of YF4 *in vitro* and a 5 days long-term antihypertensive effect *in vivo*. In summary, the lipid nanoparticles for oral antihypertensive peptide delivery were successfully constructed, which might have a promising future for hypertension treatment.

Keywords: lipid nanoparticles, antihypertensive peptide, hypertension, oral administration, sustained release, continuously antihypertensive effect

INTRODUCTION

Nanotechnology has been widely used to improve the oral absorption and therapeutic efficacy of small molecule peptide drugs, which have shown tremendous potentials but great challenges (Olbrich et al., 2001; Tan et al., 2009; Li et al., 2013; Yang et al., 2013; Thi et al., 2015; Wang et al., 2018). Poly-(lactic-co-glycolic) acid (PLGA) nanoparticles have attracted much attention, owing to the unique properties of biodegradability, biocompatibility, and sustained release (Musumeci et al., 2006). Liposomes also have been applied for drug delivery due to the superior biocompatibility, drug absorption and nontoxicity (Wang and Liu, 2013). Unfortunately, both of them have some unsatisfied disadvantages in peptide delivery, such as leakage and safety issues, which seriously limited the delivery efficiency. It is necessary to deal with these problems for improving the oral delivery efficiency of peptides (Luo et al., 2006).

Lipid coating PLGA nanoparticles system (lipid nanoparticles, LNPs) has not only combined the advantages of polymer nanoparticles and liposomes but efficiently avoided the defects of them (Muller and Keck, 2004; Alavi et al., 2017). The dual advantages of the particles and vesicle make it an excellent oral drug carrier with high biocompatibility and sustained release (Xie et al., 2018). In this system, drugs can be efficiently encapsulated in the nanoparticles core and/or the lipid bilayers, resulted in increased drug load capability. The drug diffusion rate can be delayed by the polymer core. Additionally, the stability of the LNPs can be further increased by the lipid shell (Nogués et al., 2006). However, it is still challenging to achieve high encapsulation efficiency (EE) and decent particle size when incorporating hydrophilic drugs into LNPs.

Hypertension has become a strong risk factor for cardiovascular disease and affected almost 2 billion people. In detail, it has highly correlated with the heart attack, cerebral hemorrhage, stroke, kidney failure and blindness (Kjeldsen, 2017). Angiotensin-converting enzyme (ACE), located in various tissues, is potent to affect the cascade of process that trigger the increasing of blood pressure. Hence, ACE inhibitors (ACEIs) are commonly used to decrease blood pressure (Girgih et al., 2016). However, the synthetic ACEIs were reported to produce negative side effects such as dry cough, angioedema, itch, diarrhea (Tenenbaum et al., 2000; Abassi et al., 2009), and renal impairment. Alternatively, natural antihypertensive peptide fragments have gradually entered the field of human vision due to the sound security.

YF4, a polypeptide extracted from milk protein, has been reported for the opioid activity for the first time in 1986 (Yoshikawa et al., 1986). Other research groups have conducted other pharmacological studies and found that it had hypotensive activity as well (Espejo-Carpio et al., 2013). However, the antihypertensive peptides are usually accompanied by extremely poor stability and easily degraded by gastric acid and pepsin in the gastrointestinal (GI). At present, the existing peptide drugs in clinical are given mainly by injection (Boelsma and Kloek, 2010; Majumder et al., 2013). Because of the short circulation time (Agrawal et al., 2015) and degradation of polypeptide drugs in the GI, the patients need to be injected frequently which results in the poor compliance (Cleland et al., 2012). To address these issues, novel oral peptide delivery systems are urged to improve their stability in the stomach and intestines in order to improve its therapy effect with a convenient and economic way (Niu et al., 2018).

In the present study, we chose the antihypertensive peptide YF4 as a model drug to systematically optimize the lipid nanoparticles and investigate it's potential in oral peptide delivery. The formulation parameters of YF4-LNPs were systematically investigated. The physic-chemical properties including particle size, surface charge, EE, Transmission electron microscope (TEM), Differential scanning calorimeter (DSC), and *in vitro* release profile were then characterized systemically. Additionally, the *in vivo* antihypertensive efficacy was assessed on spontaneously hypertensive rats.

MATERIALS AND METHODS

Materials

YF4 (purity > 99%) was gained from Phtdpeptides Co., Ltd. (Zhengzhou, China). PLGA (MW = 15 kDa; LA/GA = 75:25) was purchased from Jinan Daigang Biomaterial Co., Ltd. (Jinan, China). Poly (vinyl alcohol) (PVA, MW = 30–70 kDa, HD, 80%) and TPGS were obtained from Sigma-Aldrich (St. Louis, MO, United States). Soybean phosphatidylcholine (SP) was gained from Shanghai A.V.T. Pharmaceutical Co., Ltd (Shanghai, China). Carbomer 996 was supplied by Hang Zhou Carbokar Import & Export Co., Ltd. (Hang Zhou, China). Poloxamer 188 was acquired from BASFSE (Germany). $mPEG_{2000}$-Chol (purity > 98.6%) was synthesized by State Key Laboratory of Biotherapy, Sichuan University. Cholesterol was purchased from Shanghai source poly Biotechnology Co., Ltd.). All other reagents were of analytical grade and were used unless otherwise stated.

Animals

Twelve weeks old male spontaneously hypertensive rats (SHRs) with a circa weight between 250 and 320 g were purchased from Beijing Vital River Laboratory Animal Technology Co., Ltd. After a week of adaption, animals were admitted to experiments (six per group). Animals were maintained under 12 h dark and light cycles at controlled temperature, 55% humidity, 22°C. The rats were free access to food and water. All the experiments were approved and supervised by the State Key Laboratory of Biotherapy Animal Care and Use Committee (Sichuan University, Chengdu, Sichuan, China). In this study, groups of rats were used for the oral administration of saline group, Captopril group vs. YF4 group, YF4 vs. YF4-NPs vs YF4-LNPs.

Preparation of YF4-LNPs

YF4-NPs were prepared by an easy and controllable method. The YF4-NPs were further coated by membrane hydration-ultrasonic dispersion method to obtain the lipid nanoparticles (YF4-LNPs). Firstly, the core of YF4-LNPs (YF4-NPs) was prepared by a double-emulsion internal phase/organic phase/external phase (W1/O/W2) solvent evaporation method (Yu et al., 2016). In brief, 50 μL YF4 (10 mg/mL) deionized water solution was used to form the inner aqueous phase. The 1 mL organic phase (mixed solution of acetone and acetonitrile, initial volume ratio was 5:1) containing PLGA was used as the organic phase, and then mixed with the inner aqueous phase by probe sonication in ice bath to form the primary W1/O emulsion. The primary emulsion was then added to the 4 mL external phase solution and further sonicated to obtain the final W1/O/W2 double emulsion. The organic phase in the ultimate emulsion was rapidly removed by evaporation under vacuum at 37°C to get YF4-NPs. At the same time, SP (lipid), cholesterol (Chol) and $mPEG_{2000}$-cholmixture (the mass ratio was 4:1:0.25) were dissolved in 2 mL chloroform at a certain proportion. The organic solvents were subsequently removed using a rotary evaporator (R-201Shanghai Shen Shun Biological Technology Co., Ltd.) to produce a thin film of lipid at 37°C. The lipid film was hydrated with 4 mL prepared YF4-NPs for 1 h at 60°C to obtain a suspension. YF4-LNPs were finally acquired by Ultrasonic cell crushing and isolating machine (VCX130, American Systems on ICs).

Characterization of YF4-LNPs

Particle Size and Zeta Potential

The mean particle size, size distribution and ζ potential were measured by Zetasizer (Zetasizer Nano-ZS 90; Malvern Instruments Ltd., Malvern, United Kingdom) at 25°C. The prepared YF4-LNPs were diluted with deionized water and experiments were conducted in triplicate. All the data were presented as mean ± SD.

Entrapment Efficiency and Drug Loading

Briefly, the obtained supernatant by ultrafiltration centrifuging the colloidal suspension during the preparation of YF4-LNPs was stored to determine the EE and drug loading capacity (DL) of YF4-LNPs as previously described (Yu et al., 2016). The untrapped YF4 in supernatant was determined by high performance liquid chromatography (HPLC, Waters Alliance 2695) to calculate the amount of YF4 unpackaged into YF4-LNPs. Analyses were performed in triplicate and the values were expressed as mean ± SD. EE and DL of YF4 were calculated as following formulas:

$$EE\% = \left(\frac{\text{TotalYF4amount} - \text{AmountofYF4insupernatant}}{\text{TotalYF4amount}}\right) \times 100$$

$$DL\% = \left(\frac{\text{TotalYF4amount} - \text{AmountofYF4insupernatant}}{\text{Totalweightoflipidnanoparticles}}\right) \times 100$$

Stability

YF4-LNPs were stored at 4°C for two weeks to investigate the preliminary stability. The changes of particle size and EE of YF4-LNPs were examined by the methods described above. Analyses were performed in triplicate and the values were expressed as mean ± S.D.

Appearance and Morphology

The appearance and Tyndall effect of YF4-LNPs were observed by a digital camera. The morphology of the YF4-LNPs was examined by TEM (H-600, Hitachi, Japan). In brief, the prepared samples were diluted to proper concentration by deionized water and then were placed on a copper electron microscopy grid and negatively stained with 2wt% phosphotungstic acid solution for 30 s for observation.

Differential Scanning Calorimetry (DSC)

The physical state of YF4 loaded in YF4-LNPs was verified by DSC (200PC, Netzsch, Karlsruhe, Germany). Freeze-dried YF4-LNPs, blank LNPs, YF4, and the physical mixture of blank LNPs and free YF4 with the same mass ratio as those in YF4-LNPs were heated from 75 to 250°C at a heating ramp of 20°C/min under nitrogen atmosphere at a flow rate of 50 mL/min.

In vitro Release Studies

The *in vitro* release profiles of YF4-LNPs were investigated in PBS buffer at pH 1.0 (simulated gastric fluid), pH 4.5, pH 6.8 (simulated different intestinal fluids), and pH 7.4 (physiological pH condition) by dynamic dialysis method (Boelsma and Kloek, 2010). In brief, free YF4 solution, YF4-NPs, and YF4-LNPs were first dispersed in release media in dialysis bags (MWCO 3000) and then were shaken at 37°C with a speed of 100 rpm. One milliliter buffer was removed and replaced with equal volume fresh release medium at 0, 2, 4, 8, 12 h, respectively. The content of YF4 was measured by HPLC after centrifugation for 10 min at 13,000 rpm as described in section of "Entrapment efficiency and drug loading." Analyses were performed in triplicate and the values were expressed as mean ± S.D.

In vivo Antihypertensive Efficacy

Before the experiment, we first verified the antihypertensive activity of YF4 in SHRs. Simultaneously, the captopril and the saline water were used as the positive control and control group, respectively. SHRs were randomly divided into three groups (n = 6). Control group were treated with 0.9% saline water, and the other groups were treated with captopril (5 mg/kg) or the same dose of YF4 dissolved in saline water. All rats were administered at a single oral dose. Blood pressure was indirectly recorded using the tail-cuff method (BP-2010A, Softron Beijing Biotechnology, China) at each of the following times: 0, 2, 4, 8, 12, and 24 h after administration.

In YF4-LNPs pharmacodynamics study, the SHRs were randomly divided into three groups (n = 6). Control group were treated with 0.9% saline water, the other groups of SHRs were treated withYF4 and YF4-LNPs. All the groups of rats were given the same dose at 0.8 mg/kg body weight. Blood pressure was indirectly recorded as described above. Aside from free YF4 group, all the other groups were needed to detect blood pressure at more time points every day after administration until the pressure reached to normal level. All the SBP were measured for three times to get the average value at each time point.

Statistical Analysis

The obtained data were analyzed using the Graph Pad Prism 5. Data were analyzed by one-way analysis of variance. $p < 0.05$ was considered a statistically difference, and $p < 0.01$ was considered a statistically significant difference.

RESULTS

Characterization of YF4-LNPs

Several factors that could affect the features of YF4-LNPs were systematically optimized to produce the desirable YF4-LNPs, including the PLGA concentration, the volume of acetone in the organic phase, the volume of the inner aqueous medium, the pH of the aqueous medium, the external water phase, the PVA concentration, the PVA volume, the ultrasonic time, PLGA to lipid material ratio, and the ultrasound power. Firstly, the influence of PLGA concentration on the EE and particle size was investigated in **Figure 1A**.The EE and the particle size were positively correlated with the PLGA amount within the range of 10–50 mg. **Figure 1B** showed that the EE was dually increased and then suddenly decreased when acetone volume was above 200 μL while the particle size was negatively correlated with the increasing of acetone volume in the organic phase. In **Figure 1C**, the EE firstly increased and then decreased dramatically with the increase of inner aqueous volume, whereas the particle size was negligibly affected by the volume of internal phase. As seen in **Figure 1D**, the EE occurred a sudden enlargement when the pH reached 13, whereas there were no obvious changes in particle size. As shown in **Figure 1E**, the PVA was used as the external water phase, both the EE and the particle size were desirable. **Figure 1F** illustrated the influence of the PVA concentration on EE and particle size. As PVA concentration increased, the EE firstly increased dramatically and then decreased over 1%. Simultaneously, the particle size was observed to slightly fluctuate as PVA concentration changed. As the volume of PVA increased, a slight downward trend of EE and a fluctuation of particle size were observed in the **Figure 1G**. In **Figure 1H**, as internal phase/organic phase (W1/O) ultrasonic time was prolonged, the EE increased dually firstly and then dropped, while particle size was relatively stable. Furthermore, the effect of the ultrasonic time of internal phase/organic phase/external phase (W1/O/W2) on EE and particle size was also investigated in **Figure 1I**. EE was firstly increased under short-term ultrasound condition, but was suddenly compromised when the ultrasonic time was beyond 45 s, while the particle size decreased with the ultrasonic time prolonged. Different ratios of PLGA vs. lipid bilayer materials (PLGA/LPs) were investigated in **Figure 1J**. The EE was also significantly affected by the PLGA/LPs ratio, while the particle size was relatively stable. **Figure 1J** showed that the formulations exhibited a better size and higher EE when the PLGA/LPs ratio was 1:1.5. It was shown in **Figure 1K** that with the ultrasound power increased from 100 to 500 W, both the EE and particle size exhibited a rapidly decreasing tendency. Overall, the optimal YF4-LNPs were demonstrated to significantly improve the drug incorporation with an EE of 89.88 ± 1.23% (n = 3) and DL of 2.18 ± 0.25%. The average particle size was 227.3 ± 3.8 nm with a narrow size distribution (PDI = 0.09 ± 0.02) (**Figure 2A**). The zeta potential of YF4-LNPs was slightly negative, with the value of −7.27 ± 0.85 mV (**Figure 2B**). The colloidal suspension was observed as slightly blue opalescence with strong Tyndall effect (**Figure 2C**).

As shown in the TEM image in **Figure 3A**, YF4-LNPs were generally spherical, homogeneous and the lipid bilayer

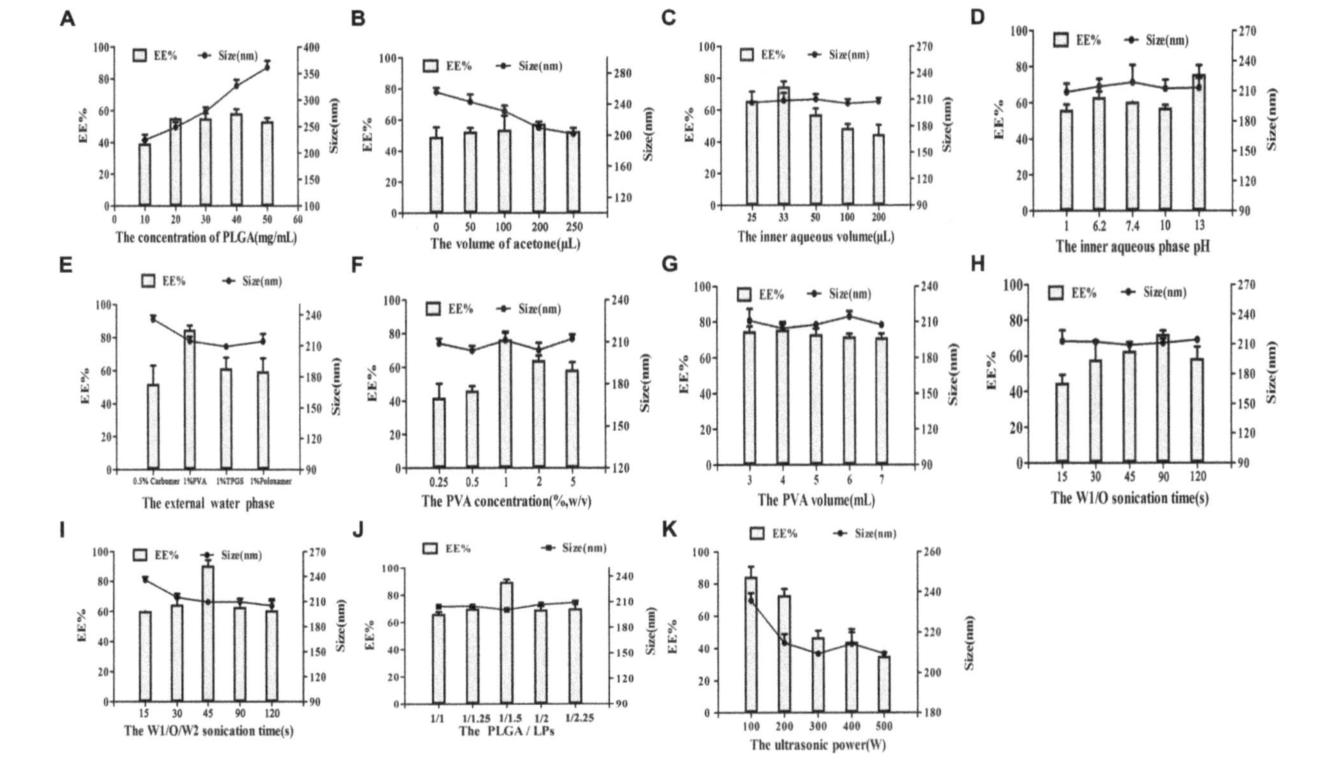

FIGURE 1 | Effect of various processing parameters on the particle size (nm) and EE of YF4-LNPs. **(A)** The concentration of PLGA, **(B)** The volume of acetone, **(C)** The volume of the inner aqueous medium, **(D)** The pH, **(E)** The external water phase, **(F)** The concentration and **(G)** The volume of PVA, **(H)** The ultrasonic time of W1/O and **(I)**W1/O/W2, **(J)** The ratio of PLGA/LPs, and **(K)** The ultrasonic power.

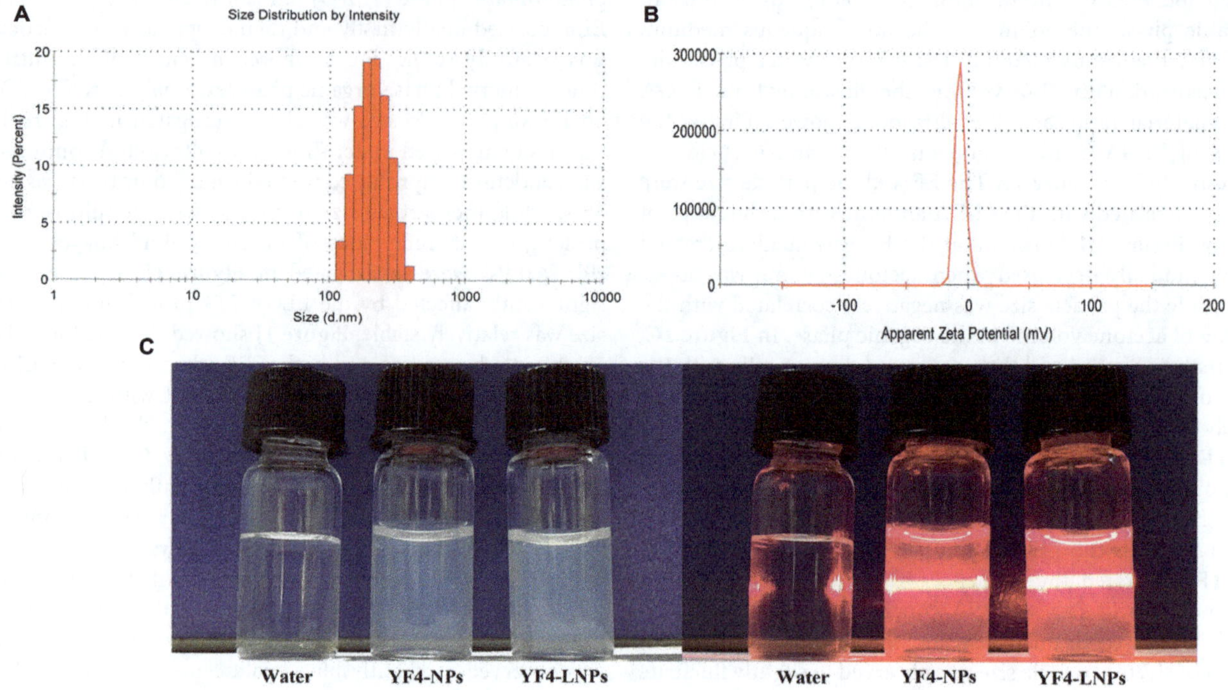

FIGURE 2 | Physical-chemical properties of YF4-LNPs. **(A)** Size distribution. **(B)** Zeta potential. **(C)** The appearance of YF4-LNPs.

was well coated on the nanoparticles. In **Figure 3B**, the DSC analysis showed that the free YF4 displayed an obviously sharp endothermic peak at 225.6°C. The YF4-LNPs only presented two smooth endothermic peaks at 140.1°C, 205.2°C, with the absent sharp endothermic peak of free YF4. However, in the physical mixture group, there were three endothermic peaks at 145.3°C, 202.3°C, and the peak at 226.9°C, which represented the free YF4.All the obtained statistics suggested that YF4 was successfully encapsulated into the YF4-LNPs. The stability study displayed that YF4-LNPs remained stable without change of EE and size for at least 1 week (**Figure 3C**). When YF4-LNPs were stored for 2 weeks, the EE of YF4 got a sharp drop and the particle size became larger, which illustrated that YF4-LNPs could keep stable in 4°C for 1 week and were suitable for developing an oral administration.

In vitro Release

In vitro release profiles of YF4 from YF4-LNPs were presented in **Figure 4** and **Supplementary Figure S2**, the free YF4 exhibited a burst release, and over 80% of YF4 released in 6 h, while those loaded in YF4-LNPs were released gradually without apparent burst release in all of the release media. Within a 12 h period, compared with the approximately total release of free YF4 at pH 4.5, 6.8, only less than 40% of YF4 was released from YF4-LNPs. Besides, over more than 40% of YF4 was still packed in the YF4-LNPs while the free YF4 was quickly released in the acid-like solution in the stomach (pH 1.0). All the results illustrated that YF4 was efficiently packed in YF4-LNPs and might achieve a sustained release in small intestine.

In vivo Antihypertensive Efficacy

To investigate the blood pressure lowing (BPL) effect of YF4, captopril was chosed as the positive control. As seen in the **Figure 5**, compared with saline group, the BPL effect of YF4 at a dose of 5 mg/kg presented at 2 h after a single oral administration was 23.0 mmHg, which was equal to captopril with the same dose. However, both of them showed the short BPL effect.

Then we prepared the lipid nanoparticles encapsulated YF4 and further investigated the BPL effect of YF4-LNPs in SHRs. As **Figure 6** showed, compared with saline group, YF4 and YF4-LNPs at a dose of 0.8 mg/kg all emerged a BPL effect. Administration of 0.8 mg/kg of YF4 signicantly decreased SBP by 15.6 mmHg at 4 h post-administration and SBP returned to the untreated level at 12 h post administration. And the decreased SBP between 2 and 120 h post administration was observed after treated by 0.8 mg/kg YF4 LNPs. YF4-LNPs at a dose of 0.8 mg/kg strikngly decreased the blood pressureby 43.5 mmHg about 2 h post administration. Amazingly, even after 120 h, obviously BPL effect was still seen as a significantly reduction of 20.5 mmHg. The SBP returned to the initial level at 144 h post administration.

DISCUSSION

The hypertension patients are required to lifelong medication, which severely affects the living quality. Oral administration is preferred due to its convenience and safety. However, the oral antihypertensive peptides still face enormous difficulties, such as the inactivation by acid and enzyme in the GI (Richard, 2017), low effienciency in penetrateing the mucous layer of the intestinal

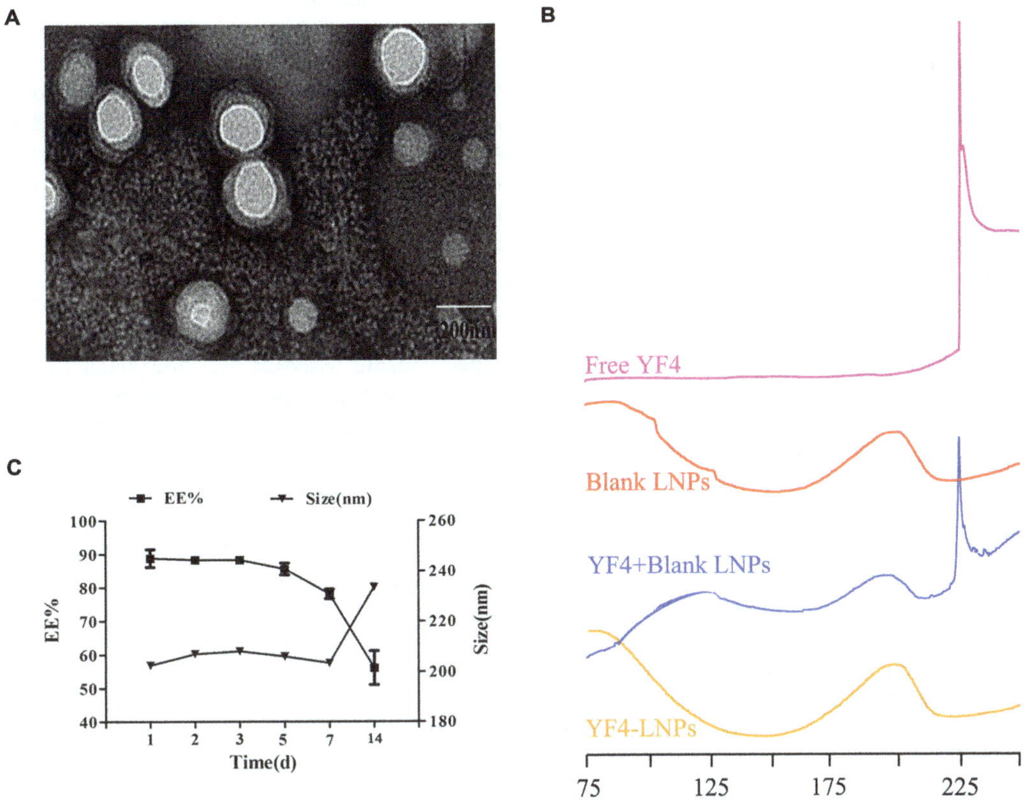

FIGURE 3 | Characterization of optimal YF4-LNPs. **(A)** TEM image of YF4-LNPs. **(B)** DSC curves of Free YF4, Blank LNPs, Blank LNPs, and YF4 mixture and YF4-LNPs. **(C)** Change in EE and size of YF4-LNPs in 2 weeks stored at 4°C.

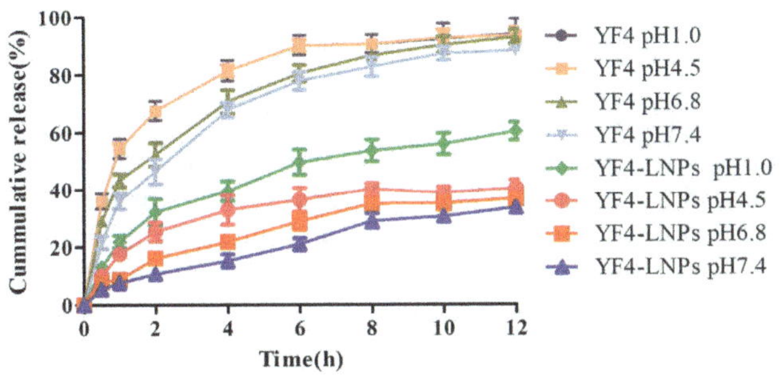

FIGURE 4 | Release profiles of free YF4 and YF4-LNPs in different phosphate buffers (pH1.0, 4.5, 6.8, and 7.4).

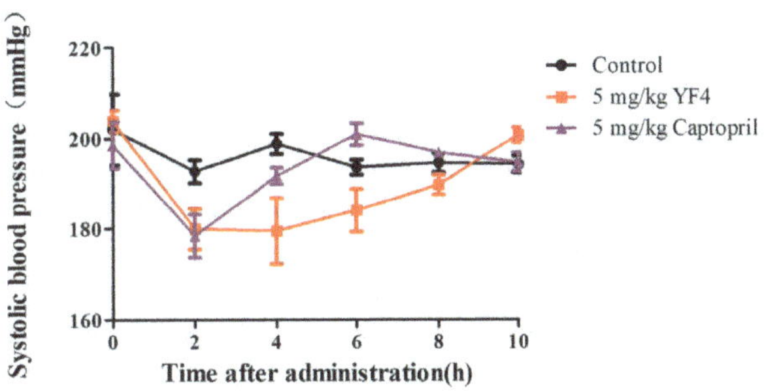

FIGURE 5 | Antihypertensive effects of Free YF4 and Captopril in SHRs within 10 h by a single oral administration of 5 mg/kg.

(Lai et al., 2009), and unable to be efficiently absorbed by small intestinal epithelial cells, which result in the depressing therpeacy effect (Ensign et al., 2012). These defects seriously limit the application of antihypertensive peptides, thus it is essential to develop a new oral antihypertensive peptide system to solve the problem of poor stability (Chen et al., 2015) and achieve the goal of long-term effect of blood pressure reduction.

PLGA nanoparticles, as a safe drug-loading system, can effectively slow the drug release and protect drugs from gastrointestinal degradation (Lozoya-Agullo et al., 2017; Mustafa et al., 2017). Then coating the lipid membrane on the particles can further protect the drugs from GI and improve the contact between the nanoparticles and the small intestinal epithelial cells, which may achieve the goal of prolonging the circulation in the blood. The formed LNPs are potential to increase the stability, permeability and bioavailability of drugs (Zhang et al., 2010; Fang et al., 2014) in the GI.

The formed YF4-LNPs were prepared by a simple and controllable method (Yu et al., 2016). It was reported that EE and partice size both have enormous influence on the quality

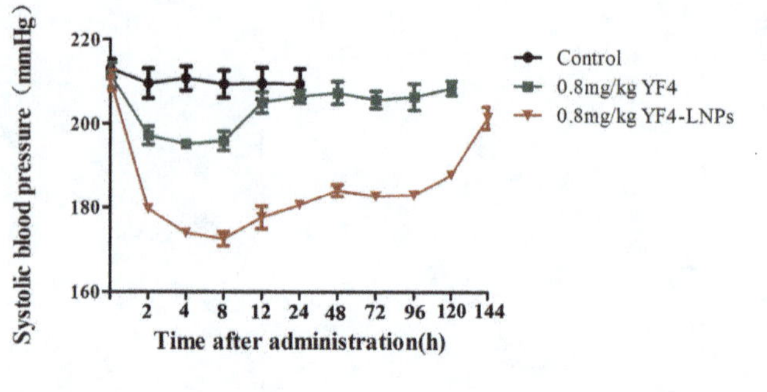

FIGURE 6 | Antihypertensive effects of same doses of YF4and YF4-LNPs in SHRs within 144 h by a single oral administration.

of nano-preparions (Johnstone et al., 2013). The utilization and absorption of drug can be improved by nano-preparions with higher EE and smaller particle size (Yu et al., 2016). Hence, factors which might influent the EE and size were optimized systemically, including the PLGA concentration, the volume of acetone in the organic phase, the pH of the aqueous medium, the volume of the inner aqueous medium, the external water phase, the PVA concentration, the PVA volume, the ultrasonic time, lipid material to nanomaterial ratio, and the ultrasound power. The an ever-growing PLGA viscosity in the organic phase caused droplets became larger and net shear stress became less, which would limit the free YF4 in inner aqueous diffuse into organic phase (**Figure 1**; Kiss et al., 2011; Turk et al., 2014). Therefore, the increasing PLGA concentration was indicated to lead to higher EE and larger particle size. The addition of acetone in the organic phase plays a great role in the nanoparticles forming (Anarjan et al., 2011). The addition of acetone in the organic phase could significantly affect the EE and particle size. The presence of acetone promoted organic phase to diffuse to inner phase (Luo et al., 2016), causing the carrier materials PLGA quickly precipitated and contained YF4 in the water phase, attributing to the EE increased. Whereas, too much acetone in the organic phase could also increase the opportunity of diffusion from inner to organic phase, which might result in the drug leakage (Yu et al., 2016). In addition, the interfacial energy at the oil/water interface was also reduced by the addition of acetone in the organic phase and thereby the stability of droplets was enhanced, which contributed to the smaller sizes of nanoparticles (Wang and Anderko, 2013). The opportunity of entrapment of the internal phase by the organic phase was enhanced as the W1/O volume ratio increased (Sang, 1999), which attribute to an excellent EE and a smaller particle size. However,when the W1/O volume ratio is too low or high, the W1/O emulsion structure was not complete, causing the poor EE and particle size. There is no doubt that the pH and ionizing status of peptide was highly related with the solubility of peptide (Ragab et al., 2004), which could affect the peptide loading state in the nanoparticles. When the pH was in isoelectric point (pI) of the YF4 peptide (Silva et al., 2013), in alkaline state, the state of charge distribution and the ionization state changed, the EE was significantly improved.

The effect of external water phase was also investigated. As an emulsifying agent, different external water phases make a great difference on the EE and particle size (Peng et al., 2007), which mainly related to viscosity and surface tension (Rayat and Feyzi, 2011). Although these surfactants can significantly reduce the surface tension, it is easy to lead to excessive viscosity of the aqueous phase, eventually leading to a larger particle size, the drug is not easy to be encapsulated, and the encapsulation efficiency is very low. Therefore, the optimal external aqueous media must possess these comprehensive properties to obtain higher EE and more appropriate particle size. According to above analysis, PVA was selected as the externalwater phase. Then we further evaluated the impacts of the concentration and volume of PVA. When the concentration of PVA was below 1%, the outer aqueous viscosity was too small to stable the droplet, the EE and the particle size were both unsatisfyed. However, the EE was declined as the increase of PVA concentration and volume (Song et al., 2008; Moralescruz et al., 2012; Sun et al., 2016), which might be attributed to the increase viscosity. In addition, the corresponding shear stress decreased as the increase viscosity, and led to the diffusion of YF4 from the inner aqueous phase into outside hampered, which might explain the lagrer particle size.

Ultrasonic duration might affect the drug leakage and the homogeneity of particle size in the preparation of LNPs. Moreover, peptides are generally denatured under high intensity ultrasonic shear systems (Gentile et al., 2012). Consequently, the proper ultrasonic duration was seemed as vital in the preparation of YF4-LNPs. The EE was increased firstly and suddenly decreased with longer ultrasonic time, which might be attributed by the broken coarse emulsion drops into nano-droplets (Fricker et al., 2010). However, too long ultrasonic time would lead to the leakage of YF4 from the internal phase to the external phase, causing a decrease in EE. Besides, prolonging W1/O/W2 ultrasonic time for a short time could significantly enhance the EE and decrease the particle size, caused by the increasing net sheer force, which is similar to the changes of ultrasonic power.

Ultimately, the ratio of PLGA/lipid materials was further optimized. As a result, a higher EE and a better particle size of YF4-LNPs were gained at 1:1.5 ratio of PLGA/lipid materials, which might result from the increased affinity between drug and the formulation (Luo et al., 2006).

To investigate the entrapment state of YF4 into lipid nanoparticles, DSC analysis were performed. The DSC showed that the YF4 was successfully entrapped in the YF4-LNPs. Additionally, the YF4-loaded nanoparticles were coated with lipid film according to TEM images, indicating the successful construction of lipid nanoparticles.

The release of YF4 from lipid nanoparticles was dramatically lower than the unincorporated YF4, which might be attributed to the surprising core-shell structure that could result in the tunable and sustained drug release profiles (Zhang et al., 2008; Fang et al., 2014). Although, our results are unsatisfactory, there is no obvious gastric protective and obviously sustained release in the intestinal tract, our study does protect the free drug from degradation in the stomach to a certain extent, providing more possibilities for its slow release in the intestinal tract and so as to prolonging the circulation in the blood and exerting its efficacy. Our result showed that only less than 30% of YF4 diffused into the dispersed medium after 12 h in all pH conditions, indicating a prolonged release of YF4-LNPs, which might lead to a potent and prolonged therapeutic efficacy of YF4-LNPs. For YF4-LNPs, the release percentages in media with different pH can provide some evidence that YF4-LNPs could provide sustainable release of YF4 in both stomach and intestine and protect YF4 from degradation.

It has been reported that ACEI peptides have amazing hypotensive activity *in vitro* (Escudero et al., 2012). We then firstly verified the BPL effect of YF4 compared with ACEI positive drug captopril shown in **Figure 5** (Nurminen et al., 2000). However, the oral duration is short and the dosage of antihypertensive peptides is far higher than that in literature (Yu et al., 2016). Oral delivery of peptides has enormously continuous challenge due to its poor stability in the GI tract and low permeability through the intestinal epithelium membrane (Friedman and Amidon, 1991). The pharmacokinetics of YF4 in rats was studied and showed in the **Supplementary Figure S1** and **Supplementary Table 1**. The results showed that the half-life of YF4 was only 2.91 h, just like that of conventional polypeptide and protein drugs. Thus, the new oral peptide delivery systems need to be developed. LNPs exhibit a wide range of erosion times, tunable biodegradation and mechanical properties, such as improving the connection between the nano-preparations and the intestinal epithelium cells, protecting the drugs from the GI, which might explain the antihypertensive effect in SHRs of YF4-LNPs. The YF4-LNPs exhibited a much better antihypertensive efficiency, especially YF4-LNPs showed a ten-time prolonged BPL effect. Currently, the mechanism of enhancement in therapeutic efficacy is still under investigation. The efficiency of YF4-LNPs being absorbed into systemic circulation requires further quantification. The association between elevated therapeutic efficacy and the increase in AUC or bioavailability needs further elucidation.

Over all, we systematically optimized the factors that could affect the features of LNPs, and finally constructed YF4-LNPs with a high entrapment efficiency and small particle size. Then, we evaluated its antihypertensive efficiency *in vivo*, and found that YF4-LNPs displayed stronger BPL effect and prolonged the effect up to 120 h. This may be explained by the controlled release of YF4 and the protection effect of the nanoparticles core and lipid membrane avoiding enzymatic degradation. This may provide some methodological clues and insights for the therapy of hypertension.

CONCLUSION

In this study, we have developed uniform-sized PLGA lipid nanoparticles for oral delivery of peptides. The LNPs was successfully prepared by thin-film membrane hydration-ultrasonic dispersion method and systematically optimized. Then, the properties of YF4-LNPs were investigated, including the stability, the *in vitro* release profile. To our surprise, YF4-LNPs were considerable stable and showed a sustained release profile. Then the DSC curves and TEM illustrated that the successfully loading of YF4 and the coating of lipid bilayer. YF4-LNPs exhibited an enhanced antihypertensive function with a longer duration (up to 120 h in SHRs), which suggested the sustained release. In summary, all these data supported the belief that YF4-LNPs would be a promising platform for oral hypertension treatment. However, the preparation process of YF4-LNPs was relatively complex, which might be difficult to be scaled up. Hence, a simplified process is worthy of being further investigated to fabricateYF4-LNPs for the clinical translation study. Moreover, the pharmacokinetics of YF4-LNPs is also necessary to be investigated in the future.

AUTHOR CONTRIBUTIONS

JY conceived the project. XG, CF, and JY designed the experiments. SZ, JL, and YZ conducted most of the experiments. SZ and JL drafted the manuscript. LH performed some preliminary experiments. YL and JX participated in literature searching. JY, XG, and CF finished manuscript editing. All authors reviewed and approved the manuscript.

FUNDING

This work was financially supported from the Science and Technology Project of Shenzhen (JCYJ20170413155047512), Sichuan Province Science and Technology Support Program (16ZC2698) and National Natural Science Foundation of China (No. 81472162).

REFERENCES

Abassi, Z., Winaver, J., and Feuerstein, G. Z. (2009). The biochemical pharmacology of renin inhibitors: implications for translational medicine in hypertension, diabetic nephropathy and heart failure: expectations and reality. *Biochem. Pharm.* 78, 933–940. doi: 10.1016/j.bcp.2009.05.018

Agrawal, A., Kulkarni, S., Sharma, S. B., and Jain, A. (2015). Development and characterization of nanoparticle based oral delivery of insulin. *J. Mater. Sci.* 44, 3349–3355.

Alavi, M., Karimi, N., and Safaei, M. (2017). Application of various types of liposomes in drug delivery systems. *Adv. Pharm. Bull.* 7, 3–9. doi: 10.15171/apb.2017.002

Anarjan, N., Tan, C. P., Ling, T. C., Lye, K. L., Malmiri, H. J., Nehdi, I. A., et al. (2011). Effect of organic-phase solvents on physicochemical properties and cellular uptake of astaxanthin nano dispersions. *J. Agric. Food Chem.* 59, 8733–8741. doi: 10.1021/jf201314u

Boelsma, E., and Kloek, J. (2010). Ipp-rich milk protein hydrolysate lowers blood pressure in subjects with stage 1 hypertension, a randomized controlled trial. *Nutr. J.* 9:52. doi: 10.1186/1475-2891-9-52

Chen, J., Liu, C., Shan, W., Xiao, Z., Guo, H., and Huang, Y. (2015). Enhanced stability of oral insulin in targeted peptide ligand trimethyl chitosan nanoparticles against trypsin. *J. Microencapsul.* 32, 632–641. doi: 10.3109/02652048.2015.1065920

Cleland, J. L., Geething, N. C., Moore, J. A., Rogers, B. C., Spink, B. J., Wang, C., et al. (2012). A novel long-acting human growth hormone fusion protein (vrs-317), enhanced *in vivo* potency and half-life. *J. Pharm. Sci.* 101, 2744–2754. doi: 10.1002/jps.23229

Ensign, L. M., Cone, R., and Hanes, J. (2012). Oral drug delivery with polymeric nanoparticles: the gastrointestinal mucus barriers. *Adv. Drug Deliv. Rev.* 64, 557–570. doi: 10.1016/j.addr.2011.12.009

Escudero, E., Aristoy, M. C., Nishimura, H., Arihara, K., and Toldrá, F. (2012). Antihypertensive effect and antioxidant activity of peptide fractions extracted from spanish dry-cured ham. *Meat Sci.* 91, 306–311. doi: 10.1016/j.meatsci.2012.02.008

Espejo-Carpio, F. J., Gobba, C. D., Guadix, A., Guadix, E. M., and Otte, J. (2013). Angiotensin I-converting enzyme inhibitory activity of enzymatic hydrolysates of goat milk protein fractions. *Int. Dairy J.* 32, 175–183. doi: 10.1016/j.idairyj.2013.04.002

Fang, D. L., Chen, Y., Xu, B., Ren, K., He, Z. Y., He, L. L., et al. (2014). Development of lipid-shell and polymer core nanoparticles with water-soluble salidroside for anti-cancer therapy. *Int. J. Mol. Sci.* 15, 3373–3388. doi: 10.3390/ijms15033373

Fricker, G., Kromp, T., Wendel, A., Blume, A., Zirkel, J., Rebmann, H., et al. (2010). Phospholipids and lipid-based formulations in oral drug delivery. *Pharm. Res.* 27, 1469–1486. doi: 10.1007/s11095-010-0130-x

Friedman, D. I., and Amidon, G. L. (1991). Oral absorption of peptides: influence of pH and inhibitors on the intestinal hydrolysis of leu-enkephalin and analogues. *Pharm. Res.* 8, 93–96. doi: 10.1023/A:1015842609565

Gentile, P., Nandagiri, V. K., Pabari, R., Daly, J., Tonda-Turo, C., Ciardelli, G., et al. (2012). Influence of parathyroid hormone-loaded PLGA nanoparticles in porous scaffolds for bone regeneration. *Int. J. Mol. Sci.* 16, 20492–20510. doi: 10.3390/ijms160920492

Girgih, A. T., Nwachukwu, I. D., Onuh, J. O., Malomo, S. A., and Aluko, R. E. (2016). Antihypertensive properties of a pea protein hydrolysate during short- and long-term oral administration to spontaneously hypertensive rats. *J. Food Sci.* 81, 1281–1287. doi: 10.1111/1750-3841.13272

Johnstone, T. C., Kulak, N., Pridgen, E. M., Farokhzad, O. C., Langer, R., and Lippard, S. J. (2013). Nanoparticle encapsulation of mitaplatin and the effect thereof on/ *in vivo* properties. *ACS Nano* 7, 5675–5683. doi: 10.1021/nn401905g

Kiss, N., Brenn, G., Pucher, H., Wieser, J., Scheler, S., Jennewein, H., et al. (2011). Formation of o/w emulsions by static mixers for pharmaceutical applications. *Chem. Eng. Sci.* 66, 5084–5094. doi: 10.1016/j.ces.2011.06.065

Kjeldsen, S. E. (2017). Hypertension and cardiovascular risk: general aspects. *Pharm. Res.* 129, 95–99. doi: 10.1016/j.phrs.2017.11.003

Lai, S. K., Wang, Y. Y., and Hanes, J. (2009). Mucus-penetrating nanoparticles for drug and gene delivery to mucosal tissues. *Adv. Drug Deliv. Rev.* 61, 158–171. doi: 10.1016/j.addr.2008.11.002

Li, X., Chen, Y., Wang, M., Ma, Y., Xia, W., and Gu, H. (2013). A mesoporous silica nanoparticle–PEI–Fusogenic peptide system for siRNA delivery in cancer therapy. *Biomaterials* 34, 1391–1401. doi: 10.1016/j.biomaterials.2012.10.072

Lozoya-Agullo, I., Araújo, F., González-álvarez, I., Merino-Sanjuán, M., González-Álvarez, M., Bermejo, M., et al. (2017). PLGA nanoparticles are effective to control the colonic release and absorption on ibuprofen. *Eur. J. Pharm. Sci.* 115, 119–125. doi: 10.1016/j.ejps.2017.12.009

Luo, L., Zheng, S., Huang, Y., Qin, T., Xing, J., Niu, Y., et al. (2016). Preparation and characterization of Chinese yam polysaccharide PLGA nanoparticles and their immunological activity. *Int. J. Pharm.* 511, 140–150. doi: 10.1016/j.ijpharm.2016.06.130

Luo, Y., Chen, D., and Ren, L. (2006). Solid lipid nanoparticles for enhancing vinpocetine's oral bioavailability. *J. Control. Release* 114, 53–59. doi: 10.1016/j.jconrel.2006.05.010

Majumder, K., Chakrabarti, S., Morton, J. S., Panahi, S., Kaufman, S., Davidge, S. T., et al. (2013). Egg-derived tri-peptide IRW exerts antihypertensive effects in spontaneously hypertensive rats. *PLoS One* 8:82829. doi: 10.1371/journal.pone.0082829

Moralescruz, M., Floresfernández, G. M., Moralescruz, M., Orellano, E. A., Rodriguezmartinez, J. A., Ruiz, M., et al. (2012). Two-step nanoprecipitation for the production of protein-loaded PLGA nanospheres. *Results Pharma Sci.* 2, 79–85. doi: 10.1016/j.rinphs.2012.11.001

Muller, R. H., and Keck, C. M. (2004). Challenges and solutions for the delivery of biotech drugs – a review of drug nanocrystal technology and lipid nanoparticles. *J. Biotechnol.* 113, 151–170. doi: 10.1016/j.jbiotec.2004.06.007

Mustafa, S., Devi, V. K., and Pai, R. S. (2017). Effect of PEG and water-soluble chitosan coating on moxifloxacin-loaded PLGAlong-circulating nanoparticles. *Drug Deliv. Transl. Res.* 7, 27–36. doi: 10.1007/s13346-016-0326-7

Musumeci, T., Ventura, C. A., Giannone, I., Ruozi, B., Montenegro, L., Pignatello, R., et al. (2006). PLA/ PLGA nanoparticles for sustained release of docetaxel. *Int. J. Pharm.* 325, 172–179. doi: 10.1016/j.ijpharm.2006.06.023

Niu, Z., Samaridou, E., Jaumain, E., Coëne, J., Ullio, G., Shrestha, N., et al. (2018). PEG-PGA enveloped octaarginine-peptide nanocomplexes: an oral peptide delivery strategy. *J. Control. Release* 276, 125–139. doi: 10.1016/j.jconrel.2018.03.004

Nogués, J., Skumryev, V., Sort, J., Stoyanov, S., and Givord, D. (2006). Shell-driven magnetic stability in core-shell nanoparticles. *Phys. Rev. Lett.* 97:157203. doi: 10.1103/PhysRevLett.97.157203

Nurminen, M. L., Sipola, M., Kaarto, H., Pihlanto-Leppälä, A., Piilola, K., Korpela, R., et al. (2000). α-lactorphin lowers blood pressure measured by radiotelemetry in normotensive and spontaneously hypertensive rats. *Life Sci.* 66, 1535–1543. doi: 10.1016/S0024-3205(00)00471-9

Olbrich, C., Bakowsky, U., Lehr, C. M., Müller, R. H., and Kneuer, C. (2001). Cationic solid-lipid nanoparticles can efficiently bind and transfect plasmid DNA. *J. Control. Release* 77, 345–355. doi: 10.1016/S0168-3659(01)00506-5

Peng, H. S., Hu-Lun, L. I., and Gui-Xiang, L. V. (2007). Preparation of insulin micro-/nanoparticles: effect of external water phase on dispersion of particles in colloid. *Chin. J. Biologicals* 20, 15–18. doi: 10.1504/PCFD.2007.013013

Ragab, D. M., Babiker, E. E., and Eltinay, A. H. (2004). Fractionation, solubility and functional properties of cowpea (Vigna unguiculata) proteins as affected by pH and/or salt concentration. *Food Chem.* 84, 207–212. doi: 10.1016/s0308-8146(03)00203-6

Rayat, K., and Feyzi, F. (2011). Influence of external electric field on the polarity of water droplets in water-in-oil emulsion phase transition. *Colloids Surf A Physicochem. Eng. Asp.* 375, 61–67. doi: 10.1016/j.colsurfa.2010.11.056

Richard, J. (2017). Challenges in oral peptide delivery: lessons learnt from the clinic and future prospects. *Ther. Deliv.* 8, 663–684. doi: 10.4155/tde-2017-0024

Sang, C. L. (1999). Effect of volume ratio of internal aqueous phase to organic membrane phase (w/o ratio) of water-in-oil emulsion on penicillin g extraction by emulsion liquid membrane. *J. Memb. Sci.* 163, 193–201. doi: 10.1016/S0376-7388(99)00182-9

Silva, A. L., Rosalia, R. A., Sazak, A., Carstens, M. G., Ossendorp, F., Oostendorp, J., et al. (2013). Optimization of encapsulation of a synthetic long peptide in plga nanoparticles: low-burst release is crucial for efficient CD8(+) T cell activation. *Eur. J. Pharm. Biopharm.* 83, 338–345. doi: 10.1016/j.ejpb.2012.11.006

Song, X., Zhao, Y., Wu, W., Bi, Y., Cai, Z., Chen, Q., et al. (2008). PLGA nanoparticles simultaneously loaded with vincristine sulfate and verapamil hydrochloride: systematic study of particle size and drug entrapment efficiency. *Int. J. Pharm.* 350, 320–329. doi: 10.1016/j.ijpharm.2007.08.034

Sun, D., Xue, A., Zhang, B., Xia, X., Jie, Z., and Liu, W. (2016). Enhanced oral bioavailability of acetylpuerarin by poly(lactide-co-glycolide) nanoparticles optimized using uniform design combined with response surface methodology. *Drug Des. Devel. Ther.* 10, 2029–2039. doi: 10.2147/DDDT.S108185

Tan, M. L., Choong, P. F., and Dass, C. R. (2009). Recent developments in liposomes, microparticles and nanoparticles for protein and peptide drug delivery. *Peptides* 31, 184–193. doi: 10.1016/j.peptides.2009.10.002

Tenenbaum, A., Grossman, E., Shemesh, J., Fisman, E. Z., Nosrati, I., and Motro, M. (2000). Intermediate but not low doses of aspirin can suppress angiotensin-converting enzyme inhibitor-induced cough. *Am. J. Hypertens.* 13, 776–782. doi: 10.1016/S0895-7061(00)00268-5

Thi, E. P., Mire, C. E., Lee, A. C., Geisbert, J. B., Zhou, J. Z., Agans, K. N., et al. (2015). Lipid nanoparticle sirna treatment of ebola-virus-makona-infected nonhuman primates. *Nature* 521, 362–365. doi: 10.1038/nature14442

Turk, C. T., Oz, U. C., Serim, T. M., and Hascicek, C. (2014). Formulation and optimization of nonionic surfactants emulsified nimesulide-loaded PLGA-based nanoparticles by design of experiments. *AAPS PharmsciTech.* 15, 161–176. doi: 10.1208/s12249-013-0048-9

Wang, F., Bao, X., Fang, A., Li, H., Zhou, Y., Liu, Y., et al. (2018). Nanoliposome-encapsulated brinzolamide-hydropropyl-β-cyclodextrin inclusion complex: a potential therapeutic ocular drug-delivery system. *Front. Pharmacol.* 9:91. doi: 10.3389/fphar.2018.00091

Wang, F., and Liu, J. (2013). Nanodiamond decorated liposomes as highly biocompatible delivery vehicles and a comparison with carbon nanotubes and graphene oxide. *Nanoscale* 5, 12375–12382. doi: 10.1039/C3NR04143C

Wang, P., and Anderko, A. (2013). Modeling interfacial tension in liquid–liquid systems containing electrolytes. *Ind. Eng. Chem. Res.* 52, 6822–6840. doi: 10.1021/ie303460c

Xie, B., Liu, Y., Guo, Y., Zhang, E., Pu, C., He, H., et al. (2018). Progesterone PLGA/mPEG-PLGA hybrid nanoparticle sustained-release system by intramuscular injection. *Pharm. Res.* 35:62. doi: 10.1007/s11095-018-2357-x

Yang, L., Luo, J., Shi, S., Zhang, Q., Sun, X., Zhang, Z., et al. (2013). Development of a pulmonary peptide delivery system using porous nanoparticle-aggregate particles for systemic application. *Int. J. Pharm.* 451, 104–111. doi: 10.1016/j.ijpharm.2013.04.077

Yoshikawa, M., Tani, F., Yoshimura, T., and Chiba, H. (1986). Opioid peptides from milk proteins. *J. Agric. Chem. Soc. Jpn* 50, 2419–2421. doi: 10.1080/00021369.1986.10867763

Yu, T., Zhao, S., Li, Z., Wang, Y., Xu, B., Fang, D., et al. (2016). Enhanced and extended anti-hypertensive effect of VP5 nanoparticles. *Int. J. Mol. Sci.* 17:1977. doi: 10.3390/ijms17121977

Zhang, L., Chan, J. M., Gu, F. X., Rhee, J. W., Wang, A. Z., Radovic-Moreno, A. F., et al. (2008). Self-assembled lipid-polymer hybrid nanoparticles: a robust drug delivery platform. *ACS Nano* 2, 1696–1702. doi: 10.1021/nn800275r

Zhang, Z., Bu, H., Gao, Z., Huang, Y., Gao, F., and Li, Y. (2010). The characteristics and mechanism of simvastatin loaded lipid nanoparticles to increase oral bioavailability in rats. *Int. J. Pharm.* 394, 147–153. doi: 10.1016/j.ijpharm.2010.04.039

18

Polypeptide Nanogels with Different Functional Cores Promote Chemotherapy of Lung Carcinoma

Kai Niu[1†], Nan Li[2†], Yunming Yao[3†], Chunjie Guo[4], Yuanyuan Ge[5] and Jianmeng Wang[5]*

[1] Department of Otorhinolaryngology Head and Neck Surgery, The First Hospital of Jilin University, Changchun, China, [2] Department of Neonatology, The First Hospital of Jilin University, Changchun, China, [3] Department of Abdominal Ultrasound, The First Hospital of Jilin University, Changchun, China, [4] Department of Radiology, The First Hospital of Jilin University, Changchun, China, [5] Department of Geriatrics, The First Hospital of Jilin University, Changchun, China

***Correspondence:**
Jianmeng Wang
jmwang1981@126.com

† These authors have contributed equally to this work

Two kinds of tumor microenvironment-responsive polypeptide nanogels were developed for intracellular delivery of cytotoxics to enhance the antitumor efficacies and reduce the side effects in the chemotherapy of lung carcinoma. The sizes of both doxorubicin (DOX)-loaded nanogels methoxy poly(ethylene glycol)–poly(L-phenylalanine-*co*-L-cystine) [mPEG–P(LP-*co*-LC)] and methoxy poly(ethylene glycol)–poly(L-glutamic acid-*co*-L-cystine) [mPEG–P(LG-*co*-LC)] (NGP/DOX and NGG/DOX) were less than 100 nm, which was appropriate for the enhanced permeability and retention (EPR) effect. The bigger and smaller scale of nanoparticle could induce the elimination of reticuloendothelial system (RES) and decrease the *in vivo* circulating half-life, respectively. The loading nanogels were stable in the neutral environment while quickly degraded in the mimic intracellular microenvironment. Furthermore, the DOX-loaded reduction-responsive nanogels showed significantly higher tumor cell uptake than free DOX·HCl as time went on from 2 to 6 h. In addition, these DOX-loaded nanogels showed efficient antitumor effects *in vivo*, which was verified by the obviously increased necrosis areas in the tumor tissues. Furthermore, these DOX-loaded nanogels efficiently reduced the side effects of DOX. In conclusion, these reduction-responsive polypeptides based nanogels are suitable for the efficient therapy of lung carcinoma.

Keywords: nanogel, reduction-responsive, controlled drug delivery, lung carcinoma, antitumor

INTRODUCTION

Lung carcinoma has been the most common malignancy in both men and women with high mortality (Kanodra et al., 2015; Kernstine, 2017). Chemotherapy, as a traditional treatment, is important to the treatment of lung cancer. However, the main therapeutic platforms available for chemotherapy drugs currently have the disadvantages of not being able to effectively aggregate in tumor cells and causing various systemic side effects. Due to these deficiencies, various nanomedicine delivery systems have been studied such as micelles (Feng et al., 2017; Shen et al., 2017; Xu et al., 2017; Kosakowska et al., 2018; Li et al., 2018b; Sun et al., 2018), nanogels (Ding et al., 2011; Guo et al., 2017, 2018; Jiang et al., 2018b; Li et al., 2018d; Zhang et al., 2018; Zhu et al., 2018), polymer–drug conjugates (Zhao et al., 2017; Cong et al., 2018; Li et al., 2018a; Yang et al., 2018), liposomes (Allen and Cullis, 2013; Zhao et al., 2013; Piffoux et al., 2018), and so forth

(Ding et al., 2014; Tao et al., 2015, 2017; Chen et al., 2017a; Armstrong and Stevens, 2018; Ji et al., 2018; Jiang et al., 2018a; Li et al., 2018b,c; Xiao et al., 2018), which help to improve the drug accumulation in the tumor, to achieve the effective control of drug release in the tumor lesions, and to reduce the side effects (Yu et al., 2016; Zhang et al., 2017). Among them, nanogels have the strong core–shell structures by cross-linking, which enables them not only to exhibit high drug loading capacity, but also to prevent drug leakage (Ye et al., 2016; Chen et al., 2017b). In addition, the suitable sizes of the nanogels made them can efficiently accumulate at the tumor lesions by the enhanced permeability and retention (EPR) effect (Acharya and Sahoo, 2011). More importantly, additional functionality is given to crosslinkers to achieve "switch on/off" release of drugs from nanogels in tumor cells (Mura et al., 2013). In addition, the stability of nanogels is one of the major obstacles, which handers the *in vivo* application of them. Fortunately, the chemistry crosslinking has been widely used to enhance the stability and functionality of nanogels, which is more stable than non-covalent interactions (Ryu et al., 2010; Jiang et al., 2018a). Furthermore, cross-linking nanoparticles with different functional chemical crosslinkers could controllably release the laden drugs according to the redox, low pH, and high enzyme level of tumor microenvironments (Zha et al., 2011).

Due to the different metabolic pathways of tumor cells, the microenvironments of tumor tissues show hypoxia, low sugar, and low pH (Parks et al., 2013). It is worth noting that malignant cells show the reductive intracellular microenvironment (Ge and Liu, 2013). Therefore, the reduction-sensitive polymeric nanoparticles have attracted more and more attention in the realm of smart antitumor drug delivery (Cheng et al., 2013; Phillips and Gibson, 2014).

Herein, we reported the drug delivery potential of reduction-sensitive polypeptide nanogels formulations, which could suppress lung carcinoma cell proliferation at low dose and reduce unwanted adverse effects. The reduction-responsive methoxy poly(ethylene glycol)–poly(L-phenylalanine-*co*-L-cystine) (mPEG–P(LP-*co*-LC)) and methoxy poly(ethylene glycol)–poly(L-glutamic acid-*co*-L-cystine) mPEG–P(LG-*co*-LC) nanogels were prepared to selectively deliver chemotherapy agents (**Scheme 1**). Typically, nanogels loaded with doxorubicin (DOX) were used as models for clinical antitumor drug. Results showed that both DOX-loaded nanogels exhibited satisfactory antitumor activity and higher safety than free DOX·HCl. These DOX-loaded nanogels are able to serve as satisfactory nanoplatforms for the therapy of lung carcinoma.

MATERIALS AND METHODS

Methoxy (ethylene glycol) (mPEG) was purchased from Aladdin Industrial Co., Ltd. (Shanghai, China) and mPEG-NH_2 was synthesized by trimethylamine modified. L-Glutamic acid (LC), L-phenylalanine (LP), and L-cystine (LC) were obtained from GL Biochem, Ltd. (Shanghai, China). LG NCA, LP NCA, and LC NCA were prepared as reported in previous work (Huang et al., 2015; Shi et al., 2017). Doxorubicin hydrochloride (DOX·HCl) was bought from Beijing Huafeng United Technology Co., Ltd. (Beijing, China). Glutathione (GSH) (used for cell culture) was bought from Aladdin Reagent Co., Ltd. (Shanghai, China). Both 4,6-Diamidino-2-phenylindole (DAPI) and methyl thiazolyl tetrazolium (MTT) were obtained from Sigma–Aldrich (Shanghai, China). Hematoxylin and eosin were purchased from Merck Company (Darmstadt, Germany).

Characterizations

Proton Nuclear Magnetic Resonance (^1H NMR) spectra were detected on a Bruker AV 600 NMR spectrometer (Billerica, MA, United States) using deuterated dimethyl sulfoxide (DMSO-d_6) as the solvent. Fourier-transform infrared spectroscopy (FT-IR) was performed on a Bio-Rad Win-IR instrument (Bio-Rad Laboratories Inc., Cambridge, MA, United States) by using potassium bromide method. The morphology of NGP/DOX and NGG/DOX nanogels were visualized on JEM-1011 transmission electron microscope (TEM; JEOL, Tokyo, Japan). Sizes of NGP/DOX and NGG/DOX were determined by dynamic laser scattering (DLS) measurement on a WyattQELS instrument (DAWN EOS, Wyatt Technology Corporation, Santa Barbara, CA, United States), and the scattering angle was set at 90°.

Syntheses and Characterizations of mPEG–P(LP-*co*-LC) and mPEG–P(LG-*co*-LC)

The reduction-responsive mPEG–P(LP-*co*-LC) nanogel was synthesized through the one-step ROP of LP NCA and LC NCA with amino-terminated mPEG (mPEG–NH_2) as a macroinitiator according to the reports in our previous works. Firstly, 2 g of mPEG-NH_2, 2.3 g of NCA LP NCA and 0.9 g of LC NCA were dissolved in 100 mL of DMF and stirred for three days. The obtained solution was poured into 700 mL of the ethyl ether twice, and the white precipitate was collected. After vacuum drying, mPEG–P(LP-*co*-LC) was obtained with the yield of 75.2%. mPEG–P(BLG-*co*-LC) was prepared in a similar route. mPEG—P(LG-*co*-LC) was generated by removing the benzyl group from mPEG–P(BLG-*co*-LC). mPEG–P(BLG-*co*-LC) was dissolved in dichloroacetic acid (100 mg mL^{-1}) and a 33 wt. % solution of HBr in acetic acid was added subsequently (20 mL for 1 g copolymer). After stirring for 1 h at 30°C, the mixture was precipitated into diethyl ether (10 times volume of the reaction solution). The obtained product was further dried under vacuum at room temperature for 24 h after washing twice with diethyl ether (Yield: 80.5%). The products were characterized by proton nuclear magnetic resonance (^1H NMR), Fourier-transform infrared (FT-IR), inductively coupled plasma optical emission spectroscopy (ICP-OES), and elemental analysis.

DOX Encapsulation

Nanogel was loaded with DOX by nanoprecipitation method. Firstly, 50 mg of nanogel was dispersed in 20 mL of N,N-dimethylformamide (DMF). After adding 10 mg of DOX·HCl, the solution was further stirred for 12 h at room temperature. Then, 2 mL of phosphate buffered saline (PBS; 0.01 M) was slowly mixed into the above solution, along with 18 mL of MilliQ water.

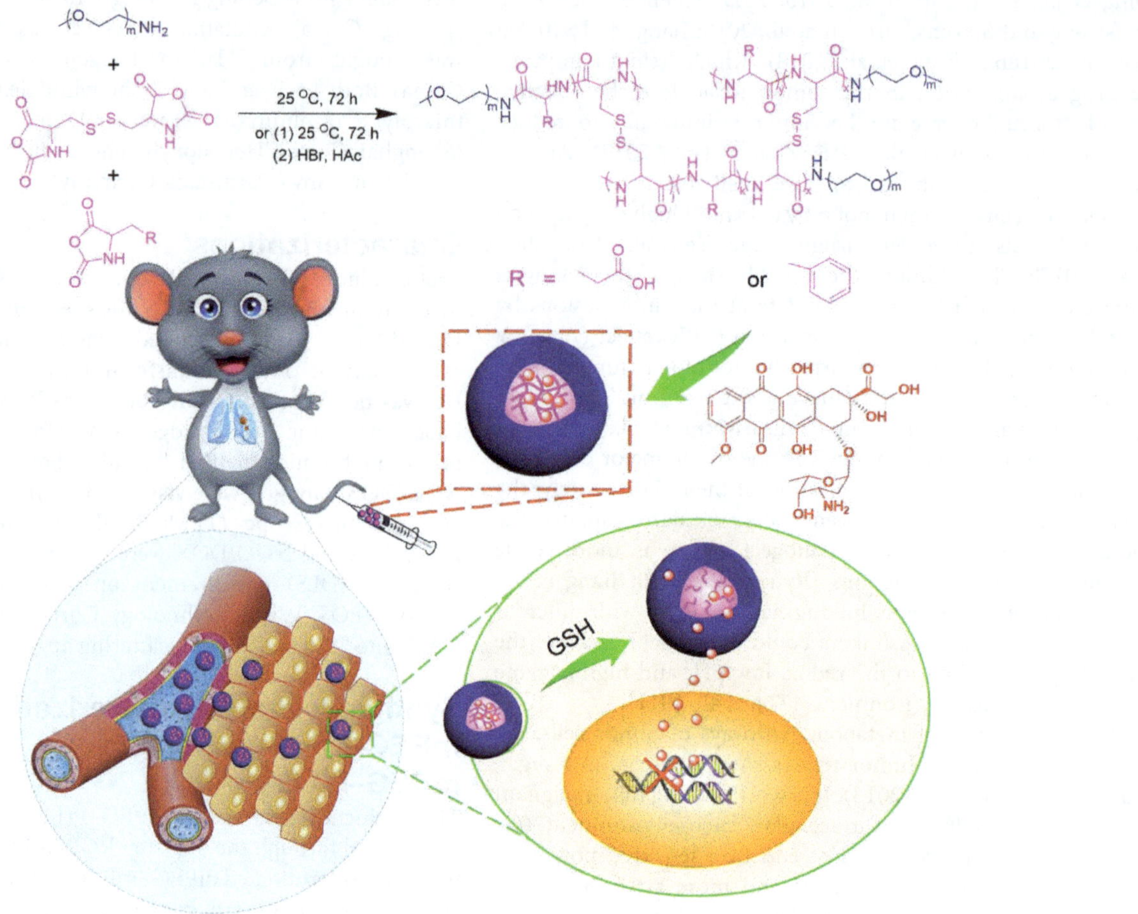

SCHEME 1 | Synthetic pathway for mPEG–P(LP-*co*-LC) and mPEG–P(LG-*co*-LC) nanogel, illustrations of DOX encapsulation by nanogel, and its circulation, intratumoral accumulation, endocytosis, and targeting intracellular DOX release after intravenous injection.

The final mixture was dialyzed against MilliQ water for 24 h (molecular weight cut-off (MWCO) = 3500 Da) after stirring for 12 h at room temperature. The MilliQ water was changed every 2 h. Finally, NGP/DOX and NGG/DOX nanogels were obtained by filtration and lyophilization.

The drug loading content (DLC) and drug loading efficiency (DLE) were detected by standard curve method, using fluorescence spectroscopy on a Photon Technology International (PTI) Fluorescence Master System with Felix 4.1.0 software (PTI, Lawrenceville, NJ, United States; kex = 480 nm). The DLC and DLE of NGP/DOX and NG/DOX were calculated according to Eqs. (1) and (2), respectively.

$$\mathrm{DLC}(\%) = \frac{\text{Weight of Drug in Nanogel}}{\text{Weight of Drug} - \text{Loaded Nanogel}} \times 100\% \quad (1)$$

$$\mathrm{DLE}(\%) = \frac{\text{Weight of Drug in Nanogel}}{\text{Weight of Feeding Drug}} \times 100\% \quad (2)$$

In vitro DOX Release

In vitro drug release profiles of DOX from NGP/DOX and NGG/DOX nanogels were performed in PBS (pH 7.4) with or without 10 nM GSH. 10 mL of nanogel (0.1 mg mL^{-1}) aqueous solution was transferred into an end-sealed dialysis bag (MWCO = 3500 Da). The release experiment was carried out by putting the end-sealed dialysis bag into the corresponding release medium (100 mL) at 37°C with continuous shaking at 75 rpm in the dark. At fixed time intervals, 2 mL of release medium was removed and an equal volume of fresh medium was added. The amount of released DOX was measured by the fluorescence spectrophotometer (kex = 480 nm).

Cell Culture

Under the conditions of 37°C and 5% (V/V) carbon dioxide (CO_2), the human lung Lewis cells were cultured in RPMI-1640, which was supplemented with 10% (V/V) fetal bovine serum (FBS), penicillin (100 IU mL^{-1}), and streptomycin (100 IU mL^{-1}).

Intracellular DOX Release

The intracellular DOX release from NGP/DOX and NGG/DOX were measured by confocal laser scanning microscopy (CLSM) toward Lewis cells. The cells (15,000 cells) were seeded in disks, incubated in 1 mL of RPMI-1640 medium containing 10% FBS for 24 h, and pretreated with 10 mM GSH or buthionine sulfoximine (BSO) for 2 h. After removing the medium and subsequently washing three times with PBS (pH 7.4) solution, 1 mL of NGP/DOX and NGG/DOX solution in RPMI-1640 was added, with a final DOX dose of 10 μg mL^{-1}. The cells treated with equivalent free DOX without GSH pretreatment were used as control. After another 2 h of incubation, the cells were washed with PBS for five times, and fixed with 4% (W/V) PBS-buffered paraformaldehyde at room temperature for 30 min. The cellular nuclei were then stained at 37°C for 3 min using DAPI. A CLSM (Carl Zeiss, LSM 780, Jena, Germany) was used to view the intracellular localization of DOX.

Cytotoxicity Assays

The cytotoxicities of NGP/DOX, NGG/DOX and free DOX were evaluate din Lewis cells at different conditions. The cells were planted in 96-well plates (7×10^3 cells per well) in 200 μL of RPMI-1640 medium supplemented with 1X penicillin/streptomycin and 10% fetal bovine serum. After incubation for 24 h at 37°C, the cells were pretreated with 10 mM GSH or BSO for 2 h. Subsequently, each culture medium was replaced by 180 μL of RPMI-1640 containing NGP/DOX, NGG/DOX and free DOX at equivalent concentrations, respectively, with the DOX ranging from 0.3 to 18.4 μM. After a further 24, 48, and 72 h incubation, 20 μL MTT (5 mg mL^{-1}) in PBS was added to each well, followed by another 4°h incubation at 37°C. Then the sediment was dissolved in 150 μL DMSO after the medium was removed. The absorbance at 490 nm of the above solution was determined on an ELx808 microplate reader (Bio-Tek Instruments, Inc., Winooski, VT, United States). The percentage of cell viability was determined by comparing the absorbance of the sample cells and the control cells [Eq. (3)].

$$\text{Cell}(\%) = \frac{A_{\text{Sample}}}{A_{\text{Control}}} \times 100\% \quad (3)$$

Animal Procedures

5-Week-old male BALB/c mice weighting 18 ± 0.2 g were supplied by the Jilin University Experiment Animal Center (Changchun, China). All animal experiments were performed according to the Guidelines for Animal Care and Use of Jilin University. The tumor grafted mouse model was established by subcutaneous injection of 100 μL of cell suspension containing 2×10^6 Lewis cells in PBS into the armpit of right anterior forelimb.

In vivo Antitumor Assessments

The tumor volumes and mice's body weights were monitored every two days from the second day after the inoculation of Lewis cells (that was, Day 1). When tumor volume increased to about 100 mm^3 after 8 days of inoculation, the nude mice were randomly divided into 7 groups (n = 10), that was, free DOX, NGP/DOX or NGG/DOX at a DOX dose of 3 or 6 mg $(\text{kg BW})^{-1}$ and normal saline (control group). The formulations of DOX were recorded as DOX/3, DOX/6, NGP/DOX/3, NGP/DOX/6, NGG/DOX/3 and NGG/DOX/6, respectively. At the same time, the treatments began with injecting100 μL of normal saline and various DOX preparations in normal saline into the tail vein of mice for four times every 5 days. The tumor sizes were measured every day, and the body weights were measured every subsequent day. Tumor volumes [Eq. (4)] and body weights were used to evaluate the antitumor efficacy and security *in vivo*.

$$V(\text{mm}^3) = \frac{\text{L} \times \text{S}^2}{2} \quad (4)$$

In Eq. (4), L (mm) was the largest diameter of tumor, and S (mm) was the smallest diameter.

The following formula was used to calculate the tumor inhibition ratio:

$$\text{Tumor inhibition rate } (\%) = (V_{\text{control}} - V_{\text{sample}})/V_{\text{control}} \quad (5)$$

In Eq. (5), V_{control} and V_{sample} represented the tumor volumes of control groups and sample groups, respectively.

The weights of the major organs were recorded. The organ indices of all the organs of mice were calculated by [Eq. (6)].

$$\text{Organ}(\%) = \frac{W_{\text{Organ}}}{W_{\text{Body}}} \times 100\% \quad (6)$$

Immunohistochemical Analyses of Tumor Tissues

On day 27, the Lewis lung carcinoma-grafted BALB/c mice were killed by cervical dislocation 5 days after the last injections. The tumors and major organs (heart, liver, spleen, lung, kidney, thymus, and marrow) were isolated at first, and then fixed with 4% (W/V) paraformaldehyde overnight, followed by dehydration, clearing, wax infiltration, and embedding. The paraffin-embedded tumors and organ tissues were cut at a thickness of 5 μm for hematoxylin and eosin (H&E) staining. Paraffin sections with a thickness of 3 μm were used for immunohistochemical staining (including caspase-3, survivin, Bax, and Bcl-2) to assess the pathological and immunological characteristics of tumor tissues. The instruments used included Leica RM 2245 paraffin machine (Leica, Germany), Leica HI1210 fishing machine (Leica, Germany), Leica EG1150H embedding machine (Leica, Germany), Leica HI1220 booth machine (Leica, Germany), Olympus BX51 microscope (Olympus, Japan), and Motic image analysis system (Motic Industrial Group Co., Ltd., Xiamen, China).

Histopathological and Biochemical Analyses of Organs

The major internal organs and tissues (heart, liver, spleen, lung, kidney, thymus, and marrow) were collected at the same time. The organs from healthy mice were used as controls. All the organs involved were divided into two parts as follows: (i) one part (excluding marrow) fixed with 4% (*W*/*V*) PBS-buffered paraformaldehyde was prepared for the histopathological analyses by H&E staining. (ii) The other part was used to detect the organ function-related biochemical indicators, including blood urea nitrogen (BUN), creatinine (Cr), alanine aminotransferase (ALT), aspartate aminotransferase (AST), creatine kinase (CK), creatine kinase-MB (CK-MB) and lactate dehydrogenase (LDH), by commercial enzyme-linked immunosorbent assay (ELISA) kits. The biochemical indicators in serum were also tested. Briefly, 300 μL of blood without anticoagulant was centrifuged at 3000 rpm for 10 min. The serum was then collected to detect the clinical biochemical parameters. The data from healthy nude mice were used as controls. The histopathological results were detected and analyzed by Olympus BX51 microscope and Motic image analysis system, respectively.

Detections of White Blood Cell (WBC) Count and Bone Marrow Cell Micronucleus Rates (BMMRs)

On day 27, 20 μL of blood (anticoagulated through enucleation method) was taken from each nude mouse to count the WBCs. The sternums from BALB/c mice were decalcified and fixed for 10 days after being placed in 10% (V/V) formic acid-formalin solution. The data from normal nude mice were used as controls. Then, the tissues were dehydrated, cleared, wax infiltrated, and embedded. For each sternum, paraffin sections with a thickness of 5 μm were collected for H&E staining, with an interval of 50 μm. The H&E-stained section was used to evaluate the BMMR.

Statistical Analyses

All tests were carried out at least three times, and the relevant data were expressed as mean ± standard deviation (SD). Statistical analysis was performed using SPSS 13.0 statistical software (SPSS Inc., Chicago, IL, United States), $^{***}P < 0.05$ was considered statistically significant, and $^{**}P < 0.01$ and $^{*}P < 0.001$ were as considered significant differences.

RESULTS AND DISCUSSION

Characterizations of NGP/DOX and NGG/DOX

These reduction-responsive nanogels consisted of mPEG (hydrophilic shell) and disulfide-cross-linked P(LP-*co*-LC) or P(LG-*co*-LC) (hydrophobic core). The disulfide bond of the LC segment endowed the nanogels with reduction-responsiveness (Huang et al., 2015; Shi et al., 2017). These DOX-loaded nanogels were prepared through a modified nanoprecipitation method

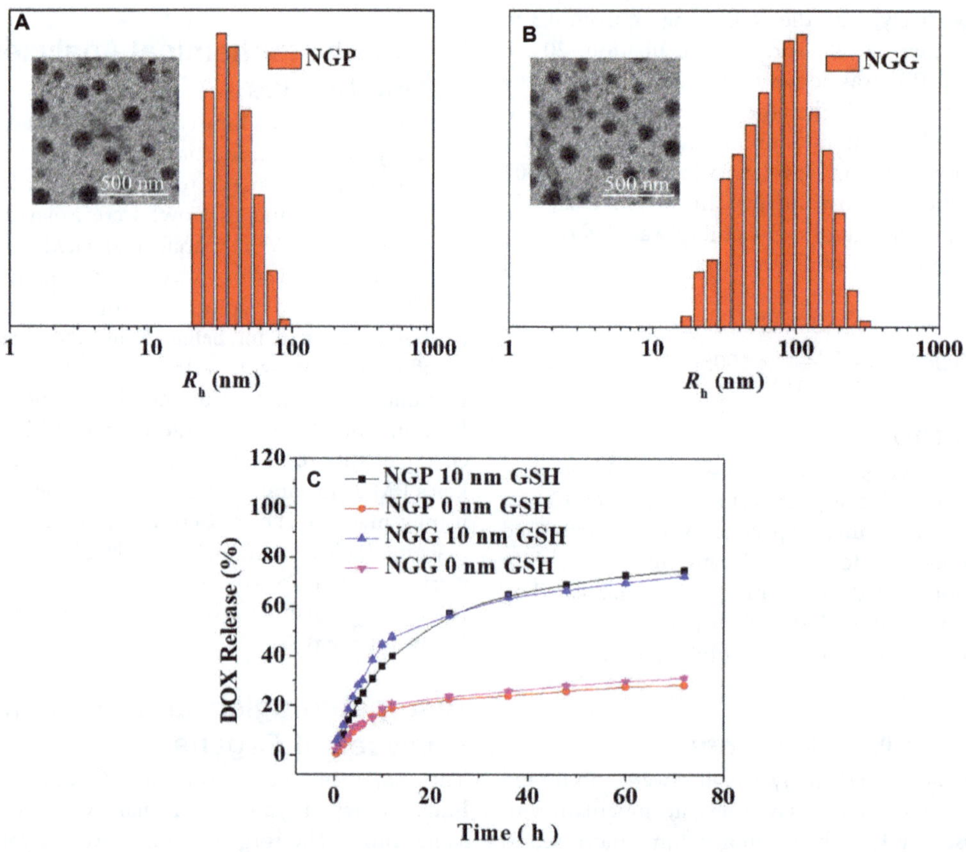

FIGURE 1 | Chemo-Physical Characterizations. Typical TEM micrograph and R_h detected by DLS of NGP/DOX **(A)** and NGG/DOX **(B)**. *In vitro* DOX release from NGP/DOX and NGG/DOX **(C)** in PBS of pH 7.4 and 7.4 with 10 nm GSH at 37°C. Scale bar in B represents 500 nm. The statistical data are represented as mean ± standard deviation (*SD*; *n* = 3).

by adding DOX aqueous solution to dimethylformamide (DMF) solution containing NGP or NGG nanogel (**Scheme 1**) (Ding et al., 2013a; Huang et al., 2015; Liu et al., 2015; Shi et al., 2017). The drug loading content (DLCs) and drug loading efficiency (DLEs) of NGP/DOX and NGG/DOX were calculated to be 9.8, 54.7 and 15.2, 91.5 wt.%, respectively. As shown in the TEM images, NGP/DOX, and NGG/DOX showed a spherical morphology at a diameter of about 80 and 93 nm, respectively (**Figures 1A,B**). The R_h of NGP/DOX and NGG/DOX detected by dynamic laser scattering (DLS) were 78.1 ± 3.5 and 93.3 ± 3.5 nm, respectively (**Figures 1A,B**). The hydrodynamic size of NGP/DOX and NGG/DOX was slightly larger than the diameter detected by TEM due to the swelling of nanogels in the aqueous condition (Huang et al., 2015; Shi et al., 2017). Appropriate size facilitated the efficient accumulation of nanogels in the tumors (Ding et al., 2013b,c, 2015).

In vitro Release Performance and Tumor Cell Inhibition

The DOX release performances of NGP/DOX and NGG/DOX were carried out in PBS with 0 or 10.0 mM glutathione (GSH). As shown in **Figure 1C**, during the 72 h test, only around 30%

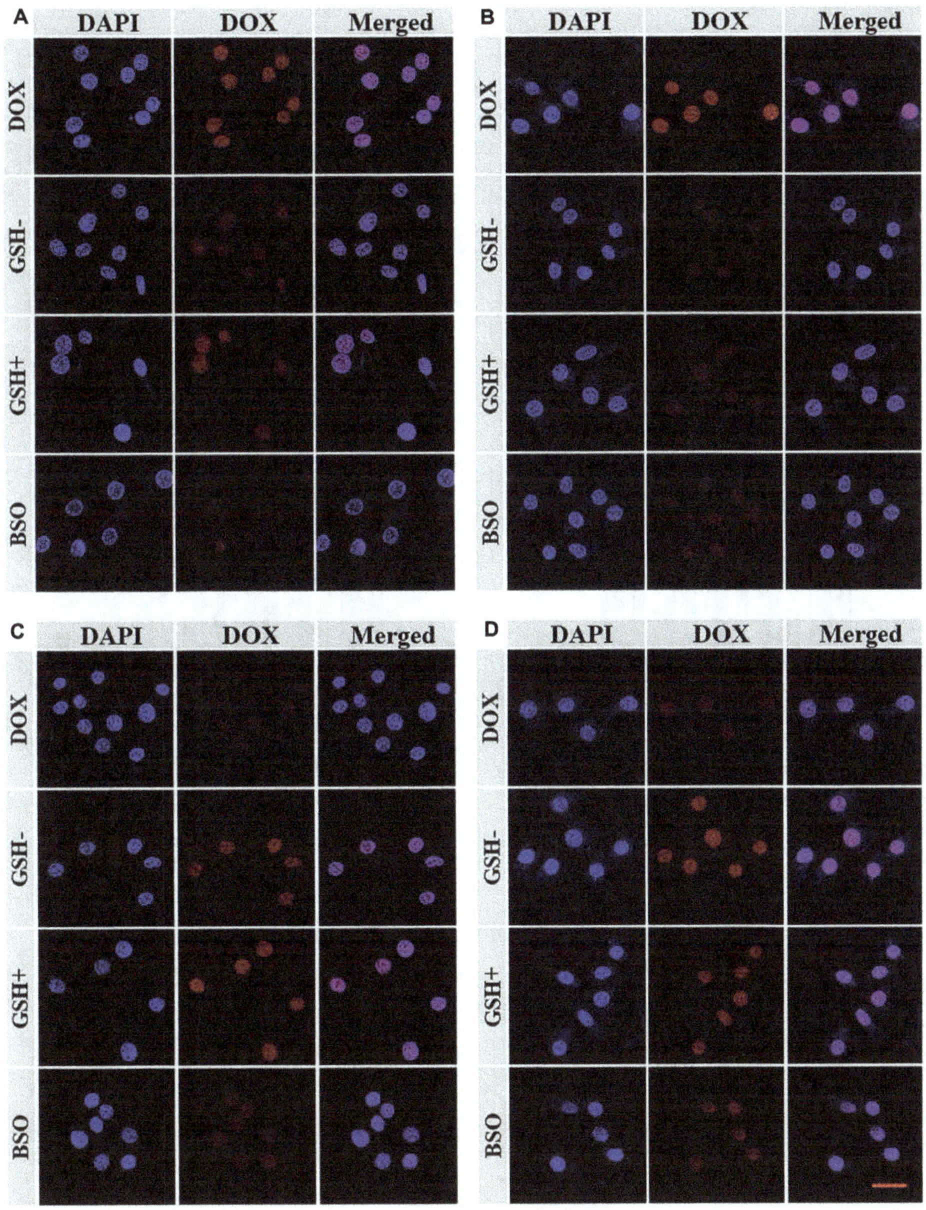

FIGURE 2 | The CLSM microimages analyses for cell internalization of NGP **(A,C)** and NGG **(B,D)** after incubation with Lewis cells for 2 h **(A,B)** and 6 h **(C,D)**. Scale bar =50 μm.

of DOX was released in the PBS with 0 mM GSH. In contrast, an obviously increased DOX release was observed in the PBS with 10.0 mM GSH. In detail, the proportions of cumulative released DOX from NGP/DOX and NGG/DOX in the initial 12 h were 47.8 and 39.8% in PBS with GSH (GSH+), respectively. After 72 h of incubation, the DOX released from NGP/DOX and NGG/DOX in the GSH+ medium (72.4 and 74.7%) were more than twice that in the GSH− medium (31.0 and 28.1%), respectively. The accelerated release of DOX should be due to GSH breaking the disulfide bond of nanogels (Huang et al., 2015). After 24 h, the drug release of nanogels was relatively decelerated and sustained. The release results indicated the NGP/DOX and NGG/DOX could efficiently release the DOX in tumor cells according to the different redox potential between intracellular and extracellular microenvironments, which might have more obvious antitumor activity.

Confocal laser scanning microscopy (CLSM) assays were performed toward Lewis lung carcinoma cells pretreated without (GSH−), with 10.0 mM GSH (GSH+) or buthionine sulfoximine (BSO) to verify the satisfactory intracellular DOX release of NGP/DOX and NGG/DOX. NG/DOX with a dosage of 10.0 μg mL^{-1} DOX·HCl was used to co-cultured with the GSH− or GSH+ cells for 2 and 6 h. The unpretreated cells co-cultured with equivalent free DOX·HCl were prepared as a control. As shown, the DOX fluorescence was shown in all the Lewis lung carcinoma cells treated with DOX formulations (**Figure 2**). As

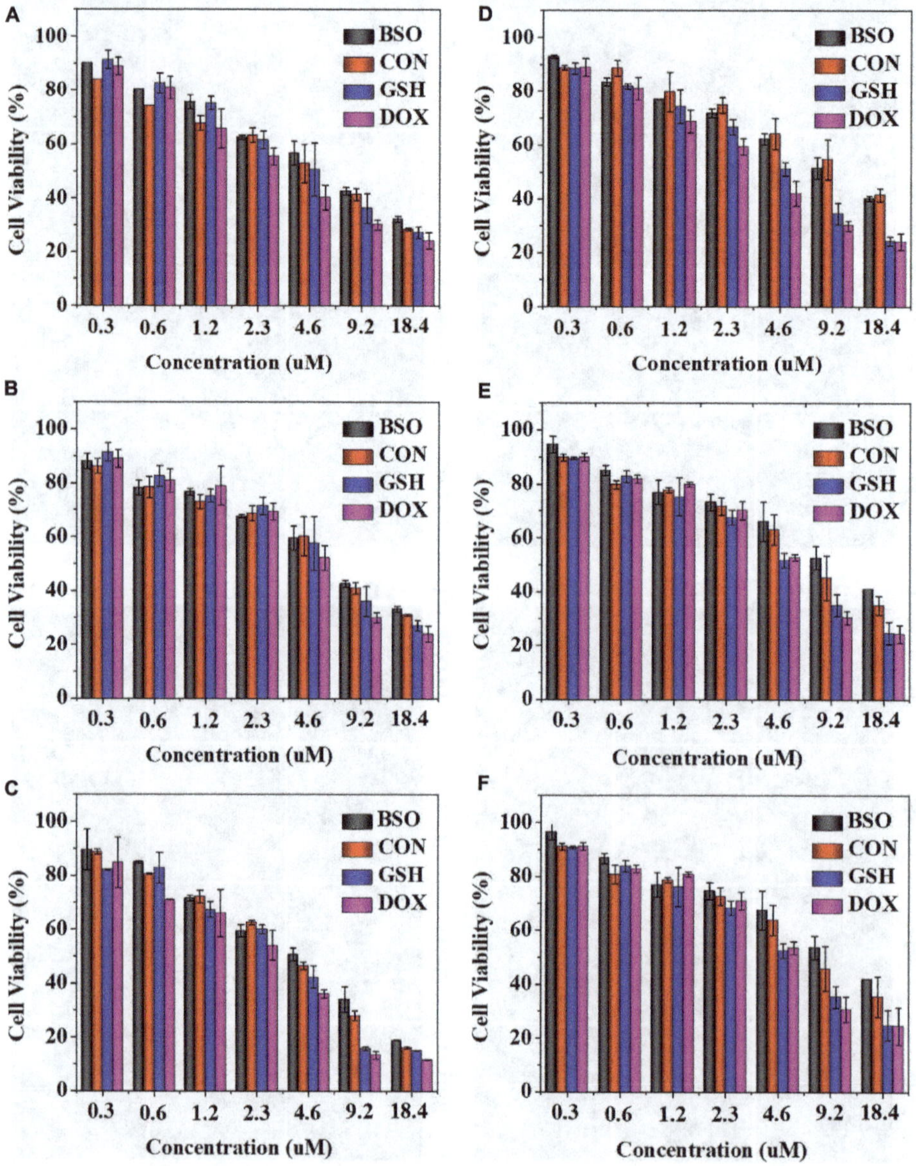

FIGURE 3 | *In vitro* cytotoxicity of NGP **(A–C)** and NGG **(D–F)** after incubation with Lewis cells for 24, 48, and 72 h. The statistical data are presented as a mean ± *SD* (*n* = 6).

time went on, the DOX fluorescence in the nanogels with GSH pretreatment groups were higher than that of the free DOX·HCl and BSO pretreated groups. As far as we knew, only the DOX released from nanogels in the cells could be detected by CLSM (Ding et al., 2013c). These results verified the efficient endocytosis as well as the reduction-responsive intracellular DOX release of NGG/DOX and NGP/DOX. These results might be related to that with the pretreatment of GSH, the intracellular GSH content was increased, which facilitated the rapid release of DOX from nanogels. Moreover, the results were consistent with the *in vitro* DOX release kinetics in PBS (**Figure 1C**). It was interesting that the tumor cells incubated with free DOX·HCl exhibited the strongest DOX fluorescence at 2 h. This result was related to the way of free DOX·HCl entered cells was diffusion, which was faster than the endocytosis of nanogels (Ding et al., 2013b,c).

The *in vitro* antitumor activities of NGG/DOX and NGP/DOX were estimated by MTT assay at 24, 48, and 72 h. As shown in **Figure 3**, compared with the BSO pretreated and unpretreated groups, GSH pretreated nanogels showed obviously higher growth inhibition efficiency in Lewis cells during the test time. This more satisfactory inhibition of GSH pretreated nanogels might be related to the intracellular GSH content was increased after GSH pretreatment, which facilitated the rapid release of DOX from nanogels and showed stronger tumor killing effect. As time went on, the half maximal inhibitory concentrations (IC_{50}s) of NGP/DOX decreased, but the order was constant: BSO < GSH− < GSH+. At 72 h, the IC_{50}s of BSO, GSH−, and GSH+ pretreated groups were calculated to be 3.78, 3.30, and 2.61 $\mu M\ mL^{-1}$, respectively. The NGG/DOX groups showed similar results, and the IC_{50}s of BSO, GSH−, and GSH+ pretreated groups were calculated to be 12.12, 7.92, and 4.65 $\mu M\ mL^{-1}$ at 72 h. The NGP/DOX and NGG/DOX groups pretreated by GSH had the lowest IC_{50}, demonstrating their enhanced suppressor capability against the tumor cells and their advantage as potential antitumor drug formulations.

In vivo Antitumor Efficacy

The most important indicators of drug use *in vivo* were efficacy and safety, which must be rigorously evaluated before any newly formulations could be used clinically. Tumor-grafted animal models are the main method to evaluate the antitumor activities of drug delivery systems. As shown, compared with free DOX·HCl, DOX-loaded nanogels exhibited stronger antitumor effect (**Figure 4A**). This result was related to two factors: one was related to the EPR effect (Huang et al., 2015; Shi et al., 2017), which resulted more DOX-loaded nanogels accumulated in tumor sites, the other was due to the more controlled release of DOX from nanogels, which resulted less DOX was released in circulation and more DOX accumulated in tumor sites. The tumor inhibition rates of NGP/DOX/3, NGP/DOX/6, NGG/DOX/3, and NGG/DOX/6 groups were 98.9 ± 0.2%, 99.4 ± 0.03%, 97.15 ± 0.4%, and 99.1 ± 0.1%, which were much stronger than that of DOX/3 and DOX/6 groups (i.e., 87.4 ± 2.1% and 95.8 ± 3.0%; $P < 0.001$). Despite DOX also showed antitumor effect, the weight loss of mice was very obvious during the therapy (**Figure 4B**), especially in the DOX/6 group, indicating the severe systemic toxicity of DOX. In contrast, the groups treated with DOX-loaded nanogels showed tiny body weight loss, indicating the effective attenuation effect DOX-loaded nanogels. Furthermore, organ indices were provided to offer a general impression of the system toxicity of DOX. The tumor index was also calculated. As shown, the organ indices exhibited no obvious difference except the tumor indices (**Figure 5**), indicating these nanogels would efficiently suppress the tumor growth while not cause systemic toxicities *in vivo*.

In addition, the histopathological and immunohistochemical tests were performed to further confirm the antitumor efficacy of DOX-loaded nanogels (**Figure 6**). In this study, four immunohistochemical stainings caspase-3, survivin, Bax, and Bcl-2 were performed (**Figure 6**). It is well known that the process of cell apoptosis is regulated and controlled by various apoptotic genes. Notably, the caspase family plays a crucial role in the process of apoptosis (Huang et al., 2015; Shi et al., 2017). The activation of apoptosis-inducing factor caspase-3 is the key pathway for a variety of stimuli-induced apoptosis (Huang et al., 2015; Shi et al., 2017). As shown, the signals of pro-apoptotic protein Bax (brown) and caspase-3 (brown) of the nanogels treatment groups were much stronger than those of the free DOX·HCl treatment groups. In contrast, the anti-apoptotic protein Bcl-2 (brown)

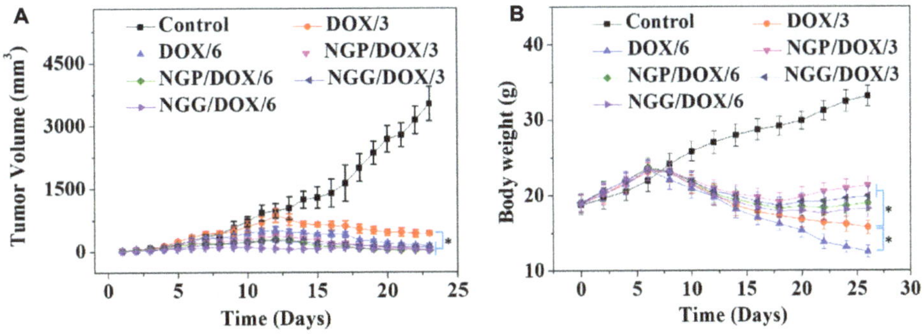

FIGURE 4 | Tumor volume **(A)** and body weight **(B)** changes of Lewis lung carcinoma-bearing BALB/c mice in the course of treatment with control, or free DOX·HCl, or NGP/DOX, or NGG/DOX at a dosage of 3.0 or 6.0 mg DOX·HCl equivalent per kg body weight. Each set of data is represented as mean ± *SD* ($n = 10$; $^*P < 0.001$).

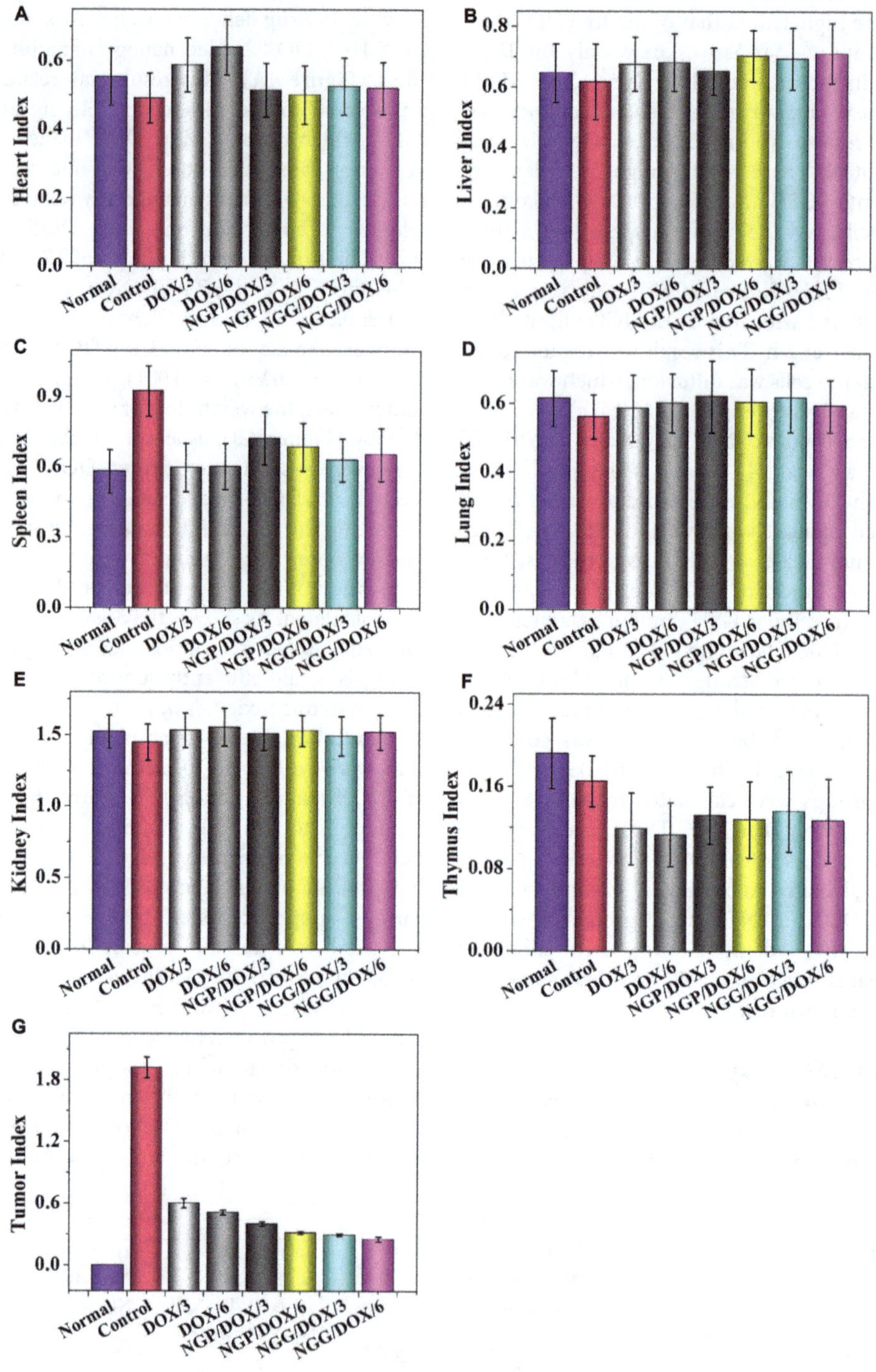

FIGURE 5 | Evaluations of heart **(A)**, liver **(B)**, spleen **(C)**, lung **(D)**, kidney **(E)**, thymus **(F)**, and tumor **(G)** indexes of Lewis lung carcinoma-allografted mice after injected with NS, DOX/3, DOX/6, NGP/DOX/3, NGP/DOX/6, NGG/DOX/3, or NGG/DOX/6. Each set of data is represented as mean ± *SD* (*n* = 8).

showed an obvious decline in the nanogels treatment groups. Furthermore, survivin was also tested to evaluate the cell survival (Huang et al., 2015; Shi et al., 2017). As shown, the signals of survivin (brown) were obviously reduced in the DOX-loaded nanogels treatment groups. These results fully verified that our DOX-loaded nanogels, especially NGP/DOX/6 and NGG/DOX/6, could be served as efficient nano-therapeutic agents.

As shown in **Figure 6**, H&E staining showed universal mitosis and mild hemorrhagic necrosis in the control

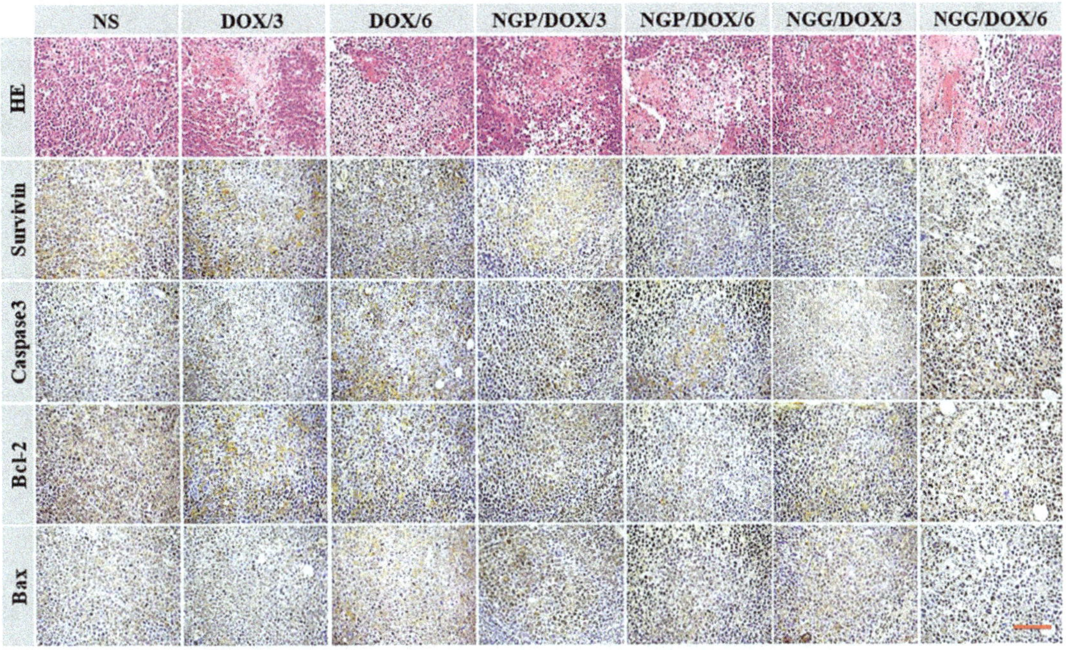

FIGURE 6 | Immunohistochemical (i.e., caspase-3, survivin, Bax, and Bcl-2) analyses of tumor tissue sections after treatments with NS, free DOX·HCl at a dose of 3 and 6 mg (DOX/3, DOX/6), NGP/DOX, and NGG/DOX at a dose of 3.0 or 6.0 mg DOX·HCl equivalent per kg body weight. Scale bar = 50 μm, magnification: 200×.

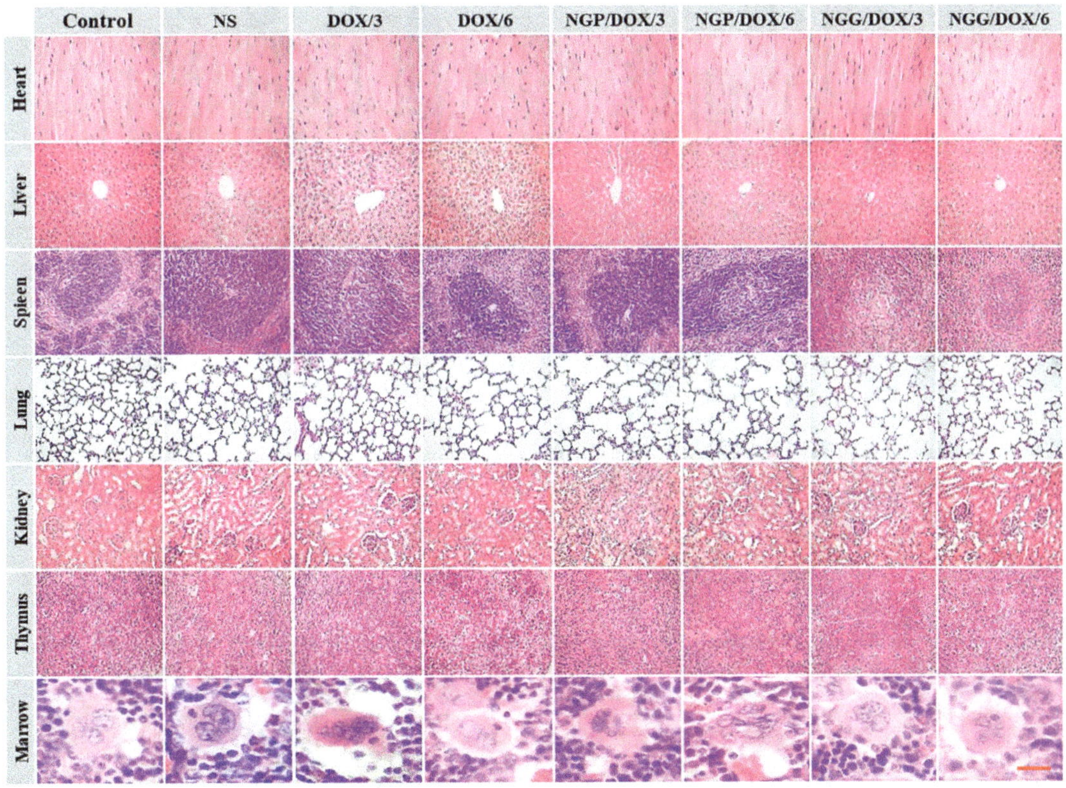

FIGURE 7 | *Ex vivo* histopathological analyses (i.e., H&E) of lung tumor, visceral organ, thymus, and marrow sections after all treatments with control, NS, free DOX 3 and 6 mg (DOX/3, DOX/6), NGP/DOX, and NGG/DOX at a dose of 3.0 or 6.0 mg DOX·HCl equivalent per kg body weight (NG/DOX/3, NG/DOX/6). Magnification: 200×.

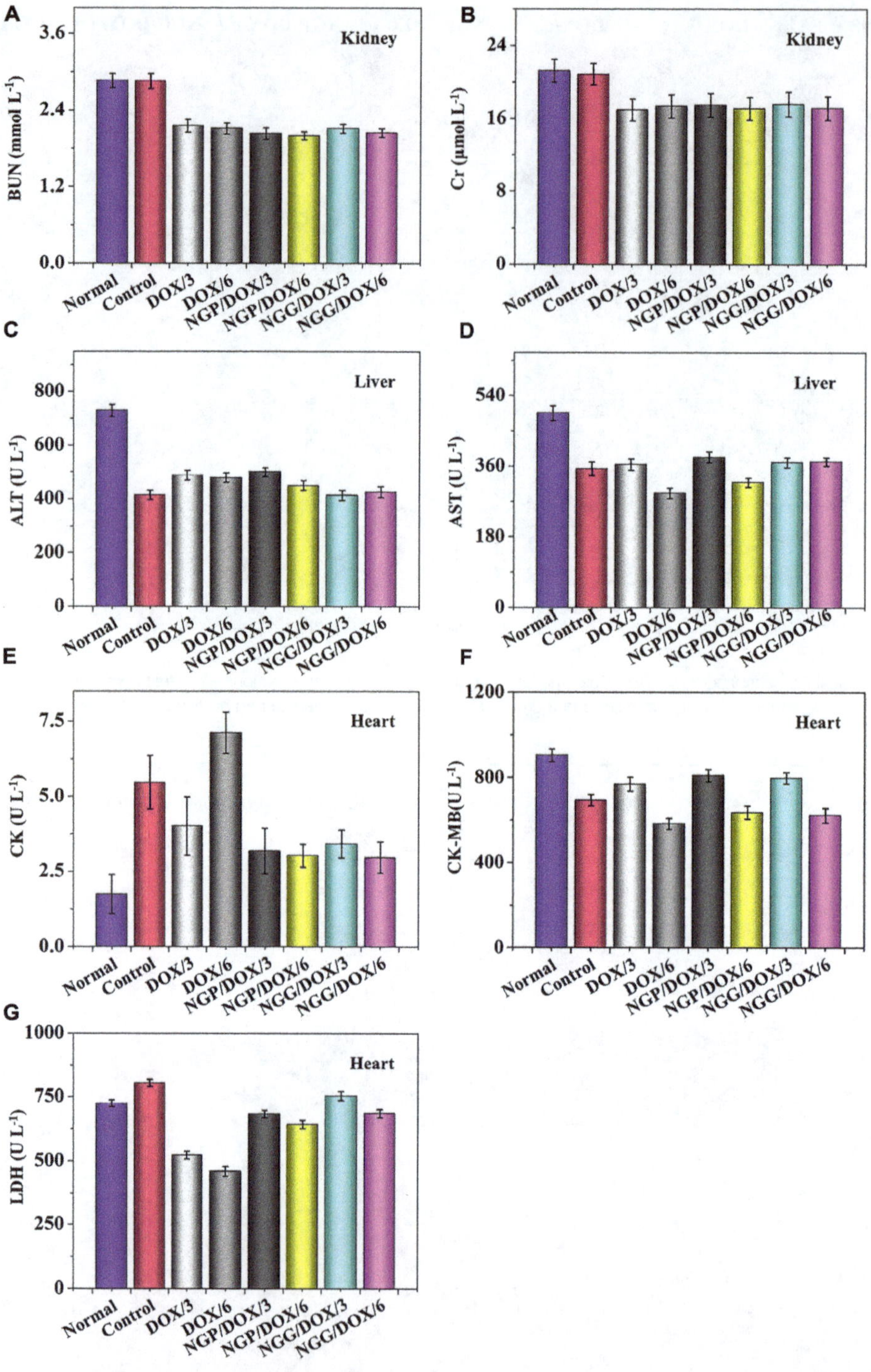

FIGURE 8 | Biochemical parameter assays for safety evaluation. Evaluations of BUN **(A)**, Cr **(B)**, ALT **(C)**, AST **(D)**, CK **(E)**, CK-MB **(F)**, and LDH **(G)** in corresponding internal organs of normal mice or Lewis lung carcinoma-allografted BALB/c mice after treatment with NS, free DOX·HCl at a dose of 3 and 6 mg (DOX/3, DOX/6), NGP/DOX, and NGG/DOX at a dose of 3.0 or 6.0 mg DOX·HCl equivalent per kg body weight. Each set of data is represented as mean ± *SD* (*n* = 3).

group, indicating the rapid cell growth. In contrast, all the DOX formulations treatment groups showed varying degrees of tumor growth suppression. Specifically, DOX formulations caused a reduction in mitosis and extensive hemorrhage and necrosis. The treatment groups were ranked as follows according to the relative amount of necrotic tissues: NGP/DOX/6.0 > NGG/DOX/6.0 > DOX/6.0 > NGP/DOX/3.0 > NGG/DOX/3.0 > DOX/3.0. Furthermore, the results of semi-quantitative in **Figures 10C,F** showed the necrotic areas of NGP/DOX/6 and NGP/DOX/6 treatment groups were 1.4 and

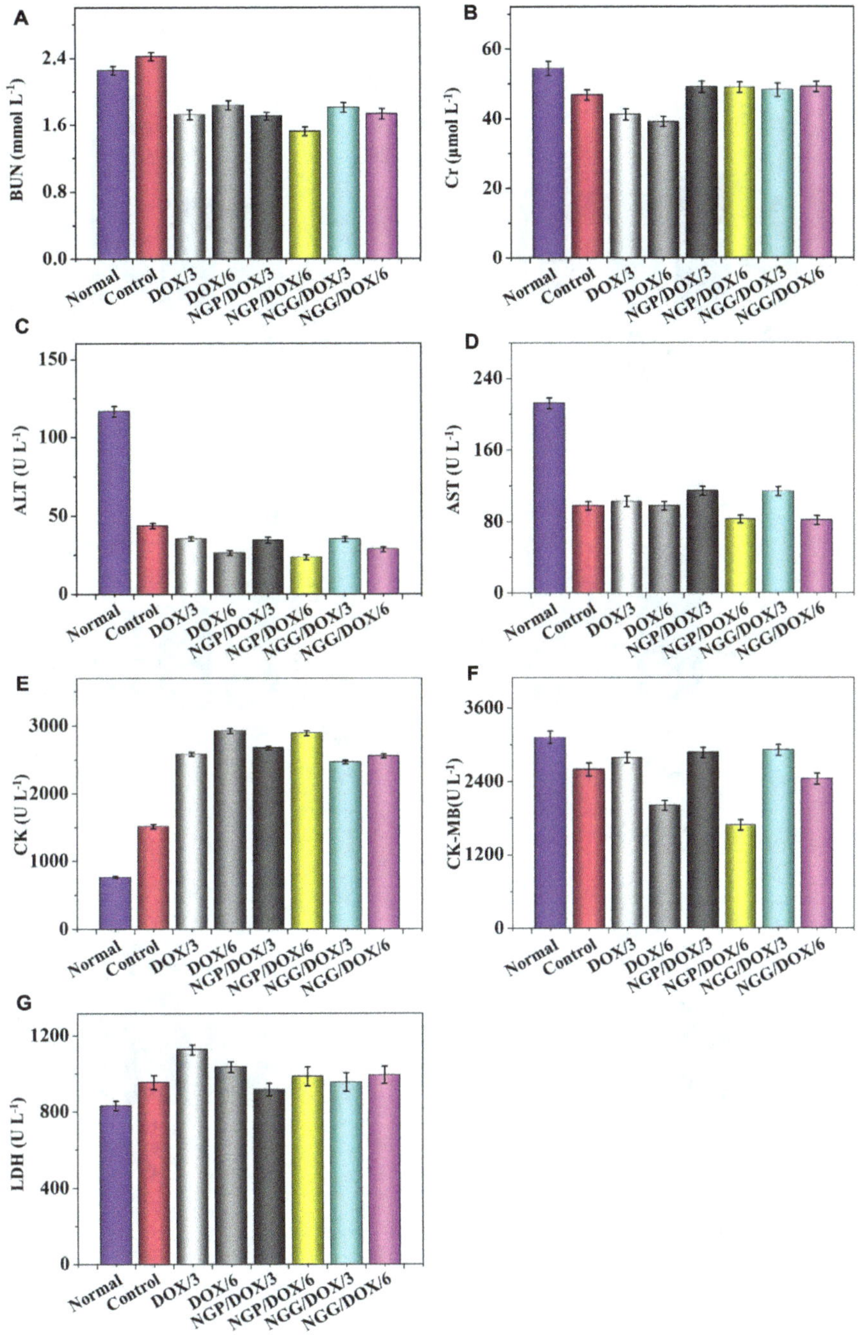

FIGURE 9 | Biochemical parameter assays for safety evaluation. Evaluations of BUN **(A)**, Cr **(B)**, ALT **(C)**, AST **(D)**, CK **(E)**, CK-MB **(F)**, and LDH **(G)** in serum of normal mice or Lewis lung carcinoma-allografted BALB/c mice after treatment with NS, free DOX·HCl at a dose of 3 and 6 mg (DOX/3, DOX/6), NGP/DOX, and NGG/DOX at a dose of 3.0 or 6.0 mg DOX·HCl equivalent per kg body weight. Each set of data is represented as mean ± *SD* (*n* = 3).

1.2 times larger than those of the free DOX·HCl/6 treatment group, respectively.

In vivo Security Evaluation

In this study, systematic safety was evaluated by monitoring the physical conditions and body weights changes, by analyzing the pathological morphology of various organs, by detecting the biological parameters from organs and serum, and by examining the BMMR and WBC levels after therapeutics. The *in vivo* systematic toxicity of DOX was reflected by body weight and histopathology of organs. Similar body weight gain trends were observed in each group of nude mice within the initial 1–10 days (**Figure 4B**). After that, the body weights of the nanogels treatment groups still showed similar

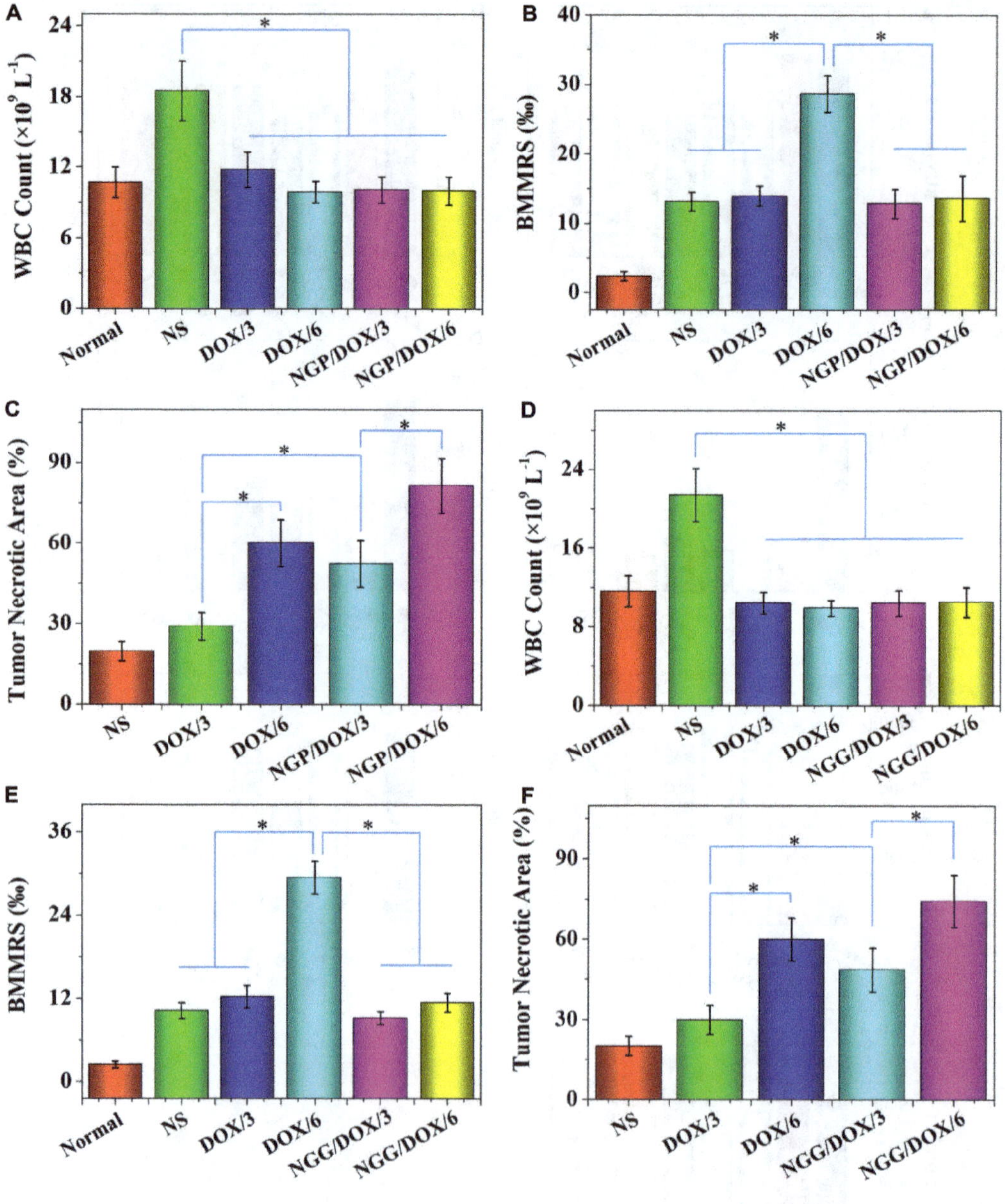

FIGURE 10 | WBC counts **(A,D)**, BMMRs **(B,E)** and tumor necrotic area from H&E **(C,F)**, normal mice (as control), or Lewis lung carcinoma-allografted BALB/c nude mice after treatment with NS, or free DOX·HCl or NGP/DOX **(A–C)** or NGG/DOX **(D–F)** at a dose of 3.0 or 6.0 mg DOX·HCl equivalent per kg body weight. Normal BALB/c nude mice serve as controls (Normal). Each set of data is represented as mean ± SD (n = 10; *P < 0.001).

growth trends on day 11–26. This result might be related to that controlled release of nanogels, which resulted less DOX release in the circulation. On the contrary, the body weights of free DOX·HCl treated groups showed significant downward trends within the same time interval, and larger doses cause more weight loss (P < 0.001). Especially the dose of 6.0 mg (kg BW)$^{-1}$ DOX treatment group caused severe weight loss, indicating the toxicity of DOX were dose-dependent.

The histopathological analyses of major organs were shown in **Figure 7**. Significant neutrophil accumulation and myocardial fiber breakage were observed in the showed in the free DOX·HCl treatment groups. In contrast, the neutrophil accumulation did not occur in the nanogels treatment groups, the myocardial cells were arranged orderly, and the sarcolemma-maintained integrity, probably relate to the reduced accumulation of free DOX·HCl in heart. Moreover, the microregional necrosis of hepatocytes in the free DOX·HCl treatment group indicated that free DOX·HCl had significant hepatotoxicity. On the contrary, less structural interferences were observed in the nanogels treatment groups. Moreover, the nephrotoxicity of free DOX·HCl was also reduced by the nanogels, which was verified by the intact structure of the kidneys in the nanogels treatment groups. These results indicated that the DOX-loaded nanogels could effectively reduce systematic toxicity, probably due to the satisfactory stability of DOX-loaded nanogels. All the results confirmed that the DOX-loaded nanogels had good biocompatibility.

The relevant clinical parameters of heart (CK, CK-MB, and LDH), liver (ALT and AST), and kidney (BUN and Cr) can reflect the function of corresponding organs. In this work, these clinical parameters were detected to verify the safety of DOX-loaded nanogels *in vivo*. As shown, the parameters of all organs except heart in each treated group were within the normal range (**Figure 8**). Free DOX·HCl/6 could cause serious damage to the heart (**Figure 8E**). The relevant parameters in serum were also tested by the commercial ELISA kits. All the clinical parameters of mice treated with DOX-loaded nanogels were equal or lower than normal nude mice treated with NS except CK (**Figure 9**). These results indicated that DOX-loaded nanogels did not cause serious organ dysfunction.

The number of WBC was tested to reflect the influence of chemotherapy drugs on the immune system. As shown in **Figures 10A,D**, the WBC counts of the NS treatment group was increased obviously. On the contrary, the DOX formulation treatment groups did not show increased WBC counts. The results indicated that the treatments with DOX formulations could effectively reduce the inflammation induced by tumor ($P < 0.01$).

The genotoxicity caused by chemotherapy drugs can be quantified by BMMR (Wang et al., 2018). As shown in **Figures 10B,E**, H&E-stained marrow sections were used to observe bone marrow mononuclear cells. These histopathological sections were also used to calculate BMMRs. Compared with normal mice, the BMMRs increased obviously in Lewis lung-grafted mice. For the mice treated with DOX formulations, a dose-related increase in BMMR was observed. Moreover, the BMMRs of the groups treated with free DOX·HCl were significantly greater than those of groups treated with DOX-loaded nanogels ($P < 0.001$). These results demonstrated that the physiological damage caused by free DOX was dose-dependent. Fortunately, DOX-loaded nanogels could effectively mitigate this injury.

CONCLUSION

In this work, reduction-responsive DOX-loaded nanogels (NGP/DOX and NGG/DOX) were prepared by classical nanoprecipitation method. *In vitro* studies showed that both NGP/DOX and NGG/DOX groups exhibited stronger cellular uptake of Lewis cells compared with free DOX treatment groups. Furthermore, all the NGP/DOX and NGG/DOX groups exhibited more efficient antitumor efficacy than the free DOX·HCl treatment groups in the Lewis lung carcinoma grafted nude mouse model. Importantly, all the DOX-loaded nanogels could significantly reduce the systemic toxicity of DOX. Therefore, these polypeptides nanogels with high systemic safety could serve as promising nanodrug delivery platforms for the future lung carcinoma chemotherapy.

AUTHOR CONTRIBUTIONS

All authors conceived and designed the study. KN, NL, and YY performed the experiments. KN, NL, YY, CG, YG, and JW analyzed and interpreted the data, and prepared the manuscript.

REFERENCES

Acharya, S., and Sahoo, S. K. (2011). PLGA nanoparticles containing various anticancer agents and tumour delivery by EPR effect. *Adv. Drug Deliv. Rev.* 63, 170–183. doi: 10.1016/j.addr.2010.10.008

Allen, T. M., and Cullis, P. R. (2013). Liposomal drug delivery systems: from concept to clinical applications. *Adv. Drug Deliv. Rev.* 65, 36–48. doi: 10.1016/j.addr.2012.09.037

Armstrong, J. P. K., and Stevens, M. M. (2018). Strategic design of extracellular vesicle drug delivery systems. *Adv. Drug Deliv. Rev.* 130, 12–16. doi: 10.1016/j.addr.2018.06.017

Chen, J., Ding, J., Wang, Y., Cheng, J., Ji, S., Zhuang, X., et al. (2017a). Sequentially responsive shell-stacked nanoparticles for deep penetration into solid tumors. *Adv. Mater.* 29:1701170. doi: 10.1002/adma.201701170

Chen, J., Ding, J., Xu, W., Sun, T., Xiao, H., Zhuang, X., et al. (2017b). Receptor and microenvironment dual-recognizable nanogel for targeted chemotherapy of highly metastatic malignancy. *Nano Lett.* 17, 4526–4533. doi: 10.1021/acs.nanolett.7b02129

Cheng, R., Meng, F., Deng, C., Klok, H.-A., and Zhong, Z. (2013). Dual and multi-stimuli responsive polymeric nanoparticles for programmed site-specific drug delivery. *Biomaterials* 34, 3647–3657. doi: 10.1016/j.biomaterials.2013.01.084

Cong, Y., Xiao, H., Xiong, H., Wang, Z., Ding, J., Li, C., et al. (2018). Dual drug backboned shattering polymeric theranostic nanomedicine for synergistic eradication of patient-derived lung cancer. *Adv. Mater.* 30:1706220. doi: 10.1002/adma.201706220

Ding, J., Chen, L., Xiao, C., Chen, L., Zhuang, X., and Chen, X. (2014). Noncovalent interaction-assisted polymeric micelles for controlled drug delivery. *Chem. Commun.* 50, 11274–11290. doi: 10.1039/C4CC03153A

Ding, J., Li, C., Zhang, Y., Xu, W., Wang, J., and Chen, X. (2015). Chirality-mediated polypeptide micelles for regulated drug delivery. *Acta Biomater.* 11, 346–355. doi: 10.1016/j.actbio.2014.09.043

Ding, J., Shi, F., Xiao, C., Lin, L., Chen, L., He, C., et al. (2011). One-step preparation of reduction-responsive poly(ethylene glycol)-poly (amino acid)s nanogels as efficient intracellular drug delivery platforms. *Polym. Chem.* 2, 2857–2864. doi: 10.1039/c1py00360g

Ding, J., Shi, F., Xiao, C., Zhuang, X., He, C., and Chen, X. (2013a). Facile preparation of pH and reduction responsive PEGylated polypeptide nanogel for efficient doxorubicin loading and intracellular delivery. *J. Control. Release* 172, E40–E41. doi: 10.1016/j.jconrel.2013.08.087

Ding, J., Xiao, C., Li, Y., Cheng, Y., Wang, N., He, C., et al. (2013b). Efficacious hepatoma-targeted nanomedicine self-assembled from galactopeptide and doxorubicin driven by two-stage physical interactions. *J. Control. Release* 169, 193–203. doi: 10.1016/j.jconrel.2012.12.006

Ding, J., Xu, W., Zhang, Y., Sun, D., Xiao, C., Liu, D., et al. (2013c). Self-reinforced endocytoses of smart polypeptide nanogels for "on-demand" drug delivery. *J. Control. Release* 172, 444–455. doi: 10.1016/j.jconrel.2013.05.029

Feng, X.-R., Ding, J.-X., Gref, R., and Chen, X.-S. (2017). Poly(β-cyclodextrin)-mediated polylactide-cholesterol stereocomplex micelles for controlled drug delivery. *Chin. J. Polym. Sci.* 35, 693–699. doi: 10.1007/s10118-017-1932-7

Ge, Z., and Liu, S. (2013). Functional block copolymer assemblies responsive to tumor and intracellular microenvironments for site-specific drug delivery and enhanced imaging performance. *Chem. Soc. Rev.* 42, 7289–7325. doi: 10.1039/c3cs60048c

Guo, H., Li, F., Xu, W., Chen, J., Hou, Y., Wang, C., et al. (2018). Mucoadhesive cationic polypeptide nanogel with enhanced penetration for efficient intravesical chemotherapy of bladder cancer. *Adv. Sci.* 5:1800004. doi: 10.1002/advs.201800004

Guo, H., Xu, W., Chen, J., Yan, L., Ding, J., Hou, Y., et al. (2017). Positively charged polypeptide nanogel enhances mucoadhesion and penetrability of 10-hydroxycamptothecin in orthotopic bladder carcinoma. *J. Control. Release* 259, 136–148. doi: 10.1016/j.jconrel.2016.12.041

Huang, K., Shi, B., Xu, W., Ding, J., Yang, Y., Liu, H., et al. (2015). Reduction-responsive polypeptide nanogel delivers antitumor drug for improved efficacy and safety. *Acta biomater.* 27, 179–193. doi: 10.1016/j.actbio.2015.08.049

Ji, X. Y., Kong, N., Wang, J. Q., Li, W. L., Xiao, Y. L., Gan, S. T., et al. (2018). A novel top-down synthesis of ultrathin 2D boron nanosheets for multimodal imaging-guided cancer therapy. *Adv. Mater.* 30:e1803031. doi: 10.1002/adma.201803031

Jiang, Z., Chen, J., Cui, L., Zhuang, X., Ding, J., and Chen, X. (2018a). Advances in stimuli-responsive polypeptide nanogels. *Small Methods* 2:1700307. doi: 10.1002/smtd.201700307

Jiang, Z. Y., Chen, J. J., Cui, L. G., Zhuang, X. L., Ding, J. X., and Chen, X. S. (2018b). Advances in stimuli-responsive polypeptide nanogels. *Small Methods* 2:1700307. doi: 10.1002/smtd.201700307

Kanodra, N. M., Silvestri, G. A., and Tanner, N. T. (2015). Screening and early detection efforts in lung cancer. *Cancer* 121, 1347–1356. doi: 10.1002/cncr.29222

Kernstine, K. (2017). "Treatment of small cell lung neoplasms by surgery," in *Modern.Thoracic Oncology*, eds R. B. Cameron, O. Olevsky, and D. Gage (Singapore: World Scientific Publishing Company), 189–196.

Kosakowska, K. A., Casey, B. K., Kurtz, S. L., Lawson, L. B., and Grayson, S. M. (2018). Evaluation of amphiphilic star/linear–dendritic polymer reverse micelles for transdermal drug delivery: directing carrier properties by tailoring core versus peripheral branching. *Biomacromolecules* 19, 3163–3176. doi: 10.1021/acs.biomac.8b00680

Li, D., Feng, X., Chen, L., Ding, J., and Chen, X. (2018a). One-step synthesis of targeted acid-labile polysaccharide prodrug for efficiently intracellular drug delivery. *ACS Biomater. Sci. Eng.* 4, 539–546. doi: 10.1021/acsbiomaterials.7b00856

Li, J., Xu, W., Li, D., Liu, T., Zhang, Y. S., Ding, J., et al. (2018b). A locally deployable nanofiber patch for sequential drug delivery in treatment of primary and advanced orthotopic hepatomas. *ACS Nano* 12, 6685–6699. doi: 10.1021/acsnano.8b01729

Li, S., Dong, S., Xu, W., Tu, S., Yan, L., Zhao, C., et al. (2018c). Antibacterial hydrogels. *Adv. Sci.* 5:1700527. doi: 10.1002/advs.201700527

Li, S., Zhang, T., Xu, W., Ding, J., Yin, F., Xu, J., et al. (2018d). Sarcoma-targeting peptide-decorated polypeptide nanogel intracellularly delivers shikonin for upregulated osteosarcoma necroptosis and diminished pulmonary metastasis. *Theranostics* 8, 1361–1375. doi: 10.7150/thno.18299

Liu, X., Wang, J., Xu, W., Ding, J., Shi, B., Huang, K., et al. (2015). Glutathione-degradable drug-loaded nanogel effectively and securely suppresses hepatoma in mouse model. *Int. J. Nanomed.* 10, 6587–6602. doi: 10.2147/IJN.S90000

Mura, S., Nicolas, J., and Couvreur, P. (2013). Stimuli-responsive nanocarriers for drug delivery. *Nat. Mater.* 12, 991–1003. doi: 10.1038/nmat3776

Parks, S. K., Chiche, J., and Pouysségur, J. (2013). Disrupting proton dynamics and energy metabolism for cancer therapy. *Nat. Rev. Cancer* 13, 611–623. doi: 10.1038/nrc3579

Phillips, D. J., and Gibson, M. I. (2014). Redox-sensitive materials for drug delivery: targeting the correct intracellular environment, tuning release rates, and appropriate predictive systems. *Antioxid. Redox Signal.* 21, 786–803. doi: 10.1089/ars.2013.5728

Piffoux, M., Silva, A. K. A., Wilhelm, C., Gazeau, F., and Tareste, D. (2018). Modification of extracellular vesicles by fusion with liposomes for the design of personalized biogenic drug delivery systems. *ACS Nano* 12, 6830–6842. doi: 10.1021/acsnano.8b02053

Ryu, J.-H., Jiwpanich, S., Chacko, R., Bickerton, S., and Thayumanavan, S. (2010). Surface-functionalizable polymer nanogels with facile hydrophobic guest encapsulation capabilities. *J. Am. Chem. Soc.* 132, 8246–8247. doi: 10.1021/ja102316a

Shen, K., Li, D., Guan, J., Ding, J., Wang, Z., Gu, J., et al. (2017). Targeted sustained delivery of antineoplastic agent with multicomponent polylactide stereocomplex micelle. *Nanomed. Nanotechnol. Biol. Med.* 13, 1279–1288. doi: 10.1016/j.nano.2016.12.022

Shi, B., Huang, K., Ding, J., Xu, W., Yang, Y., Liu, H., et al. (2017). Intracellularly swollen polypeptide nanogel assists hepatoma chemotherapy. *Theranostics* 7, 703–716. doi: 10.7150/thno.16794

Sun, X., Wang, G., Zhang, H., Hu, S., Liu, X., Tang, J., et al. (2018). The blood clearance kinetics and pathway of polymeric micelles in cancer drug delivery. *ACS Nano* 12, 6179–6192. doi: 10.1021/acsnano.8b02830

Tao, W., Zhang, J., Zeng, X., Liu, D., Liu, G., Zhu, X., et al. (2015). Blended nanoparticle system based on miscible structurally similar polymers: a safe, simple, targeted, and surprisingly high efficiency vehicle for cancer therapy. *Adv. Healthcare Mater.* 4, 1203–1214. doi: 10.1002/adhm.201400751

Tao, W., Zhu, X. B., Yu, X. H., Zeng, X. W., Xiao, Q. L., Zhang, X. D., et al. (2017). Black phosphorus nanosheets as a robust delivery platform for cancer theranostics. *Adv. Mater.* 29:1603276. doi: 10.1002/adma.201603276

Wang, J., Xu, W., Li, S., Qiu, H., Li, Z., Wang, C., et al. (2018). Polylactide-cholesterol stereocomplex micelle encapsulating chemotherapeutic agent for improved antitumor efficacy and safety. *J. Biomed. Nanotechnol.* 14, 2102–2113. doi: 10.1166/jbn.2018.2624

Xiao, H., Yan, L., Dempsey, E. M., Song, W., Qi, R., Li, W., et al. (2018). Recent progress in polymer-based platinum drug delivery systems. *Prog. Polym. Sci.* 87, 70–106. doi: 10.7497/j.issn.2095-3941.2015.0063

Xu, W., Ding, J., and Chen, X. (2017). Reduction-responsive polypeptide micelles for intracellular delivery of antineoplastic agent. *Biomacromolecules* 18, 3291–3301. doi: 10.1021/acs.biomac.7b00950

Yang, N., Ding, Y., Zhang, Y., Wang, B., Zhao, X., Cheng, K., et al. (2018). Surface functionalization of polymeric nanoparticles with umbilical cord-derived mesenchymal stem cell membrane for tumor-targeted therapy. *ACS Appl. Mater. Interfaces* 10, 22963–22973. doi: 10.1021/acsami.8b05363

Ye, Y., Yu, J., and Gu, Z. (2016). Versatile protein nanogels prepared by in situ polymerization. *Macromol. Chem. Phys.* 217, 333–343. doi: 10.1002/macp.201500296

Yu, J., Zhang, Y., Sun, W., Wang, C., Ranson, D., Ye, Y., et al. (2016). Endosome-mimicking nanogels for targeted drug delivery. *Nanoscale* 8, 9178–9184. doi: 10.1039/C5NR08895J

Zha, L. S., Banik, B., and Alexis, F. (2011). Stimulus responsive nanogels for drug delivery. *Soft Matter* 7, 5908–5916. doi: 10.1039/c0sm01307b

Zhang, X., Liang, X., Gu, J., Chang, D., Zhang, J., Chen, Z., et al. (2017). Investigation and intervention of autophagy to guide cancer treatment with nanogels. *Nanoscale* 9, 150–163. doi: 10.1039/c6nr07866d

Zhang, Y., Cai, L., Li, D., Lao, Y.-H., Liu, D., Li, M., et al. (2018). Tumor microenvironment-responsive hyaluronate-calcium carbonate hybrid nanoparticle enables effective chemotherapy for primary and advanced osteosarcomas. *Nano Res.* 11, 4806–4822. doi: 10.1007/s12274-018-2066-0

Zhao, K., Li, D., Xu, W., Ding, J., Jiang, W., Li, M., et al. (2017). Targeted hydroxyethyl starch prodrug for inhibiting the growth and metastasis of prostate cancer. *Biomaterials* 116, 82–94. doi: 10.1016/j.biomaterials.2016.11.030

Zhao, Y., Alakhova, D. Y., Kim, J. O., Bronich, T. K., and Kabanov, A. V. (2013). A simple way to enhance Doxil (R) therapy: drug release from liposomes at the tumor site by amphiphilic block copolymer. *J. Control. Release* 168, 61–69. doi: 10.1016/j.jconrel.2013.02.026

Zhu, Q., Chen, X., Xu, X., Zhang, Y., Zhang, C., and Mo, R. (2018). Drug delivery: tumor-specific self-degradable nanogels as potential carriers for systemic delivery of anticancer proteins (Adv. Funct. Mater. 17/2018). *Adv. Func. Mat.* 28:1870109. doi: 10.1002/adfm.201870109

19

Human Albumin Fragments Nanoparticles as PTX Carrier for Improved Anti-Cancer Efficacy

Liang Ge[1,2†], Xinru You[3†], Jun Huang[3†], Yuejian Chen[4], Li Chen[2], Ying Zhu[1], Yuan Zhang[5], Xiqiang Liu[6], Jun Wu[3*] and Qian Hai[1*]*

[1] State Key Laboratory of Natural Medicines, China Pharmaceutical University, Nanjing, China, [2] School of Pharmacy, Xinjiang Medical University, Ürümqi, China, [3] Key Laboratory of Sensing Technology and Biomedical Instruments of Guangdong Province, School of Biomedical Engineering, Sun Yat-sen University, Guangzhou, China, [4] Nanjing iPharma Technology, Co., Ltd., Nanjing, China, [5] Department of Orthopedics, Xinqiao Hospital, Third Military Medical University, Chongqing, China, [6] Guangdong Provincial Key Laboratory of Stomatology, Guanghua School of Stomatology, Hospital of Stomatology, Sun Yat-sen University, Guangzhou, China

***Correspondence:**
Xiqiang Liu
xiqiangliu@aliyun.com
Jun Wu
wujun29@mail.sysu.edu.cn
Qian Hai
qianhai24@163.com

† These authors have contributed equally to this work.

For enhanced anti-cancer performance, human serum albumin fragments (HSAFs) nanoparticles (NPs) were developed as paclitaxel (PTX) carrier in this paper. Human albumins were broken into fragments via degradation and crosslinked by genipin to form HSAF NPs for better biocompatibility, improved PTX drug loading and sustained drug release. Compared with crosslinked human serum albumin NPs, the HSAF-NPs showed relative smaller particle size, higher drug loading, and improved sustained release. Cellular and animal results both indicated that the PTX encapsulated HSAF-NPs have shown good anti-cancer performance. And the anticancer results confirmed that NPs with fast cellular internalization showed better tumor inhibition. These findings will not only provide a safe and robust drug delivery NP platform for cancer therapy, but also offer fundamental information for the optimal design of albumin based NPs.

Keywords: human serum albumin fragments, nanoparticle, paclitaxel, drug delivery, anticancer

INTRODUCTION

With the fast growing of material chemistry and nanomedicine, biodegradable nanoscale drug delivery platforms, including nanoparticles, micelles (Wang et al., 2014a; Li W. et al., 2016; Qu et al., 2017) and liposomes, have been widely utilized for biomedical diagnosis (Park et al., 2009; Morral-Ruiz et al., 2013; Wang et al., 2014b; Hu et al., 2018) and therapy (Boussif et al., 1995; Ding et al., 2013; Xing et al., 2013; Bertrand et al., 2014; You et al., 2016; Ge et al., 2017; Li et al., 2017; Pan et al., 2018; Yang et al., 2018). Recently, a great number of functional delivery systems (Liu and Lu, 2006; Cho et al., 2011; Shrestha et al., 2012; Wu et al., 2012, 2014; Li et al., 2013; Wu and Chu, 2013; Yu et al., 2013; Hai et al., 2014; Li H. et al., 2016; Hao et al., 2017; Xu et al., 2017) have been studied. But even the nanoparticles (NPs) based on FDA approved materials, such as the poly-ε-caprolactone (PCL), poly(DL-lactic acid), poly(lactide-cocaprolactone), and poly(lactide-co-glycolide) (PLGA), are still toxic for high dosage treatment (Singh and Ramarao, 2013). Then, NP systems with improved biocompatibility are highly desired (Maiti, 2011; Wang et al., 2016, 2018).

Albumin, as a biodegradable, non-toxic and non-immunogenic protein, has been used to prepare NPs (Elzoghby et al., 2012). Albumin based nanocarriers (Shimanovich et al., 2011; Altintas et al., 2013; Bakare et al., 2014; Rosenberger et al., 2014; Watcharin et al., 2014) have been reported and the albumin-bound paclitaxel (Abraxane®) had been proved to be safe and efficient (Saif, 2013; Cecco et al., 2014). The crosslinked albumin NPs were able to increase their physical stabilities, but the drug encapsulation efficiencies and sustained release still need to be improved (Kratz, 2008; Li et al., 2010, 2014; Elzoghby et al., 2012; Kou et al., 2018). For this goal, we hypothesized that albumin fragments based NPs could have better drug loading/release performance, which would result improved anti-cancer performance. Non-toxicity, biodegradability and preferential uptake in tumor and inflamed tissues make human serum albumin fragments (HSAFs) an ideal drug delivery system. Due to these advantages, it's motivated to develop a novel and safety nanoplatform based on HASF.

Therefore, in this report, as a model platform, a HSAF NP platform was developed as drug carriers with different crosslinking degrees and diameters using genipin as a very biocompatible crosslinker (**Figure 1A**). HSAFs were obtained via the degradation and the natural genipin crosslinker is expected to significantly reduce the toxicity while keep the similar crosslinking capability, comparing to the widely used glutaraldehyde. HSAF NPs were screened by a quantitative method based on FRET theory (**Figure 1B**) following previous report to obtain faster cellular uptake for further evaluations (Jiang et al., 2015).

MATERIALS AND METHODS

HSAF NPs Preparation

Human serum albumin (HSA) was dissolved deionized water before 70% formic acid was added. CNBr was then added to degrade the HSA into fragment products (McMenamy et al., 1971). HSA degradation products were separated and purified by Superdex75 (Lapresle and Doyen, 1975; Yuan et al., 2014), and the three main peptide fragments are Fraction $A_{299-585}$, Fraction B_{1-123}, and Fraction $C_{124-298\ (46-48)}$ (w : w = 3.5:1:2.2), then the purified HSAF was used to prepare HSAF NPs. HSAF NPs were prepared and characterized according to the published protocols (Jiang et al., 2013). Then HSAF NPs with different crosslinking degrees and diameters were developed using a disulfide bond reducing method established in the previous work (Jiang et al., 2013). Briefly, a predeterminded amount of cysteine was added into the HSAF PBS solution under pH 8.0 at 37°C. The final concentration is 5 mg/mL. After dialysis, the remaining cysteine was removed and genipin was used to do second crosslinking (1 h). The genipin residue was cleaned by same method as above and the HSAF NPs were collected by lyophilization. The HSAF NP library with formulation parameters is summarized in **Table 1**.

Preparation and Characterization of Paclitaxel (PTX)-Loaded HSAF NPs

The PTX-loaded HSAF NPs with serious of crosslinking densities and diameters (PLC40S70, PLC70S70, PLC90S70, PLC40S160, and PLC40S260) were prepared following the same method preparing the above NPs. Briefly, the certain amount of HSAF was dissolved in PBS 8.0 at 37°C, and then PTX were dissolved in ethanol (PTX/HSAF50 mg/g) and genipin were added. Then system was incubated for 30 min to complete the crosslinking. The NP solution was purified and concentrated using Amicon Ultra Centrifugal Filters (MWCO 100,000). The size and zeta potential of PTX-loaded HSAF NPs were evaluated by a zeta potential and particle size analyser (ZetaPlus, Brookhaven, NY, United States). The morphology of nanoparticle was verified by transmission electron microscope (H-7650, HITACHI, Japan).

PTX Drug Release Profiles of HSAF NPs

Dialysis was used to determine the release behavior of paclitaxel from nanoparticles. 3 mL of the nanoparticle suspension

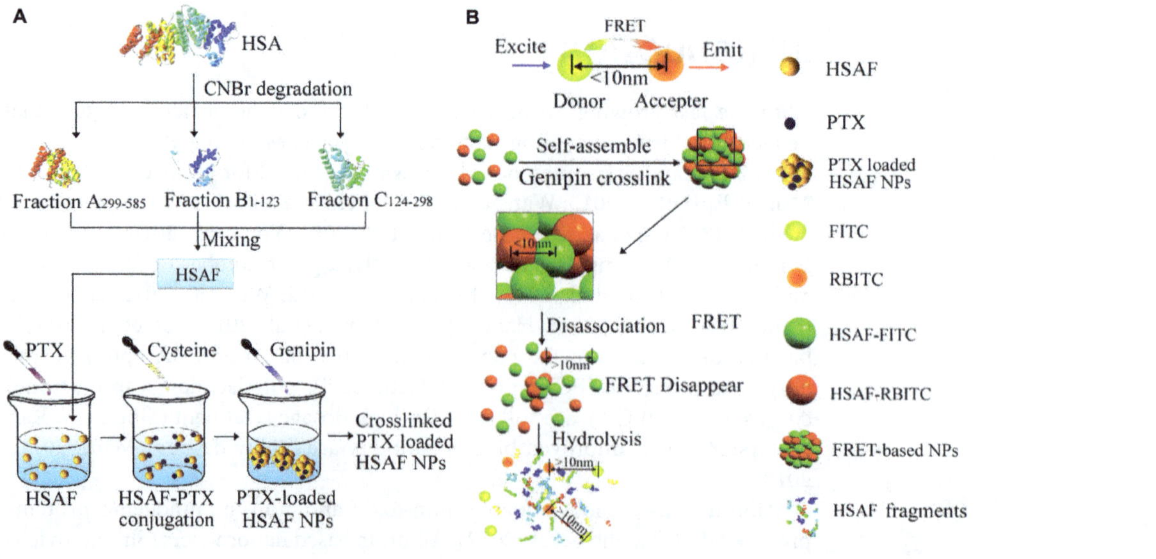

FIGURE 1 | The illustration of nanoparticle preparation procedures and the related FRET phenomenon and the degradation process of NPs. **(A)** The fabrication of PTX-loaded HSAF NPs. **(B)** The degradation process of FRET-based NPs.

TABLE 1 | Physical and chemical properties of HSAF and HSA NPs.

	Crosslinking degree (%)	Diameter (nm)	Zeta potential (mV)	FRET Index (%)
$C40S70_{HSAF}$	40.9 ± 1.5	65.9 ± 2.1	−20.86 ± 1.53	23.6 ± 0.9
$C70S70_{HSAF}$	65.2 ± 2.0	68.0 ± 3.3	−24.09 ± 1.66	27.0 ± 2.8
$C90S70_{HSAF}$	90.1 ± 0.9	74.7 ± 1.4	−27.12 ± 1.57	31.9 ± 0.4
$C40S160_{HSAF}$	41.3 ± 1.0	157.3 ± 2.3	−23.58 ± 1.33	23.1 ± 0.3
$C40S260_{HSAF}$	40.8 ± 1.1	255.9 ± 1.2	−20.13 ± 1.05	23.4 ± 1.3
$C40S70_{HSA}$	38.8 ± 0.8	78.1 ± 0.3	−20.91 ± 1.51	23.7 ± 0.8
$C70S70_{HSA}$	57.8 ± 1.9	80.1 ± 0.6	−23.09 ± 1.68	27.1 ± 1.7
$C90S70_{HSA}$	85.8 ± 1.8	83.1 ± 1.1	−28.17 ± 1.59	30.6 ± 0.7
$C40S160_{HSA}$	38.8 ± 1.1	182.7 ± 2.3	−24.11 ± 1.13	23.4 ± 0.6
$C40S260_{HSA}$	37.6 ± 0.8	264.4 ± 3.1	−20.86 ± 1.53	23.5 ± 0.9

(containing 10 mg PTX) was placed in a dialysis bag (molecular weight cut-off: 13 kDa). The dialysis bags were placed in 80 mL of 1 M salicylic acid solution. Shaking was performed at a shaking speed of 100 rpm and a temperature of 37°C. 0.5 mL of dialysate was collected at 0.5, 1, 2, 4, 6, 8, 12, 24, 36, and 48 h, respectively, and an equal volume of fresh dialyzing media was added.

Pharmacokinetic Studies

The PTX NPs (PLC40S70, PLC70S70, and PLC90S70) had similar diameters of about 70 nm but different crosslinking densities (41, 65, and 90%). And the NPs (PLC40S70, PLC40S160, and PLC40S260) prepared with albumin had similar crosslinking degrees around 42% but different diameters (65.9, 157.3, and 255.9 nm). The NPs (PLC40S70, PLC70S70, PLC90S70, PLC40S160, and PLC40S260) was i.v. administrated to Sprague-Dawley rats at a dose of 1 mg/kg as PTX. The blood sample was collected (100 μL) from rats into heparinized tubes at scheduled time (0, 0.083, 0.167, 0.333, 0.5, 1, 2, 4, 8, 12, and 24 h). Plasma was separated via centrifuging (4000 rpm, 10 min) and stored under −70°C until analysis. The drug concentrations were measured by LC–MS/MS (Wang et al., 2013) as previous study. For details, the analytes were eluted with at 5% mobile phase A methanol and 95% B water phase (containing 0.1% formic acid). The flow rate was 0.3 mL/min, and the temperature of column was 30°C. Mass analysis was operated in the positive ionization mode. Quantification was accomplished by monitoring the transition of m/z 876.0→307.8 for paclitaxel and m/z 830.3→549.0 for docetaxel (the internal standard). The spray voltage, the temperature of capillary, sheath gas pressure and auxiliary gas pressure were set at 4000 V, 350°C, 35 and 25 Arb, respectively. The pharmacokinetic parameters were estimated via a non-compartmental analysis (WinNonlin computer program, Version 4.0; Pharsight Corporation). All the experiments were performed in accordance with the recommendations of "guidelines of the Experimental Laboratory Animal Committee of China Pharmaceutical University and the National Institutes of Health's Guide for the Care and Use of Laboratory Animals." The protocol was approved by the "Experimental Laboratory Animal Committee of China Pharmaceutical University."

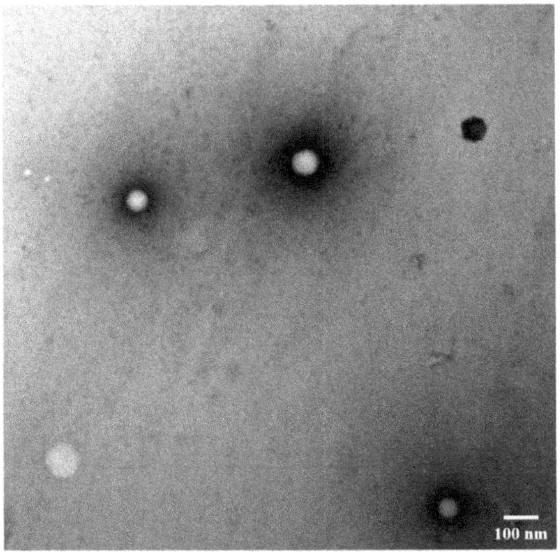

FIGURE 2 | TEM image of C90S70 (length bar = 100 nm).

In Vivo Imaging Study of HSAF Nanoparticles in Tumor-Bearing Mice

The NPs (C40S70, C70S70, and C90S70) had similar diameters around 70 nm but different crosslinking densities (42, 66, and 91%). And the NPs (C40S70, C40S160, and C40S260)

TABLE 2 | The diameters and drug loading efficiencies of the PTX-loaded HSAF and/or HSA NPs (n = 3).

	Diameter (nm)		PTX loading efficiencies (%)	
	HSAF NPs	HAS NPs	HSAF NPs	HSA NPs
C40S70	70.9 ± 3.3	87.2 ± 2.4	7.4	5.1
C70S70	74.0 ± 4.7	94.0 ± 3.6	7.2	5.3
C90S70	81.7 ± 3.2	95.7 ± 5.9	7.0	5.2
C40S160	172.3 ± 7.5	201.2 ± 15.8	8.3	6.5
C40S260	269.5 ± 14.6	295.1 ± 12.1	7.5	5.7

prepared with various protein fragment concentrations had similar degrees of crosslinking around 40% but different size (65.9, 157.3, and 255.9 nm). DLC40S70, DLC70S70, DLC90S70, DLC40S160, and DLC40S260 expressed (DL means Dir was loaded) was made as the method as the NPs above, and the crosslinking densities and diameters differs not as the NPS without Dir. The certain amount of HSAF (Dir/protein 50 mg/g) was dissolved in PBS 8.0, and then the ethanol Dir was added at 37°C water bath. 5 mg/mL Cys was added. The system was cooled for 10 min. Genipin cross-linking was completed after dialysis. The configuration of the concentration of 50 μg/mL Dir which was dissolved in the polyoxyethylene castor oil and ethanol (50:50, V/V) solution was made as a control group. DLC40S70, DLC70S70, DLC90S70, DLC40S160, DLC40S260, and Dir solution formulation (0.5 mg/kg) was injected into the tumor-bearing mice via the tail vein. After intravenous injection, intraperitoneal injection of sodium pentobarbital solution (1%, 50 mg/kg) was given to anesthetize the mice. After the anesthetization, the whole body fluorescence images were acquired using small animal *in vivo* near-infrared imaging system at 0.5, 1, 2, 4, and 8 h.

In Vivo Anticancer Evaluation in Breast Cancer Models

To evaluate *in vivo* anticancer activity of PTX-loaded HSAF and HSA NPs, PTX-loaded HSAF and HSA NPs were made by the method as C90S70 NPs whose particle size is the smallest and the crossing link degree is the highest. The 1 × 10^7/ml MCF-7 cells were re-suspended in 9% saline, and 0.1 ml cells suspension was injected to nude mice on the right axillary subcutaneous. Tumor volumes were determined on alternate day by a vernier caliper, and the tumor volumes were calculated by an equation: V (cm^3) = a × b^2/2 (a: largest diameter; b: smallest diameter), meanwhile, mice weights were monitored three times per week. Fourteen days after tumor implantation, the volumes of tumor size were allowed to reach no less than 0.1 cm^3, and mice groups (n = 8) were designed to have paclitaxel at dose of 5 mg/kg

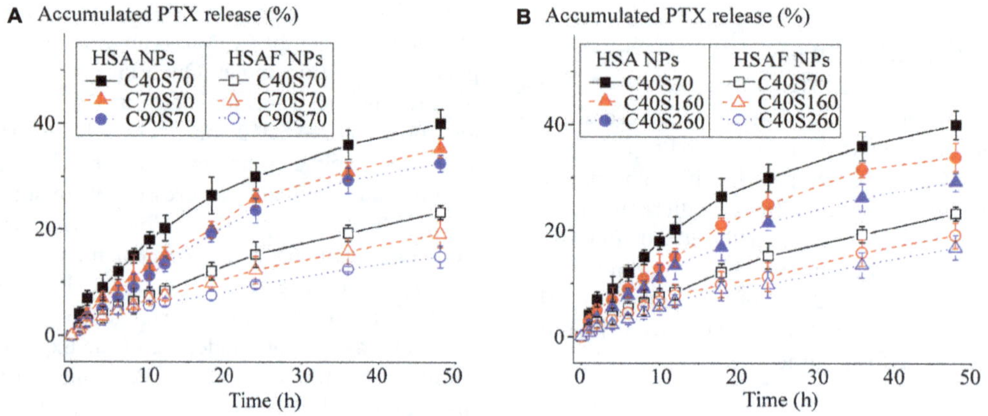

FIGURE 3 | The cumulative release profiles of PTX from HSA NPs and HSAF NPs with various crosslinking degrees **(A)** and diameters **(B)** (n = 3).

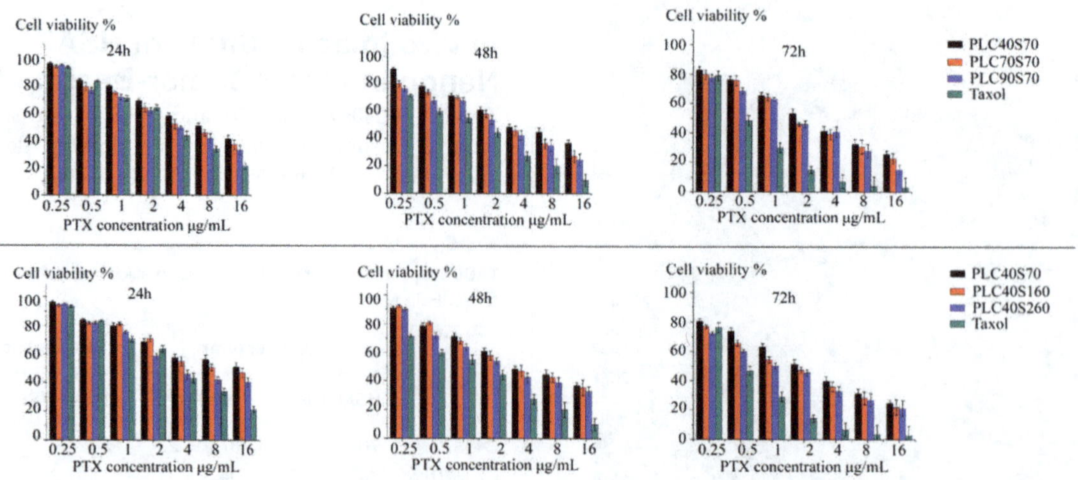

FIGURE 4 | Cytoxicity of PTX-loaded HSAF NPs with different crosslinking degrees and diameters (PLC40S70, PLC70S70, PLC90S70, PLC40S160, and PLC40S260) against MCF-7 cells at 24, 48, and 72 h. The commercial product Taxol® was used as the positive control (n = 6). PL, paclitaxel loading.

intravenously, (A) control group received 0.9% NaCl every 2 day (B) PTX Injection (PTX equivalent of 5 mg/kg) every 2 day; (C) HSA NPs (PTX equivalent of 5 mg/kg) every 2 day; (D) HSAF NPs (PTX equivalent of 5 mg/kg) every 2 day; After 28 days of initial treatment, mice were sacrificed and tumor tissues were collected. The tumor volume and weight were used for assessment of the therapeutic activity.

RESULTS AND DISCUSSION

Synthesis and Characterization of Human Albumin Based NPs

To figure out how physical and chemical properties of NPs may affect the cellular behavior of HSAF NPs, a HSAF NP platform was prepared using genipin as crosslinker with different crosslinking degrees and sizes, but similar surface charge (zeta potentials: $-20 \sim -30$ mV). The physical and chemical properties are summarized in **Table 1**. The NPs with different crosslinking degrees from 40.9 to 90.1% (C40S70, C70S70, and C90S70) were obtained by reacting with predetermined genipin. The NPs (C40S70, C40S160, and C40S260) prepared from different amount of albumin had similar crosslinking degrees around 41% but different sizes (65.9, 157.3, and 255.9 nm). These NPs are named as $CxSy_Z$: C means crosslinking; x means the crosslinking density; S means size; y means the NP size is around that number; z means is HSA or HSAF. A HSA or HSAF library could be obtained by varying the x and y. **Figure 2** showed the one example of TEM image of $C70S70_{HSAF}$. The FRET indices of these NPs were in the range of 23 ~ 32%, indicating that the NPs formulated in this study have significant FRET effects.

Preparation and Characterization of PTX-Loaded HSAF NPs

The PTX-loaded HSAF and/or HSA NPs were prepared as the method as the NPs above. As shown in **Table 2**, compared to the HSA NPs, the smaller diameters and higher drug loading efficiencies were obtained by the HSAF NPs when using the same formulations.

PTX Drug Release Profiles of HSAF NPs

In vitro PTX release profiles from HSA NPs and HSAF NPs were shown in **Figure 3**. Palitaxel release from NPs was detected by dialysis (Cho et al., 2004), the drug released was calculated at scheduled time (0.5, 1, 2, 4, 6, 8, 12, 24, 36, and 48 h). Compared with HSA NPs, PTX was released more slowly from HSAF NPs: within 48 h less than 50% of PTX was released from HSA NPs, but for HSAF NPs less than 25% PTX was released within the same time, indicating HSAF NPs could provide more possibility to delivery of PTX to specific organs and tissues than HAS NPs. For all HSA and HSAF NPs with comparable diameters, the increase of crosslinking degree decreased PTX release, perhaps because the compact structure of NPs, which was brought in by the chemical crosslink, hindered diffusion of PTX from NPs. F or NPs with comparable crosslinking degrees, the small NPs (C40S70 and C40S160) possessed faster PTX release behaviors, perhaps because small NPs possessed short drug diffusion distances.

In Vitro Anti-cancer Evaluation of HSAF NPs

The cytotoxicity profiles of PTX-loaded HSAF NPs were compared in MCF-7 cells by MTT assay over a range of concentrations (0.25, 0.5, 1, 2, 4, 8, and 16 μg/mL). As shown in the **Figure 4**, the viability of the cells was dose-dependently decreased by the PTX-loaded HSAF NPs. Furthermore, the inhibitory effects of the NPs were increased with the NPs crosslinking density or diameter increasing at 24, 48, and 72 h, and this may result from the more efficient endocytosis brought in by the increased crosslinking degree and diameter. In comparison to the commercial product Taxol®, the weaker inhibitory effect of the PTX-loaded HSAF NPs was believed to associate with the sustained release and/or the relatively slower endocytosis of the NPs (Jia et al., 2014).

Pharmacokinetic Studies of HSAF NPs

The major pharmacokinetic parameters of i.v. administration of HSAF PTX NPs have been summarized in **Table 3**. PTX NPs with lower particle size (C40S70, C70S70, C90S70) showed an obvious increasing in the AUC, MRT, $t^1/_2$ ($P < 0.05$), which correlated with an obvious decreasing in the Cl ($P < 0.05$). The results could be due to the lower particle size decrease the uptake of NPs by the mononuclear phagocyte system (Dobrovolskaia et al., 2008). The increasing of AUC, MRT, $t^1/_2$b and Cl could be achieved from C40S70, C70S70 and C90S70 as compared with C40S160 and C40S260 ($P < 0.05$), but the increment for C40S160 was not

TABLE 3 | Pharmacokinetic parameters of PTX after i.v. administration of NPs in mice (1 mg/kg).

Pharmacokinetic parameters	C40S260	C40S160	C40S70	C70S70	C90S70	C90S70HSA
AUC $_{0-t}$ (μg h/L)	423.2 ± 95.3	441.2 ± 105.1	543.1 ± 95.1*#	563.2 ± 108.2*#	573.2 ± 115.7*#	513.9 ± 105.1
A UC $_{0-\infty}$ (μg h/L)	523.1 ± 131.3	541.2 ± 137.3	649.1 ± 147.3*#	680.4 ± 146.1*#	691.3 ± 141.3*#	619.9 ± 145.4
MRT $_{0-t}$ (h)	2.3 ± 0.4	2.6 ± 0.7	4.40 ± 0.9*#	4.54 ± 1.2*#	4.58 ± 1.3*#	4.13 ± 1.1
Cl (L/h/kg)	1.9 ± 0.4	2.0 ± 0.5	1.4 ± 0.5*#	1.3 ± 0.4*#	1.2 ± 0.6*#	1.5 ± 0.5
V_d (L/kg)	28.4 ± 9.7	29.4 ± 12.1	31.4 ± 12.4	32.48 ± 11.9	38.4 ± 12.1	30.4 ± 11.3
C_{max} (μg/L)	1051.3 ± 221.9	1067.3 ± 233.9	1089.3 ± 224.3	1099.31 ± 224.6	1100.3 ± 249.2	1087.1 ± 219.8
$t_{1/2}$ (h)	9.14 ± 2.9	10.1 ± 3.1	13.1 ± 3.0*#	14.1 ± 3.4*#	14.9 ± 3.9*#	12.6 ± 3.2

*Each value is the mean ± SD, n = 6. *P < 0.05, compared with C90S260; #P < 0.05, compared with C70S160.*

higher than C40S260. This result indicate that the NP size which is lower than 100 nm may be due to the inhibiting the fast uptake of NPs via the reticulo-endothelial system (RES) (Dobrovolskaia et al., 2008). The HAS PTX NPs which was made by the same method as C90S70 (C90S70HSA) was also studied, and the AUC, MRT, $t_{1/2}$ of HAS PTX NPs is lower than that of HSAF PTX NPs (C90S70). There are significant difference between C90S70 and C90S70HSA ($P < 0.05$). The drug loading rate of C90S70 is higher than that of C90S70HSA, and the drug circulation time is longer than that of C90S70HSA too.

In Vivo Imaging Study of HSAF NPs in Tumor-Bearing Mice

As shown in **Figure 5**, most of the HSAF NPs containing the near-infrared fluorescent probe Dir clearly enriched in the liver after

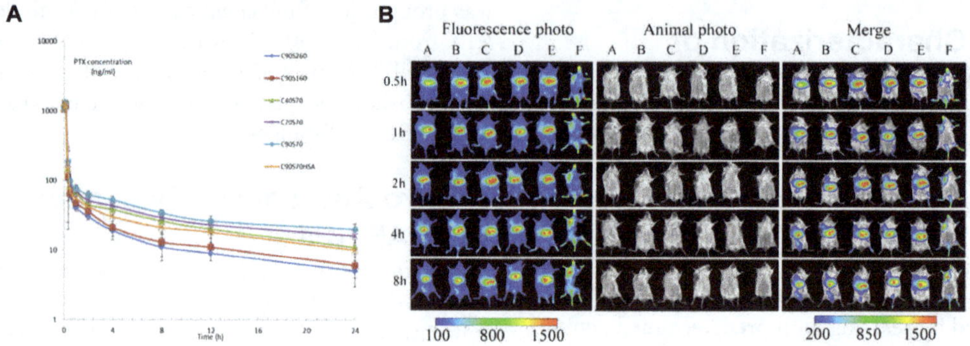

FIGURE 5 | Paclitaxel plasma concentration profiles after intravenous administration of 1 mg/kg drug to Sprague-Dawley rats **(A)** and *in vivo* distribution of Dir labeled HSAF nanoparticles DLC90S70 $_{(A)}$, DLC70S70 $_{(B)}$, DLC 40S70$_{(C)}$, DLC40S160 $_{(D)}$, DLC40S260 $_{(E)}$, and Dir solution $_{(F)}$ in tumor-bearing mice **(B)**. Results are expressed with the mean ± SD (n = 6). DL, Dir loading.

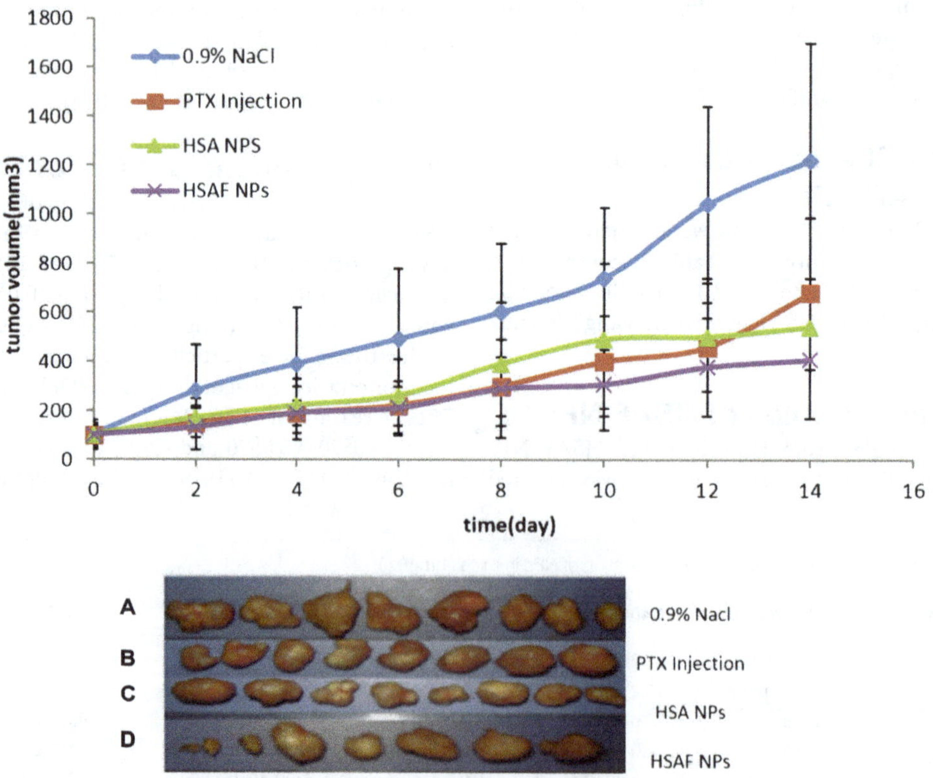

FIGURE 6 | Picture of tumor and tumor size of four groups, **(A)** control group received 0.9% NaCl every other day **(B)** PTX Injection (PTX equivalent of 5 mg/kg) every other day; **(C)** HSA NPs (PTX equivalent of 5 mg/kg) every other day; **(D)** HSAF NPs (PTX equivalent of 5 mg/kg) every other day.

three kinds of HSAF NPs were delivered to tumor-bearing mice *in vivo*, indicating that the liver is still the barrier for NP system to achieve maximum efficient drug delivery to tumor, and how to avoid the NPs to be taken up by the liver is still priority problem for the drug delivery systems. The NPs with higher crosslinking densities or particle size distribute more to the liver. In addition to the liver, the right forelimb solid tumors in mice are the main distribution area of the HSAF NPs. From the graph, it could be observed that DLC40S70, DLC70S70, DLC90S70, DLC40S160, and DLC40S260 significantly concentrated in the tumor site at 4, 1, 0.5, 1, and 0.5 h, respectively. This difference suggests that NPs with higher size and the degree of crosslinking have the higher biodistribution to the tumor site. In this experiment, polyoxyethylene castor oil and ethanol (50:50, V/V) were used for preparing solutions. Dir was used as control, and we find Dir solutions distribute quickly to the mouse head, limbs, and solid tumors. The Dir solutions disappeared in the mice quickly and much faster than the nanoparticles.

In Vivo Anticancer Evaluation of HSAF NPs for Breast Cancer Models

After 14 days of tumor inoculation, the average tumor volume was around 101 ± 23.19 mm^3. Then administration was continued for a total of 28 days after tumor implantation. The results (**Figure 6**) showed that tumors were significantly ($*P < 0.01$) inhibited after being treated with HSA NPs and HSAF NPs compared to PTX injection. Tumor inhibitory rate (tab.) in mice treated with HSA NPs and HSAF NPs were 63.3 and 71.4 respectively, which showed a significant ($*P < 0.01$) compared to PTX injection and control groups. There was observed a non-significant ($P > 0.05$) change in tumor inhibitory rate for HSA NPs and HSAF NPs, and the tumor Inhibitory rate of HSAF NPs is higher than that of HSA NPs. There is no observable weight loss or other cytotoxicity in HSA NPs and HSAF NPs mice groups. Also, the tumor volume showed the same trend as the tumor weight, and the tumor volume of HSAF NPs group is the smallest. The dose of HSAF used in the NPS is lower than that of HSA, but the effect is better.

CONCLUSION

In this report, a HSAF NP system with controllable crosslinking density and size were developed for better biosafety and anticancer efficacy. The HSAF NP library with a series of crosslinking degrees and particle sizes were developed, and the results showed that the similar particle size of HSAF NPs had different crosslinking densities, and the highest crosslinking density combined with the smallest particle size. This may lead to a higher drug loading rate and longer drug circulation time and further higher biodistribution in tumor site. Drug loading and release tests confirmed that the HSAF NPs have better drug loading and release performance than HSA NPs. *In vivo* anticancer evaluations confirmed that the NPs with fast cellular uptake showed better tumor accumulation and tumor inhibition. The results provide basic information not only for the biochemical effects and biosafety of albumin based NPs, but also for regulating the physicochemical properties which are important for the *in vivo* delivering of drugs.

AUTHOR CONTRIBUTIONS

LG, JW, and QH conceived and directed the study. YC and LC prepared NPs and obtained spectroscopic results. LG and XY co-wrote the paper. LG, XY, and JH contributed to the results analysis and discussion. YiZ and YuZ provided technical support and corrections of manuscript. XL, JW, and QH oversaw the project. All authors reviewed and approved the final paper.

FUNDING

This work was supported by the National Natural Science Foundation of China (Grant Nos. 81760638 and 81572978), the Natural Science Foundation of Xinjiang Province (Grant No. 2017D01C200), the Thousand Talents Plan for Young Professionals and the Science and Technology Planning Project of Guangdong Province (Grant No. 2016A010103015), and the Science and Technology Program of Guangzhou (Grant No. 201707010094). Guangdong Innovative and Entrepreneurial Research Team Program (Grant Nos. 2016ZT06S029 and 2013S086). The National Natural Science Foundation of China (Grant Nos. 81372885 and 81772889) and the Major Special Research Collaborative Innovation of Guangzhou (Grant No. 201604020160).

REFERENCES

Altintas, I., Heukers, R., van der Meel, R., Lacombe, M., Amidi, M., van Bergen En Henegouwen, P. M., et al. (2013). Nanobody-albumin nanoparticles (NANAPs) for the delivery of a multikinase inhibitor 17864 to EGFR overexpressing tumor cells. *J. Control. Release* 165, 110–118. doi: 10.1016/j.jconrel.2012.11.007

Bakare, R. A., Bhan, C., and Raghavan, D. (2014). Synthesis and characterization of collagen grafted poly(hydroxybutyrate-valerate) (PHBV) scaffold for loading of bovine serum albumin capped silver (Ag/BSA) nanoparticles in the potential use of tissue engineering application. *Biomacromolecules* 15, 423–435. doi: 10.1021/bm401686v

Bertrand, N., Wu, J., Xu, X., Kamaly, N., and Farokhzad, O. C. (2014). Cancer nanotechnology: the impact of passive and active targeting in the era of modern cancer biology. *Adv. Drug Deliv. Rev.* 66, 2–25. doi: 10.1016/j.addr.2013.11.009

Boussif, O., Lezoualc'h, F., Zanta, M. A., Mergny, M. D., Scherman, D., Demeneix, B., et al. (1995). A versatile vector for gene and oligonucleotide transfer into cells in culture and in vivo: polyethylenimine. *Proc. Natl. Acad. Sci. U.S.A.* 92, 7297–7301. doi: 10.1073/pnas.92.16.7297

Cecco, S., Aliberti, M., Baldo, P., Giacomin, E., and Leone, R. (2014). Safety and efficacy evaluation of albumin-bound paclitaxel. *Expert Opin. Drug Saf.* 13, 511–520. doi: 10.1517/14740338.2014.893293

Cho, N. H., Cheong, T. C., Min, J. H., Wu, J. H., Lee, S. J., Kim, D., et al. (2011). A multifunctional core-shell nanoparticle for dendritic cell-based cancer immunotherapy. *Nat. Nanotechnol.* 6, 675–682. doi: 10.1038/nnano.2011.149

Cho, Y. W., Lee, J., Lee, S. C., Huh, K. M., and Park, K. (2004). Hydrotropic agents for study of in vitro paclitaxel release from polymeric micelles. *J. Control. Release* 97, 249–257. doi: 10.1016/j.jconrel.2004.03.013

Ding, Y., Zhou, Y. Y., Chen, H., Geng, D. D., Wu, D. Y., Hong, J., et al. (2013). The performance of thiol-terminated PEG-paclitaxel-conjugated gold nanoparticles. *Biomaterials* 34, 10217–10227. doi: 10.1016/j.biomaterials.2013.09.008

Dobrovolskaia, M. A., Aggarwal, P., Hall, J. B., and McNeil, S. E. (2008). Preclinical studies to understand nanoparticle interaction with the immune system and its potential effects on nanoparticle biodistribution. *Mol. Pharm.* 5, 487–495. doi: 10.1021/mp800032f

Elzoghby, A. O., Samy, W. M., and Elgindy, N. A. (2012). Albumin-based nanoparticles as potential controlled release drug delivery systems. *J. Control. Release* 157, 168–182. doi: 10.1016/j.jconrel.2011.07.031

Ge, L., You, X., Zhang, Y., Huang, K., Lu, X., Ren, Y., et al. (2017). Development of self-emulsifying nanoplatform as anti-diabetic sulfonylurea carrier for oral diabetes therapy. *J. Biomed. Nanotechnol.* 13, 931–945. doi: 10.1166/jbn.2017.2385

Hai, W., Sujuan, M., Xueqin, C., Junwei, Z., Ming, L., Jianxin, T., et al. (2014). Facile synthesis of Pt/Pd nanodendrites for the direct oxidation of methanol. *Nanotechnology* 25:195702. doi: 10.1088/0957-4484/25/19/195702

Hao, Y., Li, W., Zhou, X., Yang, F., and Qian, Z. (2017). Microneedles-based transdermal drug delivery systems: a review. *J. Biomed. Nanotechnol.* 13, 1581–1597. doi: 10.1166/jbn.2017.2474

Hu, D., Chen, L., Qu, Y., Peng, J., Chu, B., Shi, K., et al. (2018). Oxygen-generating hybrid polymeric nanoparticles with encapsulated doxorubicin and chlorin e6 for trimodal imaging-guided combined chemo-photodynamic therapy. *Theranostics* 8, 1558–1574. doi: 10.7150/thno.22989

Jia, H. Z., Zhu, J. Y., Wang, X. L., Cheng, H., Chen, G., Zhao, Y. F., et al. (2014). A boronate-linked linear-hyperbranched polymeric nanovehicle for pH-dependent tumor-targeted drug delivery. *Biomaterials* 35, 5240–5249. doi: 10.1016/j.biomaterials.2014.03.029

Jiang, L., Xu, Y., Liu, Q., Tang, Y., Ge, L., Zheng, C., et al. (2013). A nontoxic disulfide bond reducing method for lipophilic drug-loaded albumin nanoparticle preparation: formation dynamics, influencing factors and formation mechanisms investigation. *Int. J. Pharm.* 443, 80–86. doi: 10.1016/j.ijpharm.2012.12.035

Jiang, L., Zhao, X., Zheng, C., Li, F., Maclean, J. L., Chen, F., et al. (2015). The quantitative detection of the uptake and intracellular fate of albumin nanoparticles. *RSC Adv.* 5, 34956–34966. doi: 10.1039/C5RA01683E

Kou, L., Bhutia, Y. D., Yao, Q., He, Z., Sun, J., and Ganapathy, V. (2018). Transporter-guided delivery of nanoparticles to improve drug permeation across cellular barriers and drug exposure to selective cell types. *Front. Pharmacol.* 9:27. doi: 10.3389/fphar.2018.00027

Kratz, F. (2008). Albumin as a drug carrier: design of prodrugs, drug conjugates and nanoparticles. *J. Control. Release* 132, 171–183. doi: 10.1016/j.jconrel.2008.05.010

Lapresle, C., and Doyen, N. (1975). Isolation and properties of a fragment of human serum albumin demonstrating the absence of a methionine residue from some of the albumin molecules. *Biochem. J.* 151, 637–643. doi: 10.1042/bj1510637

Li, C., Li, Y., Gao, Y., Wei, N., Zhao, X., Wang, C., et al. (2014). Direct comparison of two albumin-based paclitaxel-loaded nanoparticle formulations: is the crosslinked version more advantageous? *Int. J. Pharm.* 468, 15–25. doi: 10.1016/j.ijpharm.2014.04.010

Li, H., Li, X., Zhang, C., Sun, Q., Yi, W., Wang, X., et al. (2016). Regulated pH-Responsive polymeric micelles for doxorubicin delivery to the nucleus of liver cancer cells. *J. Biomed. Nanotechnol.* 12, 1258–1269. doi: 10.1166/jbn.2016.2247

Li, Q., Liang, J., You, X., Liu, X., Wu, H., Gao, W., et al. (2017). A novel reactive oxygen species triggered polymeric nanoplatform for controlled drug delivery and cancer therapy. *J. Biomed. Nanotechnol.* 13, 513–521. doi: 10.1166/jbn.2017.2370

Li, S., Zheng, J., Chen, D., Wu, Y., Zhang, W., Zheng, F., et al. (2013). Yolk-shell hybrid nanoparticles with magnetic and pH-sensitive properties for controlled anticancer drug delivery. *Nanoscale* 5, 11718–11724. doi: 10.1039/c3nr04032a

Li, W., Peng, J., Tan, L., Wu, J., Shi, K., Qu, Y., et al. (2016). Mild photothermal therapy/photodynamic therapy/chemotherapy of breast cancer by Lyp-1 modified Docetaxel/IR820 Co-loaded micelles. *Biomaterials* 106, 119–133. doi: 10.1016/j.biomaterials.2016.08.016

Li, Y., Xiao, K., Luo, J., Lee, J., Pan, S., and Lam, K. S. (2010). A novel size-tunable nanocarrier system for targeted anticancer drug delivery. *J. Control. Release* 144, 314–323. doi: 10.1016/j.jconrel.2010.02.027

Liu, J., and Lu, Y. (2006). Preparation of aptamer-linked gold nanoparticle purple aggregates for colorimetric sensing of analytes. *Nat. Protoc.* 1, 246–252. doi: 10.1038/nprot.2006.38

Maiti, S. (2011). Nanotoxicity of gold and iron nanoparticles. *J. Biomed. Nanotechnol.* 7, 65–65. doi: 10.1166/jbn.2011.1203

McMenamy, R. H., Dintzis, H. M., and Watson, F. (1971). Cyanogen bromide fragments of human serum albumin. *J. Biol. Chem.* 246, 4744–4750.

Morral-Ruiz, G., Melgar-Lesmes, P., Solans, C., and Garcia-Celma, M. J. (2013). Multifunctional polyurethane-urea nanoparticles to target and arrest inflamed vascular environment: a potential tool for cancer therapy and diagnosis. *J. Control. Release* 171, 163–171. doi: 10.1016/j.jconrel.2013.06.027

Pan, Y., Xue, P., Liu, S., Zhang, L., Guan, Q., Zhu, J., et al. (2018). Metal-based hybrid nanoparticles as radiosensitizers in cancer therapy. *Colloid Interface Sci. Commun.* 23, 45–51. doi: 10.1016/j.colcom.2018.01.004

Park, J. S., Cho, M. K., Lee, E. J., Ahn, K. Y., Lee, K. E., Jung, J. H., et al. (2009). A highly sensitive and selective diagnostic assay based on virus nanoparticles. *Nat. Nanotechnol.* 4, 259–264. doi: 10.1038/nnano.2009.38

Qu, Y., Chu, B., Shi, K., Peng, J., and Qian, Z. (2017). Recent progress in functional micellar carriers with intrinsic therapeutic activities for anticancer drug delivery. *J. Biomed. Nanotechnol.* 13, 1598–1618. doi: 10.1166/jbn.2017.2475

Rosenberger, I., Schmithals, C., Vandooren, J., Bianchessi, S., Milani, P., Locatelli, E., et al. (2014). Physico-chemical and toxicological characterization of iron-containing albumin nanoparticles as platforms for medical imaging. *J. Control Release* 194, 130–137. doi: 10.1016/j.jconrel.2014.08.017

Saif, M. W. (2013). U.S. Food and drug administration approves paclitaxel protein-bound particles (Abraxane(R)) in combination with gemcitabine as first-line treatment of patients with metastatic pancreatic cancer. *JOP* 14, 686–688. doi: 10.6092/1590-8577/2028

Shimanovich, U., Tkacz, I. D., Eliaz, D., Cavaco-Paulo, A., Michaeli, S., and Gedanken, A. (2011). Encapsulation of RNA molecules in BSA microspheres and internalization into *Trypanosoma Brucei* parasites and human U2OS cancer cells. *Adv. Funct. Mater.* 21, 3659–3666. doi: 10.1002/adfm.201100963

Shrestha, R., Elsabahy, M., Florez-Malaver, S., Samarajeewa, S., and Wooley, K. L. (2012). Endosomal escape and siRNA delivery with cationic shell crosslinked knedel-like nanoparticles with tunable buffering capacities. *Biomaterials* 33, 8557–8568. doi: 10.1016/j.biomaterials.2012.07.054

Singh, R. P., and Ramarao, P. (2013). Accumulated polymer degradation products as effector molecules in cytotoxicity of polymeric nanoparticles. *Toxicol. Sci.* 136, 131–143. doi: 10.1093/toxsci/kft179

Wang, J., Li, S., Han, Y., Guan, J., Chung, S., Wang, C., et al. (2018). Poly(Ethylene Glycol)–polylactide micelles for cancer therapy. *Front. Pharmacol.* 9:202. doi: 10.3389/fphar.2018.00202

Wang, X., Song, L., Li, N., Qiu, Z., Zhou, S., Li, C., et al. (2013). Pharmacokinetics and biodistribution study of paclitaxel liposome in Sprague–Dawley rats and beagle dogs by liquid chromatography-tandem mass spectrometry. *Drug Res.* 63, 603–606. doi: 10.1055/s-0033-1349126

Wang, Y., Chen, L., Tan, L., Zhao, Q., Luo, F., Wei, Y., et al. (2014a). PEG–PCL based micelle hydrogels as oral docetaxel delivery systems for breast cancer therapy. *Biomaterials* 35, 6972–6985. doi: 10.1016/j.biomaterials.2014.04.099

Wang, Y., Li, C., Yao, C., Ding, L., Lei, Z., and Wu, M. (2016). Techniques for investigating molecular toxicology of nanomaterials. *J. Biomed. Nanotechnol.* 12, 1115–1135. doi: 10.1166/jbn.2016.2220

Wang, Y., Xu, H., Wang, J., Ge, L., and Zhu, J. (2014b). Development of a thermally responsive nanogel based on chitosan-poly(N-isopropylacrylamide-co-acrylamide) for paclitaxel delivery. *J. Pharm. Sci.* 103, 2012–2021. doi: 10.1002/jps.23995

Watcharin, W., Schmithals, C., Pleli, T., Koberle, V., Korkusuz, H., Huebner, F., et al. (2014). Biodegradable human serum albumin nanoparticles as contrast agents for the detection of hepatocellular carcinoma by magnetic resonance imaging. *Eur. J. Pharm. Biopharm.* 87, 132–141. doi: 10.1016/j.ejpb.2013.12.010

Wu, J., and Chu, C.-C. (2013). Water insoluble cationic poly(ester amide)s: synthesis, characterization and applications. *J. Mater. Chem. B* 1, 353–360. doi: 10.1016/j.actbio.2014.04.002

Wu, J., Kamaly, N., Shi, J., Zhao, L., Xiao, Z., Hollett, G., et al. (2014). Development of multinuclear polymeric nanoparticles as robust protein nanocarriers. *Angew. Chem. Int. Ed.* 53, 8975–8979. doi: 10.1002/anie.201404766

Wu, J., Yamanouchi, D., Liu, B., and Chu, C.-C. (2012). Biodegradable arginine-based poly(ether ester amide)s as a non-viral DNA delivery vector and their structure-function study. *J. Mater. Chem.* 22, 18983–18991. doi: 10.1039/C2JM33753C

Xing, R., Liu, G., Zhu, J., Hou, Y., and Chen, X. (2013). Functional magnetic nanoparticles for non-viral gene delivery and MR imaging. *Pharm. Res.* 31, 1377–1389. doi: 10.1007/s11095-013-1205-2

Xu, X., Wu, J., Liu, Y., Saw, P. E., Tao, W., Yu, M., et al. (2017). Multifunctional envelope-type siRNA delivery nanoparticle platform for prostate cancer therapy. *ACS Nano* 11, 2618–2627. doi: 10.1021/acsnano.6b07195

Yang, Q., Peng, J., Xiao, Y., Li, W., Tan, L., Xu, X., et al. (2018). Porous Au@Pt nanoparticles: therapeutic platform for tumor chemo-photothermal co-therapy and alleviating doxorubicin-induced oxidative damage. *ACS Appl. Mater. Interfaces* 10, 150–164. doi: 10.1021/acsami.7b14705

You, X., Kang, Y., Hollett, G., Chen, X., Zhao, W., Gu, Z., et al. (2016). Polymeric nanoparticles for colon cancer therapy: overview and perspectives. *J. Mater. Chem. B* 4, 7779–7792. doi: 10.1039/C6TB01925K

Yu, Z., Schmaltz, R. M., Bozeman, T. C., Paul, R., Rishel, M. J., Tsosie, K. S., et al. (2013). Selective tumor cell targeting by the disaccharide moiety of bleomycin. *J. Am. Chem. Soc.* 135, 2883–2886. doi: 10.1021/ja311090e

Yuan, Z. X., He, X. K., Wu, X. J., Gao, Y., Fan, M., Song, L. Q., et al. (2014). Peptide fragments of human serum albumin as novel renal targeting carriers. *Int. J. Pharm.* 460, 196–204. doi: 10.1016/j.ijpharm.2013.10.041

20

Tumor-Associated Fibronectin Targeted Liposomal Nanoplatform for Cyclophilin A siRNA Delivery and Targeted Malignant Glioblastoma Therapy

Phei Er Saw[1,2†], Ao Zhang[1,2†], Yan Nie[1,2], Lei Zhang[1,3], Yingjie Xu[4*] and Xiaoding Xu[1,2*]*

[1] Guangdong Provincial Key Laboratory of Malignant Tumor Epigenetics and Gene Regulation, Medical Research Center, Sun Yat-sen Memorial Hospital, Sun Yat-sen University, Guangzhou, China, [2] RNA Biomedical Institute, Sun Yat-sen Memorial Hospital, Sun Yat-sen University, Guangzhou, China, [3] Department of Hepatobiliary Surgery, Sun Yat-sen Memorial Hospital, Sun Yat-sen University, Guangzhou, China, [4] Department of Biochemistry and Molecular Cell Biology, Shanghai Key Laboratory for Tumor Microenvironment and Inflammation, Shanghai Jiao Tong University School of Medicine, Shanghai, China

***Correspondence:**
Lei Zhang
zhanglei646@126.com
Yingjie Xu
xuyingjie@shsmu.edu.cn
Xiaoding Xu
xuxiaod5@mail.sysu.edu.cn

† These authors have contributed equally to this work

Malignant glioblastoma (GBM) is the most aggressive brain cancer that has a very low survival rate. With the rapid development of nanotechnology in the past few decades, the use of nanoparticles (NPs) for nucleic acid delivery is expected to have a revolutionary impact on GBM therapy. However, clinical success in GBM therapy remains a formidable challenge, mainly due to suboptimal *in vivo* delivery of therapeutics to glioma cells. Herein, we developed an aptamer-like peptide (aptide)-decorated liposomal nanoplatform for systemic small interfering RNA (siRNA) delivery and targeted GBM therapy. This nanoplatform is mainly composed of the following key components: (i) classic liposome structure with an aqueous core that can encapsulate therapeutic siRNA; (ii) hydrophilic polyethylene glycol (PEG) chains on the outer shell to prolong blood circulation; and (iii) surface-encoded aptide to specifically target the extra-domain B (EDB) of fibronectin that over-expressed on glioma cells. After systemic administration of these new siRNA delivery NPs, they can target the glioma cells and efficiently inhibit the GBM tumor growth by silencing the expression of cyclophilin A (CypA), which is up-regulated in brain cancer and plays an important role in malignant transformation of brain cancer and maintaining glioma cell stemness. These results suggest that the reported RNA interference (RNAi) NP platform herein could become an effective tool for targeted GBM therapy.

Keywords: nanoparticle, aptide, siRNA, targeted delivery, glioblastoma

INTRODUCTION

Glioblastoma (GBM) is the most common and aggressive form of brain cancer with poor diagnosis, difficult management, and low survival rate. Even when detected early, less than 5% of GBM patients are alive 5 years after diagnosis and the median survival rate is around 14.6 months (Behin et al., 2003; Brandsma and van den Bent, 2007; Johnson and O'Neill, 2012). Currently, multimodality treatment approach including surgical resection, radiotherapy, and chemotherapy is the standard care for GBM patients (Meyers et al., 2013; Cheng et al., 2014; Mahmoudi and Hadjipanayis, 2014; Krizbai et al., 2016). However, the development of resistance to therapies (e.g., radiotherapy and chemotherapy) has emerged as a persistent clinical problem and ultimately induces the failure of GBM treatment. Multiple reasons have been demonstrated to contribute to this disappointed outcome, including (i) the complex structure of the brain, (ii) the heterogeneous and invasive nature of GBM, and (iii) difficulty in delivering therapeutics specifically to glioma cells (Lesniak and Brem, 2004; Pardridge, 2005; Ozdemir-Kaynak et al., 2018; Shergalis et al., 2018). Therefore, there is a critical need to develop alternative strategies for more effective GBM treatment.

Since the discovery of RNA interference (RNAi) by Fire et al. (1998), RNAi technology has demonstrated significant potential for disease treatment by silencing the expression of target gene(s), especially those encoding "undruggable" proteins (Whitehead et al., 2009; Xu et al., 2016). However, the safe and effective delivery of RNAi agents such as siRNA to target cells remains a major hurdle for the widespread clinical application of RNAi technology. RNAi agents are biomacromolecules with polyanionic characteristics, which are easily attacked by serum nucleases and cannot readily cross cell membrane. Therefore, specific delivery vehicles are required to facilitate the intracellular uptake and cytosolic delivery of RNAi agents (Yang et al., 2012; Kanasty et al., 2013; Liu et al., 2017; Xu et al., 2017a,b). Over the past decades, nanoparticles (NPs) have been demonstrated as a powerful tool toward this end, especially showing hepatocyte-specificity in non-human primates and clinical trials (Zimmermann et al., 2006; Tseng et al., 2009; Jhaveri and Torchilin, 2014; Shi et al., 2017; Durymanov and Reineke, 2018). Nevertheless, it is still challenged to accomplish the systemic delivery of RNAi agents to a particular non-liver diseased tissue (e.g., solid tumor) and cell type, followed by sufficient intra-cytosolic transport. While several RNAi NP platforms have entered into early phase clinical trials for cancer treatment (Zuckerman and Davis, 2015), substantial obstacles still remain, including long blood circulation, selective accumulation at tumor site, and efficient tumor cell internalization. Specifically, these challenges are amplified by the structural complex of the brain (Pardridge, 2005; Mahmoudi and Hadjipanayis, 2014; Shergalis et al., 2018).

To address these issues, we herein developed a liposome-based extra-domain B (EDB)-targeting nanoplatform for systemic siRNA delivery and GBM therapy. As shown in **Figure 1**, this nanoplatform is composed of a classic liposome structure (i.e., one phospholipid bilayer surrounding an aqueous core), hydrophilic polyethylene glycol (PEG) chains on the outer shell, and surface-encoded aptamer-like peptide (aptide) to specifically target the EDB of fibronectin that over-expressed on glioma cells (Borsi et al., 1992; Castellani et al., 2002; Han and Lu, 2017; Saw et al., 2017). After loading siRNA and then systemic administration, the resulting nanoplatform shows the following unique functions: (i) the hydrophilic PEG chains allow the NPs to escape immunological recognition, thus improving blood circulation; (ii) the surface-encoded aptide moieties can enhance the GBM targeting ability and intracellular siRNA delivery; and (iii) commercial available of the NP compositions and robust NP formulation enables the scale-up of this NP platform. As a proof of concept, we chose cyclophilin A (CypA) as a therapeutic target and systemically evaluated the EDB-targeting NPs for CypA siRNA (siCypA) delivery and its anticancer efficacy. CypA is a ubiquitously distributed protein belonging to the immunophilin family, which shows an activity of peptidylprolyl *cis trans* isomerase and plays an important role in regulation of protein folding (Wang and Heitman, 2005), trafficking (Shieh et al., 1989; Luban, 1996), assembly (Pan et al., 2008; Tanaka et al., 2011), immune-modulator and cell signaling (Jin et al., 2000; Satoh et al., 2008). It has been demonstrated that CypA is up-regulated in many cancers (e.g., liver, brain, and lung cancers) and is a key determinant for malignant transformation, epithelial to mesenchymal transition (EMT) and cancer metastasis (Yang et al., 2007; Qi et al., 2008). Recent research demonstrated that over-expressed CypA in GBM involves in maintaining glioma cell stemness via Wnt/β-catenin signaling pathway (Wang et al., 2017). Our *in vivo* results show that the systemic delivery of siCypA with the EDB-targeting NP platform can efficiently inhibit CypA expression in the tumor tissue and significantly inhibit GBM tumor growth.

MATERIALS AND METHODS

Materials

CypA siRNA (siCypA) and Cy5.5-labeled CypA siRNA (Cy5.5-siCypA) were acquired from Dharmacon (United States). The siRNA sequences are as follows: 5′-UGA CUU CAC ACG CCA UAA UdTdT-3′ (sense); 5′-AUU AUG GCG UGU GAA GUC AdTdT-3′ (antisense). Protamine sulfate and sepharose CL-4B column were purchased from Sigma Aldrich (United States). 1-Palmitoyl-2-oleoyl-*sn*-glycero-3-phosphocholine (POPC), 1-palmitoyl-2-oleoyl-*sn*-glycero-3-phospho-(10-rac-glycerol) (POPG), 1,2-distearoyl-*sn*-glycero-3-phosphoethanolamine (DSPE), and PEG (2000)-DSPE (ammonium salt) (PEG_{2000}-DSPE) were purchased from Avanti Polar Lipids (United States) and used as received. *N*-Maleimide-PEG_{2000}-DSPE (ammonium salt) (Mal-PEG_{2000}-DSPE) and plant cholesterol (Chol) were purchased from A.V.T. (Shanghai) Pharmaceuticals (China). EDB-targeting aptide (APT_{EDB}) with an additional cysteine in the β-hairpin constant loop region (sequence from *N* to *C* terminal, CSSPIQGSWTWENGK(C)WTWGIIRLEQ) was synthesized by Guangzhou IGE biotechnology Co., Ltd (China). Lipofectamine 2000 (Lipo2000) was provided by Thermofisher Scientific (United States). Real-time PCR assay kit was procured from Promega (United States). All antibodies were purchased from Abcam (United States) and used according to the manufacturer's protocol. All other chemicals were of reagent grade and used directly.

Methods

Synthesis of APT_{EDB} Conjugated PEG_{2000}-DSPE (APT_{EDB}-PEG_{2000}-DSPE)

The APT_{EDB}-PEG_{2000}-DSPE was synthesized via the reaction between the thiol group of APT_{EDB} and maleimide terminal

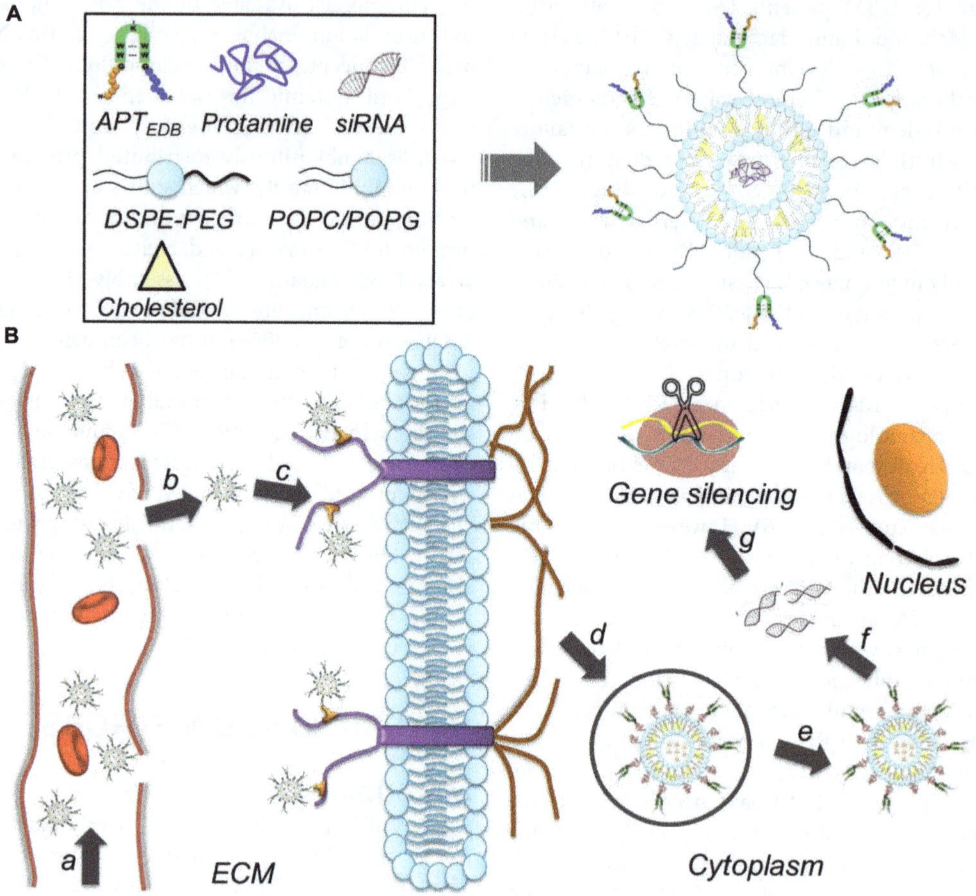

FIGURE 1 | (A) Formulation of the aptide-decorated liposomal nanoplatform (APT-$_{EDB}$ NPs); **(B)** schematic illustration of the APT-$_{EDB}$ NPs for systemic siRNA delivery and targeted GBM treatment. After intravenous injection (a), the long-circulating NPs can accumulate in the GBM tumor tissues (b) and subsequently target the glioma cells via the specific recognition between aptide and EDB (c). After targeted cellular uptake (d,e), the APT-$_{EDB}$ NPs can release the siRNA in the cytoplasm (f), leading to effective silencing of GBM-associated CypA expression and ultimate inhibition of GBM tumor growth (g).

group of Mal- PEG_{2000}-DSPE. In brief, APT_{EDB} and Mal- PEG_{2000}-DSPE were dissolved in dimethyl sulfoxide (DMSO) and chloroform, respectively. Subsequently, these two solutions were mixed in a molar ratio (APT_{EDB}: Mal-PEG_{2000}-DSPE) of 1:2. Under nitrogen atmosphere, the mixture was stirred at room temperature for 12 h. Thereafter, the mixture was transferred to dialysis membrane (MWCO 3500) and dialyzed against deionized water for 3 days. After freeze-drying under vacuum, the APT_{EDB}-PEG_{2000}-DSPE was collected as a white powder.

Preparation and Characterizations of EDB-Targeting siRNA-Loaded NPs

The classic rehydration method was employed to prepare the EDB-targeting siRNA-loaded NPs (Saw et al., 2015). POPC, Chol, and POPG were dissolved in chloroform in a molar ratio of 4:3:3 and APT_{EDB}-PEG_{2000}-DSPE (2.5 wt% of the total lipid) was then added. The mixture was stirred at room temperature for 10 min to form a homogenous solution. Subsequently, the solvent was removed by using rotary evaporator and a thin lipid film was thus generated. Then, HEPES-buffered 5% glucose (HBG) containing siCypA/protamine complexes was added and the resulting mixture (2 mg/mL) was briefly sonicated to accelerate the formation of siRNA-loaded liposomes. Thereafter, extrusions were performed by using a 100 nm polycarbonate membrane to ensure the formation of uniform liposomes, which were then passed over sepharose CL-4B column to obtain the purified siRNA-loaded NPs. To prepare the siRNA-loaded NPs without EDB-targeting ability, the POPC, Chol, and POPG were dissolved in chloroform in a molar ratio of 4:3:3 and then the siRNA-loaded NPs were prepared and purified according to the method described above.

The siRNA-loaded NPs were characterized in terms of size, zeta potential, and morphology. The particle size and zeta potential were examined by dynamic light scattering (DLS, Malvern Instruments Corporation). The morphology of siRNA loaded NPs was visualized by transmission electron microscopy (TEM, Tecnai G^2 Spirit BioTWIN). To determine the siRNA encapsulation efficiency (EE), Cy5.5-siCypA was used to prepare the siRNA-loaded NPs according to the method aforementioned and the obtained NPs were dispersed in 1 mL of PBS. Subsequently, a small volume (5 μL) of the NP solution was withdrawn and mixed with 20-fold DMSO. The standard was prepared by mixing 5 μL of naked Cy5.5-siCypA solution with 20-fold DMSO. The fluorescence intensity of Cy5.5-siCypA was measured using a Synergy HT multimode microplate reader (BioTek Instruments), and the siRNA EE% is calculated as EE% = $(FI_{NPs} / FI_{Standard}) \times 100$.

In vitro siRNA Release

Cy5.5-siCypA-loaded NPs were dispersed in 1 mL of PBS (pH 7.4) and then transferred to a Float-a-lyzer G2 dialysis device (MWCO 100 kDa, Spectrum) that was immersed in PBS (pH 7.4) at 37°C. At a predetermined interval, 5 μL of the NP solution was withdrawn and mixed with 20-fold DMSO. The fluorescence intensity of Cy5.5-siCypA was determined by Synergy HT multi-mode microplate reader.

Cell Culture

Human glioma cells (U87MG and U251MG), skin melanoma cells (A375), prostate cancer cells (PC3), breast cancer cells (MCF-7), and Jurkat leukemic T cells were incubated in DMEM medium with 10% FBS at 37°C in a humidified atmosphere containing 5% CO_2.

Evaluation of the Expression of EDB and CypA in Glioma Cells

Real-time qPCR was used to evaluate the mRNA level of EDB and CypA in the glioma cells. The intracellular RNA was isolated with RiboEx using an RNA isolation kit (Geneall, South Korea). cDNA was then synthesized using reverse transcription technique using 1 μg of total RNA from each sample. The primers used for detecting the EDB domain of fibronectin were 5′-AAC TCA CTG ACC TAA GCT TT-3′ (forward) and 5′-CGT TTG TTG TGT CAG TGT AG-3′ (reverse). The primers for detecting the CypA were 5′-TAT CTG CAC TGC CAA GAC TGA GTG-3′ (forward) and 5′-CTT CTT GCT GGT CTT GCC ATT CC-3′ (reverse).

Targeted Cellular Uptake

Glioma cells (20,000 cells) were seeded in disks and incubated in 2 mL of DMEM medium containing 10% FBS for 24 h. Subsequently, the Cy5.5-siCypA-loaded NPs were added at a siRNA concentration of 5 nM, and the cells were allowed to incubate at 37°C for 4 h. After removing the medium and subsequently washing with PBS buffer thrice, the nuclei were stained with Hoechst 33342 and the cells were then viewed under a FV1000 confocal laser scanning microscope (CLSM, Olympus).

In vitro Gene Silencing

Glioma cells were seeded in 6-well plates (50,000 cells per well) and incubated in 2 mL of DMEM medium containing 10% FBS for 24 h. Subsequently, the cells were incubated with the siCypA-loaded NPs for 24 h. After washing the cells with PBS buffer thrice, the cells were further incubated in fresh medium for another 48 h. Thereafter, the cells were digested by trypsin and the intracellular RNA was isolated for real-time qPCR to examine the CypA expression. As a positive control, Lipo2000/siCypA complexes were prepared according to manufacturer's protocol and then incubated with the glioma cells for 4 h. After washing the cells thrice with PBS, the cells were further incubated for another 48 h and then collected for real-time qPCR analysis.

In vitro Cell Viability Assay

Glioma cells were seeded in 96-well plates (5,000 cells per well) and incubated in 0.1 mL of DMEM medium with 10% FBS for 24 h. Thereafter, the siCypA-loaded NPs were added at predetermined concentration and the cells were allowed to incubate for 48 h. After removing the medium and washing the cells with PBS thrice, the cell viability was measured using the AlamarBlue assay according to the manufacturer's protocol.

Animals

Healthy female BALB/c normal mice and nude mice (4–5 weeks old) were purchased from Sun Yat-sen University experimental animal center. All *in vivo* studies were performed in accordance with a protocol approved by the Institutional Animal Care and Use Committee at Sun Yat-sen University.

Pharmacokinetics

Healthy female BALB/c normal mice were randomly divided into three groups (n = 3) and given an intravenous injection of either (i) naked Cy5.5-siCypA, (ii) Cy5.5-siCypA-loaded NPs, or (iii) EDB-targeting NPs at a 1 nmol siRNA dose per mouse. At predetermined time intervals, 20 μL of blood was withdrawn and the wound was pressed for several seconds to stop bleeding. The fluorescence intensity of Cy5.5-siCypA in the blood was determined by Synergy HT multi-mode microplate reader. The blood circulation half-life ($t_{1/2}$) was calculated according to previous report (Winter et al., 2013; Xu et al., 2017a).

GBM Xenograft Tumor Model

The tumor model was constructed by subcutaneous injection with 200 μL of glioma cell suspension (1:1 mixture of medium and Matrigel) with a density of 2×10^6 cells/mL into the back region of healthy female nude mice. When the volume of the tumor xenograft reached ~100 mm^3, the mice were used for the *in vivo* experiments.

Evaluation of EDB Expression in GBM Xenograft Tumor Model

The tumor tissues were excised from the GBM xenograft tumor-bearing mice and then sectioned using Leica CM 1950 Research Cyrostat (Leica Biosystems, IL, United States) at a 5 μm thickness. Subsequently, the tumor sections were washed in PBS and fixed with 4% (w/v) paraformaldehyde. After blocking with 2% bovine serum albumin (BSA) for 1 h, the tumor sections were incubated with anti-BC-1 antibody (EDB specific antibody) overnight at 4°C. Then, the tumor sections were washed in PBS and Alexa Fluor 594-conjugated goat anti-mouse IgG was added. After 1 h incubation at room temperature, the tumor sections were washed with PBS thrice and mounted with DAPI containing mounting medium. The tumor sections were finally viewed under CLSM to examine the EDB expression.

Inhibition of Tumor Growth

GBM xenograft tumor-bearing nude mice were randomly divided into three groups ($n = 4$) and intravenously injected with (i) PBS, (ii) siCypA-loaded NPs or (iii) EDB-targeting NPs at a 1 nmol siRNA dose per mouse once every two days. All the mice were administrated four consecutive injections and the tumor growth was monitored every two days by measuring perpendicular diameters using a caliper and tumor volume was calculated as follows:

$$V = W^2 \times L/2$$

where W and L are the shortest and longest diameters, respectively.

Histology

After the aforementioned treatment, the mice in each group were sacrificed at end of the evaluation period, and the tumor tissues and main organs (heart, liver, spleen, lung, and kidney) were collected. After fixing with 4% paraformaldehyde and then embedding in paraffin, the tissue was sectioned and stained with hematoxylin-eosin (H&E) and then viewed under an optical microscope. In addition, the apoptosis in the tumor tissues was examined by terminal deoxynucleotidyl transferase dUTP nick-end labeling (TUNEL) assay according to manufacturer's protocol.

RESULTS AND DISCUSSION

Preparation and Characterizations of the NPs

EDB of fibronectin has been demonstrated to be highly expressed in the aggressive and malignant GBM (Borsi et al., 1992; Castellani et al., 2002). Therefore, EDB-targeting nanoplatform could be used a robust vehicle to deliver various therapeutics for GBM treatment. Arising from the excellent targeting ability of aptamer, we previously developed aptamer-like peptide (aptide) and demonstrated its strong ability to specifically bind EDB with high affinity (K_d ~16 nM) (Saw et al., 2013, 2015, 2017). Based on the high EDB expression in GBM and strong targeting ability of aptide, we herein conjugated the EDB-targeting aptide (APT-$_{EDB}$) to PEG$_{2000}$-DSPE, which was then formulated with other lipids (POPC, Chol, and POPG) to obtain the APT-$_{EDB}$-decorated liposomes (denoted APT-$_{EDB}$ NPs) for the systemic siRNA delivery and targeted GBM treatment (**Figure 1**). In this work, we employed this nanoplatform to deliver siCypA because it can specifically silence the expression of cancer-associated CypA that over-expressed in GBM (Yang et al., 2007; Qi et al., 2008).

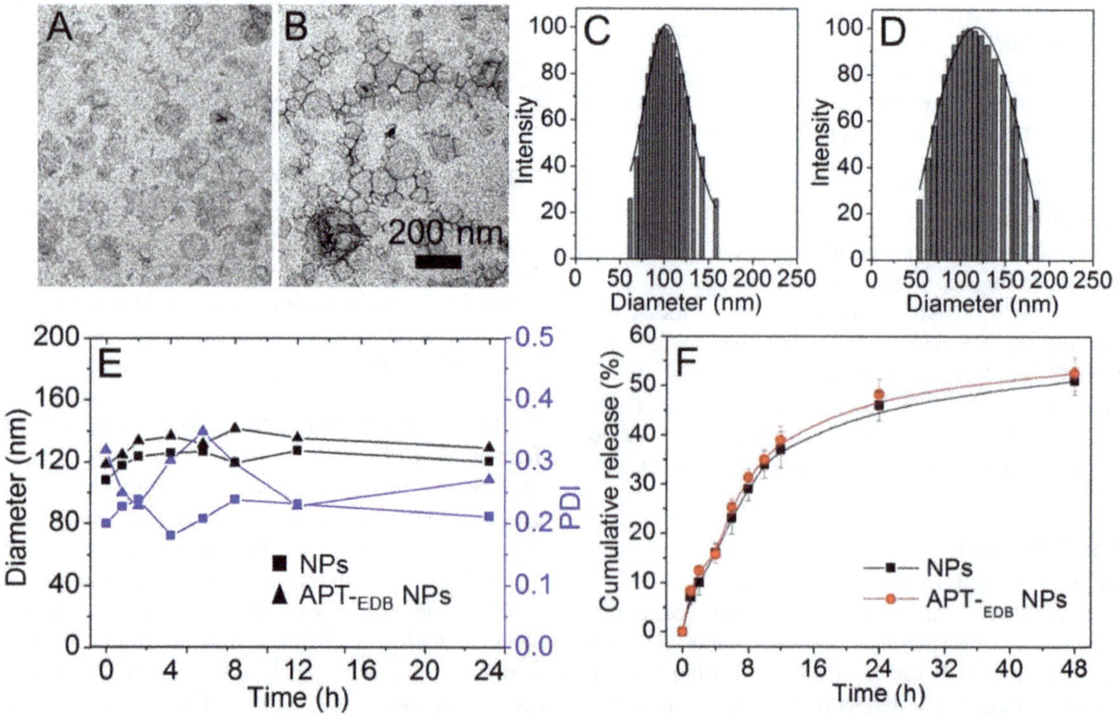

FIGURE 2 | (A–D) TEM images **(A,B)** and size distribution **(C,D)** of the siCypA-loaded NPs without aptide decoration **(A,C)** and the APT-$_{EDB}$ NPs **(B,D)**. **(E)** Size and polydispersity (PDI) of the siCypA-loaded NPs with (APT-$_{EDB}$ NPs) or without aptide decoration (NPs) incubated in PBS buffer containing 10% FBS for different time. **(F)** Cumulative siRNA release from the Cy5.5-siCypA-loaded NPs with (APT-$_{EDB}$ NPs) or without aptide decoration (NPs) incubated in PBS buffer at 37°C.

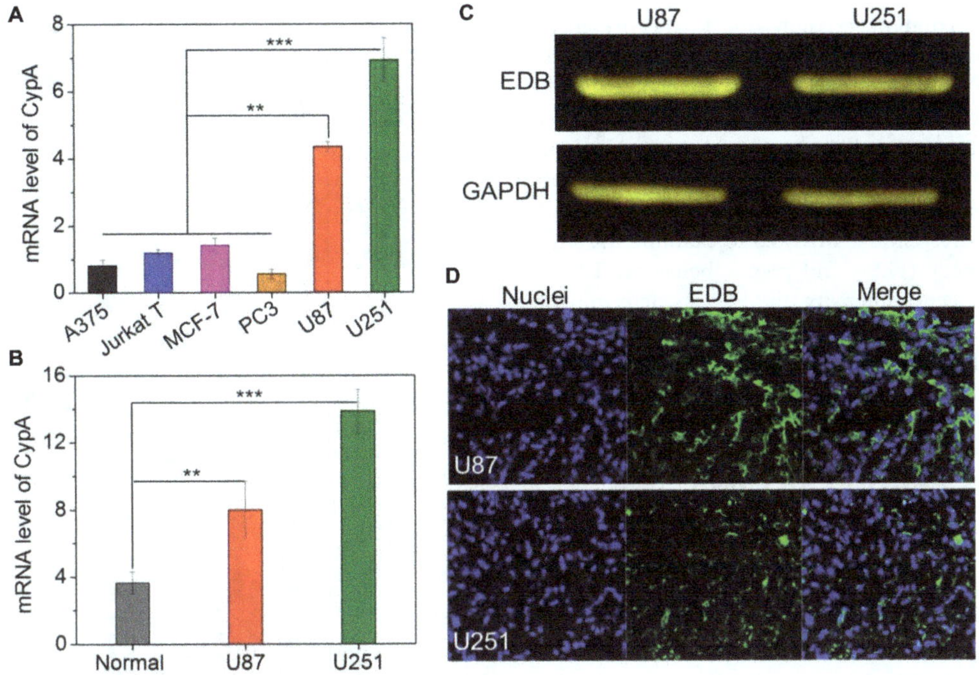

FIGURE 3 | (A) The mRNA level of CypA in the skin melanoma cells (A375), Jurkat leukemic T cells, prostate cancer cells (PC3), breast cancer cells (MCF-7), and glioma cells (U87 and U251). **(B)** The mRNA level of CypA in the normal brain tissues and GBM xenograft tumor tissues of nude mice. **(C)** Western blot analysis of the EDB expression in the glioma cells (U87 and U251). **(D)** Immunofluorescence analysis of the EDB expression in the GBM xenograft tumor tissues of nude mice. The nuclei and EDB were stained with blue and green fluorescence, respectively. $^{**}P < 0.01$; $^{***}P < 0.001$.

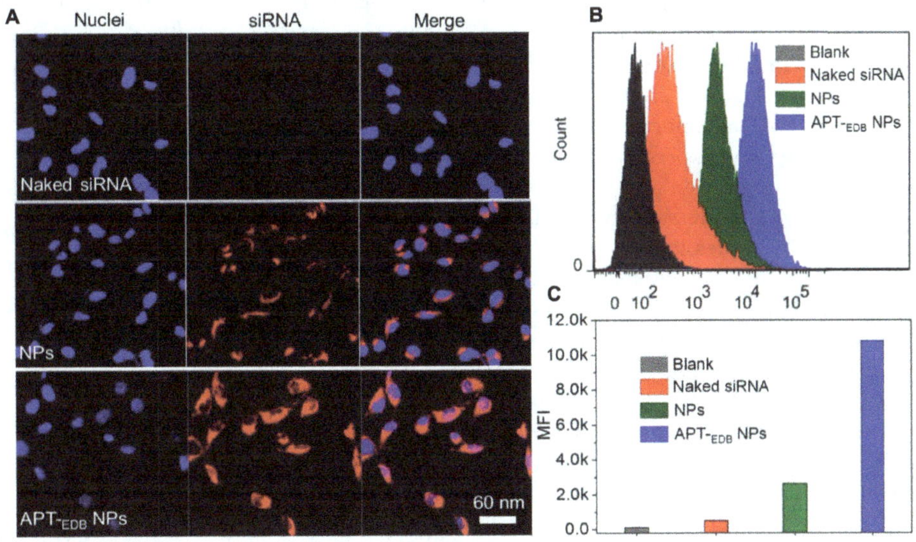

FIGURE 4 | (A) Fluorescent images of U251 cells incubated with the Cy5.5-siCypA-loaded NPs with (APT-$_{EDB}$ NPs) or without aptide decoration (NPs) for 4 h. The nuclei and siRNA were labeled with blue and red fluorescence, respectively. **(B,C)** Flow cytometry analysis **(B)** and mean fluorescence intensity [MFI, **(C)**] of U251 cells incubated with the Cy5.5-siCypA-loaded NPs with (APT-$_{EDB}$ NPs) or without aptide decoration (NPs) for 4 h.

Figure 2 shows the morphology of the siCypA-loaded APT-$_{EDB}$ NPs. Similar as other reported liposomes (Saw et al., 2013, 2015, 2017), the APT-$_{EDB}$ NPs show a spherical morphology with an average size of ~112 nm determined by DLS (**Figure 2D**). Compared to the NPs without APT-$_{EDB}$ decoration (~104 nm, **Figure 2C**), there is around 10 nm increase after APT-$_{EDB}$ decoration, suggesting the success in the APT$_{EDB}$ decoration because APT-$_{EDB}$ shows a hydrodynamic size of ~5 nm (Kim et al., 2012). Moreover, due to the presence of PEG chains on the outer layer, these siRNA-loaded NPs show a high stability. As shown in **Figure 2E**, either with or without APT-$_{EDB}$ decoration, possibly due to the presence of weak interaction between the particles and protein, there is a slight change in the particle size and polydispersity density (PDI) when incubating the NPs in 10% FBS-containing PBS solution for 8 h. However, this interaction will become stable as the incubation time increases and therefore there is no obvious size change after 8 h incubation. After obtaining these stable NPs, we next labeled the siCypA with fluorescent dye of Cy5.5 to examine the siRNA encapsulation efficiency (EE%) and release behavior. Through analyzing the fluorescence intensity, the EE was determined as ~90%. The siRNA release profile is shown in **Figure 2F**. As can be seen, the NPs show a sustained siRNA release behavior. Around 35% of loaded siRNA can be released within 12 h and the cumulative release reaches ~50% 48 h later.

Determination of EDB and CypA Expression

The main purpose of this work is to develop EDB-targeting siRNA delivery nanoplatform for GBM treatment by silencing the CypA expression. Prior to evaluating the gene silencing efficacy of the APT-$_{EDB}$ NPs, we first examined the CypA and EDB expression in the glioma cells. We chose different cancer cell lines and examined the corresponding CypA expression using real-time qPCR. As shown in **Figure 3A**, compared to skin melanoma cells (A375), Jurkat leukemic T cells, prostate cancer cells (PC3), and breast cancer cells (MCF-7), glioma cells (U87 and U251) show a much higher CypA expression. This encouraging result suggests that CypA is organ-specific over-expressed. To further verify this result, we compared the CypA expression in U87 and U251 xenograft tumors with normal brain tissues. As can be seen, the U87 or U251 xenograft tumors show around twofold or fourfold higher CypA expression that that of normal brain tissues (**Figure 3B**), implying that silencing CypA expression can be used as a potential strategy for GBM treatment.

After validation of the high CypA expression in the glioma cells, we next examined the EDB expression on these cells. As shown in **Figure 3C**, western blot analysis demonstrates that both U87 and U251 cells have a high EDB expression. Moreover, if using these two cell lines to construct xenograft tumor model, EDB is also highly expressed in the tumor tissues (green fluorescence, **Figure 3D**). All these results are consistent with previous reports (Yang et al., 2007; Qi et al., 2008) and indicate that EDB is indeed a suitable biomarker for targeted GBM therapy. Combining with results of PCR analysis (**Figures 3A,B**), because U251 cells show a relatively higher level of CypA and EDB expression compared to U87 cells, we chose U251 cells to evaluate the targeting and gene silencing ability of the APT-$_{EDB}$ NPs.

Evaluation of GBM-Targeting Ability and *in vitro* Gene Silencing

The GBM-targeting ability was evaluated by incubating U251 cells with the siCypA-loaded NPs. From the fluorescent images shown in **Figure 4A**, compared to naked siRNA, higher amount of siRNA can be observed and distributed in the cytoplasm of the cells incubated with the siRNA-loaded NPs. More importantly, due to the presence of specific recognition between aptide and EDB, the cellular uptake of APT-$_{EDB}$ NPs is much higher than that of the NPs without aptide decoration. This result is further proven by the flow cytometry analysis. As shown in **Figure 4B**, U251 cells show stronger ability to internalize the APT-$_{EDB}$ NPs and intracellular mean fluorescence intensity (MFI) is more than fivefold stronger than the cells incubated with the NPs without aptide decoration (**Figure 4C**).

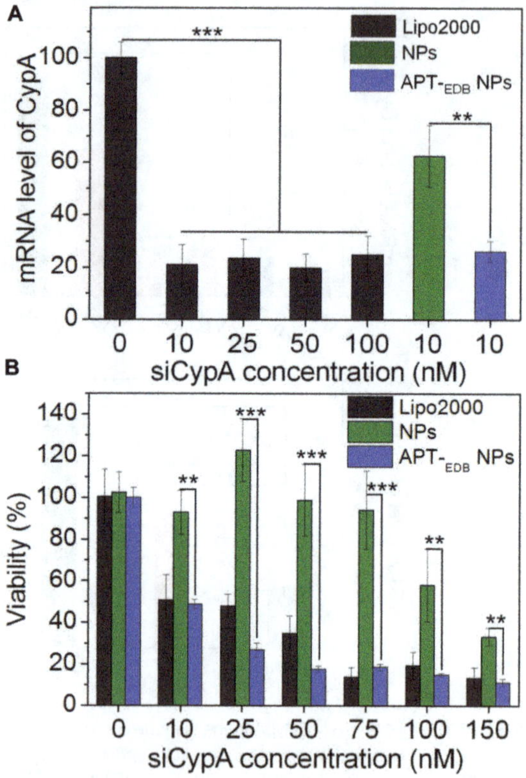

FIGURE 5 | (A) The mRNA level of CypA in U251 cells treated with the Lipo2000/siCypA complexes at various siRNA concentrations, and the siCypA-loaded NPs with (APT-$_{EDB}$ NPs) or without aptide decoration (NPs) at a 10 nM siRNA concentration. **(B)** Viability of U251 cells treated with the Lipo2000/siCypA complexes, and the siCypA-loaded NPs with (APT-$_{EDB}$ NPs) or without aptide decoration (NPs) at different siRNA concentrations. $^{**}P < 0.01$; $^{***}P < 0.001$.

After validation of the GBM-targeting ability of the APT-$_{EDB}$ NPs, we next examined their *in vitro* gene silencing efficacy. **Figure 5A** shows the mRNA level of CypA in U251 cells treated with the siCypA-loaded NPs. With the GBM-targeting ability to improve the cellular uptake, the APT-$_{EDB}$ NPs shows an effective gene silencing and there is around 80% decrease in the mRNA level of CypA in the cells at a siRNA concentration of 10 nM. This high gene silencing efficacy is similar as the commercial available Lipo2000 and is more than twofold higher than that of the NPs without aptide decoration. With this suppressed CypA expression, the cells have a very low viability. As shown in **Figure 5B**, lower than 50% of the cells are alive when treated with

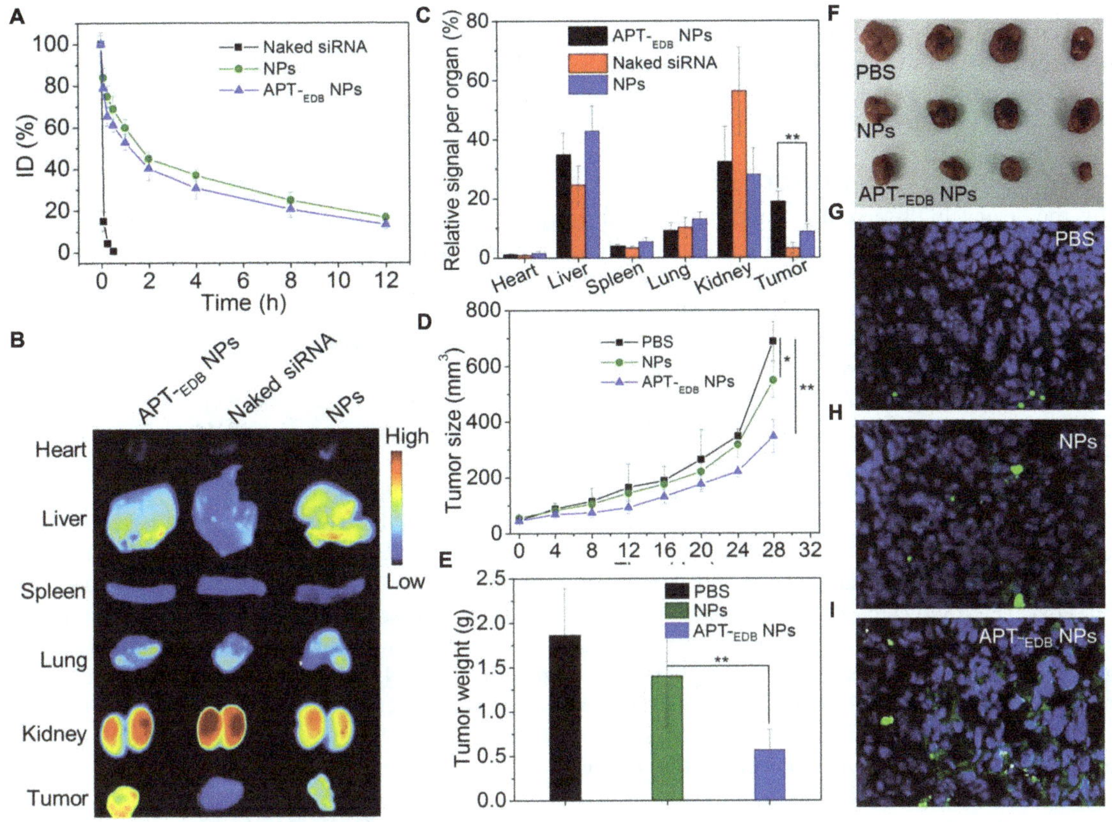

FIGURE 6 | (A) Blood circulation profile of the naked Cy5.5-siCypA and the Cy5.5-siCypA-loaded NPs with (APT_{EDB} NPs) or without aptide decoration (NPs). **(B)** Overlaid fluorescent image of the main organs of the GBM xenograft tumor-bearing mice treated with naked siRNA, and the siCypA-loaded NPs with (APT_{EDB} NPs) or without aptide decoration (NPs). **(C)** Biodistribution of the siRNA obatined from **(B)**. **(D)** Tumor growth profile of the GBM xenograft tumor-bearing mice treated with PBS, and the siCypA-loaded NPs with (APT_{EDB} NPs) or without aptide decoration (NPs). Intravenous injections are indicated by the arrows. **(E,F)** Weight **(E)** and representative photograph **(F)** of the tumor tissues from the mice in each group after 28 day evaluation period. **(G–I)** TUNEL staining of the collected tumor tissues in **(F)**. TUNEL-positive apoptotic cells were stained with green fluorescence. $^*P < 0.05$; $^{**}P < 0.01$.

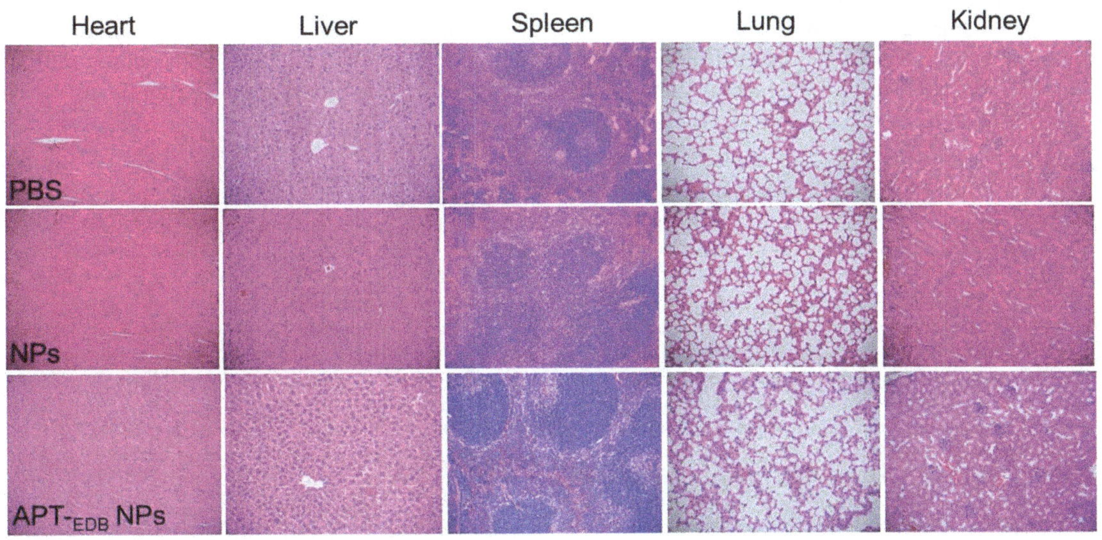

FIGURE 7 | Histological section of the main organs of the GBM xenograft tumor-bearing mice after systemic treatment with PBS, and the siCypA-loaded NPs with (APT_{EDB} NPs) or without aptide decoration (NPs). H&E; magnification 100×.

the APT-$_{EDB}$ NPs at a siRNA concentration of 10 nM. In contrast, at the same siRNA concentration, around 90% of the cells are still alive when treated with the NPs without aptide decoration. This result highlights the importance of the GBM-targeting ability of the siRNA-loaded NPs to their gene silencing in glioma cells.

Evaluation of *in vivo* Anti-tumor Efficacy

Encouraged by the strong EDB-targeting ability and effective gene silencing of the APT-$_{EDB}$ NPs, we finally evaluated their *in vivo* anti-tumor efficacy. The pharmacokinetics was first examined by intravenously injecting the Cy5.5-siCypA-loaded NPs to normal adult mice. As shown in **Figure 6A**, the naked siRNA is rapidly cleared from the blood and its half-life ($t_{1/2}$) is less than 10 min. In contrast, the APT-$_{EDB}$ NPs show much longer blood circulation with blood $t_{1/2}$ of around 4.68 h, which is comparable to the $t_{1/2}$ of the NPs without aptide decoration (~5.12 h). This long circulation feature is mainly attributed to protection by the PEG chains on the outer layer (Knop et al., 2010) and will ensure the accumulation of the APT-$_{EDB}$ NPs in the tumor tissues via enhance and permeable retention (EPR) effect (Bertrand et al., 2014). The biodistribution results in **Figures 6B,C** also demonstrate our statement. As shown in **Figure 6B**, the siRNA loaded NPs show higher tumor accumulation than that of naked siRNA. Moreover, due to the presence of APT-$_{EDB}$ targeting ligand, the APT-$_{EDB}$ NPs show more than twofold higher tumor accumulation than that of the NPs without aptide decoration (**Figure 6C**).

The *in vivo* anti-tumor efficacy was examined by intravenous injection of the siCypA-loaded APT-$_{EDB}$ NPs to GBM xenograft tumor-bearing mice once every two days at a 1 nmol siRNA dose per mouse. As shown in **Figures 6D–F**, after four consecutive injections, the tumor growth is obviously inhibited compared to the mice treated with PBS or NPs without aptide decoration. There is around sevenfold increase in the tumor size (from ~50 to ~350 mm^3) (**Figure 6B**). However, for the mice treated with PBS or the NPs without aptide decoration, there is around 14-fold (from ~50 to ~690 mm^3) or 11-fold (from ~50 to ~550 mm^3) increase in the tumor size. This tendency is further supported by the result of TUNEL assay. From the images shown in **Figures 6G–I**, more apoptotic cells can be observed in the tumor section of the mice treated with the siCypA-loaded APT-$_{EDB}$ NPs (**Figure 6I**). Noting that, the administration of the NPs does not induce apparent *in vivo* toxicity. As shown in **Figure 7**, no noticeable histological changes can be found in the tissues from heart, liver, spleen, lung, or kidney of the mice treated with PBS or siRNA-loaded NPs. All these results indicate that the NP platform developed in this work could be potentially used as a safe and efficient gene delivery system for GBM treatment.

CONCLUSION

In summary, we have developed a robust liposome-based NP platform for systemic siRNA delivery and targeted GBM treatment. This NP platform can target the glioma cells through the specific recognition between their surface-encoded aptide and over-expressed EDB on glioma cells, thereby leading to improved intracellular siRNA delivery and more effective gene silencing in glioma cells. *In vivo* results show that this long-circulating NP platform can target the GBM tumor tissues and obviously inhibit the tumor growth by silencing the CypA expression. Taken together, the NP platform developed herein could potentially serve as an effective delivery tool for non-invasive GBM treatment.

AUTHOR CONTRIBUTIONS

PS and XX conceived and designed the experiments. PS, AZ, YN, and YX performed the experiments. PS, YN, LZ, YX, and XX analyzed the data and co-wrote the paper.

FUNDING

This work was supported by the National Natural Science Foundation of China (81874226 and 81803020) and the Thousand Talents Program for Distinguished Young Scholars.

REFERENCES

Behin, A., Hoang-Xuan, K., Carpentier, A. F., and Delattre, J. Y. (2003). Primary brain tumours in adults. *Lancet* 361, 323–331. doi: 10.1016/s0140-6736(03)12328-8

Bertrand, N., Wu, J., Xu, X., Kamaly, N., and Farokhzad, O. C. (2014). Cancer nanotechnology: the impact of passive and active targeting in the era of modern cancer biology. *Adv. Drug Deliv. Rev.* 66, 2–25. doi: 10.1016/j.addr.2013.11.009

Borsi, L., Balza, E., Allemanni, G., and Zardi, L. (1992). Differential expression of the fibronectin isoform containing the ED-B oncofetal domain in normal human fibroblast cell lines originating from different tissues. *Exp. Cell Res.* 199, 98–105. doi: 10.1016/0014-4827(92)90466-L

Brandsma, D., and van den Bent, M. J. (2007). Molecular targeted therapies and chemotherapy in malignant gliomas. *Curr. Opin. Oncol.* 19, 598–605. doi: 10.1097/CCO.0b013e3282f0313b

Castellani, P., Borsi, L., Carnemolla, B., Biro, A., Dorcaratto, A., Viale, G. L., et al. (2002). Differentiation between high- and low-grade astrocytoma using a human recombinant antibody to the extra domain-B of fibronectin. *Am. J. Pathol.* 161, 1695–1700. doi: 10.1016/s0002-9440(10)64446-x

Cheng, Y., Morshed, R. A., Auffinger, B., Tobias, A. L., and Lesniak, M. S. (2014). Multifunctional nanoparticles for brain tumor imaging and therapy. *Adv. Drug Deliv. Rev.* 66, 42–57. doi: 10.1016/j.addr.2013.09.006

Durymanov, M., and Reineke, J. (2018). Non-viral Delivery of nucleic acids: insight into mechanisms of overcoming intracellular barriers. *Front. Pharmacol.* 9:971. doi: 10.3389/fphar.2018.00971

Fire, A., Xu, S., Montgomery, M. K., Kostas, S. A., Driver, S. E., and Mello, C. C. (1998). Potent and specific genetic interference by double-stranded RNA in *Caenorhabditis elegans*. *Nature* 391, 806–811. doi: 10.1038/35888

Han, Z., and Lu, Z.-R. (2017). Targeting fibronectin for cancer imaging and therapy. *J. Mater. Chem. B Mater. Biol. Med.* 5, 639–654. doi: 10.1039/C6TB02008A

Jhaveri, A. M., and Torchilin, V. P. (2014). Multifunctional polymeric micelles for delivery of drugs and siRNA. *Front. Pharmacol.* 5:77. doi: 10.3389/fphar.2014.00077

Jin, Z. G., Melaragno, M. G., Liao, D. F., Yan, C., Haendeler, J., Suh, Y. A., et al. (2000). Cyclophilin A is a secreted growth factor induced by oxidative stress. *Circ. Res.* 87, 789–796. doi: 10.1161/res.87.9.789

Johnson, D. R., and O'Neill, B. P. (2012). Glioblastoma survival in the United States before and during the temozolomide era. *J. Neurooncol.* 107, 359–364. doi: 10.1007/s11060-011-0749-4

Kanasty, R., Dorkin, J. R., Vegas, A., and Anderson, D. (2013). Delivery materials for siRNA therapeutics. *Nat. Mater.* 12, 967–977. doi: 10.1038/nmat3765

Kim, S., Kim, D., Jung, H. H., Lee, I. H., Kim, J. I., Suh, J. Y., et al. (2012). Bio-inspired design and potential biomedical applications of a novel class of high-affinity peptides. *Angew. Chem. Int. Ed. Engl.* 51, 1890–1894. doi: 10.1002/anie.201107894

Knop, K., Hoogenboom, R., Fischer, D., and Schubert, U. S. (2010). Poly(ethylene glycol) in drug delivery: pros and cons as well as potential alternatives. *Angew. Chem. Int. Ed. Engl.* 49, 6288–6308. doi: 10.1002/anie.200902672

Krizbai, I. A., Nyul-Toth, A., Bauer, H. C., Farkas, A. E., Traweger, A., Hasko, J., et al. (2016). Pharmaceutical targeting of the brain. *Curr. Pharm. Des.* 22, 5442–5462. doi: 10.2174/1381612822666160726144203

Lesniak, M. S., and Brem, H. (2004). Targeted therapy for brain tumours. *Nat. Rev. Drug Discov.* 3, 499–508. doi: 10.1038/nrd1414

Liu, Y., Xu, C. F., Iqbal, S., Yang, X. Z., and Wang, J. (2017). Responsive nanocarriers as an emerging platform for cascaded delivery of nucleic acids to cancer. *Adv. Drug Deliv. Rev.* 115, 98–114. doi: 10.1016/j.addr.2017.03.004

Luban, J. (1996). Absconding with the chaperone: essential cyclophilin-Gag interaction in HIV-1 virions. *Cell* 87, 1157–1159. doi: 10.1016/S0092-8674(00)81811-5

Mahmoudi, K., and Hadjipanayis, C. G. (2014). The application of magnetic nanoparticles for the treatment of brain tumors. *Front. Chem.* 2:109. doi: 10.3389/fchem.2014.00109

Meyers, J. D., Doane, T., Burda, C., and Basilion, J. P. (2013). Nanoparticles for imaging and treating brain cancer. *Nanomedicine* 8, 123–143. doi: 10.2217/nnm.12.185

Ozdemir-Kaynak, E., Qutub, A. A., and Yesil-Celiktas, O. (2018). Advances in glioblastoma multiforme treatment: new models for nanoparticle therapy. *Front. Physiol.* 9:170. doi: 10.3389/fphys.2018.00170

Pan, H., Luo, C., Li, R., Qiao, A., Zhang, L., Mines, M., et al. (2008). Cyclophilin A is required for CXCR4-mediated nuclear export of heterogeneous nuclear ribonucleoprotein A2, activation and nuclear translocation of ERK1/2, and chemotactic cell migration. *J. Biol. Chem.* 283, 623–637. doi: 10.1074/jbc.M704934200

Pardridge, W. M. (2005). The blood-brain barrier: bottleneck in brain drug development. *NeuroRx* 2, 3–14. doi: 10.1602/neurorx.2.1.3

Qi, Y. J., He, Q. Y., Ma, Y. F., Du, Y. W., Liu, G. C., Li, Y. J., et al. (2008). Proteomic identification of malignant transformation-related proteins in esophageal squamous cell carcinoma. *J. Cell. Biochem.* 104, 1625–1635. doi: 10.1002/jcb.21727

Satoh, K., Matoba, T., Suzuki, J., O'Dell, M. R., Nigro, P., Cui, Z., et al. (2008). Cyclophilin A mediates vascular remodeling by promoting inflammation and vascular smooth muscle cell proliferation. *Circulation* 117, 3088–3098. doi: 10.1161/CIRCULATIONAHA.107.756106

Saw, P. E., Kim, S., Lee, I.-H., Park, J., Yu, M., Lee, J., et al. (2013). Aptide-conjugated liposome targeting tumor-associated fibronectin for glioma therapy. *J Mater. Chem. B* 1, 4723–4726. doi: 10.1039/C3TB20815J

Saw, P. E., Park, J., Jon, S., and Farokhzad, O. C. (2017). A drug-delivery strategy for overcoming drug resistance in breast cancer through targeting of oncofetal fibronectin. *Nanomedicine* 13, 713–722. doi: 10.1016/j.nano.2016.10.005

Saw, P. E., Park, J., Lee, E., Ahn, S., Lee, J., Kim, H., et al. (2015). Effect of PEG pairing on the efficiency of cancer-targeting liposomes. *Theranostics* 5, 746–754. doi: 10.7150/thno.10732

Shergalis, A., Bankhead, A. III, Luesakul, U., Muangsin, N., and Neamati, N. (2018). Current challenges and opportunities in treating glioblastoma. *Pharmacol. Rev.* 70, 412–445. doi: 10.1124/pr.117.014944

Shi, J., Kantoff, P. W., Wooster, R., and Farokhzad, O. C. (2017). Cancer nanomedicine: progress, challenges and opportunities. *Nat. Rev. Cancer* 17, 20–37. doi: 10.1038/nrc.2016.108

Shieh, B. H., Stamnes, M. A., Seavello, S., Harris, G. L., and Zuker, C. S. (1989). The ninaA gene required for visual transduction in *Drosophila* encodes a homologue of cyclosporin A-binding protein. *Nature* 338, 67–70. doi: 10.1038/338067a0

Tanaka, H., Shimazaki, H., Kimura, M., Izuta, H., Tsuruma, K., Shimazawa, M., et al. (2011). Apoptosis-inducing factor and cyclophilin A cotranslocate to the motor neuronal nuclei in amyotrophic lateral sclerosis model mice. *CNS Neurosci. Ther.* 17, 294–304. doi: 10.1111/j.1755-5949.2010.00180.x

Tseng, Y. C., Mozumdar, S., and Huang, L. (2009). Lipid-based systemic delivery of siRNA. *Adv. Drug Deliv. Rev.* 61, 721–731. doi: 10.1016/j.addr.2009.03.003

Wang, G., Shen, J., Sun, J., Jiang, Z., Fan, J., Wang, H., et al. (2017). Cyclophilin A maintains glioma-initiating cell stemness by regulating Wnt/beta-catenin signaling. *Clin. Cancer Res.* 23, 6640–6649. doi: 10.1158/1078-0432.CCR-17-0774

Wang, P., and Heitman, J. (2005). The cyclophilins. *Genome Biol.* 6:226. doi: 10.1186/gb-2005-6-7-226

Whitehead, K. A., Langer, R., and Anderson, D. G. (2009). Knocking down barriers: advances in siRNA delivery. *Nat. Rev. Drug Discov.* 8, 129–138. doi: 10.1038/nrd2742

Winter, H., Ginsberg, A., Egizi, E., Erondu, N., Whitney, K., Pauli, E., et al. (2013). Effect of a high-calorie, high-fat meal on the bioavailability and pharmacokinetics of PA-824 in healthy adult subjects. *Antimicrob. Agents Chemother.* 57, 5516–5520. doi: 10.1128/aac.00798-13

Xu, X., Saw, P. E., Tao, W., Li, Y., Ji, X., Yu, M., et al. (2017a). Tumor microenvironment-responsive multistaged nanoplatform for systemic RNAi and cancer therapy. *Nano Lett.* 17, 4427–4435. doi: 10.1021/acs.nanolett.7b01571

Xu, X., Wu, J., Liu, Y., Saw, P. E., Tao, W., Yu, M., et al. (2017b). Multifunctional envelope-type siRNA delivery nanoparticle platform for prostate cancer therapy. *ACS Nano* 11, 2618–2627. doi: 10.1021/acsnano.6b07195

Xu, X., Wu, J., Liu, Y., Yu, M., Zhao, L., Zhu, X., et al. (2016). Ultra-pH-responsive and tumor-penetrating nanoplatform for targeted siRNA delivery with robust Anti-cancer efficacy. *Angew. Chem. Int. Ed. Engl.* 55, 7091–7094. doi: 10.1002/anie.201601273

Yang, H., Chen, J., Yang, J., Qiao, S., Zhao, S., and Yu, L. (2007). Cyclophilin A is upregulated in small cell lung cancer and activates ERK1/2 signal. *Biochem. Biophys. Res. Commun.* 361, 763–767. doi: 10.1016/j.bbrc.2007.07.085

Yang, X. Z., Du, J. Z., Dou, S., Mao, C. Q., Long, H. Y., and Wang, J. (2012). Sheddable ternary nanoparticles for tumor acidity-targeted siRNA delivery. *ACS Nano* 6, 771–781. doi: 10.1021/nn204240b

Zimmermann, T. S., Lee, A. C., Akinc, A., Bramlage, B., Bumcrot, D., Fedoruk, M. N., et al. (2006). RNAi-mediated gene silencing in non-human primates. *Nature* 441, 111–114. doi: 10.1038/nature04688

Zuckerman, J. E., and Davis, M. E. (2015). Clinical experiences with systemically administered siRNA-based therapeutics in cancer. *Nat. Rev. Drug Discov.* 14, 843–856. doi: 10.1038/nrd4685

Permissions

All chapters in this book were first published by Frontiers; hereby published with permission under the Creative Commons Attribution License or equivalent. Every chapter published in this book has been scrutinized by our experts. Their significance has been extensively debated. The topics covered herein carry significant findings which will fuel the growth of the discipline. They may even be implemented as practical applications or may be referred to as a beginning point for another development.

The contributors of this book come from diverse backgrounds, making this book a truly international effort. This book will bring forth new frontiers with its revolutionizing research information and detailed analysis of the nascent developments around the world.

We would like to thank all the contributing authors for lending their expertise to make the book truly unique. They have played a crucial role in the development of this book. Without their invaluable contributions this book wouldn't have been possible. They have made vital efforts to compile up to date information on the varied aspects of this subject to make this book a valuable addition to the collection of many professionals and students.

This book was conceptualized with the vision of imparting up-to-date information and advanced data in this field. To ensure the same, a matchless editorial board was set up. Every individual on the board went through rigorous rounds of assessment to prove their worth. After which they invested a large part of their time researching and compiling the most relevant data for our readers.

The editorial board has been involved in producing this book since its inception. They have spent rigorous hours researching and exploring the diverse topics which have resulted in the successful publishing of this book. They have passed on their knowledge of decades through this book. To expedite this challenging task, the publisher supported the team at every step. A small team of assistant editors was also appointed to further simplify the editing procedure and attain best results for the readers.

Apart from the editorial board, the designing team has also invested a significant amount of their time in understanding the subject and creating the most relevant covers. They scrutinized every image to scout for the most suitable representation of the subject and create an appropriate cover for the book.

The publishing team has been an ardent support to the editorial, designing and production team. Their endless efforts to recruit the best for this project, has resulted in the accomplishment of this book. They are a veteran in the field of academics and their pool of knowledge is as vast as their experience in printing. Their expertise and guidance has proved useful at every step. Their uncompromising quality standards have made this book an exceptional effort. Their encouragement from time to time has been an inspiration for everyone.

The publisher and the editorial board hope that this book will prove to be a valuable piece of knowledge for researchers, students, practitioners and scholars across the globe.

List of Contributors

Na Kong and Xiu-Na Sun
Sir Run Run Shaw Hospital, Zhejiang University School of Medicine, Hangzhou, China
Institute of Translational Medicine, Zhejiang University, Hangzhou, China

Mei Deng and Yi-Ding Chen
Department of Surgical Oncology, The Second Affiliated Hospital, Zhejiang University School of Medicine, Hangzhou, China

Xin-Bing Sui
Department of Medical Oncology, Holistic Integrative Oncology Institutes and Holistic Integrative Cancer Center of Traditional Chinese and Western Medicine, The Affiliated Hospital of Hangzhou Normal University, College of Medicine, Hangzhou Normal University, Hangzhou, China
Department of Cancer Pharmacology, Holistic Integrative Pharmacy Institutes, College of Medicine, Hangzhou Normal University, Hangzhou, China
Key Laboratory of Elemene Class Anti-cancer Chinese Medicine of Zhejiang Province and Engineering Laboratory of Development and Application of Traditional Chinese Medicine from Zhejiang Province, Hangzhou Normal University, Hangzhou, China

Zhenqiang Dong
Key Laboratory of Sensing Technology and Biomedical Instrument of Guangdong Province, School of Engineering, Sun Yat-sen University, Guangzhou, China
College of Chemical and Material Engineering, Quzhou University, Quzhou, China

Yang Kang
Key Laboratory of Mountain Ecological Restoration and Bioresource Utilization, Chengdu Institute of Biology, Chinese Academy of Sciences, Chengdu, China

Xinbing Sui
Department of Medical Oncology, Holistic Integrative Oncology Institutes and Holistic Integrative Cancer Center of Traditional Chinese and Western Medicine, The Affiliated Hospital of Hangzhou Normal University, College of Medicine, Hangzhou Normal University, Hangzhou, China
Department of Cancer Pharmacology, Holistic Integrative Pharmacy Institutes, College of Medicine, Hangzhou Normal University, Hangzhou, China

Manli Luo
Guangdong Provincial Key Laboratory of Malignant Tumor Epigenetics and Gene Regulation, Sun Yat-sen Memorial Hospital, Sun Yat-sen University, Guangzhou, China

Qijuan Yuan and Zhipeng Gu
Key Laboratory of Sensing Technology and Biomedical Instrument of Guangdong Province, School of Engineering, Sun Yat-sen University, Guangzhou, China

Wenhao Nan, Li Ding, Houjie Chen, Fahim U. Khan and Xiaojun Shi
School of Life Sciences, Tsinghua University, Beijing, China
Graduate School at Shenzhen, Tsinghua University, Shenzhen, China

Lu Yu
Shenzhen Modo Biotech Co., Ltd., Shenzhen, China

Fazhan Wang, Wen Xiao, Xingting Bao, Qian Zheng, Linhui Gong, Yang Zhou, Shuping Yang, Aiping Fang, Jinhui Wu and Xiangrong Song
State Key Laboratory of Biotherapy, Geriatrics and Cancer Center, West China Hospital and Collaborative Innovation Center for Biotherapy, Sichuan University, Chengdu, China

Mostafa A. Elbahnasawy and Mohamed M. S. Farag
Department of Botany and Microbiology, Faculty of Science, Al-Azhar University, Cairo, Egypt

Qingqing Xiong, Ge Yu and Tianqiang Song
Department of Hepatobiliary Cancer, National Clinical Research Center for Cancer, Key Laboratory of Cancer Prevention and Therapy, Tianjin's Clinical Research Center for Cancer, Tianjin Medical University Cancer Institute and Hospital, Tianjin, China

Mangmang Cui
Department of Hepatobiliary Cancer, National Clinical Research Center for Cancer, Key Laboratory of Cancer Prevention and Therapy, Tianjin's Clinical Research Center for Cancer, Tianjin Medical University Cancer Institute and Hospital, Tianjin, China
Hebei province Cangzhou Hospital of Integrated Traditional and Western Medicine, Cangzhou, China

Jian Wang
Department of Immunology, National Clinical Research Center for Cancer, Key Laboratory of Cancer Prevention and Therapy, Tianjin's Clinical Research Center for Cancer, Tianjin Medical University Cancer Institute and Hospital, Tianjin, China

Kai Niu
Department of Otorhinolaryngology Head and Neck Surgery, The First Hospital of Jilin University, Changchun, China

Yunming Yao
Department of Abdominal Ultrasound, The First Hospital of Jilin University, Changchun, China

Ming Xiu
Department of Intensive Care Unit, The First Hospital of Jilin University, Changchun, China

Chunjie Guo
Department of Radiology, The First Hospital of Jilin University, Changchun, China

Yuanyuan Ge and Jianmeng Wang
Department of Geriatrics, The First Hospital of Jilin University, Changchun, China

Xi Guo and Tong Sun
Department of Neurosurgery, West China Hospital, Sichuan University, Chengdu, China
Neurosurgery Research Laboratory, West China Hospital, Sichuan University, Chengdu, China

Rui Zhong
Institute of Blood Transfusion, Chinese Academy of Medical Sciences & Peking Union Medical College, Chengdu, China

Lu Ma and Hao Li
Neurosurgery Research Laboratory, West China Hospital, Sichuan University, Chengdu, China

Chao You and Meng Tian
Department of Neurosurgery, West China Hospital, Sichuan University, Chengdu, China
Neurosurgery Research Laboratory, West China Hospital, Sichuan University, Chengdu, China
West China Brain Research Centre, West China Hospital, Sichuan University, Chengdu, China

Chengwei Wang
Department of Integrated Traditional and Western Medicine, West China Hospital, Sichuan University, Chengdu, China

Baoyan Wang and Weijun Wu
Nanjing Drum Tower Hospital, The Affiliated Hospital of Nanjing University Medical School, Nanjing, China

Hongjin Lu and Hongliang Xin
Department of Pharmaceutics, School of Pharmacy, Nanjing Medical University, Nanjing, China

Zhi Wang
Department of Pharmacy, The Second Affiliated Hospital of Nanjing Medical University, Nanjing, China

Fazhan Wang, Xingting Bao, Huili Li, Yang Zhou, Yongmei Liu, Chunling Jiang, Jinhui Wu and Xiangrong Song
State Key Laboratory of Biotherapy, Geriatrics and Cancer Center, West China Hospital and Collaborative Innovation Center for Biotherapy, Sichuan University, Chengdu, China

Aiping Fang
State Key Laboratory of Biotherapy, Geriatrics and Cancer Center, West China Hospital and Collaborative Innovation Center for Biotherapy, Sichuan University, Chengdu, China
West China School of Public Health, Sichuan University, Chengdu, China

Shi Liang, Wei Wu, Quan Li, Jianing Chen, Herui Yao and Yandan Yao
Guangdong Provincial Key Laboratory of Malignant Tumor Epigenetics and Gene Regulation, Medical Research Center, Sun Yat-sen Memorial Hospital, Sun Yat-sen University, Guangzhou, China
RNA Biomedical Institute, Sun Yat-sen Memorial Hospital, Sun Yat-sen University, Guangzhou, China
Breast Tumor Center, Sun Yat-sen Memorial Hospital, Sun Yat-sen University, Guangzhou, China

Junmeng Zheng, Xiaoding Xu and Phei Er Saw
Guangdong Provincial Key Laboratory of Malignant Tumor Epigenetics and Gene Regulation, Medical Research Center, Sun Yat-sen Memorial Hospital, Sun Yat-sen University, Guangzhou, China
RNA Biomedical Institute, Sun Yat-sen Memorial Hospital, Sun Yat-sen University, Guangzhou, China

Jixue Wang and Shengxian Li
Department of Urology, The First Hospital of Jilin University, Changchun, China
Key Laboratory of Polymer Ecomaterials, Changchun Institute of Applied Chemistry, Chinese Academy of Sciences, Changchun, China

Jingjing Guan and Chunxi Wang
Department of Urology, The First Hospital of Jilin University, Changchun, China

Di Li
Key Laboratory of Polymer Ecomaterials, Changchun Institute of Applied Chemistry, Chinese Academy of Sciences, Changchun, China

Yuping Han
Department of Urology, China-Japan Union Hospital of Jilin University, Changchun, China

Shirley Chung
Department of Biology, University of Waterloo, Waterloo, ON, Canada

Hsiang-I Tsai, Lijuan Jiang and Jinxie Zhang
School of Life Sciences, Tsinghua University, Beijing, China

Xiaowei Zeng, Hongbo Chen, Lin Mei and Gan Liu
School of Pharmaceutical Sciences (Shenzhen), Sun Yat-sen University, Guangzhou, China

Zihuang Li
Department of Radiation Oncology, Second Clinical Medicine College of Jinan University, Shenzhen Municipal People's Hospital, Shenzhen, China

Wei Cheng and Zhenhua Xie
Division of Life and Health Sciences, Graduate School at Shenzhen, Tsinghua University, Shenzhen, China

Laiqiang Huang
School of Life Sciences, Tsinghua University, Beijing, China
Division of Life and Health Sciences, Graduate School at Shenzhen, Tsinghua University, Shenzhen, China

Jie Pan and Dong Wan
School of Environmental and Chemical Engineering, Tianjin Polytechnic University, Tianjin, China

Li Gao
Department of Urology, Affiliated Hospital of Guilin Medical University, Guilin, China

Shi-Bing Wang and Xiao-Zhou Mou
Key Laboratory of Tumor Molecular Diagnosis and Individualized Medicine of Zhejiang Province, Zhejiang Provincial People's Hospital, People's Hospital of Hangzhou Medical College, Hangzhou, China
Clinical Research Institute, Zhejiang Provincial People's Hospital, People's Hospital of Hangzhou Medical College, Hangzhou, China

Ying-Yu Ma
Clinical Research Institute, Zhejiang Provincial People's Hospital, People's Hospital of Hangzhou Medical College, Hangzhou, China

Xiao-Yi Chen and Yuan-Yuan Zhao
Key Laboratory of Tumor Molecular Diagnosis and Individualized Medicine of Zhejiang Province, Zhejiang Provincial People's Hospital, People's Hospital of Hangzhou Medical College, Hangzhou, China

Jing Wu, Jiayi Yuan, Baotong Ye, Yaling Wu, Zheng Xu, Jinghua Chen and Jingxiao Chen
Key Laboratory of Carbohydrate Chemistry and Biotechnology, Ministry of Education, School of Pharmaceutical Sciences, Jiangnan University, Wuxi, China

Xing Chen, Zhiyu He, Fei Xiong, Xiang Ling and Jun Wu
Key Laboratory of Sensing Technology and Biomedical Instrument of Guangdong Province, School of Engineering, Sun Yat-sen University, Guangzhou, China

Lili Zhao
Digestive Endoscopy Center, Jiangsu Province Hospital, Nanjing, China

Yang Kang
Key Laboratory of Mountain Ecological Restoration and Bioresource Utilization, Chengdu Institute of Biology, Chinese Academy of Sciences, Chengdu, China

Bobin Mi, Yi Liu, Jing Liu, Liangcong Hu, Guohui Liu and Wu Zhou
Department of Orthopaedics, Union Hospital, Tongji Medical College, Huazhong University of Science and Technology, Wuhan, China

Junqing Wang
State Key Laboratory of Molecular Vaccinology and Molecular Diagnostics & Center for Molecular Imaging and Translational Medicine, School of Public Health, Xiamen University, Xiamen, China

Adriana C. Panayi
Addenbrooke's Hospital, University of Cambridge School of Clinical Medicine, Cambridge, United Kingdom

Shengnan Zhao and Jian Yang
School of Applied Chemistry and Biological Technology, Shenzhen Polytechnic, Shenzhen, China

Xia Guo
Key Laboratory of Birth Defect and Related Disorders of Women and Children, Department of Pediatric Hematology/Oncology, West China Second University Hospital, Sichuan University, Chengdu, China

Jinhua Li and Yang Zhou
School of Applied Chemistry and Biological Technology, Shenzhen Polytechnic, Shenzhen, China
Key Laboratory of Birth Defect and Related Disorders of Women and Children, Department of Pediatric Hematology/Oncology, West China Second University Hospital, Sichuan University, Chengdu, China

Lingjing Huang, Yanfei Li, Juanjuan Xu and Chunmei Fu
Key Laboratory of Drug Targeting and Drug Delivery System (Ministry of Education), West China School of Pharmacy, Sichuan University, Chengdu, China

Kai Niu
Department of Otorhinolaryngology Head and Neck Surgery, The First Hospital of Jilin University, Changchun, China

Yunming Yao
Department of Abdominal Ultrasound, The First Hospital of Jilin University, Changchun, China

Chunjie Guo
Department of Radiology, The First Hospital of Jilin University, Changchun, China

Yuanyuan Ge and Jianmeng Wang
Department of Geriatrics, The First Hospital of Jilin University, Changchun, China

Liang Ge
State Key Laboratory of Natural Medicines, China Pharmaceutical University, Nanjing, China
School of Pharmacy, Xinjiang Medical University, Ürümqi, China

Xinru You, Jun Huang and Jun Wu
Key Laboratory of Sensing Technology and Biomedical Instruments of Guangdong Province, School of Biomedical Engineering, Sun Yat-sen University, Guangzhou, China

Yuejian Chen
Nanjing iPharma Technology, Co., Ltd., Nanjing, China

Li Chen
School of Pharmacy, Xinjiang Medical University, Ürümqi, China

Ying Zhu and Qian Hai
State Key Laboratory of Natural Medicines, China Pharmaceutical University, Nanjing, China

Yuan Zhang
Department of Orthopedics, Xinqiao Hospital, Third Military Medical University, Chongqing, China

Xiqiang Liu
Guangdong Provincial Key Laboratory of Stomatology, Guanghua School of Stomatology, Hospital of Stomatology, Sun Yat-sen University, Guangzhou, China

Nan Li
Department of Neonatology, The First Hospital of Jilin University, Changchun, China

Phei Er Saw, Ao Zhang, Yan Nie and Xiaoding Xu
Guangdong Provincial Key Laboratory of Malignant Tumor Epigenetics and Gene Regulation, Medical Research Center, Sun Yat-sen Memorial Hospital, Sun Yat-sen University, Guangzhou, China
RNA Biomedical Institute, Sun Yat-sen Memorial Hospital, Sun Yat-sen University, Guangzhou, China

Lei Zhang
Guangdong Provincial Key Laboratory of Malignant Tumor Epigenetics and Gene Regulation, Medical Research Center, Sun Yat-sen Memorial Hospital, Sun Yat-sen University, Guangzhou, China
Department of Hepatobiliary Surgery, Sun Yat-sen Memorial Hospital, Sun Yat-sen University, Guangzhou, China

Yingjie Xu
Department of Biochemistry and Molecular Cell Biology, Shanghai Key Laboratory for Tumor Microenvironment and Inflammation, Shanghai Jiao Tong University School of Medicine, Shanghai, China

Index

A

Acetonitrile, 2-3, 52, 86, 94-96, 102, 105, 162, 183
American Type Culture Collection, 3, 104, 127, 162
Anticoagulation Activity, 73, 78, 80
Antitumor Agents, 126
Antitumor Efficacy, 2, 4-5, 11, 37, 59-60, 62, 64, 67-68, 71, 90, 119, 129, 136-137, 142, 163, 168, 195, 199, 205-206
Apoptosis Activation, 176, 178
Autophagy, 13, 137, 145, 170-171, 173-174, 176-180, 206

B

Biocompatibility, 2, 4, 11, 17, 20, 22, 26, 70, 81-82, 91, 121, 160, 166, 179, 183, 205, 207
Biodistribution, 65, 67, 83, 87, 89, 99, 125, 147, 213-214, 223-224

C

Cardiotoxicity, 51, 69
Catabolism, 175-177, 179
Cell Apoptosis Assay, 138, 172
Cell Membranes, 74, 98
Cell Viability Assay, 138, 162, 219
Cellular Internalization, 22, 64, 162, 165, 207
Cellular Uptake, 4, 7, 9, 12-13, 21, 26-27, 29, 34, 37, 40, 44, 47, 49, 51, 53, 55-56, 62, 67, 71, 83, 86, 88, 90-91, 106, 108, 114, 126-127, 129-131, 134-137, 139, 144, 154-155, 162, 165, 168, 189, 208, 213, 218-219, 222
Centrifugation, 3-4, 20, 26, 94, 149, 184
Cervical Carcinoma, 61-62, 67, 71, 116
Chemotherapy, 1-2, 4, 8, 11-12, 50, 59, 61-62, 71-72, 81, 83, 91, 111, 120, 122, 124-125, 134-135, 137, 146-147, 153, 157, 159, 167-169, 192-193, 205-206, 214, 216-217, 224
Chitosan Oligosaccharide, 73, 81-82
Chondrocytes, 170-180
Confocal Laser Scanning Microscope, 27, 53, 150, 162, 165, 219
Conventional Liposomes, 93
Corneal Hydration, 95, 98
Corneal Permeability, 92-94, 100
Corneal Permeation, 95, 98-99
Cyclodextrins, 51, 97, 99-100
Cytokines, 117, 122, 154, 170-171, 173, 175-179
Cytotoxicity, 8, 10-11, 21, 25-27, 29, 34, 37, 40, 44, 47-48, 50-51, 53, 55-58, 63-64, 71, 81, 86, 88-90, 100, 104, 106, 114, 116, 123, 126-127, 130-131, 135-136, 141-145, 150, 152, 157, 160, 162, 164-165, 168, 171, 173, 195, 198, 211, 213-214
Cytotoxicity Assay, 40, 44, 50, 58, 116, 150, 152, 171

D

Deformability, 73-75, 77-78, 80
Dendritic Block Copolymer, 127-128, 133
Diffusion Chamber, 94
Doxorubicin, 12-13, 23, 50-52, 59-62, 71-72, 81, 91, 115, 123-124, 134, 137, 145, 148, 156-157, 192-193, 205, 214-215
Drug Encapsulation Efficiency, 26, 135
Drug Entrapment Efficiency, 94, 96, 190
Drug Loading Content, 1, 3, 26, 62, 128-129, 194, 197
Drug Release Study, 129
Drug Resistance, 51, 59-60, 91, 127, 132-133, 135, 144-145, 147, 225

E

Enhanced Permeation and Retention, 62, 126
Enzymes, 16, 51, 65, 148, 175
Extracellular Fluids, 51, 93, 115

F

Fibrinogen, 73-75, 78, 80, 82
Flow Cytometry Analysis, 50-51, 55-56, 174, 221-222

G

Gel Retardation Assay, 103, 106-107
Glaucoma, 92-93, 98-100
Glioblastoma, 72, 91, 109, 120, 125, 169, 216, 225

H

Hemocompatibility, 74, 79, 81-82
Hemolysis, 73-75, 77, 80
Hemostatic Property, 74, 78
Hepatocellular Carcinoma, 50, 59-60, 136-137, 145-147, 157, 214
Histopathological Analysis, 27-28, 66, 71, 143, 166
Homopolymer, 101-102, 105-106, 108
Host-guest Interaction, 17, 50-51
Hydrophobic Drugs, 26, 32, 34, 93, 99, 123-124, 159
Hydroxyl Groups, 74, 80

I

Immune Cells, 101, 109, 117
Immune System, 79, 101, 117, 119, 205, 214
Immunoblotting, 27-28, 30, 32-33
Immunocytochemical Staining, 27, 172, 175
Immunohistochemical Analysis, 65, 68, 143
Immunosuppression, 25, 35, 101-102
Intrinsic Coagulation Pathway, 73, 78, 80

M

Macrophages, 37, 48-49, 82, 101-109, 157, 171
Molecular Structure, 80

Morphology, 2-3, 5-6, 11, 21, 26, 31-32, 34, 40, 43, 51-54, 68, 70, 81, 83, 85, 88, 94, 103, 105, 128, 150-151, 162, 164, 184, 193, 197, 203, 208, 218, 221

Multidrug Resistance, 112, 124, 126-127, 129, 134-136, 143

N

Nanoliposomes, 92-94, 97-98

Nanoparticles, 1-2, 12-16, 20, 23, 25-26, 29, 34-35, 48-61, 71-72, 81-86, 88-91, 99-100, 102-103, 109, 116-118, 122-130, 134-137, 140, 145, 147, 156-157, 159-161, 168-169, 179-180, 182-183, 186-191, 193, 205-209, 212-217, 224-225

Nanotechnology, 13, 49, 51, 99, 112, 143-144, 147, 168, 171, 182, 213-214, 216, 224

Neovascularization, 101-102

P

Percutaneous Absorption, 25-27, 31-34

Pharmacokinetic Parameters, 163, 166, 209, 211

Pharmacokinetics, 5, 23, 48, 100, 111, 117, 125, 134, 139, 147, 163, 166-168, 189, 214, 219, 224-225

Phenotypes, 101, 109

Prothrombin Time, 73, 75

R

Radiotherapy, 112, 216-217

Reactive Oxygen Species, 16, 117, 134, 170, 172

S

Sorafenib, 50-51, 56, 58-60, 136, 138, 141-146

Spectrophotometer, 4, 53, 75-76, 94, 140, 144, 149-150, 194

Spectroscopy, 19, 39-40, 42, 74, 81, 94-95, 99, 128-129, 151, 193-194

Supramolecular Amphiphiles, 50-53, 58-59

Surgical Resection, 159, 216

T

Therapeutic Efficacy, 1-2, 7-9, 11, 32, 46, 93, 99-100, 124, 137, 143, 157, 167, 182, 189

Thrombin Time, 73-75

Transmission Electron Microscopy, 19, 40, 94, 103, 128, 151-152, 162, 164, 172, 174, 218

Tumor Cells, 51, 62-63, 67-69, 83-85, 91, 114-115, 117-119, 124-125, 129, 133, 137, 145, 168, 192-193, 198-199

U

Unimolecular Micelle, 127, 133

www.ingramcontent.com/pod-product-compliance
Lightning Source LLC
LaVergne TN
LVHW082206200926
848484LV00008B/2218